SURGERY of the SHOULDER

James E. Bateman, M.D., F.R.C.S.(C)

Surgeon-in-Chief (Emeritus),
Orthopaedic and Arthritic Hospital;
Associate Professor of Surgery
University of Toronto Faculty of Medicine
Toronto, Ontario

R. Peter Welsh, M.B., Ch.B., F.R.C.S.(C)

Orthopaedic Surgeon,
Acting Deputy Chief of Staff,
Orthopaedic and Arthritic Hospital;
Assistant Professor of Surgery
University of Toronto Faculty of Medicine
Toronto, Ontario

1984

B.C. DECKER INC. • Philadelphia • Toronto
THE C.V. MOSBY COMPANY • Saint Louis • Toronto • London

Publisher: **B.C. Decker Inc.**
3228 South Service Road
Burlington, Ontario L7N 3H8

B.C. Decker Inc.
P.O. Box 30246
Philadelphia, Pennsylvania 19103

North American and worldwide sales and distribution:

The C.V. Mosby Company
11830 Westline Industrial Drive
Saint Louis, Missouri 63141

In Canada: **The C.V. Mosby Company, Ltd.**
120 Melford Drive
Toronto, Ontario M1B 2X5

Surgery of the Shoulder   ISBN 0-941158-25-X

© 1984 by B.C. Decker Incorporated under the International Copyright Union. All rights reserved. No part of this publication may be reused or republished in any form without written permission of the publisher.

Library of Congress catalog number: 83-073017

10 9 8 7 6 5 4 3 2 1

CONTRIBUTORS

KARI A. AALTO, M.D.
Senior Orthopaedic Surgeon, University Central Hospital, Helsinki, Finland
Surgical Pathology in Chronic Shoulder Pain

IWATSUGU ANRAKU, M.D.
Associate Professor of Medicine, Department of Orthopaedic Surgery, Showa University Fujigaoka Hospital, Yokohama, Japan
Arthroscopy of the Shoulder Joint

HARUO ARAI, M.D.
Associate Professor of Medicine, Department of Orthopaedic Surgery, Showa University Fujigaoka Hospital, Yokohama, Japan
Arthroscopy of the Shoulder Joint

HARRY A. BADE, III, M.D.
Assistant Attending in Orthopaedic Surgery, Monmouth Medical Center, Long Branch, New Jersey; Orthopaedic Surgeon, Out-Patient Department, Hospital for Special Surgery; Clinical Instructor in Surgery, Cornell University Medical College, New York, New York
Long-Term Results of Neer Total Shoulder Replacement

PHILLIPE BANCEL, M.D.
The Children's Hospital Medical Center, Boston, Massachusetts
The Anteroinferior Vulnerable Point of the Glenoid Rim

GORDON CAMPBELL BANNISTER, M.Ch., Orth., F.R.C.S.(Ed)
Clinical Lecturer in Orthopaedic Surgery, University of Bristol, Bristol, England
A Prospective Study of the Treatment of Acromioclavicular Dislocation

L. K. BARTALSKY, M.D.
Senior Registrar, Department of Traumatology, A.Ö.N.Ö. Landeskrankenhaus, Mödling, Weyprechtgasser, Mödling, Austria
Experience in the Treatment of Recurrent Anterior Dislocation of the Shoulder with a Modified Version of Bankart's Procedure

MARGARET J. BARTON, M.C.S.P.
Research Assistant, Department of Orthopaedic Surgery, University of Nottingham, Nottingham, England
The Power Available During Movement of the Shoulder

JAMES E. BATEMAN, M.D., F.R.C.S.(C)
Surgeon-in-Chief, (Emeritus), Orthopaedic and Arthritic Hospital; Associate Professor, Department of Surgery, University of Toronto, Toronto, Ontario, Canada
Rotator Cuff Tears in the Young
Long Term Results of Surgical Repair of Full Thickness Rotator Cuff Tears

OMAR BAYNE, M.D.
Research Fellow, Orthopaedic and Arthritic Hospital, Toronto, Ontario, Canada
Rotator Cuff Tears in the Young
Long Term Results of Surgical Repair of Full Thickness Rotator Cuff Tears

CHRISTOPHER PAUL BEAUCHAMP, M.D.
Departments of Orthopaedics and Radiology, Royal Columbian Hospital, New Westminster, British Columbia, and Division of Orthopaedic Surgery, University of British Columbia, Vancouver, British Columbia, Canada
Shoulder Arthrotomography and Computed Axial Tomography in the Diagnosis of Recurrent Shoulder Subluxations

DENIS BERGERON, M.D., F.R.C.P.(C)
Department of Radiology, Faculté de Médecine, Université de Sherbrooke, Sherbrooke, Québec
The Place of Computed Arthrotomography in Unstable Shoulder

J. BERNAGEAU, M.D.
Attaché-Consultant CHU Henri Mondor, Creteil, France
The Anteroinferior Vulnerable Point of the Glenoid Rim

LOUIS U. BIGLIANI, M.D.
Clinical Instructor and Attending in Orthopaedic Surgery, Columbia Presbyterian Medical Center,

Columbia University College of Physicians and Surgeons, New York, New York; Chief, Adult Surgical Service, Helen Hayes Hospital, Haverstraw, New York
Analysis of Failed Repair for Shoulder Instability—A Preliminary Report

LESTER S. BORDEN, M.D.

Department of Orthopaedic Surgery, The Cleveland Clinic Foundation, Cleveland, Ohio
Experience with the Neer Total Shoulder Replacement

JOHN J. BREMS, M.D.

Department of Orthopaedic Surgery, The Cleveland Clinic Foundation, Cleveland, Ohio
Experience with the Neer Total Shoulder Replacement

EDMUND Y. S. CHAO, Ph.D.

Professor of Orthopaedics, Orthopaedic Biomechanics Laboratory, Mayo Clinic, Rochester, Minnesota
Limb Salvage Procedures for Primary Bone Tumors of the Shoulder Region

ROBERT H. COFIELD, M.D.

Consultant, Department of Orthopaedics, Mayo Clinic and Mayo Foundation; Associate Professor of Orthopaedic Surgery, Mayo Medical School, Rochester, Minnesota
The Role of Arthroscopy in Surgery of the Shoulder
Total Shoulder Arthroplasty: Associated Disease of the Rotator Cuff; Results, and Complications

STEPHEN ANDREW COPELAND, M.B., B.S., F.R.C.S.

Consultant Orthopaedic Surgeon, Royal Berkshire Hospital, Reading, Berkshire, England
Thoracoscapular Fusion for Facioscapulohumeral Dystrophy

CARLOS ALBERTO DEANQUIN, M.D.

Assistant Professor of Orthopaedic Surgery and Traumatology, Orthopaedic Department and Traumatology, Hospital de Clínicas de Córdoba–Children's Hospital, Córdoba, R. Argentina
Comparative Study of Bone Lesions in Traumatic Recurrent Dislocations of the Shoulder—Their Importance and Treatment

CARLOS E. DEANQUIN, M.D.

Emeritus Professor, University of Córdoba, Orthopaedic Department (Hospital de Clínicas); Director, Instituto de Traumatología, Córdoba, R. Argentina
Comparative Study of Bone Lesions in Traumatic Recurrent Dislocations of the Shoulder—Their Importance and Treatment

JACQUES E. DESMARCHAIS, M.D., M.Sc., F.R.C.S.(C)

Hôpital du Sacré-Coeur; Associate Professor of Surgery, Université de Montréal; Assistant to the Dean for Medical Education, Faculté de Médecine, Université de Montréal, Montréal, Québec
Treatment of Complex Fractures of the Proximal Humerus by Neer Hemiarthroplasty
Diagnosis of Rotator Cuff Tears by Double Contrast Arthrotomography: Reliability Study

E. ENGELBRECHT, M.D.

Endo-Klinik, Clinic for Bone and Joint Surgery; Chief Surgeon, Traumatologist, Holstenstrabe, Hamburg, Germany
Ten Years of Experience with Unconstrained Shoulder Replacement

SEI FUJIMOTO, M.D.

Clinical Fellow, Department of Orthopaedic Surgery, Nara Medical University; Member, Japanese Shoulder Joint Association, Kashihara, Nara, Japan
Repair of Chronic Massive Rotator Cuff Tears with Synthetic Fabrics

R. GANZ, M.D.

Professor of Orthopaedics, Orthopaedic Department, University of Bern, Bern, Switzerland
Classification and Aspects of Treatment of Fractures of the Proximal Humerus

CARL FREDRIK GENTZ, M.D.

Orthopaedic Surgery and Diagnostic Radiology, Malmö General Hospital, University of Lund, Malmö, Sweden
The Significance of Distally Pointing Acromioclavicular Osteophytes in Ruptures of the Supraspinatus Tendon

DOUGLAS GORDON, B.Sc., M.D.

Resident in Orthopaedic Surgery, Department of Orthopaedic Surgery, Faculté de Médecine,

Université de Sherbrooke, Sherbrooke, Québec
The Place of Computed Arthrotomography in Unstable Shoulder

PAUL M. GRAMMONT, M.D.

Chief of Orthopaedic Surgery, Hôpital Bocage; Professor of Orthopaedic and Traumatologic Surgery, Bourgogne University, Dijon Cedex, France
Role of the Tendon of the Long Head of the Biceps Brachii in Anterior Subluxation of the Shoulder
The Acropole Prosthesis

NORBERT GSCHWEND, M.D.

Chief Orthopaedic Surgeon, Klinik Wilhelm Schulthess; Professor of Orthopaedic Surgery, University of Zurich, Zurich, Switzerland
A Surgical Approach to Rotator Cuff Tears
Surgery of the Rheumatoid Shoulder

OLLE HÄGG, M.D.

Department of Orthopaedic Surgery, Gävle Hospital, Gävle, Sweden
Aspects of Prognostic Factors in Comminuted and Dislocated Proximal Humeral Fractures

DAVID IAN HAMMOND, M.D., F.R.C.P.(C)

Division of Orthopaedics, Ottawa General Hospital, Departments of Pathology and Radiology, University of Ottawa, Ottawa, Ontario
The Subacromial Bursae: A Clinicopathological Study

R. J. HAWKINS, M.D., F.R.C.S.(C)

Clinical Associate Professor, Department of Surgery, University of Western Ontario, St. Joseph's Hospital, London, Ontario
Missed Posterior Dislocations of the Shoulder
Surgical Management of Rotator Cuff Tears

HIROMICHI HAYASHI, M.D.

Orthopaedic Surgeon, Tokyo Metropolitan Police Hospital, Tokyo, Japan
Treatment of Acute Complete Dislocation of the Acromioclavicular Joint

SHINKICHI HIMENO, M.D.

Medical Staff, Division of Orthopaedic Surgery, Fukuoka Children's Hospital; Member of Japanese Orthopaedic Association, Fukuoka, Japan
The Role of the Rotator Cuff as a Stabilizing Mechanism of the Shoulder

Roentgenographical Examination of the Tilted Angle of the Scapula in Three Dimensions in the Relaxed Standing Position

LENNART HOVELIUS, M.D.

Orthopaedic Surgeon, Gävle Hospital, Gävle, Sweden
Operative Treatment of Recurrent Anterior Shoulder Dislocation with the Bristow-Latarjet Procedure

M.A. HUTSON, B.CHIR., M.B.

Director of Sports Clinic, General Hospital, Nottingham, England
A Prospective Study of the Treatment of Acromioclavicular Dislocation

ROLF T. IDEBERG, M.D.

Senior Surgeon, Clinic of Orthopaedic Surgery, Central Hospital, Uddevalla, Sweden
Fractures of the Scapula Involving the Glenoid Fossa

HITOSHI IKEDA, M.D.

Chief, Orthopaedic Department, Nobuhara Hospital, Tatsuno, Japan
Glenoid Osteotomy for Loose Shoulder

ALLAN E. INGLIS, M.D.

Director, CAP Service, The Hospital for Special Surgery, New York, New York
Long-Term Results of Neer Total Shoulder Replacement

KUNINARI ITO, M.D.

Orthopaedic Surgeon, Tokyo Metropolitan Police Hospital, Tokyo, Japan
Treatment of Acute Complete Dislocation of the Acromioclavicular Joint

ROLI P. JAKOB, M.D.

Assistant Professor of Orthopaedics, Orthopaedic Department, University of Bern, Bern, Switzerland
Classification and Aspects of Treatment of Fractures of the Proximal Humerus

FUMIO KATO, M.D.

Chief Orthopaedic Surgeon, Tokyo Metropolitan Police Hospital; Lecturer in Orthopaedic Surgery, University of Tokyo, Tokyo, Japan
Treatment of Acute Complete Dislocation of the Acromioclavicular Joint

AXEL KENTSCH, M.D.
Chefarzt, Klinik Wilhelm Schulthess, Zurich, Switzerland
Surgery of the Rheumatoid Shoulder

LIPMANN KESSEL, M.B.E., M.C., F.R.C.S.
Emeritus Professor of Orthopaedics, Royal National Orthopaedic Hospital, London, England
Codman Lecture

HIROSHI KIDA, M.D.
Chief, Division of Orthopaedics, Iwaki Kyoritsu General Hospital, Iwaki-City, Japan
Diagnosis and Treatment of Partial Thickness Tears of Rotator Cuff

PATRICK KINNARD, M.D., F.R.C.S.(C)
Associate Professor of Orthopaedic Surgery, Department of Orthopaedic Surgery, Centre Hospitalier Universitaire de Sherbrooke, Sherbrooke, Québec
The Place of Computed Arthrotomography in Unstable Shoulder

REINHARD KOELBEL, M.D.
Orthopadische Universitatsklinik, Martinistabe, Hamburg, Germany
Stabilization of Shoulders with Bone and Muscle Defects Using Joint Replacement Implants

MASAYUKI KONDO, M.D.
Medical Staff Fellow, Department of Orthopaedic Surgery; Medical Staff Fellow of Orthopaedic Surgery, Nagasaki University School of Medicine, Nagasaki-City, Japan
Changes of the Tilting Angle of the Scapula Following Elevation of the Arm

JOHN PHILIP KOSTUIK, M.D., F.R.C.S.(C)
Associate Professor, University of Toronto; Deputy Chief of Orthopaedic Surgery, Mount Sinai and Toronto General Hospitals, Toronto, Ontario
Shoulder Arthrodesis—A.O. Technique

H. A. KRAMPS, M.D.
Orthopädische Klinik und Poliklinik der Westfälischen, Wilhelms-Universität, Münster, West Germany
Computer Tomography of Recurrent Shoulder Dislocation

T. KRISTIANSEN, M.D.
Assistant Professor of Orthopaedics, Orthopaedics Department, University of Vermont, Burlington, Vermont
Classification and Aspects of Treatment of Fractures of the Proximal Humerus

V. PREM KUMAR, M.B., B.S., F.R.C.S.(Ed)
Clinical Fellow, Orthopaedic and Arthritic Hospital, Toronto, Ontario; Assistant Professor, Department of Surgery, University of Singapore, Singapore
Rotator Cuff Tears in the Young

YOSHIKATSU KUROKI, M.D.
Department of Orthopaedic Surgery, Showa University Fujigaoka Hospital, Yokohama, Japan
Arthroscopy of the Shoulder Joint

TOMOMITSU KUTSUMA, M.D.
Department of Orthopaedic Surgery, Kofu City Hospital, Kofu, Japan
Results of Surgical Treatment for Deltoid Muscle Contracture

UDO LAUMANN, M.D.
Orthopädische Klinik und Poliklinik der Westfälischen, Wilhelms-Universität, Münster, West Germany
Kinesiology of the Shoulder—Electromyographic and Stereophotogrammetric Studies
Computer Tomography of Recurrent Shoulder Dislocation

ROBERT E. LEACH, M.D.
Professor and Chairman, Department of Orthopaedics, Boston Universiy School of Medicine, Boston, Massachusetts
Chronic Shoulder Pain in the Athlete

RÉJEAN-YVES LÉVESQUE, M.D., F.R.C.P.(C)
Associate Professor of Radiology, Department of Radiology, Faculté de Médecine, Université de Sherbrooke, Sherbrooke, Québec
The Place of Computed Arthrotomography in Unstable Shoulder

HELGE LILLEBY, M.D.
    Orthopaedic Surgeon, Martina Hansens Hospital, Sandvika, Norway
Indications and Benefits of Arthroscopy of the Shoulder Joint

JOCHEN R. LÖHR, M.D.
    Orthopaedic Resident, University of Ottawa School of Medicine, Ottawa, Ontario, Canada
The Role of the Tendon of the Long Head of the Biceps Brachii in Anterior Subluxation of the Shoulder

RICHARD L. LOOMER, M.D., F.R.C.S.(C)
    Departments of Orthopaedics and Radiology, Royal Columbia Hospital, New Westminster, British Columbia; Division of Orthopaedic Surgery, University of British Columbia, Vancouver, British Columbia
Shoulder Arthrotomography and Computed Axial Tomography in the Diagnosis of Recurrent Shoulder Subluxations

BO J. LUNDBERG, M.D.
    Department of Orthopaedic Surgery, Gävle Hospital, Gävle, Sweden
Aspects of Prognostic Factors in Comminuted and Dislocated Proximal Humeral Fractures

KENJI MASUHARA, M.D.
    Professor and Chairman, Department of Orthopaedic Surgery, Nara Medical University; Executive Committee, Japanese Orthopaedic Association, Kashihara, Nara, Japan
Repair of Chronic Massive Rotator Cuff Tears with Synthetic Fabrics

SHOGO MASUMI, M.D.
    Professor of Orthopaedic Surgery, Department of Orthopaedic Surgery, Medical College of Oita, Hasama-cho, Oita-gun, Oita, Japan
Pyogenic Arthritis of the Glenohumeral Joint Following the Intra-articular Injection of Corticosteroid

K. MAYO, M.D.
    Assistant Professor of Orthopaedics, Harborview Hospital, Seattle, Washington
Classification and Aspects of Treatment of Fractures of the Proximal Humerus

RAINER P. MAYER, M.D.
    Chief, Department of Orthopaedic Surgery, Regionalspital, Langenthal, Switzerland
The Role of the Tendon of the Long Head of the Biceps Brachii in Anterior Subluxation of the Shoulder

MOTOHIKO MIKASA, M.D.
    Department of Orthopaedic Surgery, National Tochigi Hospital, Utsunomiya City, Japan
Trapezius Transfer for Global Tear of the Rotator Cuff

TEIJI MIYAZAKI, M.D.
    Orthopaedic Surgeon, Tokyo Metropolitan Police Hospital, Tokyo, Japan
Treatment of Acute Complete Dislocation of the Acromioclavicular Joint

MARILYN J. MODE, B.P.T.
    Director of Physical Therapy, Orthopaedic and Arthritic Hospital, Toronto, Ontario
Shoulder Rehabilitation After Rotator Cuff Surgery

G. MORAIS, M.D.
    Resident, Orthopaedics Department, Sacré Coeur Hospital, Montréal, Québec, Canada
Treatment of Complex Fractures of the Proximal Humerus by Neer Hemiarthroplasty

YUJIRO MORI, M.D.
    Associate Professor of Medicine, Showa University Fujigaoka Hospital, Yokohama, Japan
Arthroscopy of the Shoulder Joint

M. E. MÜLLER, M.D.
    Professor of Orthopaedics, Orthopaedics Department, University of Bern, Bern, Switzerland
Classification and Aspects of Treatment of Fractures of the Proximal Humerus

J. PATRICK MURNAGHAN, B.Sc., M.D., F.R.C.S.(C)
    Division of Orthopaedic Surgery, Ottawa Civic Hospital; Assistant Professor, University of Ottawa, Ottawa, Ontario, Canada
Adhesive Capsulitis of the Shoulder

RICHARD J. NASCA, M.D.

Associate Professor, Orthopaedic Surgery, University of Alabama School of Medicine, Birmingham, Alabama
Contact Areas of the "Subacromial" Joint
Surgical Treatment of Complete Rotator Cuff Tears

CHARLES S. NEER, II, M.D.

Professor of Clinical Orthopaedic Surgery, Columbia University College of Physicians and Surgeons, New York, New York
Missed Posterior Dislocations of the Shoulder
Unconstrained Shoulder Arthroplasty

ROBERT J. NEVIASER, M.D.

Professor of Orthopaedic Surgery, Department of Orthopaedic Surgery, George Washington University Medical Center, Washington, District of Columbia
Reconstruction of Chronic Tears of the Rotator Cuff

THOMAS J. NEVIASER, M.D.

Assistant Professor of Orthopaedic Surgery, Department of Orthopaedic Surgery, George Washington University Medical Center, Washington, District of Columbia
Reconstruction of Chronic Tears of the Rotator Cuff

KATSUYA NOBUHARA, M.D.

Director, Nobuhara Hospital, Tatsuno, Japan; Instructor, Orthopaedic Department, Kobe University School of Medicine, Kobe, Japan
Glenoid Osteotomy for Loose Shoulder

TOM RANDOLPH NORRIS, M.D.

Attending Staff, Orthopaedic and Hand Surgery, Presbyterian Hospital, Pacific Medical Center; Medical Director, J. Perry Yates Microsurgery Laboratory, New York, New York
C-Arm Fluoroscopic Evaluation Under Anesthesia for Glenohumeral Subluxations
Analysis of Failed Repair for Shoulder Instability—A Preliminary Report

JIRO OZAKI, M.D.

Clinical Assistant, Department of Orthopaedic Surgery, Nara Medical University; Executive Committee, Japanese Shoulder Joint Association, Kashihara, Nara, Japan
Repair of Chronic Massive Rotator Cuff Tears with Synthetic Fabrics

PEKKA PAAVOLAINEN, M.D.

Lecturer in Orthopaedics and Traumatology, University of Helsinki; Consultant in Orthopaedics and Traumatology, University Central Hospital of Helsinki, Helsinki, Finland
Surgical Pathology in Chronic Shoulder Pain

D. PATTE, M.D.

Orthopaedic Surgery, "Les Fontaines" Clinic, Melun, France
The Anteroinferior Vulnerable Point of the Glenoid Rim

CLAES J. PETERSSON, M.D.

Orthopaedic Surgery and Diagnostic Radiology, Malmö General Hospital, Malmö, Sweden; University of Lund, Sweden
The Significance of Distally Pointing Acromioclavicular Osteophytes in Ruptures of the Supraspinatus Tendon

ROBERT GREG PRINGLE, M.B., Ch.B., F.R.C.S.

Consultant Orthopaedic Surgeon, Robert Jones & Agnes Hunt Orthopaedic Hospital, Midland Spinal Injury Unit, and Royal Shrewsbury Hospital, Shrewsbury, England
Crutchwalker's Shoulder

A. PÜHRINGER, M.D.

Head of Department of Traumatology, A.Ö.N.Ö. Landeskrankenhaus, Mödling, Austria
Experience in the Treatment of Recurrent Anterior Dislocation of the Shoulder with a Modified Version of Bankart's Procedure

CHITRANJAN S. RANAWAT, M.D.

Director, Hand Service, The Hospital for Special Surgery, New York, New York
Long-Term Results of Neer Total Shoulder Replacement

MICHAEL G. ROCK, M.D.

Formerly a Special Fellow in Orthopaedic Oncology, Mayo Graduate School of Medicine, Rochester, Minnesota; now Associate Professor, Department of Orthopaedic Surgery, University of Western Ontario, London, Ontario
Limb Salvage Procedures for Primary Bone Tumors of the Shoulder Region

CARTER REDD ROWE, M.D.

Associate Professor of Orthopaedic Surgery (Emeritus), Harvard Medical School; Senior

Orthopaedic Surgeon, Massachusetts General Hospital, Boston, Massachusetts
Trends in Treatment of Complete Acromioclavicular Dislocations

MINORU SAKURAI, M.D.

Associate Professor, Department of Orthopaedic Surgery, Tohoku University School of Medicine, Sendai, Japan
Thoracic Scapulopexy for Restoration of Arm Elevation in Facioscapulohumeral Type Muscular Dystrophy

E. GEORGE SALTER, M.D.

Associate Professor, Department of Physical Therapy and Associate Professor, Division of Orthopaedic Surgery, University of Alabama, Birmingham, Alabama
Contact Areas of the "Subacromial" Joint

ROBERT L. SAMILSON, M.D.

Active Member, American Shoulder and Elbow Surgeons; Clinical Professor of Orthopaedic Surgery, University of California School of Medicine, San Francisco, California
Repair of Rotator Cuff Tears

KIRITI SARKAR, M.D., F.R.C.P.(C)

Associate Professor, Department of Pathology, University of Ottawa School of Medicine, Ottawa, Ontario, Canada
The Subacromial Bursae: A Clinicopathological Study

JOSEPH SCHATZKER, M.D., B.Sc., F.R.C.S.(C)

Staff, Wellesley Hospital; Staff, Sunnybrook Hospital; Professor of Surgery, University of Toronto Faculty of Medicine, Toronto, Ontario, Canada
Shoulder Arthrodesis—A.O. Technique

DAVID SEGAL, M.D.

Director of Orthopaedic Surgery, Boston City Hospital, Boston, Massachusetts
Chronic Shoulder Pain in the Athlete

NAOFUMI SHIMIZU, M.D.

Orthopaedic Surgeon, Tokyo Metropolitan Police Hospital, Tokyo, Japan
Treatment of Acute Complete Dislocation of the Acromioclavicular Joint

MASATERU SHINDO, M.D.

Chief Resident and Clinical Fellow, Department of Orthopaedic Surgery, Medical College of Oita, Hasama-cho, Oita-gun, Oita, Japan
Pyogenic Arthritis of the Glenohumeral Joint Following the Intra-articular Injection of Corticosteroid

FRANKLIN H. SIM, M.D.

Consultant, Department of Orthopaedics, Mayo Clinic/Mayo Foundation; Professor of Orthopaedic Surgery, Mayo Medical School, Rochester, Minnesota
Limb Salvage Procedures for Primary Bone Tumors of the Shoulder Region

PÄR SLÄTIS, M.D.

Professor and Head, Division of Orthopaedic Surgery and Traumatology, Surgical Hospital, University Central Hospital, Helsinki, Finland
Surgical Pathology in Chronic Shoulder Pain

P. G. STABLEFORTH, M.D., B.S., F.R.C.S.

Consultant-Orthopaedic Surgeon, Bristol Royal Infirmary, Bristol, England
A Prospective Study of the Treatment of Acromioclavicular Dislocation

ALFRED B. SWANSON, M.D., F.A.C.S.

Director of Orthopaedic and Hand Surgery Training Program, Blodgett & Butterworth Hospitals; Director of Orthopaedic Research, Blodgett Memorial Medical Center; Professor, Department of Surgery, Michigan State University, Lansing, Michigan
Bipolar Implant Shoulder Arthroplasty

SHIRO TABATA, M.D.

Chief, Division of Orthopaedic Surgery, Iwaki Kyoritsu General Hospital, Iwaki-City, Japan
Diagnosis and Treatment of Partial Thickness Tears of Rotator Cuff

SHIRO TAZOE, M.D.

Medical Staff Fellow, Department of Orthopaedic Surgery, Nagasaki University School of Medicine, Nagasaki, Japan
Changes of the Tilting Angle of the Scapula Following Elevation of the Arm

KAZUO TERAYAMA, M.D.

Department of Orthopaedic Surgery, Shinshu University, Matsumoto-City, Japan
Results of Surgical Treatment for Deltoid Muscle Contracture

LIVIUS TIMKO, M.D.

Departments of Orthopaedics and Radiology, Royal Columbian Hospital, New Westminster, British Columbia; Division of Orthopaedic Surgery, University of British Columbia, Vancouver, British Columbia
Shoulder Arthrotomography and Computed Axial Tomography in the Diagnosis of Recurrent Shoulder Subluxations

KATSUMASA TOMOTSUNE, M.D.

Orthopaedic Surgeon, Tokyo Metropolitan Police Hospital, Tokyo, Japan
Treatment of Acute Complete Dislocation of the Acromioclavicular Joint

TAKEHIKO TORISU, M.D.

Associate Professor of Orthopedic Surgery, Medical College of Oita, Hasama-cho, Oita-gun, Oita, Japan
Pyogenic Arthritis of the Glenohumeral Joint Following the Intra-articular Injection of Corticosteroid
Roentgenographical Examination of the Tilted Angle of the Scapula in Three Dimensions in the Relaxed Standing Position

HIROSHI TSUMURA, M.D.

Medical Staff, Division of Orthopaedic Surgery, Fukuoka Children's Hospital; Member of Japanese Orthopaedic Association, Japan
The Role of the Rotator Cuff as a Stabilizing Mechanism of the Shoulder

HIROAKI TSUTSUI, M.D.

Associate Professor of Medicine, Showa University Fujigaoka Hospital, Yokohama, Japan
Arthroscopy of the Shoulder Joint

HANS K. UHTHOFF, M.D., F.R.C.S.(C)

Professor and Head, Division of Orthopaedic Surgery, University of Ottawa School of Medicine, and Ottawa General Hospital, Ottawa, Ontario, Canada
The Subacromial Bursae: A Clinicopathological Study

MARTTI VALTTERI VASTAMÄKI, M.D.

Senior Hand Surgeon, The Orthopaedic Hospital of the Invalid Foundation, Helsinki, Finland
Pectoralis Minor Transposition in Serratus Anterior Paralysis

JEAN VEZINA, M.D.

Department of Radiology; Clinical Assistant Professor; Hôpital du Sacré-Coeur, Université de Montréal, Montréal, Québec
Diagnosis of Rotator Cuff Tears by Double Contrast Arthrotomography: Reliability Study

WILLIAM ANGUS WALLACE, F.R.C.S.

Lecturer in Orthopaedic Surgery, University of Nottingham, England; Visiting Research Fellow, Toronto Western Hospital, Toronto, Ontario, Canada
The Power Available During Movement of the Shoulder
A Prospective Study of the Treatment of Acromioclavicular Dislocation

RUSSELL F. WARREN, M.D.

Director, Sports Medicine and Shoulder Service, The Hospital for Special Surgery, New York, New York
Long-Term Results of Neer Total Shoulder Replacement

MICHAEL WATSON, M.A., M.R.C.P., F.R.C.S.

Consultant Orthopaedic Surgeon, Guy's Hospital, London, England
The Impingement Syndrome in Sportsmen

CRAIG E. WEIL, M.D.

Senior Resident in Orthopaedic Surgery, University of Alabama School of Medicine, Birmingham, Alabama
Contact Areas of the "Subacromial" Joint

ROBERT PETER WELSH, M.B., Ch.B., F.R.C.S.(C), F.A.C.S.

Acting Deputy Chief of Staff, Staff Orthopaedic Surgeon, Orthopaedic and Arthritic Hospital; Assistant Professor, University of Toronto Faculty of Medicine, Toronto, Ontario, Canada
Rotator Cuff Tears in the Young

ALAN H. WILDE, M.D.

Chairman, Department of Orthopaedic Surgery, The Cleveland Clinic Foundation, Cleveland, Ohio
Experience with the Neer Total Shoulder Replacement

A. MURRAY WILEY, M.Ch., F.R.C.S., F.R.C.S.(C)

Attending Surgeon, Toronto Western Hospital and York Finch General Hospital; Associate

Professor, Orthopaedics, University of Toronto Faculty of Medicine, Toronto, Ontario, Canada
The Power Available During Movement of the Shoulder
Arthroscopic Shoulder Surgery

MASAYUKI YAMADA, M.D.

Medical Staff Fellow, Department of Orthopaedic Surgery, Nagasaki University School of Medicine, Nagasaki, Japan
Changes of the Tilting Angle of the Scapula Following Elevation of the Arm

RYUJI YAMAMOTO, M.D.

Professor of Medicine, Department of Orthopaedic Surgery, Showa University Fujigaoka Hospital, Yokohama, Japan
Arthroscopy of the Shoulder Joint
Oudard-Iwahara's Operation for Recurrent Anterior Dislocation of the Shoulder

H. J. ZINNECKER, M.D.

Deputy Head, Department of Traumatology, A.Ö.N.Ö. Landeskrankenhaus, Weyprechtgasse, Mödling, Austria
Experience in the Treatment of Recurrent Anterior Dislocation of the Shoulder with a Modified Version of Bankart's Procedure

PREFACE

"Give me something different, for there is a chance of its being better".
Ernest Codman in his "Monumental Work"

Codman was obviously somewhat disenchanted with the current standards of practice and lack of understanding of the shoulder when he made his original statement. Taking up the challenge, his insightful observations founded the modern era of shoulder surgery. His emphasis on a full understanding of fundamental problems has led to something both different and better. Even with this inspiration, however, surgery and understanding of the shoulder have lagged somewhat behind other areas of orthopaedic management. A reawakening of interest in the shoulder has been given further impetus by the first International Shoulder Conference at London in 1980 and the second Conference in Toronto in 1983. Plans for further meetings in 1986 (Japan) and 1989 ensure a continuing forum for review of all aspects of study and clinical management of the shoulder.

The international contribution to this recent meeting with 200 registrants from 17 countries indicates the wide interest in the shoulder which we hope advances the tradition of Codman. Publication of this volume, derivative of the outstanding presentations at the second International Shoulder Conference, represents a significant contribution to the literature, containing both a distillate of current thought and inspiration to further progress. We are unaware of another book that includes such state-of-the-art information.

We are deeply grateful to the contributing authors who developed manuscripts based on the papers delivered at the Toronto assembly. We hope readers will find contained herein some useful new ideas and will be stimulated to implement improved methods for the treatment of shoulder disorders.

James E. Bateman, M.D.
R. Peter Welsh, M.B.

CODMAN LECTURE

To those of us who have thought of Ernest Codman only as a pioneer in the study of shoulder disorders, it comes as a surprise to learn that he was much more than that. Ernest Codman did indeed initiate and develop our knowledge of the shoulder joint, but his approach to clinical problems was unique. In fact, it came to constitute such a source of disagreement with his colleagues that he resigned his hospital appointment. It was his insistence on what he called the "end result" system which was primarily responsible for this antipathy. His approach to follow-up assessment was so revolutionary in his time that it was considered no less than heresy. Today, it is the basis of all good clinical practice and of a large volume of clinical research.

In the spirit of Codman, I would like to put a proposition to you which may also appear to be heretical. The proposition is that although the division of clinical practice between physician and surgeon seems to be an eternal verity, it may indeed be only a passing division of labor in the medical profession.

Some physicians think that surgeons merely practice a trade like that of plumber or carpenter; some surgeons think that physicians are an idle lot of speculators who should get down to real work. This may be mildly amusing but hardly advances our understanding. Better we realize that the ever increasing number of specialties and subspecialties which now fragment clinical medicine must eventually give way to produce a completely new type of doctor: a specialist clinician who also performs specialist manual work.

This proposition may not appeal to my geriatric contemporaries, but I hope that younger doctors will find an element of truth in it. James Addison once remarked: "A man is quickly convinced of the truth of a proposition who finds it not against his interests that it should be true."

I begin with a look at the development of the surgeon, not from any vain sense of precedence, but simply because manual work, biologically and historically, precedes intellectual development. Engels, in *The Part Played by Labor in the Transition from Ape to Man*, shows how the development of the brain is stimulated by its reaction to manual work and the use of tools. Sherrington, in his Rede Lecture, provided a more scientific model: "Some 80,000 years ago, relatively yesterday, a new thing, a tool, a stone shaped by and for the human hand, and a new animal sound, voices talking ... allowed the vast expansion of the brain to provide a gigantic combining mechanism for them."

In tracing the development of the physician, I am supported in my task by Mark Twain's observation that: "The great advantage of medicine is the large amount of conjecture that you can get from a small investment of fact." When medieval medicine became dominated by Galen and the Dark Ages descended, the separation between hand and brain had a deleterious effect. The more fashionable doctors, despising the work of the hand, began to delegate to slaves the manual attentions which they judged needful for their patients, standing over and directing them like architects. Physicians degenerated into what a contemporary graphically described as "foppish individuals with rings and carefully polished nails". The use of drugs was arbitrary and more often than not took the form of quackery. It became apparent to many enlightened contemporaries that physicians poured drugs of which they knew little into bodies of which they knew even less, and the patient was lucky if the drugs did no harm.

William Harvey pioneered the development of the clinician scientist. However, it was not until the end of the 19th Century that the scientific method was revived in clinical practice by a few doctors who showed that experimental techniques cannot be abandoned entirely to the laboratory, but that the scientific method can and must be introduced into the mainstream of clinical work.

There have been two trends in surgery: that of the journeyman-technician, and that of the surgeon-scientist. Jane Austen hinted at the social position of the surgeon as recently as the middle of the 18th Century. In one of her novels, while the doctor sips sherry in the dining room with the family, the surgeon takes his meals in the servants' quarters. In those days, the physician gave his instructions to the surgeon in simple terms: "Cut that stone; ablate that limb." This is a state of affairs which many contemporary physicians would no doubt still find enviable. The surgeon suffered much derision, as typified by Henri de Mondeville: "Many more surgeons know how to cause suppuration than to heal a wound."

The development of antiseptic and later aseptic surgery, anesthesia, and the control of shock by blood transfusion, changed all that and gave rise to a great flowering of the surgeon's art. As a result, his position in society rapidly improved to equal that of the physician, so that the two could be embraced in a single profession. In this united profession, however, their functions remain divided, and it is the nature of this division of responsibility which I would like to discuss.

Liberated from sepsis and traumatic shock, surgeons began to vie with each other in speed, dexterity, and volume of manual endeavor. The acme of this period was reached as recently as the middle of the present century in what can be termed the epoch of the great merchant surgeon, exemplified by individuals such as Halstead, impeccably dressed, elegant in pinstripe and double-breasted waistcoat, and with an assured place in society. The surgeon was regarded in awe, not only by his colleagues and his patients, but by society generally. He became the modern embodiment of the man of whom Jesus, son of Sirach, wrote in 118 B.C.: "Honor a physician according to thy need of him, and with the honor due unto him, for verily the Lord hath created him."

Although it goes without saying that a surgeon should be skilled in his operative technique, this has unfortunately often been the be-all and end-all of surgical expertise. As an undergraduate in London more than 30 years ago, I well remember Alec Bourne demonstrating an unfortunate woman to us and remarking that: "This lady has had six difficult operations; all were necessary except the first."

The range and complexity of modern surgical procedures makes entirely new intellectual demands on a surgeon, so that one may now question whether a surgeon's awareness of his own technical excellence might not in itself constitute a threat to the patient. I like to think that Ernest Codman would have been amongst the first to draw attention to this present danger.

Although physicians have perhaps been a little slow in getting their hands dirty, there are already more than a few important signposts on the way. When Avery Jones, a physician with a large gastroenterology unit in London, passed a gastroscope 30 years ago, he was starting something more than he realized. At St. Mark's Hospital for diseases of the colon, another physician, Christopher Williams, has now developed a most expert endoscopy clinic.

In this present international group of surgeons interested in disorders of the shoulder, we all know that there are many extrinsic causes of shoulder pain. Faced with this, are we going to call on the rheumatologist to diagnose the cause of the pain? Do we need a vascular surgeon to listen for a subclavian bruit? Should there not always be available in our shoulder clinics a stethoscope and a Frey hair for sensory testing? Do we rely on a psychiatrist to analyze the pattern and cause of shoulder instability?

Before bringing my argument to a conclusion, I should like to say a word about investigation, because there is a tendency to confuse scientific medicine with investigatory medicine. A clinician should not be judged by the number of investigations which he carried out, but rather by his careful selection of investigations designed to test an hypothesis based on analytical history and careful clinical examination.

I conclude by returning to my hypothesis that the present division of clinical practice into surgery and medicine is ephemeral and temporary.

Some have expressed surprise that Ernest Codman, with the whole field of clinical surgery open to him, should have chosen to focus on problems of the shoulder. I am not at all surprised. It is to my mind a natural field of activity for a person of his wide interests in the fundamentals of clinical practice. The shoulder is an area where medicine and surgery readily fuse. The best of clinical medicine is deployed in an analysis of the history, symptoms, and signs, in order to make an accurate diagnosis; and the best surgical practice is required to choose, design, and perform any necessary operative procedure. Orthopaedic surgery has very wide roots, and it would be to the honor of Codman's memory that those of us interested in the shoulder region, should lead away from the current practice of production-line surgery and introduce once more into orthopaedic practice the highest standards of clinical science based on the formulation and testing of hypotheses.

H.L. Mencken, perhaps the brightest wit and debunker of his time, warned us to be skeptical of all ideas, especially our own. I like to think that Codman, who expressed himself as disgusted with humbug, smugness, and cupidity, might well have agreed with many of the conclusions which I have made in an attempt to debunk some hallowed concepts amongst practicing orthopaedic surgeons, ideas which I believe would certainly have found favor with the stormy petrel whose name we are honoring today.

Lipmann Kessel, M.B.E., M.C., F.R.C.S.

CONTENTS

BIOMECHANICS

The Power Available During Movement of the Shoulder 1
William Angus Wallace, Margaret J. Barton, A. Murray Wiley

Kinesiology of the Shoulder—Electromyographic and Stereophotogrammetric Studies ... 6
Udo Laumann

Changes of the Tilting Angle of the Scapula Following Elevation of the Arm 12
Masayuki Kondo, Shiro Tazoe, Masayuki Yamada

The Role of the Rotator Cuff as a Stabilizing Mechanism of the Shoulder 17
Shinkichi Himeno, Hiroshi Tsumura

C-Arm Fluoroscopic Evaluation Under Anesthesia for Glenohumeral Subluxations 22
Tom Randolph Norris

Shoulder Arthrotomography and Computed Axial Tomography in the Diagnosis of Recurrent Shoulder Subluxations 26
Christopher Paul Beauchamp, Richard L. Loomer, Livius Timko

Arthroscopy of the Shoulder Joint 34
Hiroaki Tsutsui, Ryuji Yamamoto, Iwatsugu Anraku, Haruo Arai, Yujiro Mori, Yoshikatsu Kuroki

Indications and Benefits of Arthroscopy of the Shoulder Joint 38
Helge Lilleby

Arthroscopic Shoulder Surgery 41
A. Murray Wiley

The Role of Arthroscopy in Surgery of the Shoulder 45
Robert H. Cofield

TRAUMA

Aspects of Prognostic Factors in Comminuted and Dislocated Proximal Humeral Fractures 51
Olle Hägg, Bo J. Lundberg

Treatment of Complex Fractures of the Proximal Humerus by Neer Hemiarthroplasty 60
Jacques E. DesMarchais, G. Morais

Fractures of the Scapula Involving the Glenoid Fossa 63
Rolf T. Ideberg

Treatment of Acute Complete Dislocation of the Acromioclavicular Joint 67
Fumio Kato, Hiromichi Hayashi, Teiji Miyazaki, Kuninari Ito, Katsumasa Tomotsune, Naofumi Shimizu

A Prospective Study of the Treatment of Acromioclavicular Dislocation 70
Gordon Campbell Bannister, William Angus Wallace,

P. G. Stableforth,
M. A. Hutson

Trends in Treatment of
Complete Acromioclavicular
Dislocations 73
Carter Redd Rowe

SPORTS INJURIES—SHOULDER
STABILIZATION

Chronic Shoulder Pain in the
Athlete 79
Robert E. Leach,
David Segal

Computer Tomography on
Recurrent Shoulder
Dislocation 84
Udo Laumann,
H. A. Kramps

Operative Treatment of Recurrent
Anterior Shoulder Dislocation
with the Bristow-Latarjet
Procedure 87
Lennart Hovelius

Experience in the Treatment of
Recurrent Anterior Dislocation of
the Shoulder with a Modified
Version of Bankart's
Procedure 91
H. J. Zinnecker,
A. Pühringer,
L. K. Bartalsky

The Anteroinferior Vulnerable
Point of the Glenoid Rim 94
D. Patte,
J. Bernageau
Phillipe Bancel

Glenoid Osteotomy for Loose
Shoulder 100
Katsuya Nobuhara,
Hitoshi Ikeda

The Role of the Tendon of the
Long Head of the Biceps Brachii
in Anterior Subluxation of the

Shoulder 104
Paul M. Grammont,
Rainer P. Mayer,
Jochen R. Löhr

Oudard-Iwahara's Operation for
Recurrent Anterior Dislocation of
the Shoulder 106
Ryuji Yamamoto

Analysis of Failed Repair for
Shoulder Instability—A
Preliminary Report 111
Tom Randolph Norris,
Louis U. Bigliani

Missed Posterior Dislocations of
the Shoulder 117
R. J. Hawkins,
Charles S. Neer, II,

ROTATOR CUFF

The Subacromial Bursae:
A Clinicopathological
Study 121
Hans K. Uhthoff,
Kiriti Sarkar,
David Ian Hammond

Diagnosis of Rotator Cuff Tears
by Double Contrast Arthrotomography: Reliability Study ... 126
Jacques E. DesMarchais
Jean Vezina

The Significance of Distally
Pointing Acromioclavicular
Osteophytes in Ruptures of the
Supraspinatus Tendon 129
Claes J. Petersson,
Carl Fredrik Gentz

Contact Areas of the
"Subacromial" Joint 134
Richard J. Nasca,
E. George Salter,
Craig E. Weil

The Impingement Syndrome in
Sportsmen 140
Michael Watson

Diagnosis and Treatment of Partial Thickness Tears of Rotator Cuff 143
Shiro Tabata,
Hiroshi Kida

Surgical Treatment of Complete Rotator Cuff Tears 149
Richard J. Nasca

Adhesive Capsulitis of the Shoulder 154
J. Patrick Murnaghan

Rotator Cuff Tears in the Young 157
V. Prem Kumar,
Omar Bayne,
Robert Peter Welsh,
James E. Bateman

Surgical Management of Rotator Cuff Tears 161
R. J. Hawkins

Long Term Results of Surgical Repair of Full Thickness Rotator Cuff Tears 167
Omar Bayne,
James E. Bateman

Reconstruction of Chronic Tears of the Rotator Cuff 172
Robert J. Neviaser,
Thomas J. Neviaser

Shoulder Rehabilitation After Rotator Cuff Surgery 180
Marilyn J. Mode

Repair of Chronic Massive Rotator Cuff Tears with Synthetic Fabrics 185
Jiro Ozaki,
Sei Fujimoto,
Kenji Masuhara

Repair of Rotator Cuff Tears 192
Robert L. Samilson

Trapezius Transfer for Global Tear of the Rotator Cuff 196
Motohiko Mikasa

The Acropole Prosthesis 200
Paul M. Grammont

A Surgical Approach to Rotator Cuff Tears 202
Norbert Gschwend

ARTHRODESIS
ARTHROPLASTY

Shoulder Arthrodesis— A.O. Technique 207
John Philip Kostuik,
Joseph Schatzker

Bipolar Implant Shoulder Arthroplasty 211
Alfred B. Swanson

Experience with the Neer Total Shoulder Replacement, ... 224
Alan H. Wilde,
Lester S. Borden,
John J. Brems

Total Shoulder Arthroplasty: Associated Disease of the Rotator Cuff, Results, and Complications 229
Robert H. Cofield

Ten Years of Experience with Unconstrained Shoulder Replacement 234
E. Engelbrecht

Unconstrained Shoulder Arthroplasty 240
Charles S. Neer, II

NEUROMUSCULAR DISORDERS

Thoracoscapular Fusion for Facioscapulohumeral Dystrophy ... 247
Stephen Andrew Copeland

Pectoralis Minor Transposition in Serratus Anterior Paralysis 252
Martti Valtteri Vastamäki

Thoracic Scapulopexy for Restoration of Arm Elevation in Facioscapulohumeral Type

Muscular Dystrophy 255
Minoru Sakurai

Results of Surgical Treatment
for Deltoid Muscle Contracture ... 259
Tomomitsu Kutsuma,
Kazuo Terayama

ARTHRITIC DISORDERS

Surgery of the Rheumatoid
Shoulder 269
Norbet Gschwend,
A. Kentsch

Stabilization of Shoulders with
Bone and Muscle Defects
Using Joint Replacement
Implants 281
Reinhard Koelbel

Long Term Results of Neer Total
Shoulder Replacement 294
Harry A. Bade, III,
Chitranjan S. Ranawat,
Russell F. Warren,
Allan E. Inglis

SPECIAL CONSIDERATIONS

Comparative Study of Bone
Lesions in Traumatic Recurrent
Dislocations of the Shoulder—
Their Importance and Treatment .. 303
Carlos E. deAnquin,
Carlos Alberto deAnquin

The Place of Computed
Arthrotomography in Unstable
Shoulder 306
Patrick Kinnard,
Douglas Gordon,
Réjean-Yves Lévesque,
Denis Bergeron

Limb Salvage Procedures for
Primary Bone Tumors of the
Shoulder Region 310
Michael G. Rock,
Franklin H. Sim,
Edmund Y. S. Chao

Surgical Pathology in Chronic
Shoulder Pain 313
Pekka Paavolainen,
Pär Slätis,
Kari A. Aalto

Pyogenic Arthritis of the
Glenohumeral Joint Following the
Intra-articular Injection of
Corticosteroid 319
Takehiko Torisu,
Shogo Masumi,
Masateru Shindo

Crutchwalker's Shoulder 324
Robert Greg Pringle

Roentgenographical Examination
of the Tilted Angle of the Scapula
in Three Dimensions in
the Relaxed Standing Position 326
Takehiko Torisu,
Shinkichi Himeno

Classification and Aspects of
Treatment of Fractures of the
Proximal Humerus 330
R. P. Jakob,
T. Kristiansen,
K. Mayo,
R. Ganz,
M. E. Müller

BIOMECHANICS

THE POWER AVAILABLE DURING MOVEMENT OF THE SHOULDER

WILLIAM ANGUS WALLACE, F.R.C.S., MARGARET J. BARTON, M.C.S.P., and A. MURRAY WILEY, M.Ch., F.R.C.S., F.R.C.S.(C)

Patients with disorders in the region of the shoulder complain of three main symptoms—pain, stiffness and weakness of the shoulder. The most common symptom is pain but this is subjective and often difficult to assess. Stiffness of the shoulder is measured clinically with a goniometer to record active flexion and abduction movements and internal and external rotation ranges. Passive movements may also be recorded. Assessment of combined scapulothoracic and glenohumeral movements are sufficient for most clinical purposes although radiological studies will reveal the more detailed glenohumeral movements.[5]

Assessment of the weakness of the shoulder by measuring the forces produced by the arm has rarely been carried out and apart from the excellent study by van Linge and Mulder[4] and the theoretical work of Poppen and Walker[3] few other studies have been reported. Many patients report significant weakness of the shoulder, particularly those with tears of the rotator cuff and occasionally after total shoulder replacement; and a clinically applicable test of shoulder strength would be useful.

ISOKINETIC DYNAMOMETRY OF THE SHOULDER

Between 1981 and 1983 over 350 studies of the torque produced by the muscles around the shoulder during movement were carried out and a standard method for clinical use has been established.

The apparatus used for the study was a Cybex II isokinetic dynamometer fitted with an external torque cell developed by Knutsson in Sweden and described in 1980.[2] The dynamometer is mounted on a supporting platform 66 cm high as shown in Figure 1. The test is carried out with the subject standing as this is the natural position of function of the shoulder. The subject stands at right angles to the Cybex machine with the axis of rotation centered on the glenohumeral joint and the Cybex arm adjusted to an appropriate length. The speed of movement of the Cybex arm is adjusted and the patient's arm is raised in flexion with maximum force (Fig. 2) to full elevation. The arm is then brought back down again at maximum force. This test is repeated to give five times for normal shoulders and three times for symptomatic shoulders. We carry out the test on both arms in both flexion as described and abduction in the scapular plane.[1]

Although a Cybex study is usually recorded with a dual channel recorder on graph paper, the use of a computer linked to the angle and torque readings is preferable. We have a link to a Digital Minc computer with a program developed which allows a real-time analysis of the information but with a delayed (4 second) presentation of the graphical result. Figure 3 demonstrates a typical computer printout of the initial Cybex results for a left shoulder abduction test with five repetitions. The reproducibility of the graphs is excellent in the normal shoulder. In our work we have found it more appropriate to plot the angle of movement on the x-axis in 20 degree steps and the torque on the y-axis in 10 Newton-metre steps. The top half of the graph shows the forces generated during elevation of the arm in abduction, the bottom graph identifies the forces involved in bringing the arm back to the side. Before proceeding with the study, the weight of the limb is measured by resting the subject's arm on the lever arm of the Cybex

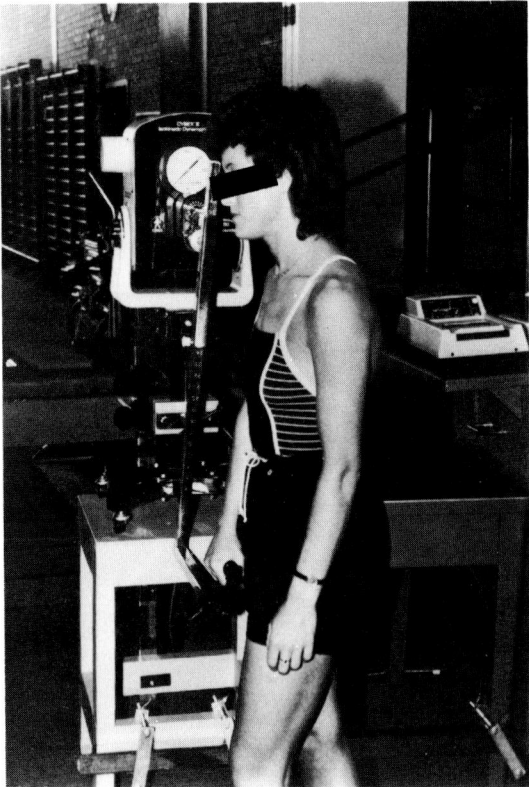

Figure 1 Positioning of the subject for Cybex shoulder study. (Torque cell omitted)

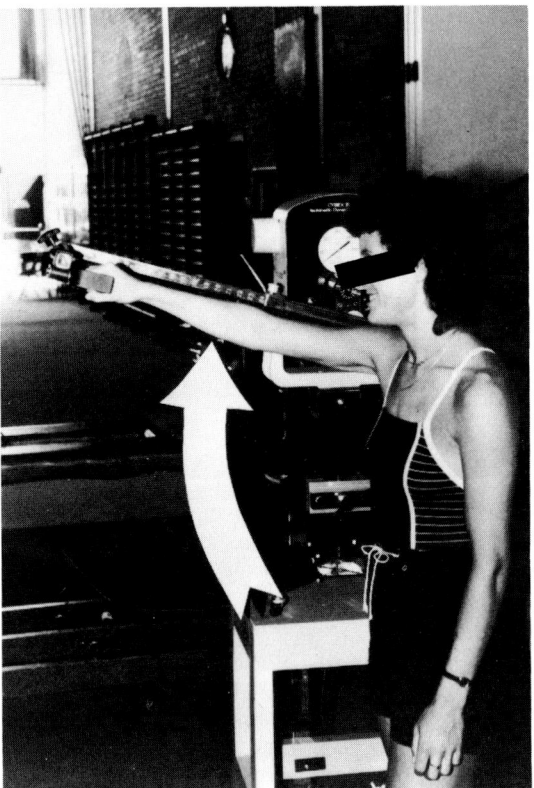

Figure 2 The arm is raised with maximum force to full elevation in flexion.

and the graph in Figure 3 includes a gravity correction factor for the weight of the limb. The information obtained from the study is analysed within one minute by the computer and the following parameters are recorded for each of the five graphs:

1. The work done during elevation
2. The peak torque value
3. The mean torque value
4. The range of movement
5. The mean and standard deviation for work done for the 5 repetitions
6. The median work done on elevation from the 5 curves
7. The median peak torque from the 5 curves.

Aims of the Study

This analysis of 350 Cybex tests of the shoulder has been carried out to identify the best speed of movement to use for the shoulder and to measure the reproducibility of the data obtained in the short and long terms, and to devise a standard method for carrying out the test. The difference between the dominant and nondominant limb was also explored.

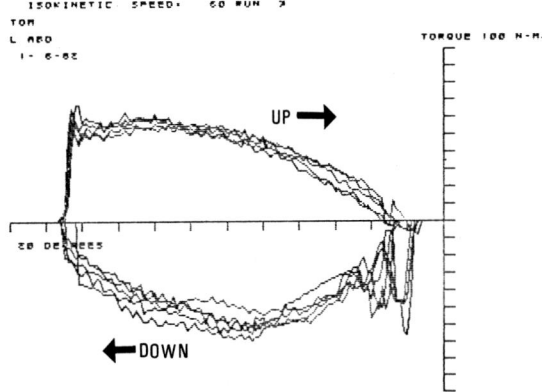

Figure 3 Typical computer printout for a Cybex study—left shoulder, abduction at 60 degrees/second. Top half elevation, bottom half returns to neutral.

Results

Speed of Movement of the Arm

Two subjects repeated the Cybex test on seven occasions at different speeds with suitable rest intervals. The speeds varied from less than 10 degrees per second (almost an isometric test) to 300 degrees per second and the results are shown in Figure 4. The graph of the man shows a plateau on an S-shaped curve at 100 to 200 degrees/sec while the woman had a more linear graph. On the basis of these tests the best speed for the normal shoulder is probably around 120 degrees/sec. However, concurrent with this study we had been testing patients with shoulder disorders and we had found that they could not tolerate speeds higher than 100 degrees/sec. Speeds of either 60 degrees per second or 30 degrees per second are therefore recommended for shoulder work.

Reproducibility of Recordings Over a Short Period

Five subjects, two male and three female, were tested daily for four days with tests carried out on both arms in flexion and abduction. In this part of the study we have analysed the work done and calculated the mean and standard deviation from the five curves on each day. Figure 5 shows the results for the right arms tested in abduction at 60 degrees/sec. The subjects were tested at both 60 and 120 degrees/sec and the results indicated better reproducibility in the 60 degrees/sec tests. We were slightly concerned at the occasional drop in torque and work done which occurred in some of our male subjects on the second or third day of testing and this was associated with mild aching in the arm perhaps indicating a soft tissue strain or impingement. It was felt a longer term study was required (see below).

Comparison of Dominant and Nondominant Arms

In the same study we were able to compare the dominant (right) and nondominant (left) arms. Figure 6 demonstrates that in some of our subjects there was little difference but in others there was a difference of as much as 30 percent in the work done, with the dominant limb more powerful. It was also noted that the nondominant limb performed less well on the third and fourth day than the dominant limb.

Reproducibility of Recordings Over a Long Period (3 Weeks)

Five subjects were studied over a period of three weeks. This study also identified an occasional sudden dip in performance as is shown in Figure 7 which we again felt might be due to a soft tissue mild injury. This "artifact" is important to record as it could introduce errors into the interpretation of Cybex performance tests in the shoulder. The overall reproducibility in the long term is acceptable, but the curves do indicate a probable early training effect from using the Cybex for testing.

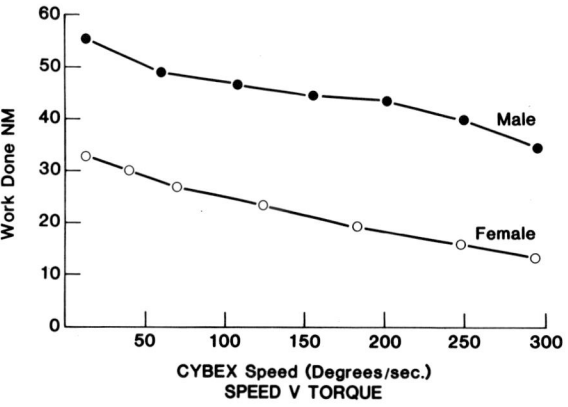

Figure 4 Effect of speed of movement of arm v. work done. Note the plateau on the male graph between 100 and 200 degrees/second.

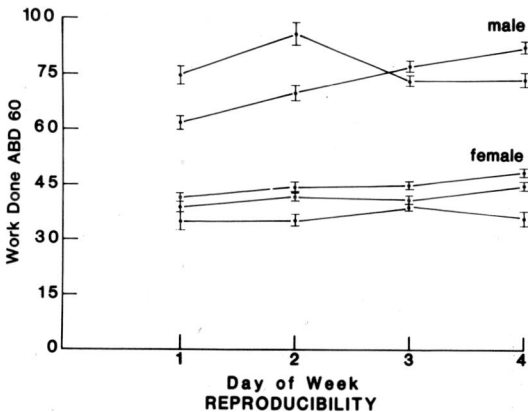

Figure 5 Five subjects, 60 degrees/second, abduction. Note the drop in performance on day 3 in one male subject.

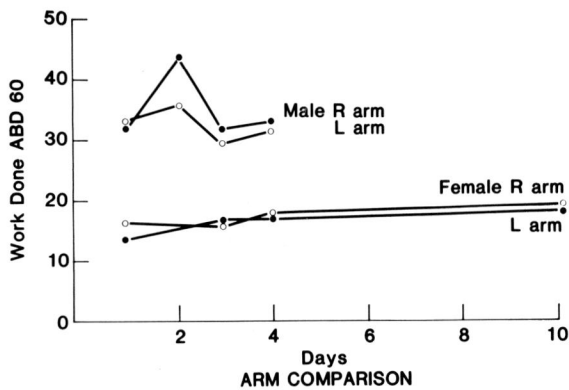
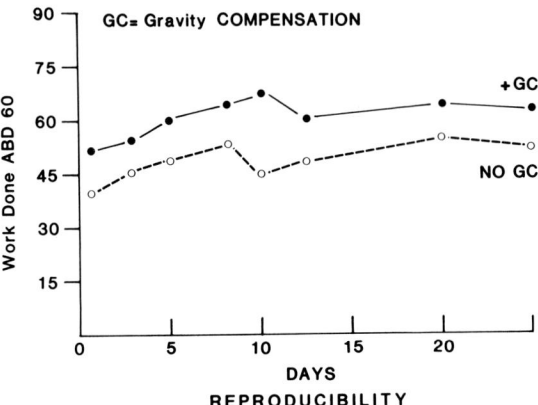

Figure 6 Comparison of dominant (R) and nondominant (L) arms.

Figure 7 One of 5 subjects monitored over a period of 3 weeks. Note the close similarity of the uncorrected (NO GC) and corrected (+GC) curves for gravity compensation.

Gravity Compensation for Torque Values

The effect of errors being introduced by adding the gravity compensation correction has been considered. Figure 7 shows the effect in one of our subjects; similar graphs were obtained for all subjects. The weight of the limb recorded using the external torque cell in a static situation is reliable and only small errors are introduced using the gravity correction. However, using the Cybex torque measurements directly from the Cybex equipment is less accurate and can only be carried out satisfactorily with the limb falling due to gravity. We see little benefit from adding gravity compensation to our curves for shoulder work and have stopped doing this. However, we still record the weight of the limb in case we should wish to reconsider this in the future.

Clinical Application of Cybex Testing

Having established the reliability and reproducibility of Cybex shoulder recordings the clinical application of this work should be considered. Which patients should be considered for Cybex testing? Figure 8 shows a patient who presented with a weak left arm and wasting of the deltoid and supraspinatus muscles. We were able to follow him for 20 weeks and monitor his progress while physiotherapy was being carried out. It was obvious at the end of the 20 weeks that he had regained no shoulder strength from the physiotherapy regime and it was abandoned. This patient demonstrates acceptable reproducibility of the "work done" during elevation of the limb. We believe this type of testing will have application to the assessment of results following surgery to the shoulder and perhaps drug treatment for shoulder pathology; both fields are being explored currently.

Conclusions

Cybex testing of strength of the shoulder is a useful reproducible test. It has application in the assessment of patients with pathology in the region of the shoulder and after surgery. We recommend the patient have the test carried out while standing as described and with a limb movement speed of 60 or 30 degrees per second. Sudden dips in performance can be expected in men but not women and are probably due to minor soft tissue injury. Gravity correction of the curves is probably not

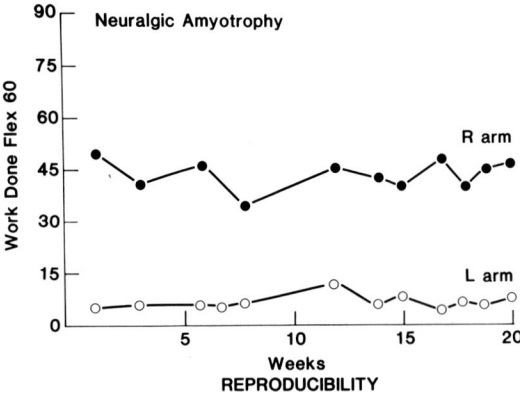

Figure 8 Clinical application of Cybex testing to a patient with neuralgic amyotrophy. There has been no improvement in the left arm despite intensive physiotherapy.

necessary. Computer linkage with the Cybex is of considerable value and should be considered for all joint assessment—not only the shoulder.

REFERENCES

1. Doody SG, Freedman L, Waterland JC. Shoulder movements during abduction in the scapular plane. Arch Phys Med Rehab 1970; 51:595–604.
2. Knutsson E, Martensson A. Dynamic Motor Capacity in Spastic Paresis and its relation to prime mover dysfunction, spastic reflexes and antagonist co-activation. Scand J Rehab Med 1980; 12:93–106.
3. Poppen NK, Walker PS. Forces at the glenohumeral joint in abduction. Clin Orthop Rel Research 1978; 135:165–170.
4. Van Linge B, Mulder JD. Function of the supraspinatus muscle and its relation to the supraspinatus syndrome. J Bone Joint Surg 1963; 45B:750–754.
5. Wallace WA. The dynamic study of shoulder movement. Berlin, Heidelberg, New York: Springer Verlag. 1982: 139–143.

KINESIOLOGY OF THE SHOULDER—ELECTROMYOGRAPHIC AND STEREOPHOTOGRAMMETRIC STUDIES

U. LAUMANN, M.D.

The aim of our study was to demonstrate the pathological variations in isolated paralyses of the shoulder muscles, in order to improve the theoretical bases for conservative and operative treatments.

The quantitative analysis of the muscle function and its coordination was performed by computer on-line electromyointegration. The movement of arm, scapula, and spine was analysed by the three-dimensional analysis of stereophotogrammetry (Fig. 1).

RESULTS

Position of the Shoulder Girdle at Rest

The capsular ligaments and the resting tone of the shoulder muscles control the position of the shoulder girdle; usually, no muscular activity is required. Isolated complete functional loss of the trapezius muscle leads to a ventrocaudal displacement of the shoulder girdle: the clavicle moves progressively in the frontal plane and drops down caudally. Of necessity, the scapula becomes more lateralized and increasingly turns in a parasagittal plane. The articular process in inclined caudally.

Isolated serratus anterior paresis also causes a disturbance of the physiological balance of the shoulder girdle. However, the direction of displacement is opposite to that of trapezius paresis: the clavicle moves away from the frontal plane in a dorsal direction, and the scapula becomes more medialised and progressively tilts in a frontal plane.

In combined functional loss of the trapezius and serratus anterior muscles, the typical shoulder displacement of trapezius paresis is present. This caudal rotation of the scapula cannot be compensated for (Fig. 2).

Antigravitational Muscle Function

Unilateral loading tests on the hanging arm with increasing weights of 10 to 200 N do not evoke any changes in shoulder girdle position in healthy subjects. The pars descendens of the trapezius muscle is progressively innervated under increasing weight loading and thus it preserves the balance of the shoulder girdle. The supraspinatus muscle holds the glenohumeral joint together.

In trapezius paresis, shoulder girdle displacement is aggravated by weight-loading on the hanging arm. This provokes pain in the arm plexus, so that the load capacity of the extremity involved is very much decreased.

In serratus anterior paresis, the attitude of the shoulder girdle does not significantly change under weight-loading; the load capacity is only scarcely diminished in comparison with healthy subjects (Fig. 3).

Dynamics of the Shoulder-Arm Complex

The dynamic electromyographic tests carried out in three definite planes of motion (frontal, scapular, and sagittal) show that only a few of the numerous shoulder muscles significantly increase their activity during arm elevation from 0 to 180 degrees. These muscles are summarized within group 1 and must be considered essential for shoulder dynamics. The functional loss of one of these muscles usually causes an evident loss of arm motility (Fig. 4, Fig. 5).

The stereophotogrammetric studies of the rotation of the scapula show that, after a short "setting phase," a linear relation between arm elevation and scapula rotation results. The setting phase is less evident during flexion than during abduction (Fig. 6).

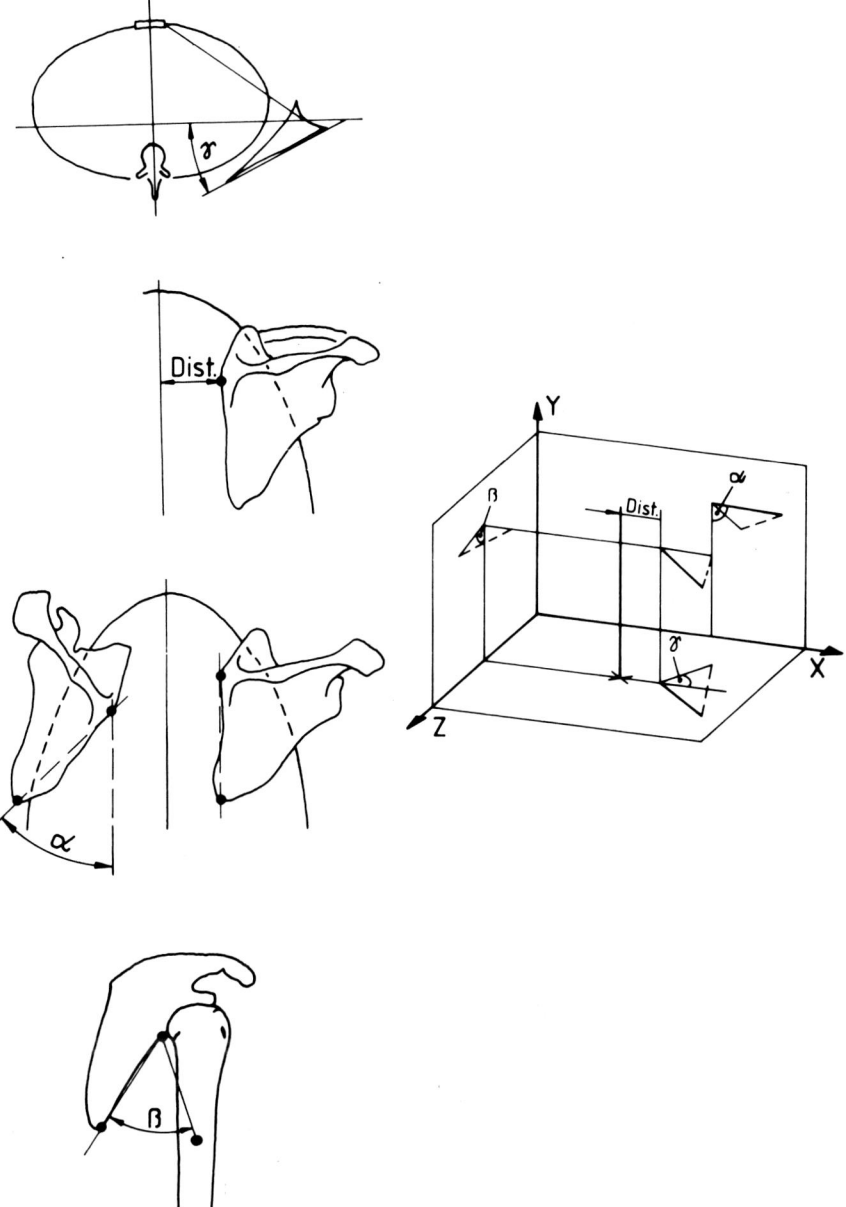

Figure 1 Determination of the changes of scapular position; three dimensional analysis.

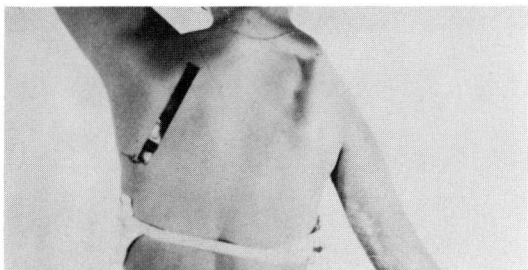

Figure 2 Combined right trapezius—serratus anterior paresis; caudal scapular rotation which cannot be compensated.

In trapezius paresis, differences in the functional capacity of arm elevation can be observed between patients, such that three groups of functional capacity were classified. Comparing these groups, the electromyographic tests show considerable differences between activity and coordination of the serratus anterior muscle on the one hand, and levator and rhomboidei muscles on the other hand. In the functionally poor group 1, change of muscle activity cannot be recognized; the scapula remains malpositioned during arm elevation. In group 3, functionally the best group, the scapula is moved by the serratus anterior muscle alone after an initial previous tension by the levator and rhomboidei muscles. In group 2, the serratus and levator and rhomboidei muscles act together until the end phase of arm elevation and fix the scapula in a middle position (Fig. 7).

In serratus anterior paresis, the scapula does not perform any rotation; it remains fixed in medium rotatory position at the thoracic wall, and motions are carried out exclusively in the glenohumeral joint. In combined trapezius—serratus anterior paresis, the rhomboideus and levator muscles are innervated when arm elevation is tried. This increases the scapular caudal rotation and leads to an adduction of the arm.

CONCLUSION

Only a few muscles are essential for the stability and dynamics of the shoulder-arm complex. The functional loss of one of these muscles always causes a disturbance of the functional unit, which, however, can be compensated in most cases by other muscles. If two essential muscles are paralysed, the result is always an important functional loss. This is evident in combined trapezius—serratus anterior paresis, which is always an absolute indication for operative treatment. By scapulothoracic fusion with fixation of the scapula in a position of 30 degrees rotation, a stable shoulder with a considerably enlarged range of motility is obtained. Isolated trapezius and serratus anterior pareses are relative indications for operative treatment.

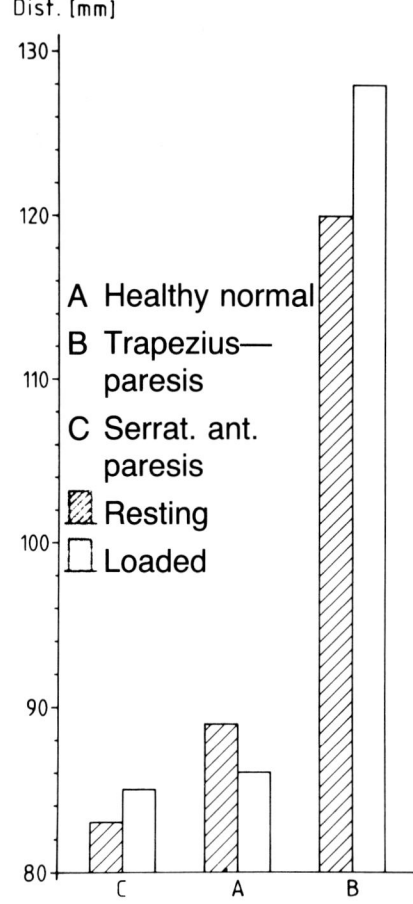

Figure 3 Changes of the distance of the medial border of the scapula towards the spine in healthy subjects (A), in cases of trapezius paresis (B), in cases of serratus anterior paresis (C). ■ → position at rest. □ → loading on the hanging arm (healthy; 200 N. pareses; possible maximum load 30–200 N).

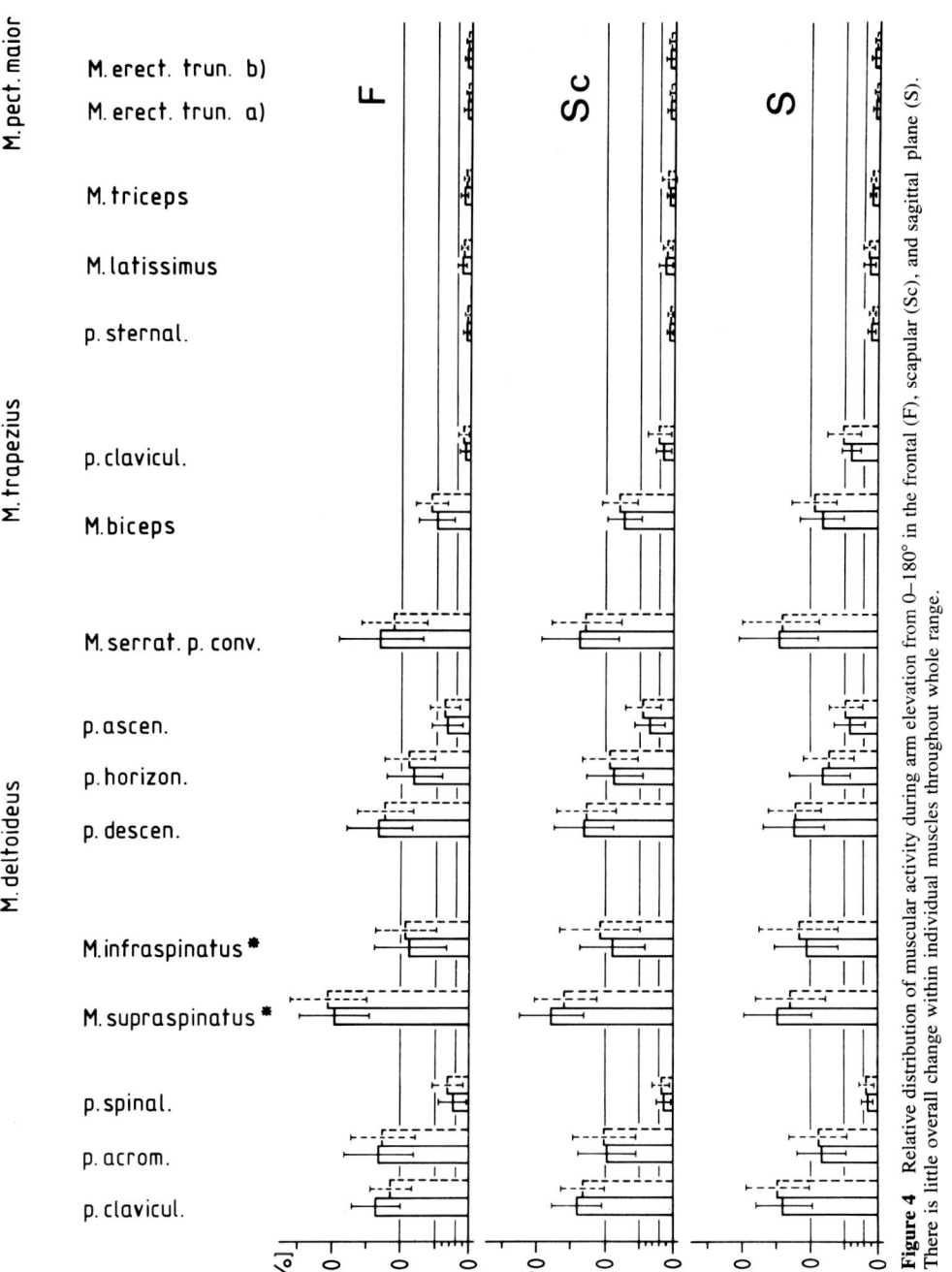

Figure 4 Relative distribution of muscular activity during arm elevation from 0–180° in the frontal (F), scapular (Sc), and sagittal plane (S). There is little overall change within individual muscles throughout whole range.

10 / Surgery of the Shoulder

Group I >10%	
1. M. deltoid. p. clavicul	13%
2. p. acrom.	10%
3. M. trap. p. descend	12%
4. M. supraspinatus ■	17%
5. M. serrat. p. converg.	13%
	65%

Group II ≧ 5 < 10%	
1. M. trap. p. horiz.	8%
2. M. infraspinatus ■	9%
3. biceps	7%
	24%

Group III ≧ 2 < 5%	
M. deltoid. p. spinalis	2%
M. pectoralis p. clav.	2%
M. trap. p. asced.	3%
	7%

Group IV ≦2%	
1. M. pectoralis p. stern	1%
2. M. latissimus	1%
3. M. triceps	1%
4. M. erector trunci	1%
	4%

Figure 5 Classification of the electromyographically tested shoulder muscles in 4 functional groups with relation to their mean activity during arm elevation. Group 1: muscles essential for shoulder dynamics.

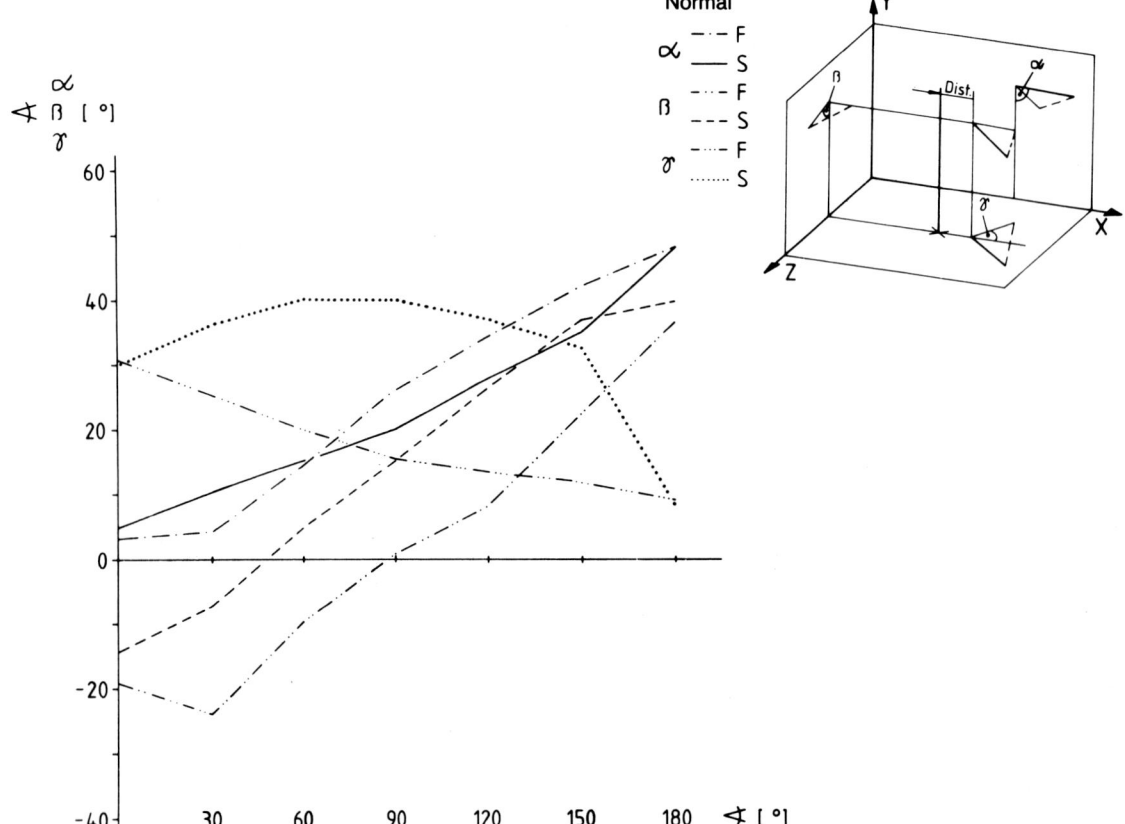

Figure 6 Changes of the scapular position during arm elevation from 0–180° in the frontal (F) and sagittal plane (S).

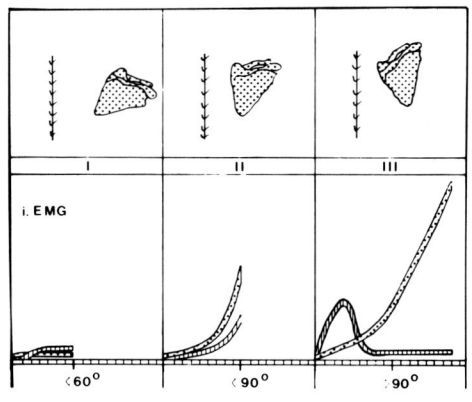

Figure 7 Different EMG patterns in the various functional groups with trapezius paresis.

CHANGES OF THE TILTING ANGLE OF THE SCAPULA FOLLOWING ELEVATION OF THE ARM

MASAYUKI KONDO, M.D., SHIRO TAZOE, M.D., and MASAYUKI YAMADA, M.D.

The shoulder is constructed of three anatomical joints and three functional joints, thus the phrase, "the shoulder complex."[2] At the scapulothoracic joint, one of the three functional joints, the scapula moves on the chest wall. However, its movement is not in one plane, but in three dimensions. There are many roentgenographic studies of the movement of the scapula during elevation of the arm, but these are almost always studied in two dimensions.[4,7] In the present study, we have devised a new method for taking roentgenograms using a specific equation of the degrees of the tilting angle of the scapula in three dimensions and calculating the degree of tilting angle of the scapula during arm elevation in a plane of 40° against the frontal plane.

MATERIALS

Roentgenographic examinations were carried out on 44 shoulders of 22 normal male subjects. Ages ranged from 20 to 34 years.

DEFINITION OF THE PLANE OF THE SHOULDER BLADE

To define the plane of the shoulder blade, three landmarks were selected on each roentgenogram (Fig. 1): A, The intersection of the vertebral border and scapular spine. B, The inferior angle. C, Infraglenoid tubercle.

METHODS

Method of Taking the Roentgenogram and Calculation

Concentrating the x-ray axis on the spinous process of the second thoracic spine, bilateral roentgenograms were taken in the postero-anterior position. In the resting position, two roentgenograms were taken at distances of one meter and two meters between the x-ray films and the source (Fig. 2). At this time, fixation of the axis of irradiation was most important. That is, the roentgenograms were taken at different distances on the same x-ray axis.

Following that, roentgenograms at 40° to the frontal plane were taken at three positions respectively, 90°, 150°, and maximum elevation.

Then X, Y coordinates of each point were measured by an X, Y coordinate processor. Using the specific equation, X, Y, Z coordinates, the degrees of the tilting angle of the scapula in three dimensions, and the lengths of the three sides (AB, BC, CA) were calculated in the resting position. Then at the arm elevation position, as only one roentgenogram was taken, respectively utilizing the lengths of the three sides (AB, BC, CA) which were already calculated in the resting position, the X, Y, Z coordinates and the degree of the tilting angle of the scapula were calculated. The tilts of the scapula in the three dimensions were termed "medially tilting angle," "downward tilting angle," and "upward rotation angle" (Fig. 3). "Medially tilting angle" refers to tilting of the scapula to the sagittal plane. At this point the frontal plane is zero. "Downward tilting angle" describes forward or backward tilts of the scapula in the complete lateral view. "Upward rotation angle" means the angle between line BC and the line of gravity.

Theory of the Calculation

Double Roentgenogram Method. Figure 4-A shows the relation between point A and the point projected on the x-ray film. As triangles OP_1A_1 and OP_2A_2 exist on the same plane, the coordinates of point A in the three dimensions can

Biomechanics / 13

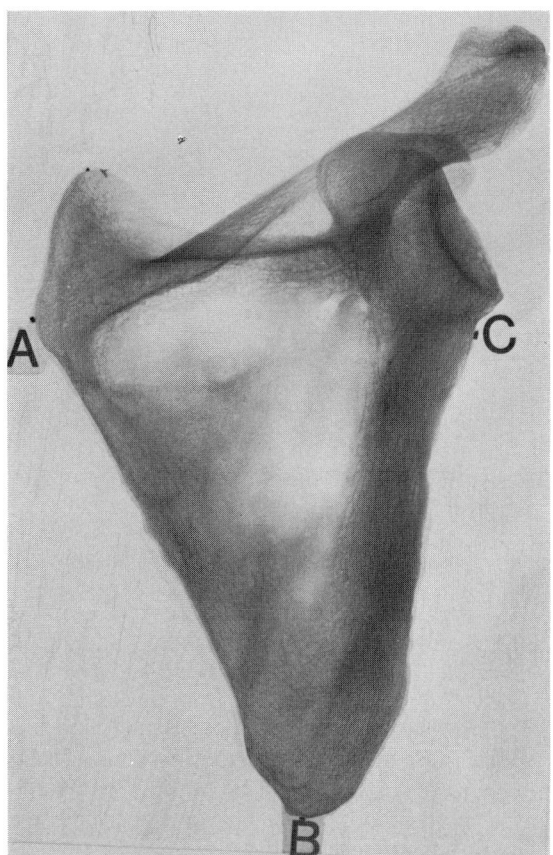

Figure 1 Definition of the plane of the shoulder blade. A. Intersection of the vertebral border and the scapular spine. B. The inferior angle. C. Infraglenoid tubercle.

be calculated by using similar figures and trigonometrical functions. From the X, Y, Z coordinates of each point of A, B, C the lengths of the three sides and the tilting angle of the scapula can be calculated.

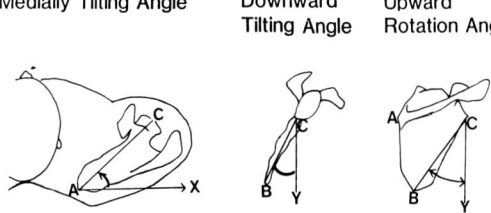

Figure 3 Tilting angle of the scapula.

Single Roentgenogram Method (Fig. 4-B). If the lengths of the three sides were already obtained and three lines were established, a triangle could be drawn by describing arcs in turn from starting point A. The lengths of the three sides were already calculated in the resting position, in addition, the lines PA', PB', PC' were established by using each X, Y coordinate. However, as our study attempted to clarify the movement of the scapula in three dimensions, computations were made by setting up the cubic equation.

In addition, X, Y coordinates of the starting point A were already obtained from the two dimensional roentgenogram. Therefore, assuming Z coordinate to be in the resting position, computations were made in the limit of plus and minus 50 mm at every millimeter. When the distance between the intersection of the line PA' and the arc described from point C and starting point A was least, we selected the final data.

Confirmation of the Method. The lengths of three sides and the tilting angles of the various plastic models, which were made to confirm the method of calculation above, were measured, and the roentgenograms of those models were taken and were calculated by "the double and single roentgenogram method." Then, measured data and calculated data were compared (Fig. 5).

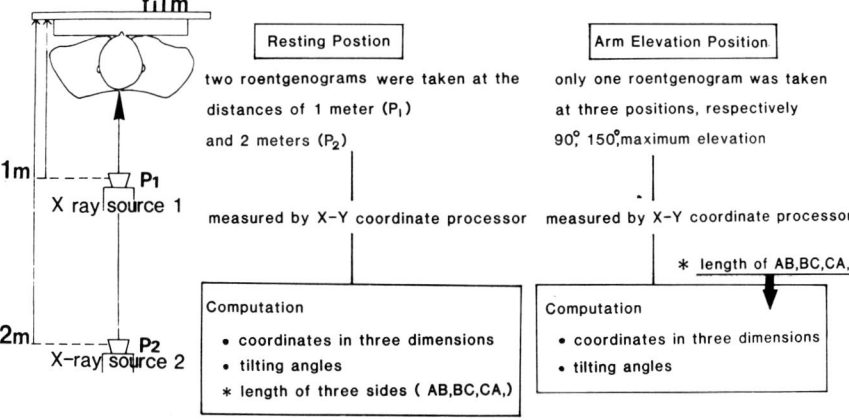

Figure 2 Plan of the study.

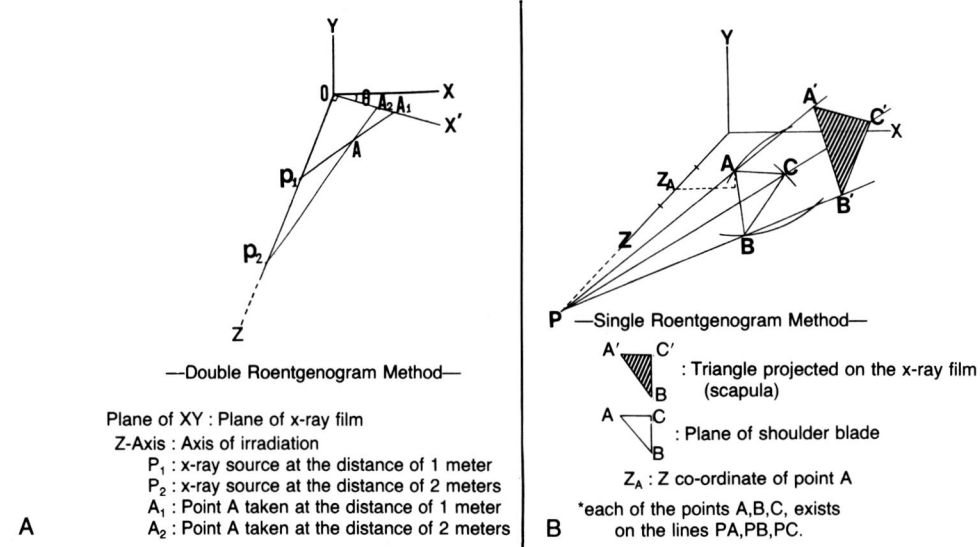

Figure 4 Theory of the calculation. A. Double roentgenogram method for calculation at the resting position. B. Single roentgenogram method for calculation at the arm elevation position.

RESULTS

Table 1 shows the correlation between calculated and measured data of various plastic models. Each correlation coefficient was above 0.916 and this reveals our method to be sufficiently reliable. The changes of the tilting angle of the scapula during elevation of the arm were as follows (Table 2):

Medially Tilting Angle. The medially tilting angle averaged 39.29° in the resting position, 39.86° at 90° of elevation, and 40.53° at 150° of elevation. That is, the medially tilting angle was nearly constant at about 40° from the resting position to 150° of elevation. In addition, there was no significant difference indicated among these three groups by the two-tailed paired T-test. However, at maximum elevation the average angle was 47.46°, a significant increase.

Downward Tilting Angle. When the superior angle of the scapula moved into the body wall and the inferior angle moved away, it was

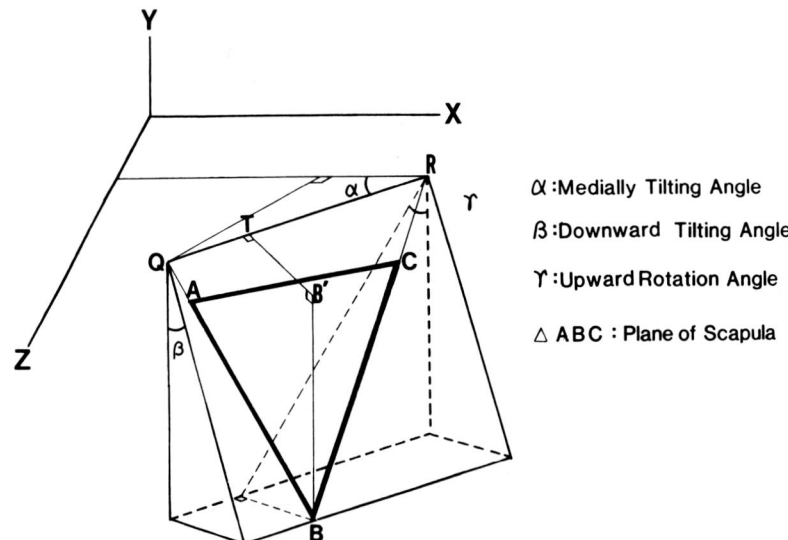

Figure 5 Plastic model to compare calculated data with measured data.

TABLE 1 Correlation Between Calculated and Measured Data		
Tilting Angle	Double Roentgenogram Method (n = 28)	Single Roentgenogram Method (n = 18)
Medially	Y = 0.95X + 2.34 r = 0.989	Y = 0.98X + 0.64 r = 0.997
Downward	Y = 1.09X − 0.13 r = 0.987	Y = 1.01X − 0.49 r = 0.994
Upward Rotation	Y = 0.91X + 3.47 r = 0.961	Y = 1.00X − 0.28 r = 0.976

Y: Regression Line
r: Correlation Coefficient

TABLE 2 Changes of the Tilting Angle of the Scapula Following Elevation of the Arm (N = 44)			
Position	Medially	Downward	Upward Rotation
Resting position	38.29 (1.45)	12.64 (1.61)	51.97 (1.88)
90° elevation	39.86 (1.51)	−0.55 (1.15)	20.59 (1.95)
150° elevation	40.53 (1.46)	−7.17 (1.41)	−0.05 (1.92)
Max. elevation	47.46 (1.30)	−11.80 (1.33)	−8.67 (1.61)

Bracketed numbers = T distribution

positively expressed. It follows that in the resting position, the average tilt of the scapula was 12.46° forward and downward. Then it gradually tilted backward, until, at 90° of elevation, it became nearly perpendicular; at the maximum elevation of the arm, it tilted 11.80° backward and downward. The movement of the scapula was about 24° in all.

Upward Rotation Angle. The negative data show that line BC exceeds the line of gravity. The average angle was 51.97° at the resting position and −8.67° at the maximum elevation. It rotated upward about 60° in all. The changes of the tilting angle of the scapula following elevation of the arm were explained above.

Now, using the X, Y, Z coordinates calculated in the present study, the motions of the scapula are depicted (Fig. 6). Figure 6-A shows changes in the frontal plane. As elevation progresses, the upward rotation angle continues to increase. Figure 6-B shows changes on the coronal plane. As elevation progresses, point B varies greatly from positive to negtive. That is, it shows that the downward tilt is inverted. Conversely, it is understood that the medially tilting angle, which is shown by line AC, varies little. Figure 6-C shows changes in the sagittal plane. As elevation progresses, the downward tilting angle continues decreasing and subsequently inverts, but the upward rotation angle continues to increase.

Discussion

When we make a roentgenographic examination of the scapular movement in three dimensions, a special method of taking the roentgenogram is necessary. In the past, the method that uses two roentgenograms of the standard antero-

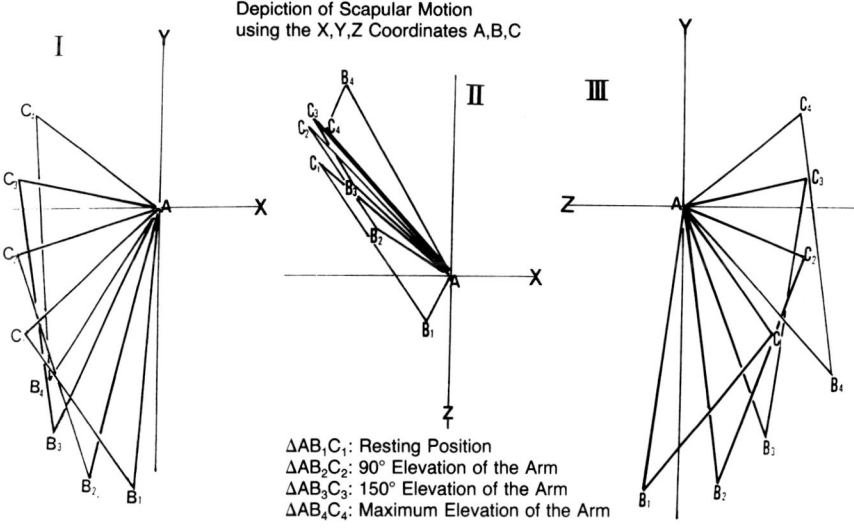

Figure 6 Anterior (I), superior (II) and lateral (III) views of the changes of the scapula following elevation of the arm.

posterior and another projection has been used. But this method produces several errors in calculation.

At the arm elevation position, in which the subjects have a tendency to move, calculation is especially difficult. Therefore, we devised the method described above. The advantages of our method are: a decrease in the dose of irradiation and resolution of the problem of errors produced by movement of the subjects.

A small variation of the degrees of the medially tilting angle in the resting position has been reported. This was described as 30° by Kapandji[5] and Steindler,[8] 40° by Lanz,[11] 32° by Torisu[10] and 40.3° by Tazoe.[9] However, some previous reports did not clarify the plane of shoulder blade. In the present study, to define its plane, we selected three points A, B, C as described above. These points were selected for two reasons. Points A and B were the clearest points on each roentgenogram of the scapula, and concerning point C, we attached great importance to the relation between the plane of the shoulder blade and the glenoid fossa.

The medially tilting angle in the resting position averaged 39.22° in our study. On the other hand, it was interesting that the medially tilting angle of the scapula following elevation of the arm from the resting position to 150° of elevation was about 40° and nearly constant.

As for the pathological states which caused increase of the medially tilting angle, Sprengel's deformity, congenital absence of the trapezius, paralysis of the accessory nerve, paralysis of the serratus anterior muscle, and contracture of the deltoid muscle are included. As Barton[1] described, in Sprengel's deformity, there is not only elevation of the scapula but also a shorter clavicle than normal. These facts suppose that the factors which participate in the medially tilting angle of the scapula are the clavicle and the muscles of the shoulder girdle. In addition, concerning the activity of the muscles of the shoulder girdle following arm elevation, Ito[3] described that, during arm elevation, the average activity pattern of the trapezius, supraspinatus, rhomboideus and deltoid muscle was virtually similar in that the intensity increased linearly in electromyography.

Therefore, we suggest that the clavicle and a cocontraction of the muscle of the shoulder girdle obstruct the increase of the medially tilting angle following elevation of the arm.

These findings suggest that the elevation at the plane of 40° against the frontal plane is very comfortable and that 40° is the exact degree of the scapular plane. As elevation progresses, the downward tilting angle continues to decrease and subsequently inverts.

There is an opinion that this depends on the external rotation of the humerus following elevation of the arm (Poppen[6]). But in our present study, subjects grasped the drip infusion stand at each arm elevation position, so changes of the amount of rotation of the humerus may be small.

Therefore, we suggest that the clavicle and a cocontraction of the muscle of the shoulder girdle obstruct the increase of the medially tilting angle following elevation of the arm.

The upward rotation angle averages 60.64°. This result was comparable to the data from the study on conventional scapular movement.

Acknowledgments

Nobuyuki Ito, M.D., Lecturer of Orthopaedic Surgery, Nagasaki University School of Medicine, Nagasaki-City, Japan

Ryohei Suzuki, M.D., Professor of Orthopaedic Surgery, Nagasaki University School of Medicine, Nagasaki-City, Japan

Nobu Ohwatari, Bachelor of Engineering, Educational Officer, Environmental Physiology, Institute for Tropical Medicine, Nagasaki University, Nagasaki-City, Japan

REFERENCES

1. Barton NJ. Anteversion of the shoulder. Shoulder Surgery 1981; 98–100.
2. Inman VT. Observations of function on shoulder joint. J. Bone and Jt. Surg 1944; 26:1–30.
3. Ito N. Electromyographic study of shoulder joint. J Jpn Ortho Ass 1980; 54:1529–1540.
4. Johnston TB. The movements of the shoulder joint. A plea for the use of the 'Plane of the Scapula' as the plane of reference for movements occurring at the humero-scapular joint. Brit J Surg 1937; 25:252–260.
5. Kapandji IA. The physiology of the joint. vol. 1. New York: Churchill Livingstone, 1970:9–79.
6. Poppen NK, Walker PS. Normal and abnormal motion of the shoulder. J. Bone and Jt. Surg 1976; 58A:195–201.
7. Saha AK. Dynamic stability of the gleno humeral joint. Acta Orthop Scand 1971; 42:491–505.
8. Steindler A. Kinesiology of human body under normal and pathological conditions. Springfield: Charles C Thomas, 1955:446–474.
9. Tazoe S. Tilting Angle of the Scapula. The Shoulder Joint, Jap Shoulder Soc 1982; 7:45–49.
10. Toris T. Roentgenographical examination on the tilted angle of the scapula in the resting position. J Jpn Ortho Ass 1981; 55:295–302.
11. Von Lanz T, Wachsmuth W. Praktische anatomie. Berlin: Springer-Verlag, 1935.

THE ROLE OF THE ROTATOR CUFF AS A STABILIZING MECHANISM OF THE SHOULDER

SHINKICHI HIMENO, M.D. and HIROSHI TSUMURA, M.D.

The shoulder joint consists of: the scapular glenoid having quite shallow bearing, the large humeral head, and abundant muscles. This structure gives the shoulder the widest range of motion in the human body. However, it also makes the shoulder susceptible to loss of stability.

This paper will analyze the role of the rotator cuff muscles in the stabilization of the shoulder using two-dimensional computer simulations. The results reveal that the rotator cuff muscles act as a "musculotendinous glenoid" which, in collaboration with the osseous glenoid, holds the humeral head stable. The deltoid muscle can abduct the upper extremity only after this stabilizing mechanism is established.

METHODS

Rigid Body Formulation

The mechanically equivalent model of the shoulder is formulated as shown in Figure 1. The scapula and the humerus are modelled as polygonal rigid plates contacting on the glenoid. Compression springs which resist compressive stress are distributed along the joint contact sides of the glenoid and also along the contact surface between the humeral head and the supraspinatus muscle. The resultant combined force of the shoulder muscles and the weight of the upper extremity is applied at the center of the humeral head. The muscle force of the supraspinatus is also applied as shown in Figure 1. Rigid body formulation, a kind of finite element method, is performed to calculate stress distribution on the compression springs. In this formulation, two kinds of springs, normal and shear, are considered on the joint contact surfaces.[4,5]

At the joint contact surface, shear stress cannot be transmitted because of its extremely low friction. As to tension, two surfaces easily separate, and transmission of tension does not take place either. Such nonlinear characteristics should be taken into account.

At the beginning of the analysis, all the joint contact areas are considered to be in contact and shear stiffness of all springs are assumed to be zero. The stiffness equation is made and solved. After the initial solution is obtained, stress on every spring is calculated. If tension is detected, the spring with tension is deleted from the model. Calculation is continued until no tension is detected.[4,5]

Joint Alignment and Muscle Force

The relative movement between the scapula and the humerus in abduction is known as the scapulo-humeral rhythm. Slight differences in the measurement of this rhythm exist in the literature.[2,3] In this analysis, the rhythm is simplified as follows:

Assumption 1. Inclination of the glenoid to the perpendicular line is zero at 30 degrees of humeral abduction and increases by 12 degrees for every 30 degrees of further humeral abduction.

Muscle forces are estimated according to the method of Poppen and Walker. Their method consists of two assumptions:

Assumption 2. The force of a muscle is proportional to: (i) its cross-sectional area, and (ii) intensity of electromyographical activity.

Assumption 3. The torque of a muscle is proportional to the product of (i) and (ii) and the lever arm of the muscle. In each phase of abduction, the torque of the weight of the upper extremity is calculated and distributed to each muscle according to Assumption 3. The distributed muscle torque is converted to the muscle force based on Assumption 1.[6,7]

The estimated loading condition is shown as Figure 2. Standardization is performed as follows. The radius of the humeral head is 22.0 mm. The enclosing angle of the glenoid is 80 degrees. The

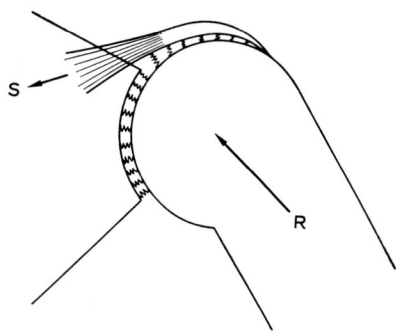

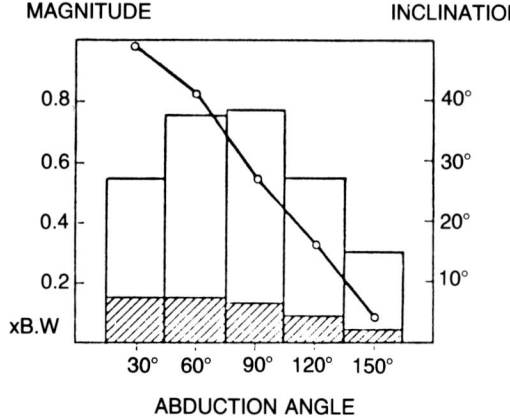

Figure 1 The mechanical model of the shoulder. Two osseous elements, the scapula and the humerus, are modelled by rigid polygonal plates contacting on the glenoid. The rotator cuff is also modelled. Compression springs are distributed along the glenoid and under the rotator cuff. R = the resultant force vector on the humeral head. S = muscle force of the rotator cuff (the supraspinatus).

Figure 2 Magnitude and direction of the resultant force and the supraspinatus muscle force. The vacant and shaded areas illustrate the magnitude of the resultant force and the supraspinatus respectively. The heavy line indicates the inclination of the resultant force to the central axis of the scapular glenoid.

upper extremity weight is 5.6 percent of body weight. The distance from the center of the humeral head to the center of gravity of the upper extremity is 334.0 mm. The insertion of the rotator cuff is at 40 degrees clockwise to the humeral shaft axis. The rotator cuff is considered to be in even contact with the humeral head.

RESULTS

Computer outputs of the analysis are shown in Figures 3a through 3c. Each arrow shows the magnitude and direction of contact stress. The large arrow at the center of the humeral head is the loading vector.

30 Degrees Abduction (Fig. 3a)

In the early phase of shoulder abduction, the direction of the loading vector is beyond the upper edge of the glenoid. The lower and middle portions of the glenoid joint become noncontacting and no load transmission takes place. Stress concentration on the upper portion of the scapular glenoid is remarkable. Contact stress distributes widely also as the rotator cuff pushes the humeral head down.

The rotator cuff acts as a kind of "musculotendinous glenoid" which collaborates with the osseous (scapular) glenoid to hold the humeral head stable.

90 Degrees Abduction (Fig. 3b)

In the middle phase of abduction, the direction of the resultant force is still eccentric but within the scapular glenoid. Stress concentration becomes moderate and just the lower portion of the scapular glenoid remains noncontacting. Stress distribution under the rotator cuff decreases in width and magnitude.

The musculotendinous glenoid becomes less important in this phase because the area of contact of the rotator cuff on the humeral head decreases due to arm abduction and the muscle force of the supraspinatus decreases slightly. The musculotendinous glenoid remains indispensable for stability (to be discussed).

150 Degrees Abduction (Fig. 3c)

In the late phase of abduction, the direction of the loading vector approaches the central axis of the scapular glenoid. Stress distribution is even and almost symmetrical over the whole scapular glenoid. The role of the rotator cuff is negligible in this phase.

The Shoulder Without a Rotator Cuff (Fig. 4a,b)

If there were no rotator cuff, to what extent could the scapular glenoid hold the shoulder sta-

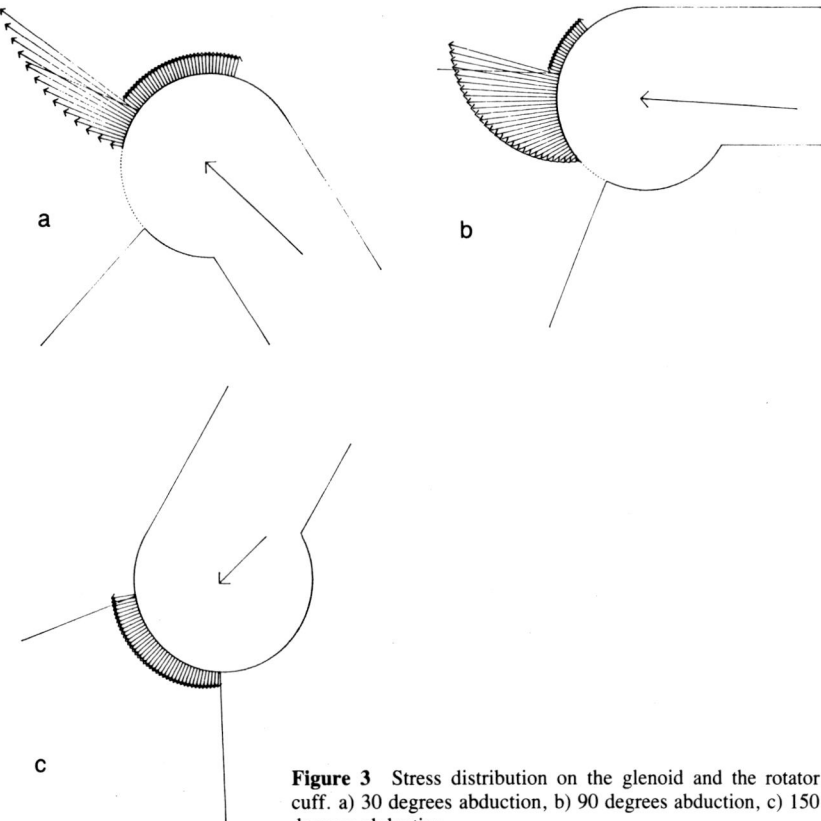

Figure 3 Stress distribution on the glenoid and the rotator cuff. a) 30 degrees abduction, b) 90 degrees abduction, c) 150 degrees abduction.

ble? To answer this question, the following simulations were performed.

From the model shown in Figure 1, the rotator cuff was removed, leaving the osseous components, the scapula and the humerus. At first, the load was applied perpendicular to the scapular glenoid. Then the load was gradually inclined and stress distribution and displacement of the humeral head were calculated in the same way as in the previous analysis.

When the load was inclined to 0 degrees, the direction of the displacement of the humerus (* in the figure) was identical with that of the loading vector. Stress distribution on the glenoid is symmetrical.

When the load is inclined 9 degrees, the displacement vector passes the edge of the glenoid. If the load is further inclined, the humeral head goes beyond the glenoid out into subluxation. If the load inclination is 9 degrees or less, both the loading vector and the displacement vector remain within the glenoidal bearings, which means absolute stability.

The scapular glenoid without the rotator cuff can maintain stability so long as the load inclination remains within $+/-$ 9 degrees, that is, when the shoulder is abducted by 120 to 130 degrees or more.

DISCUSSION

The Rotator Cuff as the "Glenoid"

The scapular glenoid has quite shallow bearings and hence poor stability of its own. Some auxiliary bearings must exist to maintain stability during shoulder movement.

The rotator cuff muscles, unlike other muscles, insert to the humerus by winding around the humeral head. A tensed soft tissue tends to become straight. If bent by the humeral head, a reactional force is generated to push back the humeral head as shown in Figure 5. When the tension of the rotator cuff is (T) and its contacting angle is (2*theta), the reactional force (R) can be calcu-

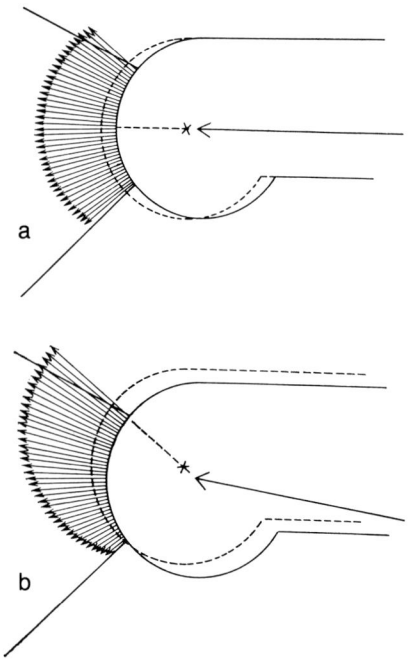

Figure 4 Analysis without the rotator cuff. * = the center of the humeral head after displacement. The dotted line = direction of the displacement. a) inclination = 0 degrees; b) inclination = 9 degrees.

lated as R = 2*T*SIN (theta), and its contact pressure (P) is P = T/r where (r) is the radius of the humeral head.

Such a mechanism acts as a musculotendinous glenoid to hold the humeral head stable. It consists of soft tissue and is retractable in abduction, which makes possible the widest range of motion without impingement of the osseous elements.

Axle-like Function of the Rotator Cuff

In a machine, an axle is usually used to hold the center of rotation rigid to ensure smooth movement. In a living body, however, there are no axles. When the humeral head moves upward, the rotator cuff muscles contract to push the humeral head down. When the humeral head is pulled down, the rotator cuff muscles contract to pull the humeral head up.[1] Thus, the center of the humeral head is retained at the same point.

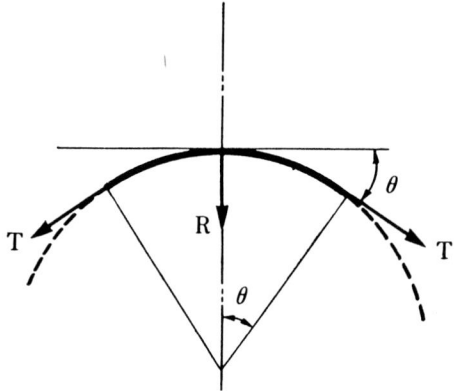

Figure 5 A representation of the way the rotator cuff pushes the humeral head down. T = tension of the rotator cuff, R = reactional force, theta = one half of the contact angle of the rotator cuff, R = 2*T*SIN (theta).

Dysfunction of the Rotator Cuff

When the rotator cuff is ruptured and the musculotendinous glenoid lost, a variety of dysfunctions take place.

In the early phase of abduction, the loading vector is beyond the upper edge of the scapular glenoid. Loss of the musculotendinous glenoid results in upward subluxation of the humeral head to impinge against the subacromial surface. Subacromial bursitis is usually observed in rotator cuff rupture. The muscle force of the deltoid is wasted for upward displacement of the humeral head and ability to abduct the arm is lost. Thus, a patient with rotator cuff rupture cannot abduct his shoulder even though his deltoid muscle remains intact and powerful.

In rare instances, the patient can abduct the shoulder completely, even though the rotator cuffs are ruptured. In such cases, the distance from the top of the humeral head to the subacromial surface is relatively short. After impingement, the deltoid muscle can contract further to abduct the arm.

In the middle phase of abduction, the musculotendinous glenoid is less important but still indispensable for stability of the humeral head. The inclination of the loading vector is 30 degrees or so, far from the stable range of +9 to −9 degrees. The osseous glenoid alone cannot maintain stability.

After the arm of a patient is passively abducted to 90 degrees or so and the support suddenly removed, the arm falls down. This phenomenon is known as 'drop arm sign'. When the rotator cuff is ruptured, contraction of the deltoid results in a slipping up of the humeral head and failure to generate abducting momentum against the weight of the upper extremity.

In the late phase of abduction, inclination of the loading vector is within the stable range of $+9$ to -9 degrees. Here the osseous glenoid can hold the humeral head stable with no help from the musculotendinous glenoid. Even a patient with complete rotator cuff tear can abduct his shoulder to the maximum (180 degrees) if his shoulder is once abducted passively to 120 to 130 degrees.

The Anterior and Posterior Rotator Cuff

The discussions above concerned the mechanics of the frontal section of the shoulder where the supraspinatus is a principal muscle of the rotator cuff. In the horizontal section, the anterior and posterior rotator cuff muscles, the subscapularis, infraspinatus, and teres minor muscles, have the same function as does the supraspinatus muscle in the frontal section.

The Scapulohumeral Rhythm in Shoulder Stability

In the final phase of abduction, the loading vector is almost perpendicular to the scapular glenoid whose stable range is from $+9$ to -9 degrees in loading inclination. If the scapulohumeral rhythm is delayed by about 15 degrees or more, inclination of the load becomes below -9 degrees. Since there is just a thin joint capsule in the axillary region, downward subluxation of the humeral head easily takes place. This pathomechanism is considered to be involved in "loose shoulder".

The scapulohumeral rhythm is intended to prevent downward subluxation rather than to increase the efficiency of the deltoid muscle. The glenoid rolls under the humeral head to support it, thus preventing downward subluxation.

REFERENCES

1. Basmajian JV et al. Factors preventing downward dislocation of the adducted shoulder joint. J Bone Joint Surg 1959; 41A:1182–1186.
2. Codman EA. *The Shoulder*. Boston: Thomas Todd, 1934:32–64.
3. Freeman L et al. Abduction of the arm in the scapular plane. Scapular and glenohumeral movement. J Bone Joint Surg. 1966; 48A:1503–1510.
4. Himeno S et al. Instability of the hip joint and its contact pressure. Proc 8th Internat Cong Biomech. 1983; 4A:132–137.
5. Kawai T et al. A new element in discrete analysis of plain strain problems. Seisan Kenkyu 1977; 29:204–207.
6. Poppen NK et al. Forces at the glenohumeral joint in abduction. Clin Orthop. 1978; 135:165–170.
7. Walker PS. Human joints and their artificial replacement. Springfield: CC Thomas, 1977:87–94.

C-ARM FLUOROSCOPIC EVALUATION UNDER ANESTHESIA FOR GLENOHUMERAL SUBLUXATIONS

TOM R. NORRIS, M.D.

Establishing the diagnosis and directions of painful shoulder instability may be difficult. The standard work-up includes an appropriate history, systematic clinical and roentgenographic evaluation, and most importantly, an examination under anesthesia prior to and even after making the operative incision. The palpable subluxation or bounce may be difficult to quantify in determining whether or not a particular patient requires surgery. In an effort to eliminate the confusion, the C-arm fluoroscopic unit has been used in the axillary and anterior posterior planes to confirm the clinical impression of instability and to document the directions and magnitude of instability of those patients with one, two or three directional instability.

The normal work-up for a patient with a dislocating or subluxing shoulder begins with the history. Instability most commonly occurs in a younger age group. The mechanism of injury may assist in determining the predominant direction. Rowe[15] has described the "dead arm syndrome" with transient neurological symptoms accompanying shoulder subluxations. The patient may even say that his shoulder feels like it is "coming out of the socket" or slipping following a surgical procedure.

Rockwood[11] and others[1,10] have reported that shoulder subluxations are often more symptomatic and disabling than intermittent shoulder dislocations. As shoulder subluxations have become a less elusive entity, roentgenographic documentation of a complete dislocation no longer is a prerequisite for surgery.[14,17] Unfortunately, this leaves room for errors.

The most frequent positive clinical finding is an apprehension against subluxation anteriorly with the arm tested overhead.[11] Guarding against shoulder extension with increasing abduction and external rotation,[12] a palpable bounce, or subluxation with the arm overhead with various stress maneuvers is a standard part of the evaluation. One clue may be an increased range of motion, particularly external rotation when measured supine with the arms at the side and in 90° of abduction. In addition, with downward traction applied to the arm, the shoulder may sublux inferiorly, leaving a large gap between the humeral head and the acromion.[7] The examiner's thumb can then push the head anterior–inferiorly or posterior–inferiorly to determine associated anterior or posterior instability. Apprehension for posterior instability is not as reliable a test to confirm direction as it is for anterior instability.

Evidence of other loose joints, such as elbows and knees that hyperextend, thumbs which can be brought back to touch the forearm, or a history of either hip or patella subluxations, is an additional finding in many patients with bilateral shoulder laxity. A differential diagnosis of subluxation includes impingement lesions, arthritic lesions of the acromioclavicular and glenohumeral joints, and snapping scapula.

There may be an overlap between instability and impingement lesions when testing for apprehension with the arm overhead. A subacromial Xylocaine^R injection test is helpful in differentiating these.[8] Likewise a Xylocaine injection to the acromioclavicular joint will differentiate lesions in this joint from the pain experienced on adduction and posterior stress when testing for posterior instability. It is important to note that not all people with shoulder instability have pain attributable to their shoulder laxity. Only a meticulous clinical and roentgenographic evaluation will ensure that another diagnosis, such as osteolysis of the distal clavicle in a patient with a lax shoulder, is not the cause of the pain.

Roentgenographic evaluation for shoulder instability begins with the standard rotational anterior posterior views and a true axillary view. Other causes for pain, such as fracture, fracture dislocations, calcific tendinitis, or arthritis, may be eliminated. A loose body or posterior lateral head defect would indicate shoulder instability. The Hill-Sachs lesion[3] is demonstrated with an internal rotation view and other angled views. Reactive bone off the glenoid rim or a bony glenoid fracture is demonstrated with special-angled axillary views such as the prone West Point[13] or the supine abduction external rotation view to visualize the anterior inferior rim without overlap of the other bony structures.

Arthrotomography and double-contrast arthrograms with CAT scans have been used to demonstrate glenoid labrum detachments in centers where radiologists have developed a special interest and competence in these otherwise confusing and elusive tests.[4,6]

The best view for inferior instability is the stress x-ray, with 20 to 25 lbs of weight strapped to each wrist, taken with the patient upright and relaxed and both shoulders captured on one cassette.[7] Downward subluxation of the humeral head relative to the glenoid alerts the physician that the standard procedures may not be successful. Special attention will be required when treating the inferior capsule to avoid residual inferior subluxation.

At times x-rays may show a small head or a hypoplastic glenoid, but in many instances they may be entirely normal. Other stress x-rays and even cineroentgenograms for instability have been tried, but apprehension may preclude subluxation in an awake patient.

Even when the diagnosis is established, the greatest direction of instability may not be certain. While abduction in external rotation with forward pressure on the proximal humerus from behind generally tests anterior instability, it may reduce a posterior subluxation back into the joint. Accurate assessment of the direction of instability is essential, for surgery to the wrong side of the shoulder will make the patient worse.[7] Evaluations may be particularly difficult for muscular patients with apprehension, litigious or compensation cases, or patients with psychiatric disorders, including voluntary dislocators.[16] Assuming that voluntary dislocators can be excluded on clinical grounds, then the special problems include confirming the diagnosis and direction(s). The C-arm fluoroscopic unit in the axillary plane with the patient under anesthesia has proved most valuable.[9] AP projections for inferior instability can also be obtained but my preferred method is to do this projection, with the patient awake, with weighted x-rays.

Attempts are first made to sublux the shoulder without the unit in place. The arm is grasped by the elbow with one hand and the other hand is placed over the anterior and posterior aspects of the humeral head near the glenoid. Attempts can then be made to sublux the shoulder anteriorly or posteriorly by positioning the elbow slightly above shoulder level and then pushing the arm along its longitudinal axis in an anterior-inferior or posterior direction. Fingertip or thumb pressure at the head can also assist in this maneuver. The arm can then be placed in what is felt to be a subluxed or dislocated position. The unit is then brought into the field.

The patient is positioned supine with a pad under the scapula. The Mayfield neurosurgical headrest replaces the normal head piece on the operating table. This allows for the receiving screen of the x-ray tube to be placed medially above the shoulder in order to see the glenoid. The technique for utilizing the C-arm is to stabilize the scapula with the patient supine at the edge of the operative table. The neck may be mildly flexed to prevent injury to the cervical spine and tilted away from the shoulder of interest (Fig. 1). Anterior-inferior and posterior stress maneuvers are applied to the humerus with documentation on a videotape (Fig. 2). Leaded apron, gloves, and special leaded glasses are recommended for the examiner.[2,5]

Normally, "stress x-rays" with maximal stress in the direction of suspected instability are performed with the arm at an obtuse angle to the glenoid. These can be difficult to interpret. With the C-arm, more information is obtained if the angle between the glenoid and the humerus is smaller and displacement of the head is measured relative to the glenoid margin. It is easy to assess posterior laxity. Anterior laxity is more difficult for two reasons. First, mild traction must be applied in the longitudinal direction of the arm to visualize the glenoid on the screen. Second, the direction of instability is often anterior-inferior rather than straight anterior. After familiarization with the technique, the x-ray exposure for an examination should be less than 30 seconds.

CLINICAL MATERIAL

Between July 1979 and October 1982, 42 shoulders in 39 patients with positive findings were examined and underwent surgical repairs. No cases with associated cuff tears or tuberosity fractures were included. Of the 42, 17 had previous surgery elsewhere—11 had failed repairs, one had

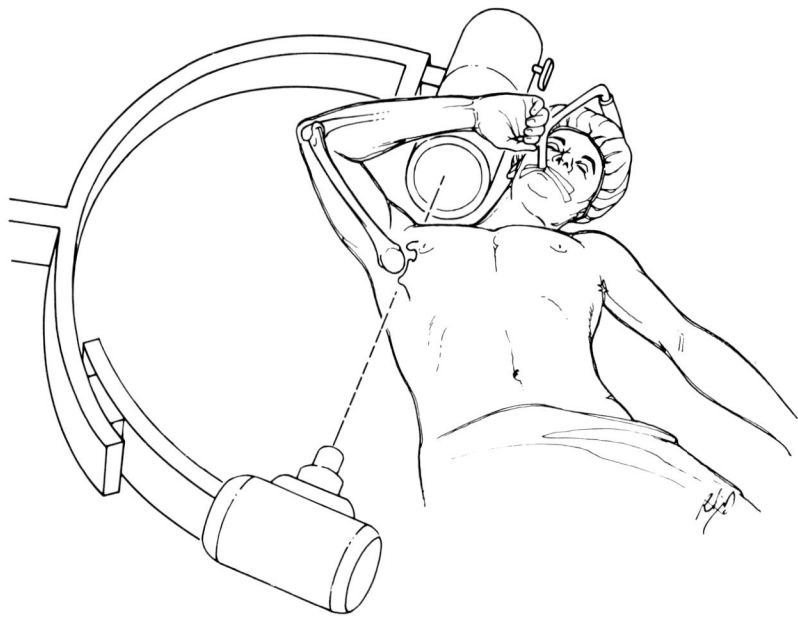

Figure 1 C-arm fluoroscopic unit positioned for an axial examination of the glenohumeral joint.

surgery to the wrong side of the shoulder, and 5 had surgery for incorrect diagnoses such as bicipital tendinitis, subluxing biceps tendon, or acromioclavicular arthritis in the face of normal roentgenograms. In patients who had had surgery to the wrong side of the shoulder or for the wrong diagnosis, excessive glenohumeral subluxation and its direction were easy to document on examination with the C-arm. In these cases examination under anesthesia might have prevented surgery for the wrong diagnosis.

For these 42 patients, the major direction of instability was anterior inferior in 22, posterior in 13, and multidirectional in 7. The C-arm was utilized in 34 of the 42 patients. The suspected clinical direction was confirmed in 24, altered from anterior to posterior in 4, and used to separate instability from other possible diagnoses in 5. In one patient with anterior instability, the examination was not felt to be helpful. Opposite shoulders were compared in selected cases. By correlating the C-arm evaluation with the operative findings, an understanding of the normal range of motion was gained. It was felt that *any* anterior subluxation was pathologic, but a posterior displacement of up to 50 percent of the humeral head diameter may be normal. Labral detachments allowed for an increase in motion in all directions, thereby mimicking a multidirectional instability. Repair of the labral detachment was usually sufficient. Additional tendon shortening procedures such as the Magnussen-Stack or Putti-Platt after repairing a labral detachment resulted in lost motion, excessive tightness and possible displacement to the opposite side.

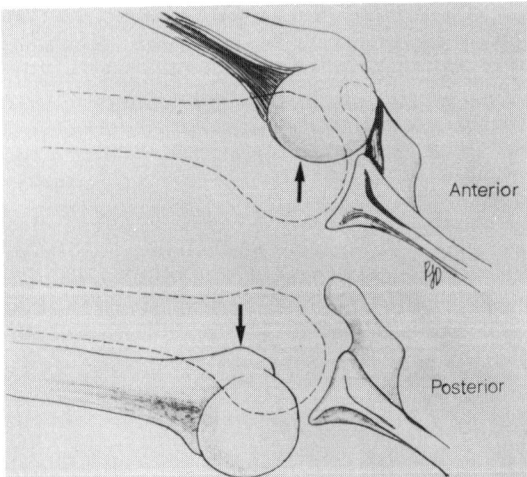

Figure 2 Axillary stress views document glenohumeral laxity. Any displacement anteriorly is pathologic. Up to 50% displacement of the humeral head posteriorly may be normal. Labral detachments may allow increased excursion in all directions.

The operation is commenced on the side of greatest instability, and if during surgery the probing and inspection of the labrum on the opposite side demonstrates the detachment, a separate incision and approach is required.[7] In none of the cases was a detachment of the posterior labrum observed. Therefore, in a situation in which there was clearly excessive motion anteriorly and posteriorly, an anterior approach would allow for inspection and repair of any labral detachments without the necessity of a posterior incision. While arthroscopy was tried in selected cases, it had the disadvantages of being an invasive procedure and not giving as clear an assessment of the amount and direction(s) of shoulder instability as the C-arm examination. It was helpful in special cases to assess the attachment of the glenoid labrum.

The C-arm has been particularly useful in measuring the palpable subluxation or bounce that otherwise has been difficult to accurately interpret. It was especially helpful in the 10 percent of these cases where its use altered the clinical impression from anterior to posterior instability. While many of the findings of the history, clinical and roentogenographic examination offer clues to the diagnosis, this technique has removed the elusive quality in the evaluation of shoulder subluxations and has provided the acid test as to whether or not the involved shoulder is unstable.

REFERENCES

1. Blazina ME, Satzman JS. Recurrent anterior subluxation of the shoulder in athletes—a distinct entity. J Bone Joint Surg. 1969; 51A:1037–1038.
2. Goldman M. Ionizing radiation and its risks. West J Med. 1982; 137:540–547.
3. Hill HA, Sachs MD. The grooved defect of the humeral head. Radiology 1940; 35:690–70.
4. McGlynn FJ, El-Khoury G, Albright JP. Arthrotomography of the glenoid labrum in shoulder instability. J Bone Joint Surg. 1982; 64A:506–518.
5. Miller ME, Davis ML, MacClean CR, Davis JG, Smith BL, Humphries JR. Radiation exposure and associated risks to operating room personnel during use of fluoroscopic guidance for selected orthopaedic surgical procedures. J Bone Joint Surg. 1983; 65A:1–4.
6. Mink JH, Richardson A, Grant TT. Evaluation of glenoid labrum by double-contrast shoulder arthrography. Am J Roentgenol. 1979; 133:883–887.
7. Neer CS II, Foster CR. Inferior capsular shift for involuntary inferior and multidirectional instability of the shoulder—a preliminary report. J Bone Joint Surg., 1980; 62A:897–908.
8. Neer CS II. Anterior acromioplasty for the chronic impingement syndrome in the shoulder—a preliminary report. J Bone Joint Surg. 1972; 54A:41–50.
9. Norris TR. C-arm fluoroscopic evaluation under anesthesia for glenohumeral subluxations. Orthopaed Trans. 1983; 7:139–140.
10. Protzman RR. Anterior instability of the shoulder. J Bone Joint Surg. 1980; 62A:909–918.
11. Rockwood CA Jr. Dislocations about the shoulder. In: Rockwood CA Jr, Green DP, eds. Fractures. Philadelphia: JB Lippincott, 1975; 1:677–680.
12. Rockwood CA Jr. Subluxation of the shoulder: diagnosis, classification and treatment. Jeff Orthop J. 1981; 10:6–12.
13. Rokous JR, Feagin JA, Abbott HG. Modified axillary roentgenogram. A useful adjunct in the diagnosis of recurrent instability of the shoulder. Clin Orthop. 1972; 82:84–86.
14. Rowe CR, Patel D, Southmayd WW. The Bankart procedure: a long-term, end-result study. J Bone Joint Surg. 1978; 60A:1–16.
15. Rowe CR, Zarins B. Recurrent transient subluxation of the shoulder. J Bone Joint Surg. 1981; 63A:863–872.
16. Rowe CR, Pierce DS, Clark JG. Voluntary dislocation of the shoulder. A preliminary report on a clinical, electromyographic and psychiatric study of 26 patients. J Bone Joint Surg. 1973; 55A:445.
17. Warren RF. Subluxation of the shoulder in athletes. Symposium on injuries to the shoulder in the athlete. Clin Sports Med. 1983; 2:339–354.

SHOULDER ARTHROTOMOGRAPHY AND COMPUTED AXIAL TOMOGRAPHY IN THE DIAGNOSIS OF RECURRENT SHOULDER SUBLUXATIONS

CHRISTOPHER BEAUCHAMP, M.D., RICHARD LOOMER, M.D., F.R.C.S.(C), and LIVIUS TIMKO, M.D.

Dead arm syndrome, recurrent subluxation, transient subluxation, and apprehension shoulder are all terms used to describe a disabling and often difficult to diagnose shoulder problem. In addition, Rockwood refers to traumatic subluxation,[10] Protzman to type I—subluxation without prior dislocation,[9] and Rowe to transient subluxation.[13] We further differentiate this entity into: traumatic subluxation, in which a specific traumatic episode is known, stress subluxation, in which this syndrome develops as a result of overuse, and congenital-developmental laxity, in which the patient often presents with multidirectional instability but is disabled by recurrent subluxations.

The reported incidence of surgically treated shoulder instability presenting as subluxation varies from Rowes' 12 percent[13] to Hastings' 30 percent[5] and Morton's 34 percent.[7] Diagnosis can often be difficult; a history of acute pain or transient instability in abduction and external rotation during sports activities is often the only clue. The only sign may be a positive apprehension test in abduction and external rotation. Careful review of x-rays may show a Hill-Sach's lesion or West Point views may show an osteophyte or small avulsion from the anterior inferior glenoid. Most authors agree with our experience that standard arthrography is usually not helpful. We noted with interest the 1979 and 1980 reports by El-Khoury[3] and McGlynn[6] of a new radiographic technique: shoulder arthrotomography specifically designed to delineate the area of the anterior inferior glenoid, labrum and capsule. These and subsequent articles, although demonstrating many of the significant radiographic findings and reporting a 95 percent positive correlation with surgical findings, left us uncertain as to the exact anatomical structures we were seeing, their normal appearance, and pathological variations. We therefore undertook a study to correlate what we see on the arthrogram/tomogram with anatomical specimens, to identify various kinds of capsular and labral lesions, and to verify the arthrotomographic findings at surgical dissection.

MATERIALS AND METHODS

We dissected two shoulders from cadavers to demonstrate the relationship between glenoid, labrum, capsule, and humeral head. The new radiographic technique was examined by taking standard A-P views of the scapular and humeral positions assumed during the tomographic exam and determining the plane in which the cuts were made through both scapula and humeral heads. The two specimens were frozen and sectioned in planes identical to those of the tomographic cuts. Two other shoulder specimens were filled with dye and air; tomographic cuts were made, and the specimens examined to correlate tomographic appearance with anatomy.

The arthrotomograms of 33 patients who had undergone surgical repair for anterior inferior subluxation or dislocation were studied in detail and the surgically described lesions correlated with radiographic appearance.

Results

The dissected anatomy was in agreement with that described in the literature, with the middle and inferior glenohumeral ligaments forming a continuous, although redundant capsule anterior and inferiorly. The anterior inferior glenoid labrum is firmly attached to the bony labrum and continuous anteriorly with the middle glenohumeral ligament.

RADIOGRAPHIC TECHNIQUE

The radiographic technique used was identical to that described by McGlynn and El-Khoury. The shoulder is prepped, a 20 gauge spinal needle is introduced into the shoulder anteriorly, and 4 cc of 60 percent Renografin and 10 cc of room air insufflated. Slow range of motion is performed and the patient carefully positioned lying with the affected side down and the arm in external rotation and full abduction, so that the articular surface of the glenoid is nearly perpendicular to the table (Fig. 1). A plain anterior radiograph shows the glenohumeral joint in this position (Fig. 2). Superior and inferior are indicated and lines on the radiograph indicate the plane of the tomographic cut.

The frozen sections (Fig. 3) cut in planes identical to those of the tomographic cuts demonstrate the bony glenoid, attached labrum and anterior capsule with adjacent subscapularis. The posterior glenoid with smaller labrum and less redundant capsule are also well seen.

After insufflation of the dye and air, tomography of the cadaver specimen in the same plane as the frozen section showed clearly the radiographic appearance of the glenoid, anterior and posterior labrum, and anterior and posterior capsule (Fig. 4A, 4B). The triangle-shaped labrum is seen continuous anteriorly with the middle glenohumeral ligament and posteriorly with the articular surface. The posterior labrum is well developed but more blunt and round than the anterior labrum. Normally an indentation is seen at the attachment of the capsule to the humerus adjacent to the greater tuberosity where Hill-Sach's lesion often occurs.

With a clear idea of the anatomic structures observed and their tomographic appearance, we carefully analyzed 31 arthrotomograms of patients who subsequently underwent surgery and had their lesions verified. From these we selected a representative sample of the variety of lesions encountered. In all examples anterior will be toward the top of the page and posterior toward the bottom. Each film reproduced is accompanied by a line drawing to demonstrate more clearly the radiographic findings.

The first patient (Fig. 5A, 5B) demonstrates a Bankart lesion with encroachment of the dye between the anterior glenoid and avulsed labrum. There is also a small Hill-Sach's lesion posteriorly. Figure 6A, 6B shows a slightly different Bankart lesion with complete separation of the labrum. Figure 7A, 7B demonstrates a Bankart lesion with a flap tear which gave the patient a painful snapping sensation during his badminton over-head shot and was removed surgically. The fourth patient (Fig. 8A, 8B) presented with pain on abduction and external rotation. An avid hockey player, he recalled many episodes of shoulder trauma but no instability. Physical examination showed only a mildly positive apprehension test. Radiographic examination showed a torn and irregular labrum with a

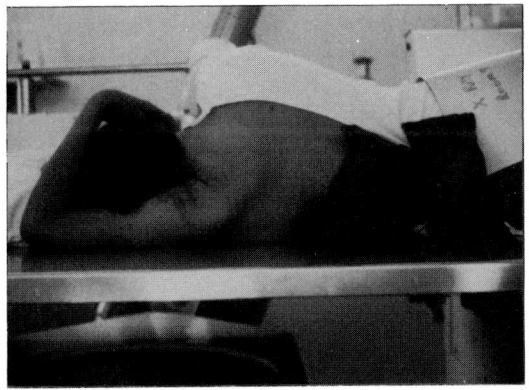

Figure 1 Patient positioned for arthrography.

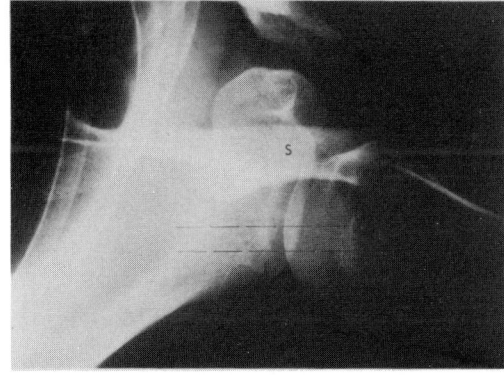

Figure 2 Plain AP radiograph with lines of tomographic cuts indicated.

28 / Surgery of the Shoulder

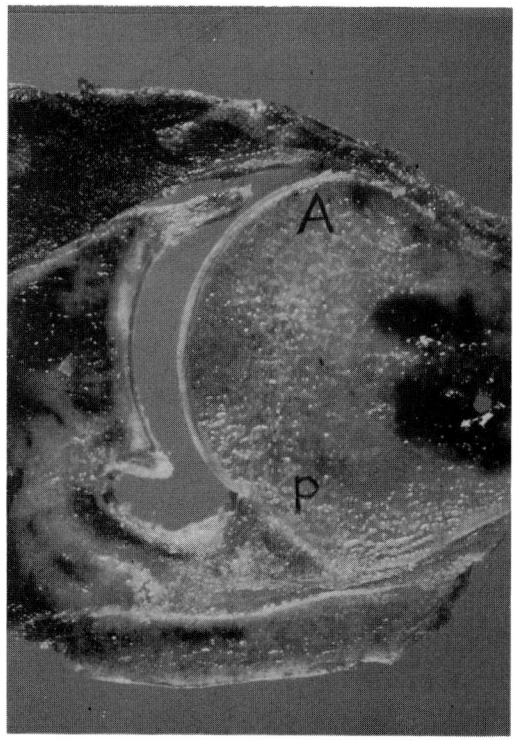

Figure 3 Frozen section cut in plane identical to those of tomographic cuts.

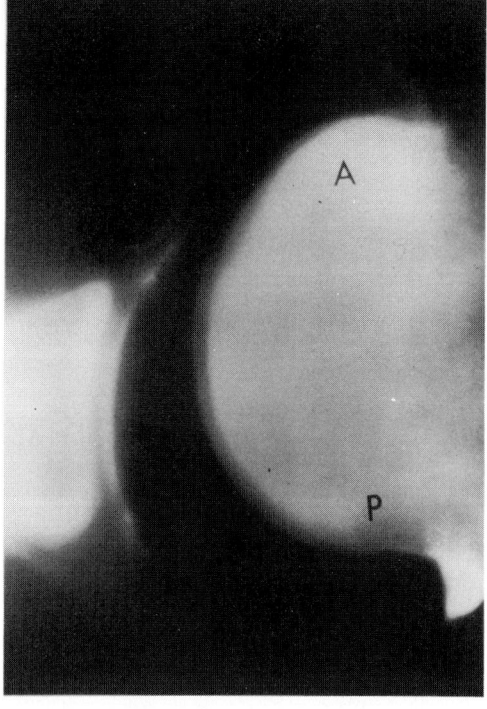

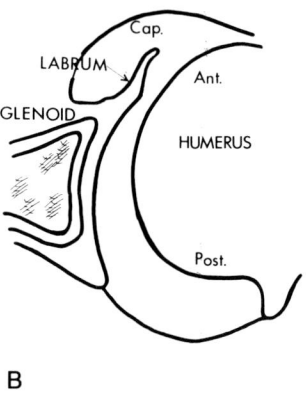

Figure 4 *A*, Arthrographic appearance—tomographic cut. *B*, Diagrammatic outline of essential features.

Biomechanics / 29

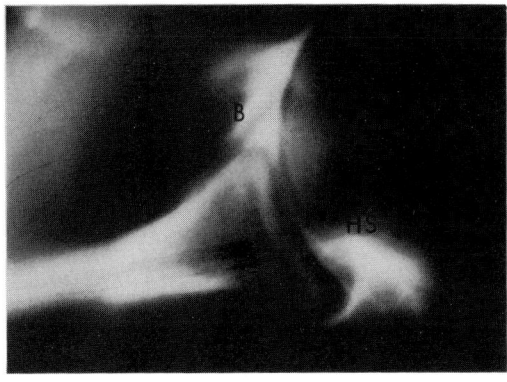 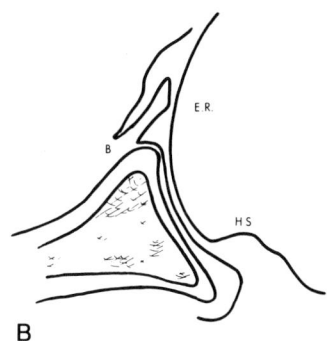

Figure 5 Bankart lesion showing encroachment of dye between labrum and glenoid.

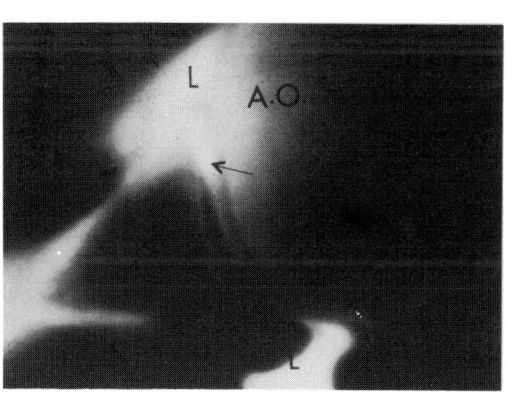 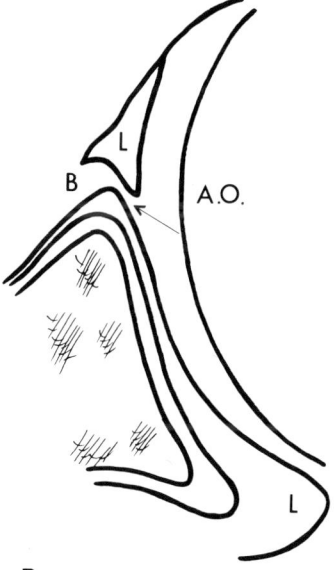

Figure 6 Bankart lesion with complete separation of the labrum.

30 / Surgery of the Shoulder

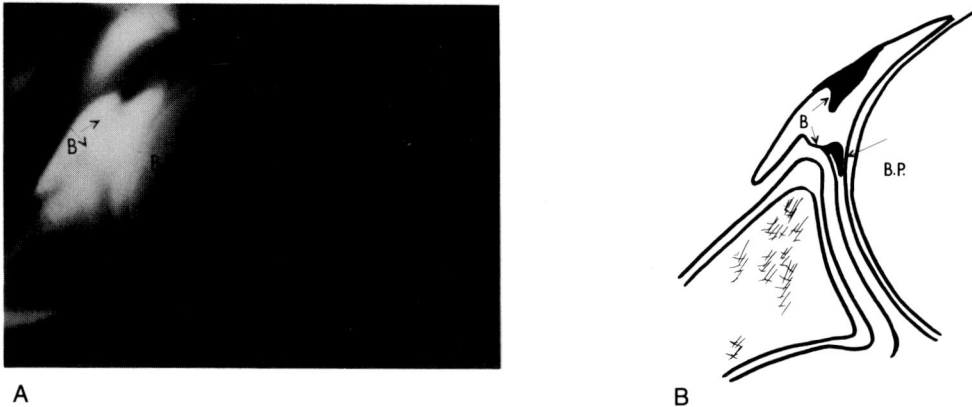

Figure 7 Bankart lesion with flap tear.

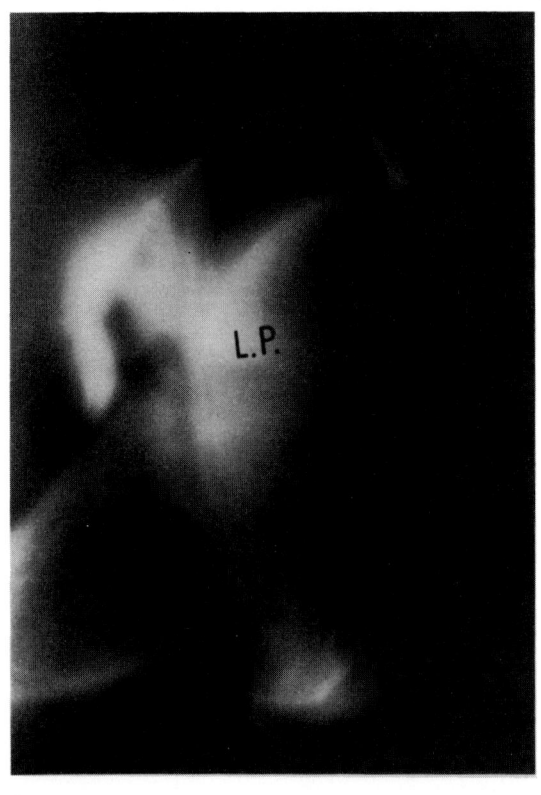
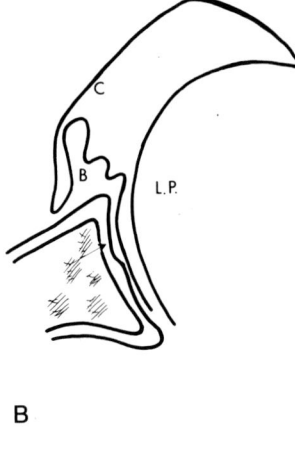

Figure 8 Redundant anterior capsule.

small impaction fracture involving the anterior glenoid surface and redundant anterior capsule. Bony avulsion is present in Figure 9A, 9B with complete labral avulsion well demonstrated by this radiographic technique.

As our expertise in diagnosing subtle instabilities has increased, the indications for double contrast tomography have narrowed. We now feel it is most useful for patients with idiopathic pain in whom instability is suspected but not demonstrable, for patients with multidirectional instability, and for patients with suspected labral flap tear in determining the presence of a Bankart lesion and assisting in planning surgery. We have begun using CT scanning in place of polytomography because it is simpler and less time-consuming, demonstrates the soft tissues better, and provides a better appreciation of humeral head contour. The CT scan is performed with the arm adducted and in neutral rotation. Inability to demonstrate fine soft tissue detail necessitates the use of air plus conray as contrast. Figure 10 shows a normal CT shoulder scan and Figure 11A, 11B shows an arthrogram CT scan of a 16-year-old male with shoulder pain and a history of anterior shoulder blow while playing hockey. He showed posterior instability on examination and a positive apprehension test in abduction and external rotation. The CT scan demonstrates an anterior Hill-Sach's or McLaughlin lesion as well as a Bankart lesion and slightly enlarged posterior capsule.

This combination of anterior and posterior findings suggests both anterior and posterior instability.

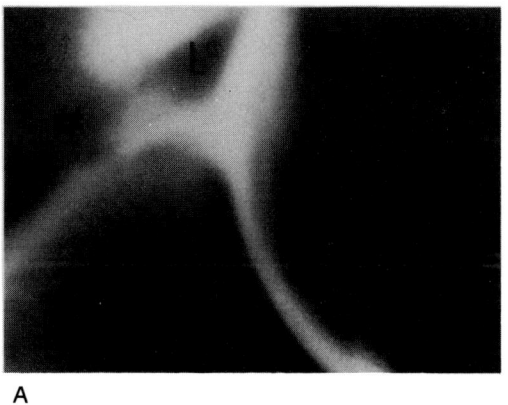
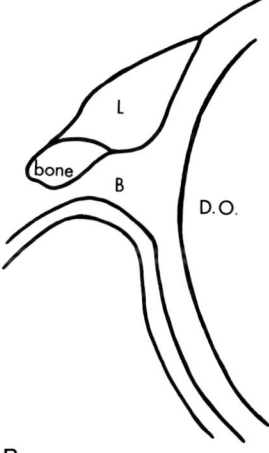

Figure 9 Avulsion of labrum with bone fragment.

32 / Surgery of the Shoulder

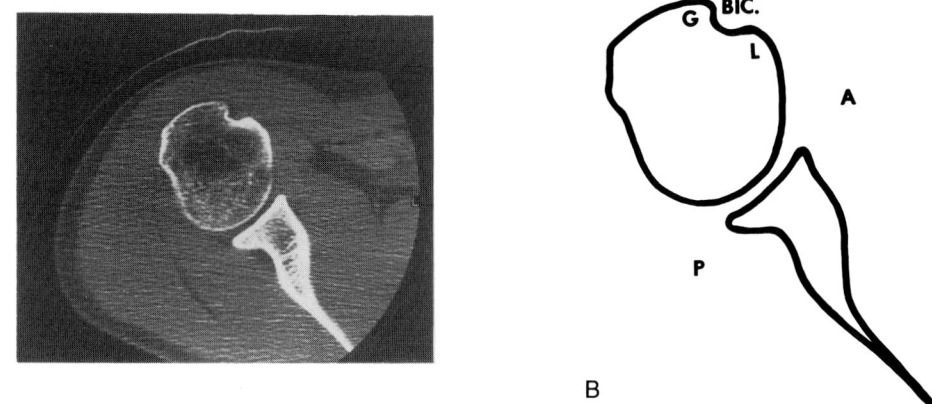

Figure 10 CT scan—normal shoulder. G = greater tuberosity; L = lesser tuberosity; BIC = biceps groove; A = anterior; P = posterior.

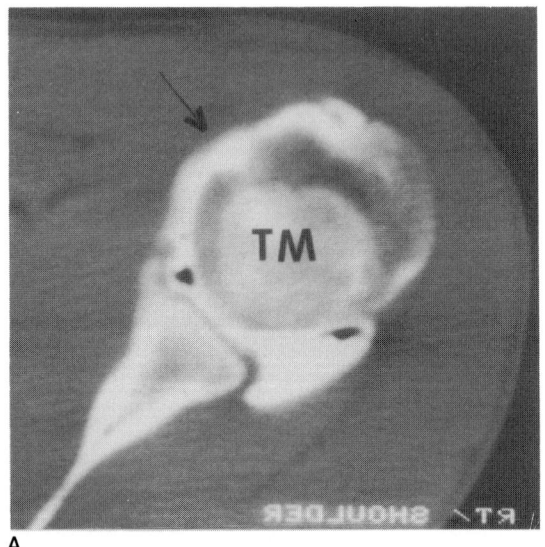
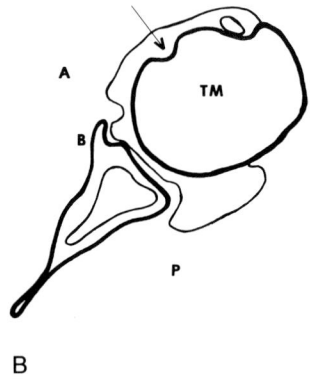

Figure 11 Patient with both anterior and posterior instability.

Summary

We have studied two new techniques to visualize the soft and bony tissues of the glenohumeral joint. In order to correctly interpret and evaluate double contrast arthrotomography and CT scanning we reviewed the cross-sectional, radiographic, and surgical anatomy in detail. The techniques have been used extensively with ease and low morbidity and have proved helpful in the diagnosis of shoulder instability and labral lesions. Our recent experience with computed tomography indicates it can demonstrate most glenohumeral structures accurately and is likely to be the preferred procedure in the future. We feel the current indications for computed tomography are:

1. Patients presenting with shoulder pain in whom instability may be suspected but not demonstrable.

2. Patients suspected or definitely known to have multidirectional instability to help both in establishing the diagnosis and determining the extent of anterior and posterior pathology and to help in planning the surgical approach.

3. Patients with a suspected torn or "snapping" anterior labrum.

REFERENCES

1. Blazina MF, Satzamn JS. Recurrent anterior subluxation of the shoulder in athletes–A distinct entity. Proceed AAOS, J Bone Joint Surg. 1969; 51A:1037–1038.
2. Deplama AF, Cooke AJ. The role of subscapularis in recurrent and anterior dislocations of the shoulder. Clin Orthop. 1967; 54:35–49.
3. El-Khoury GY, Albright JP et al. Arthrotomography of the glenoid labrum. Radiol. 1979; 131:333–337.
4. Gallie WF, Lemesurier AB. Recurring dislocation of the shoulder. J Bone Joint Surg. 1948; 30B:9–18.
5. Hastings DE, Coughlin LP. Recurrent subluxation of the glenohumeral joint. Am J Sports Med. 1981; Vol 9; 6:352–355.
6. McGlynn F, El-Khoury G, Albright J. Arthrotomography of the glenoid labrum in shoulder instability. J Bone Joint Surg. 1982; 64A:506–518.
7. Morton KS. The unstable shoulder recurring subluxation. Injury 1982; 10:304–306.
8. Neer CS II, Foster CR. Inferior capsular shift for involuntary inferior and multidirectional instability of the shoulder. A preliminary report. J Bone Joint Surg. 1980; 62A:897–908.
9. Protzman, RR. Anterior instability of the shoulder. J Bone Joint Surg. 1980; 62-A:909–918
10. Rockwood CA Jr. Dislocations about the shoulder. In: Rockwood CA Jr, Green DP, eds. Fractures. Philadelphia: JB Lippincott, 1975
11. Rokous JR, Feagin JA, Abbitt HG. Modified axillary roentgenogram. A useful adjunct in the diagnosis of recurrent instability of the shoulder. Clin Orthop. 1972; 82:84–86.
12. Rowe C, Patel D, Southmayd W. The Bankart procedure. J Bone Joint Surg. 1978; 60A:1–16.
13. Rowe CR, Zairns B. Recurrent transient subluxation of the shoulder. J Bone Joint Surg. 1981; 63-A:863–872.
14. Saha AK. Dynamic stability of the glenohumeral joint. Acta Orthop Scand. 1971; 42:491.
15. Turkel SJ, Panio MW, Marshall JL, Fakhey GC. Stabilizing mechanisms preventing anterior dislocation of the glenohumeral joint. J Bone Jone Surg. 1981; 63A:8.

ARTHROSCOPY OF THE SHOULDER JOINT

HIROAKI TSUTSUI, M.D., RYUJI YAMAMOTO, M.D.,
IWATSUGU ANRAKU, M.D., HARUO ARAI, M.D., YUJIRO MORI, M.D.,
and YOSHIKATSU KUROKI, M.D.

As a method of examining soft tissue disorders in the shoulder joint objectively, arthrography and subacromial bursography are generally used. But x-ray examinations are not sufficient to determine the exact sites of lesions in the soft tissues. Considering this point, we studied the usefulness of arthroscopy in joint disorders. Shoulder arthroscopy is a relatively difficult examination, but it is useful for diagnosis and evaluation of shoulder joint disorders even when there are no typical roentgenographical findings.

For arthroscopy of the shoulder joint, it is necessary to observe the subacromial bursa as well as the glenohumeral joint. Many shoulder joint diseases are caused by injuries of the soft tissues. Objective evaluation of these changes is essential for diagnosis and therapy of the diseases. Such disorders as tendinitis, bursitis, rotator cuff degeneration, synovitis and articular cartilage injuries are difficult to judge from contrast radiographic findings. Therefore, we have studied disorders not only in the glenohumeral joint but also in the subacromial bursa by arthroscopy.

MATERIALS AND METHODS

To examine the subacromial bursa, the patient lay on his side and saline was injected from the anterior acromion using a 19-gauge Elaster needle. The arthroscope was inserted posterolateral to the acromion (posterolateral approach). The bursal cavity was examined by moving the arthroscope back and forth, and then the inner and outer walls were examined.

For observation of the joint space, we usually employed arthroscopy with a posterior approach. With the patient lying on his side, the saline was injected into the joint space by means of a 19-gauge Elaster needle. Palpating the posterior margin with a finger, the arthroscope was introduced from the side, two fingers below the acromial angle, and directed cephalad. The arthroscope was moved up and down to examine the upper, posterior and lower aspects of the labrum. Then, the arthroscope was moved to the interior side to observe the articular cartilage of the glenoid cavity and humeral head. It was moved to the head side to observe the anterior labrum. The long head of the biceps brachii was viewed from its initial segment to the site disappearing behind the humeral head. The arthroscope was moved again to the initial segment, and the glenohumeral ligaments were observed. The foregoing procedure permitted the subacromial bursa and joint capsule to be observed.

Using the procedure mentioned above, the subacromial bursa and joint capsule were observed.

The causes of shoulder joint diseases include lesions of the suprahumeral joint, especially when the rotator cuff is sandwiched between the inner wall of the subacromial bursa and joint capsule. The rotator cuff plays an important role in the biomechanics of the shoulder, but it is difficult to observe changes in the rotator cuff by an arthroscopic approach to the joint capsule. Tears of the rotator cuff are likely to occur in the critical zone which is close to the attached site of the greater tubercle of the humerus. For this reason, it is difficult to conduct arthroscopy from the joint interior alone.

On the other hand, when arthroscopy was conducted from the subacromial bursal side, the supraspinatus tendon, especially around the critical zone, could be seen. Because arthroscopic examination of both the subacromial bursa and the joint capsule is important for some diseases, we chose one or both of these approaches depending on the disease.

The arthroscope used was a Hopkins telescope, 2.7 mm in diameter, made by Storz.

Results

Painful Arc Syndrome

The cases in this group showed almost normal findings by simple roentgenogram and arthrogram. The arthroscopy of the subacromial bursa sometimes demonstrated an irregular surface of the supraspinatus tendon; these cases were subjected to arthroscopic examination of the subacromial bursa.

Some cases showed fibrillation and irregularity of the bursal wall or bursal tears. The symptoms were alleviated following arthroscopy in some cases (Fig. 1A, 1B).

Complete Tear of the Rotator Cuff

Where tear of the rotator cuff was observed by arthroscopy, a subacromial approach was attempted to examine the tear and the changes in the bursal cavity and around the tear. Arthroscopy was effective for diagnosis of its location and for comprehension of conditions at the tear. It was possible to observe the whole of the torn part from the bursal side with arthroscope (Fig. 2A, 2B).

Recurrent Anterior Shoulder Dislocation

The patients examined had experienced dislocation. For these cases a posterior arthroscopic approach to the joint capsule was conducted. Bankart lesions, posterolateral notching, debris, and joint injuries of the articular cartilage, of the long head of the biceps brachii and of the labrum were observed (Fig. 3A, 3B).

Loose Shoulder

The patients with this condition presented with an unstable joint, and again an arthroscopic approach to the joint capsule was conducted posteriorly. In many cases, debris was found in the joint cavity. Changes in the articular cartilage of the humeral head included fissuring, which was also observed in the articular cartilage of the glenoid cavity. It was difficult to examine the changes at the bicipital groove by arthroscope. Mainly the area of biceps observed was from the glenoid to the groove. The changes at the origin included proliferation of pannus, fibrillation and edema. In some cases, growth of villi and proliferation of pannus on the tendon of the long head was considerable (Fig. 4A, 4B).

Discussion

Arthroscopy of the shoulder joint is not widely employed as routinely as arthroscopy of the

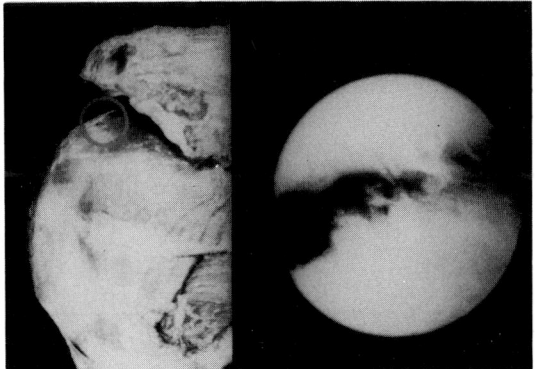

Figure 1A Fibrillation is clearly seen in the supraspinatus tendon.

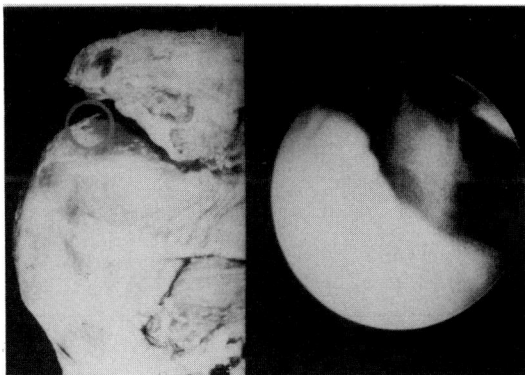

Figure 1B Degenerated and frayed supraspinatus tendon.

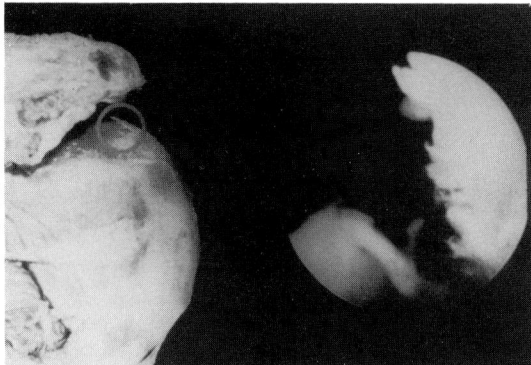

Figure 2A Fragmentation of the supraspinatus tendon.

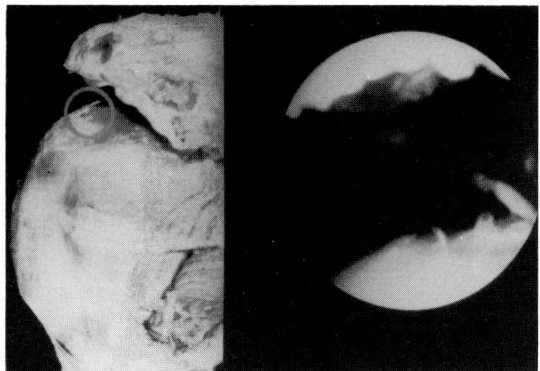

Figure 2B Torn supraspinatus with fibrillation.

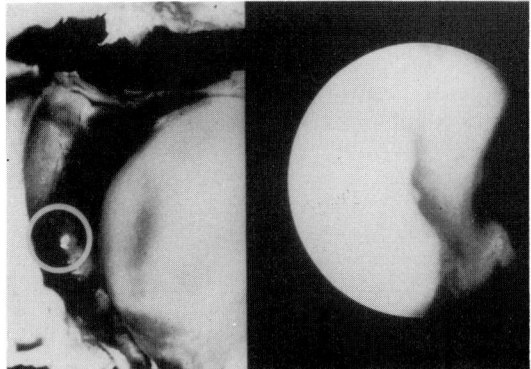

Figure 3A Bankart lesion.

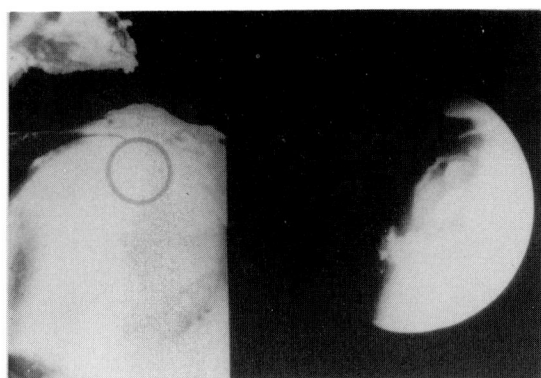

Figure 3B Posterolateral notching of the right humeral head.

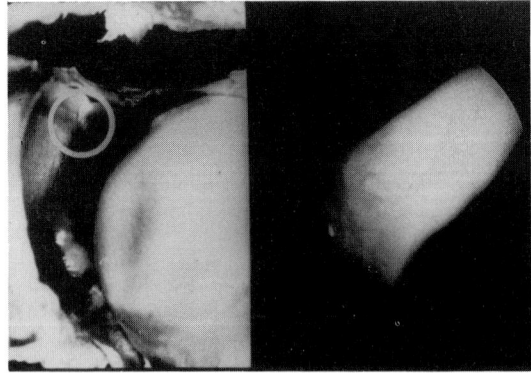

Figure 4A Proliferation of pannus around the biceps.

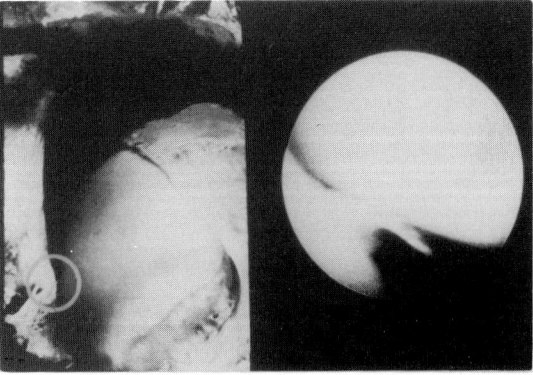

Figure 4B With downward traction, fibrillation of the labrum is demonstrated.

knee joint. This is because arthroscopy of the shoulder joint provides a limited visual field and difficult orientation resulting from the introduction of an arthroscope with narrow visual field into a joint capsule of small capacity.

Furthermore, many shoulder diseases involve changes which occur not only at the joint itself but also at the subacromial bursa. It is impossible to observe these changes by arthroscopy of the joint; arthroscopy of the subacromial bursa is required. However, there are still the problems of insertion and limitation of visual field. Sufficient data have not been obtained to establish indications for surgery and surgical method based on arthroscopic findings alone.

Based on our experience, however, arthroscopy can be used effectively is cases whose locations and grades of disorders cannot be judged objectively by roentgenographic examinations.

REFERENCES

1. Ikeuchi H. Arthroscopy of the shoulder joint. Arthroscopy 1978; 3:1–5.
2. Tsutsui H. Arthroscopic approach to shoulder disorders. Arthroscopy 1981; 7:9–12.
3. Tsutsui H. Arthroscopy of the shoulder joint. Shoulder joint 1982; 5:3–6.
4. Tsutsui H. Arthroscopy of the shoulder joint. 2nd report. Shoulder joint 1982; 6:99–101.
6. Ikeuchi H. Arthroscopy of the shoulder joint. Shoulder joint 1983; 7:123–128.

INDICATIONS AND BENEFITS OF ARTHROSCOPY OF THE SHOULDER JOINT

H. LILLEBY, M.D.

The purpose of this report is to discuss the indications of shoulder arthroscopy and the benefits of arthroscopic findings for treatment of some shoulder disorders.

Materials and Method

In 1979 a study was begun by examining cadaver specimens. Since then 70 patients with different shoulder problems have been examined by the author. Arthroscopy is performed under general or plexus anesthesia, or sometimes local anesthesia. The patient is placed on his side. A 5 mm Storz arthroscope with 30 and 70° optic is used. A posterior entry is easiest and allows excellent survey of all important structures. The joint is filled and continuously flushed with saline solution. Most of the examinations were followed by surgery; the information gained by arthroscopy was most helpful.

Rotator Cuff

Rupture of the rotator cuff is easily seen by arthroscopy. It is possible to differentiate a full thickness tear from a superficial rupture. Localization and extension can usually be determined quite well. The benefit of this information lies not only in accurate diagnosis, but also in preoperative planning. Further, the possibility of tendon transplant may be estimated.

Case Report 1. A 47-year old man presented with subacromial impingement syndrome of the right shoulder. The x-ray examination was negative. Arthroscopy showed a superficial rupture of the rotator cuff with fraying of the supraspinatus tendon. A palpating hook from the sub-

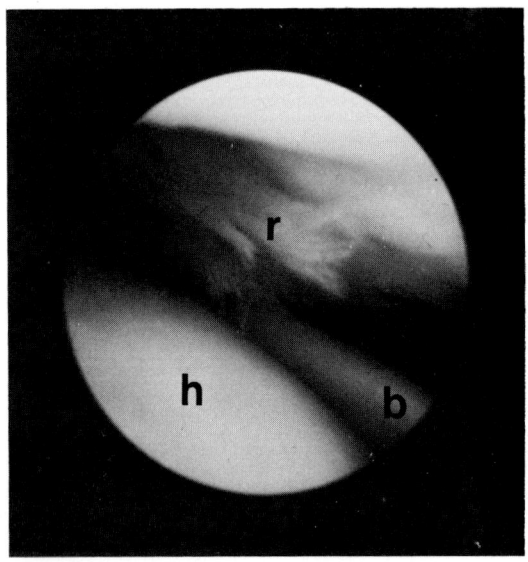

Figure 1 Superficial cuff rupture. (r) superficial rupture of the rotator cuff; (h) humeral head; (b) biceps tendon.

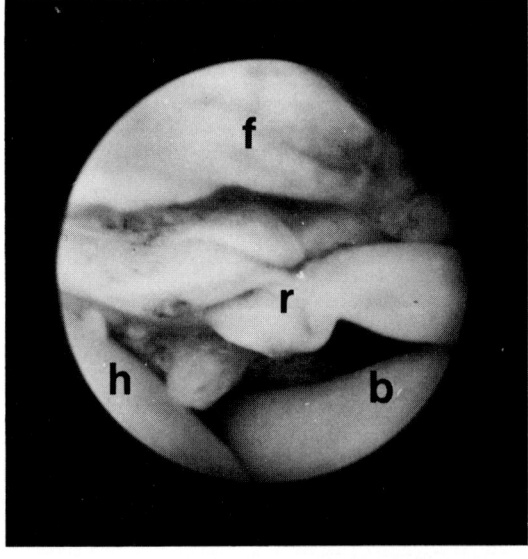

Figure 2 Full thickness cuff rupture. (r) cuff edge at rupture; (h) humeral head; (f) subacromial bursa floor; (b) biceps tendon luxated.

acromial bursa could not penetrate the cuff, proving that there was not full thickness rupture (Fig. 1). Pain was relieved after anterior acromioplasty and resection of the coracoacromial ligament through a small anterior incision.

Case Report 2. A 64-year old man with disabling shoulder pain following minor shoulder trauma presented with suspected cuff rupture. Arthroscopy revealed a large retracted full thickness rupture of the rotator cuff with luxation and partial rupture of the biceps tendon (Fig. 2). It was obvious that the necessary exposure could be achieved by a transacromial trapezius and deltoid splitting approach, and that the biceps tendon could be taken for transplant. In less extensive ruptures a much smaller anterolateral approach may be sufficient.

Head and Glenoid

The head and glenoid can be inspected for cartilage, labrum and bone lesions, and joint changes as found in arthritis can be estimated. The benefit of this inspection is accurate diagnosis. It is easy to differentiate between a posterior and an anterior habitual luxation because of the typical Hill-Sachs and Bankart lesions. An habitual subluxation of the shoulder leaves the same clear traces on the glenoid labrum and humeral head cartilage as does an habitual luxation. The information gained by arthroscopy may also help to decide whether or not arthroplasty is indicated in arthritic or post-traumatic changes.

Case Report 3. A 16-year old girl presented with habitual luxation of the left shoulder, and uncertainty as to the direction of luxation. At arthroscopy a frayed and broken anterior labrum of the glenoid was found together with a concomitant early Hill-Sachs lesion indicating an anterior habitual luxation (Fig. 3).

Case Report 4. A middle-aged woman presented with painful snapping in the right shoulder. The diagnosis was uncertain. Arthroscopy revealed a cartilage defect on the posterior part of the humeral head (early Hill-Sachs lesion) and fracture of the anterior labrum (early Bankart lesion) proving an habitual anterior subluxation of the right shoulder (Fig. 4).

Case Report 5. A 43-year old man presented with diffuse pain in the left shoulder after shoulder trauma. Clinical and x-ray examination were not helpful. Arthroscopy revealed a large cartilage lesion on the posterocranial aspect of the head. Surgery could then easily be performed from a posterolateral approach. Without arthroscopy the lesion may have gone unnoticed, or a standard arthrotomy incision might have hampered the final procedure substantially (Fig. 5).

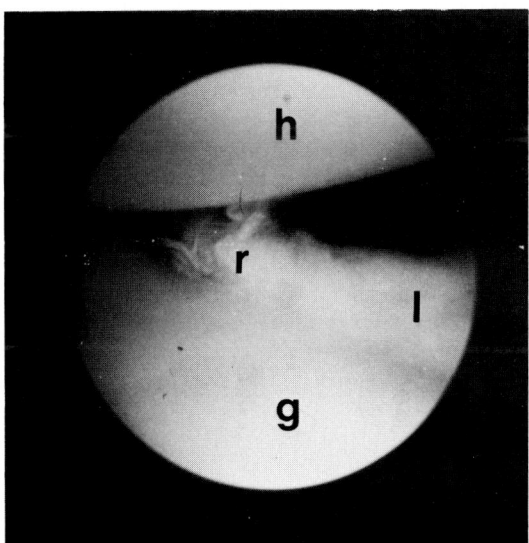

Figure 3 Anterior habitual luxation. (r) labrum rupture; early Bankart lesion; (h) humeral head; (g) glenoid fossa; (l) labrum.

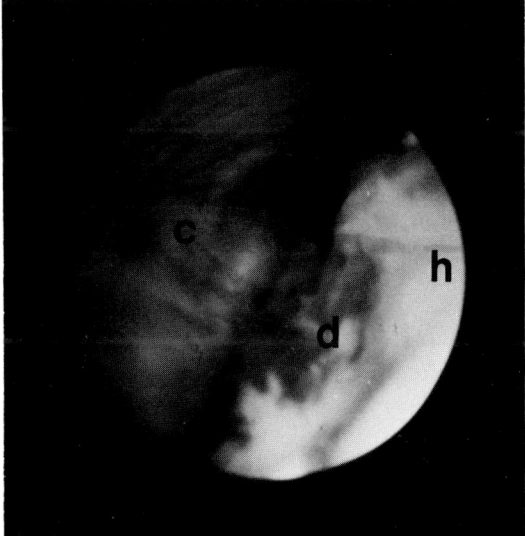

Figure 4 Anterior habitual subluxation. (d) cartilage defect, early Hill-Sachs lesion; (h) posterior part of humeral head; (c) posterior part of capsule.

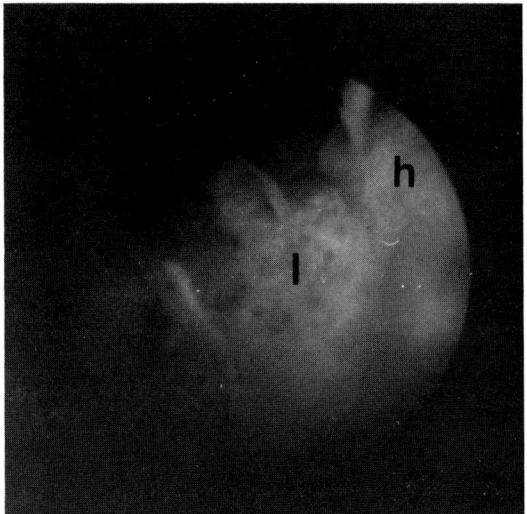

Figure 5 Traumatic lesion of the humeral head. (l) area of cartilage lesion; (h) posterocranial part of humeral head.

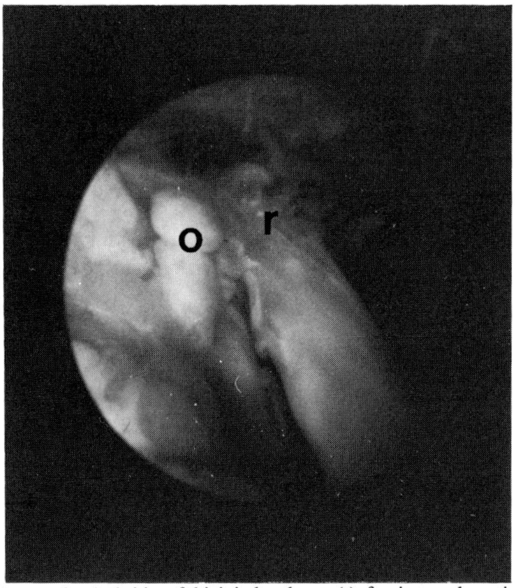

Figure 6 Arthritis of bicipital sulcus, (r) fraying and partial rupture of the biceps tendon; (o) bicipital groove osteophytes.

Synovia and Biceps

The joint can be examined for general synovitis or local changes. Biceps tendon changes are mainly found in the bicipital sulcus where ruptures, luxations, tendinitis or arthritic changes may be seen. Indications for early synovectomy of the rheumatoid shoulder may be difficult to assess with x-ray pictures and clinical examination alone, but arthroscopy will be a valuable aid to diagnosis. Arthroscopy also facilitates the follow-up of both surgical and conservative treatment. Selected biopsy may be carried during arthroscopy.

Case Report 6. A 60–year old man presented with subacromial impingement syndrome of the left shoulder. Arthroscopy revealed a superficial cuff rupture, severe bicipital arthritis with fraying and partial rupture of the tendon, and bony spurs on the sulcus edges (Fig. 6). The patient was successfully treated with transposition of the biceps tendon and removal of spurs combined with acromioplasty.

SUMMARY

Arthroscopy is an aid to exact diagnosis and satisfies a demand for better and more differentiated information in some shoulder problems. It is mainly helpful in preoperative evaluation. Surgical planning can be carried out ahead of arthrotomy, and the approach chosen need not be hampered by a badly located incision. Intra-articular survey is better in extent and detail than in arthrotomy. Arthroscopy may further contribute to our understanding of shoulder pathology; it facilitates percutaneous surgery of the shoulder joint.

Shoulder arthroscopy also has disadvantages. There is often some leaking of fluid to the soft tissue which causes swelling. This will be resorbed within a day and will not disturb surgery. The examination adds about 15 to 20 minutes to operating time. The main drawback is the need for a skilled arthroscopist.

ARTHROSCOPIC SHOULDER SURGERY

A. M. WILEY, M.Ch., F.R.C.S., F.R.C.S.(C)

It is the purpose of this chapter to review briefly the technique of shoulder arthroscopy, to discuss the endoscopic appearances of some common intra-articular lesions, and to describe techniques for bimanual and instrumental surgery. The arthroscope has proved to be of use in the diagnosis of many soft tissue lesions previously inaccessible to standard investigative techniques, and has immeasurably increased our appreciation and knowledge of shoulder pathology. As with so many relatively new techniques, the role of the instrument seems to be expanding. Skill in instrumentation is acquired by practice—sometimes a tedious and time-consuming process, which requires persistence and some patience. As visualization of the shoulder improves, the surgeon will be better able to manipulate, debride, incise, and extract.

TECHNIQUE OF ARTHROSCOPY

Posterior arthroscopy of the shoulder has been satisfactorily achieved by introducing a 5 mm Storz instrument (30° angle lens). A 3.8 mm instrument may be used in contracted shoulder and in "frozen shoulder"; the technique has been described elsewhere.[1,2] It is recommended that the patient be given a general anaesthetic to facilitate distraction of the joint by an assistant, who may later assist in a thorough examination by rotating the humerus in several directions. The instrument is inserted 2 cm below the angle of the acromion and driven into the joint just above the humeral head. It is possible to visualize all articular structures, except much of the infraspinatus as it crosses the "roof" of the joint. For teaching and recording purposes a television arm with a video recorder is a real advantage. Orientation is assisted by identifying the long head of the biceps (Fig. 1).

Common Soft Tissue Lesions

Complete and incomplete tears of the rotator cuff are readily apparent under arthroscopic visualization as are lesions of the long head of the biceps. Quite frequently after previous subacromial surgery, the long head of the biceps becomes adherent to the undersurface of the rotator cuff. The clinical implications of this are open to debate. Inspection of the mid-joint may show a torn glenoid labrum or a labrum stripped from its glenoid attachment. Bankart lesion or "clicking

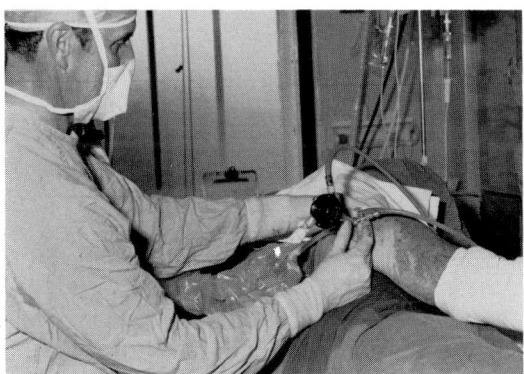

Figure 1 The arthroscope is inserted posteriorly and connected to a television arm.

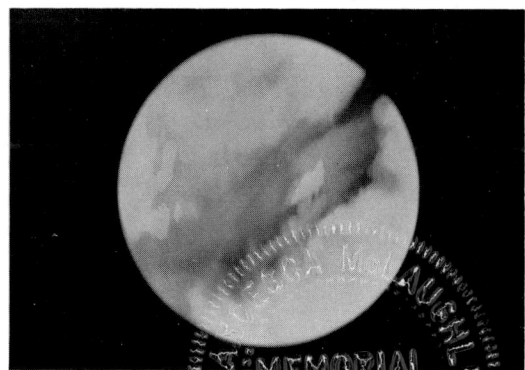

Figure 2 A "Hill-Sachs" lesion seen as an ulcer on the humeral head.

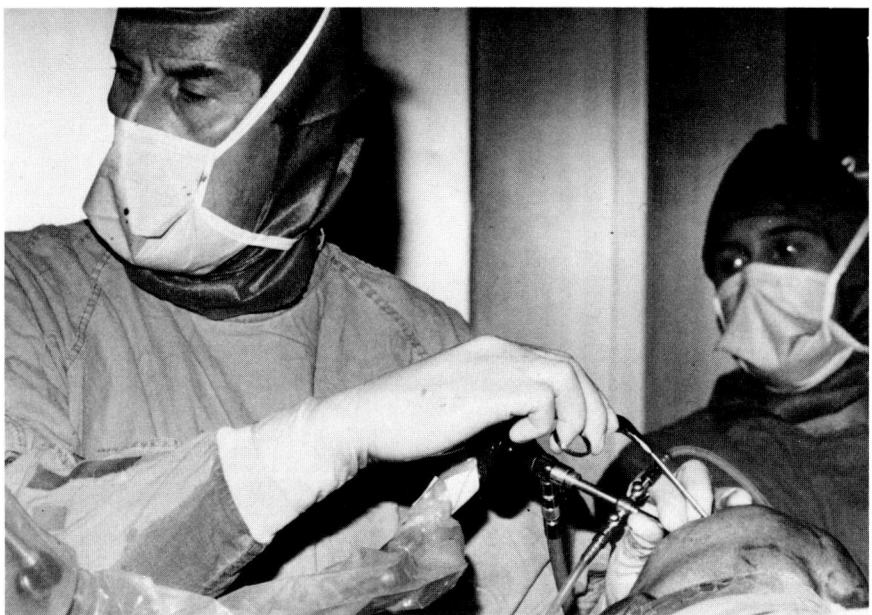

Figure 3 Posterior bimanual instrumentation of the shoulder.

shoulder" may be the clinical manifestation of a torn labrum without dislocation. Loose bodies are readily seen, especially in the infraglenoid recess. Specific forms of arthritis are readily presented for biopsy. A Hill-Sachs lesion on a humeral head may suggest an earlier dislocation (Fig. 2).

At the completion of shoulder arthroscopy it is possible to manipulate and measure the capacity of the joint.

ARTHROSCOPIC SHOULDER SURGERY

In addition to biopsy and removal of loose bodies from the shoulder, it is possible to manipulate certain soft tissue lesions, to debride, and to excise.

Technique

Operative arthroscopy may be performed using either an operating arthroscope or a bimanual technique.

Operating Arthroscope

A few appliances, such as basket forceps and a scissors, can be inserted through a special carrier within the sheath of a 5 mm Storz arthroscope. Instruments larger than this are too bulky for the shoulder and may damage the joint surfaces.

Bimanual Technique

Curved (2.4 mm) basket forceps, a scissors, a scalpel and straight curettes may be inserted 3 to 4 cm lateral to the examining instrument, again posteriorly. By triangulation the instruments may be brought into action to debride an incomplete rotator cuff tear, free a biceps tendon, and probe an apparently "incomplete" cuff tear (Fig. 3). Alternatively, using a bimanual technique, the operating instruments may be introduced anteriorly and the arthroscope posteriorly. This technique is recommended for the introduction of straight instruments, such as a curette, a (Dyonic) chondrotome (Fig. 4).

Role of Arthroscopic Shoulder Surgery

While there can be no doubt that operating techniques using the arthroscope present an attractive alternative for the patient suffering from a loose body, a loose labrum, an adhesion of the biceps tendon, and in patients with localized synovitis, the possibility of an expanded role for such techniques at this time is preliminary, even debatable.

The Torn Rotator Cuff

Incomplete Tears

These lesions are usually detectable only by the most detailed arthrography and doubtless many instances of the "impingement syndrome" may be traced to an irregularity of the rotator cuff, resulting from a partial tear. Transarticular arthroscopic debridement of such tears is not only possible but feasible. Ten such patients have been treated in this fashion and have reached an adequate follow-up period. The end result, pain relief, has not been uniformly satisfactory. Whereas this may indicate a false concept, it may also indicate that the technique must be improved and the debridement extended. Perhaps sectioning of the coracoacromial ligament is essential to the success of procedures for relief of impingement. Arthroscopic visualization of the coracoacromial ligament is feasible in some cases, when the examining instrument is placed in the subacromial space. The presence of a nearby troublesome artery (e.g., a branch of the thoracoacromial vessel) suggests a hazard in instrumental division of the ligament (Fig. 5).

Complete Tears of the Rotator Cuff

Arthroscopic examination of a complete tear of the rotator cuff offers information about the site, extent, and possible duration of the tear. During the course of such examination in 26 cases of rotator cuff tear being considered for reparative surgery, the author has been struck by the number of patients who obtained enough relief from irrigation, debridement, and manipulation to decline advice about open surgery. A host of questions have arisen about the interpretation of symptoms in this condition. For example, in 26 patients followed from three months to two years after arthroscopic debridement, 16 patients derived significant pain relief, and 17 increased the movement in the affected shoulder—surely figures that compare favorably with several series of cases treated surgically, including our own[3] and those of Cofield.[4] Relief by arthroscopic irrigation and debridement is frequently seen following instrumentation and examination of the degenerative knee. Nevertheless, the findings seem more important in the shoulder, a joint where degenerative disease is only slowly progressive (Fig. 6, 7).

Unstable Shoulder and Dislocating Shoulder

In this condition, direct examination of the pathology should facilitate more precise repair. Thus, the presence of a Bankart lesion prompts a Bankart repair. Additionally, manipulation of the

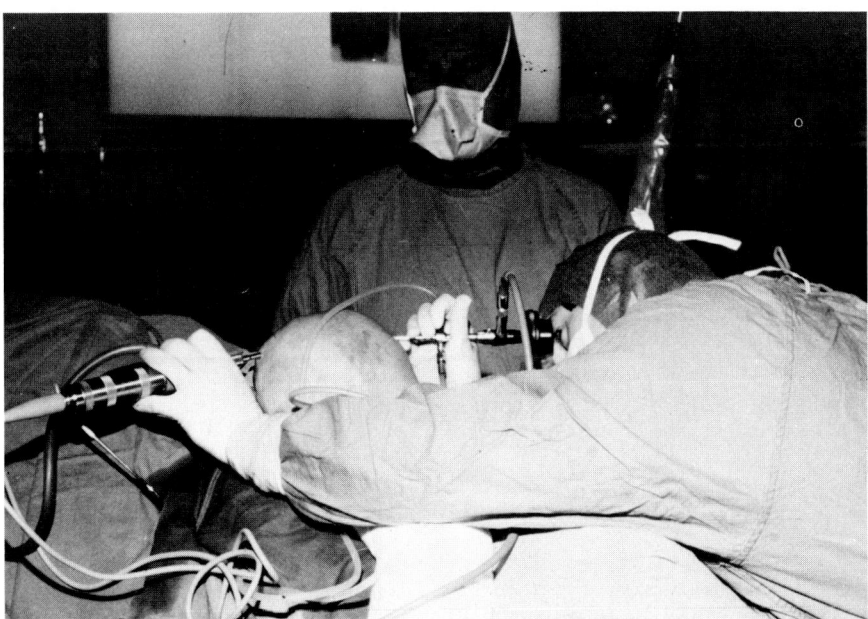

Figure 4 Anterior bimanual instrumentation using a powered "Debrider".

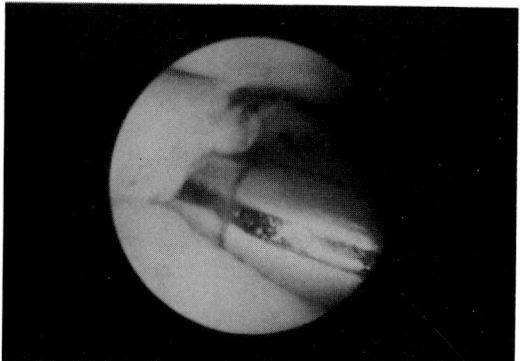

Figure 5 Debridement of an incomplete rotator cuff tear using a powered instrument.

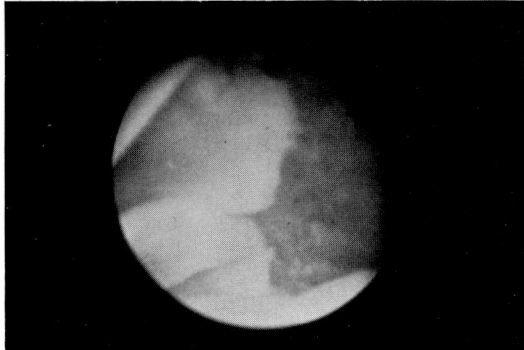

Figure 6 A complete tear of the rotator cuff.

shoulder under anaesthetic, sometimes with the C-arm of the image intensifier, has revealed a number of cases of multidirectional subluxation or dislocation.

Five patients suffering from anterior shoulder subluxation or dislocation have now been treated by arthroscopic surgery alone. In these it was found practicable to roughen the anterior glenoid with a curette and to transfix the labrum to its bony rim by means of a wire passed into the joint through a small anterior stab wound. This wire was removed three weeks later. These cases have not yet been followed long enough to justify a wider use of such endoscopic surgery.

Arthroscopy After Shoulder Surgery

Regrettably, not all surgical repairs of the rotator cuff end in a satisfactory result, nor is the cause of failure often readily apparent. Arthrography after repair of a rotator cuff is difficult to interpret.

The author has examined 15 patients with a poor result after rotator cuff repair. All were treated by a standard technique and approach, including resection of the acromioclavicular joint, section of the coracoacromial ligament, and supraspinatus advancement where indicated. In five patients the suture line was found disrupted. All have been sutured under some tension and an abduction splint or spica had been used in the recovery period.

SUMMARY

The role of the arthroscope in shoulder surgery has only just begun to be extensively explored. The potential for this instrument, espe-

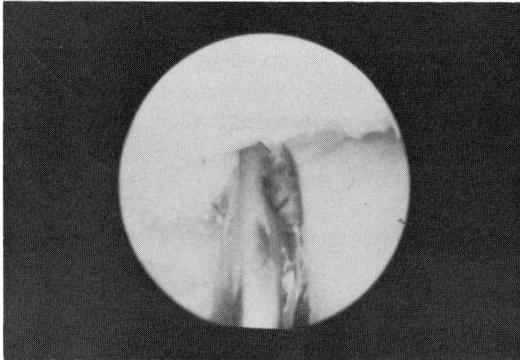

Figure 7 A curved scissors used to trim off loose fragments from the edge of a rotator cuff tear.

cially in endoscopic surgery, is apparently considerable and is comparable to that already recognized in the care of disabilities of the knee. Practice makes perfect, and the surgeon must be prepared to spend many hours with his patient (and anaesthetist). The morbidity following arthroscopic shoulder surgery is low enough to make it a worthwhile alternative to the often painful, less accurate methods of x-ray investigation and the high morbidity of open surgery.

REFERENCES

1. Wiley AM, Older MWJ. Shoulder arthroscopy: investigation with a fibro-optic instrument. Am J Sports Med. 1983; 8:30.
2. Wiley AM. Arthroscopic examination of the shoulder. Shoulder surgery. New York, Springer-Verlag, 1982; 111-118.
3. Ha'eri GB, Wiley AM. Advancement of the supraspinatus muscle in the repair of the ruptures of the rotator cuff. J Bone Joint Surg. 1981; 63A-2:232.
4. Bassett RW, Cofield RH. Acute tears of the rotator cuff: The timing of surgical repair. Clin Orthop. 1982; 175:18.

THE ROLE OF ARTHROSCOPY IN SURGERY OF THE SHOULDER

ROBERT H. COFIELD, M.D.

In 1931, in his landmark article on the use of arthroscopy, M. S. Burman[3] stated that the shoulder joint was the easiest joint to visualize consistently. In his article, he had several drawings depicting the inside of the glenohumeral joint, as seen through the arthroscope. From that time until the 1970s, very little was written about arthroscopy of the shoulder. Recently, however, Watanabe and associates,[8,9] and Johnson[7] have discussed many aspects of shoulder pathology for which arthroscopy might be useful. Conti,[5] Wiley and Older,[10] and Ha'eri and Maitland[6] have investigated the use of arthroscopy in periarthritis; Andrews and associates[1] mentioned its usefulness in the evaluation and treatment of torn glenoid labra in athletes; and Bateman[2] in 1978 and Caspari[4] in 1982 formulated some indications for arthroscopy in the shoulder.

There seems to be intense interest in arthroscopy of the shoulder. At the 1983 American Academy of Orthopaedic Surgeons Annual Meeting in Anaheim, California, six papers or exhibits were presented on this subject, and at the annual meeting of the Arthroscopy Association of North America, three presentations were given on arthroscopy and its use in the shoulder.

The present study assessed the usefulness of arthroscopy for the evaluation or treatment of shoulder problems. Is arthroscopy important for a given pathologic condition, is it optional, or is it unnecessary?

CLINICAL MATERIAL

Between December 1979 and June 1982, 71 patients with 74 involved shoulders had arthroscopic evaluation or evaluation and treatment for various clinical problems: instability in 28 shoulders, supraspinatus tendinitis in 23, arthritis in 9, rotator cuff tearing in 7, periarthritis in 3, infection in 2, and intra-articular fracture in 2. Adjunctive arthroscopic procedures were done in 8 shoulders: synovial biopsy in 2, synovectomy in 2, placement of suction-irrigation tubes in 2, removal of loose bodies in 1, and excision of the intra-articular portion of the biceps tendon in 1.

The 26 patients (11 women and 15 men) with shoulder instability were not typical of patients with that problem. The former were older, their ages averaging 26 years and ranging from 17 to 46 years. Twenty-one patients had recognized some form of injury, but only three had had a definite shoulder dislocation. Four believed they had dislocated the shoulder but were not sure. Eighteen had had one to four previous procedures on their shoulders. Four had voluntary subluxation of the shoulder at examination. In 14 shoulders, instability could not be ascertained on examination because of extreme pain. Roentgenograms of the shoulder either showed postoperative changes or were normal.

The 22 patients (5 women and 17 men) with supraspinatus tendinitis were typical of patients with that problem. Their ages averaged 49 years and ranged from 20 to 67 years. Five patients had had previous shoulder surgery. Findings on history and physical examination were diagnostic, with night pain, a painful arc of movement, a positive impingement sign, anterosuperior shoulder pain with forced internal rotation, discomfort with contraction of the supraspinatus against resistance, and tenderness over the anterosuperior rotator cuff. Roentgenograms either were normal or showed minor, nonspecific changes suggestive of chronic tendinitis. Arthrography was done in 20 shoulders; findings were normal in 15 and showed incomplete, undersurface rotator cuff tearing in five.

Nine patients (all men) were evaluated for arthritis. The patients were generally younger than those with arthritic involvement of the shoulder. Their ages averaged 40 years and ranged from 26 to 51 years. All 9 patients complained of severe symptoms and inability to work in spite of near-normal shoulder motion and strength. Routine roentgenograms did not confirm the degree of pathologic change that might be expected on the basis of the severity of symptoms. Routine roentgenograms showed mild-to-moderate loss of cartilage in eight shoulders, glenoid dysplasia in one, loose bodies in one, and osteoporosis with some resorptive changes at the junction of the synovial attachment to the humerus in one.

The ages of the 7 patients (4 women and 3 men) with rotator cuff tear averaged 50 years and ranged from 39 to 69 years. Two patients had had previous surgery. All seven patients had findings on physical examination compatible with rotator cuff tearing, and tearing was identified on the shoulder arthrogram in all seven patients.

The 3 patients (2 women and 1 man) with periarthritis had had pain and stiffness for 1.5, 3, and 4 years. The ages of the patients were 44, 48, and 51 years. One patient was believed to have cervical spondylosis as the cause of the shoulder pain and one to have recurrent supraspinatus tendinitis. In the third patient, the diagnosis was uncertain. Physical examination showed stiffness with movement, diffuse generalized muscle weakness, and pain at the extremes of motion. Roentgenograms showed osteoporosis in all three patients and mild glenohumeral arthritis in two. The arthrograms showed a contracted joint volume in all three and nonspecific synovitis in one.

In the 2 patients (both men) with intra-articular glenoid fractures, standard roentgenograms could not delineate the fracturing pattern or fragment position with enough accuracy to direct treatment. Both patients—one 19 and the other 32 years of age—had high-velocity injuries.

The two patients with infection were both men (one 44 and the other 61 years of age). One presented acutely, having had a proximal humeral prosthesis inserted previously, and the other presented subacutely three months after having an injection for tendinitis. Specimens were obtained for bacteriologic studies at the time of arthroscopy, and both grew Staphylococcus aureus.

TECHNIQUE

The procedure can be done with local anesthesia, although general anesthesia allows more ample distention of the joint and easier manipulation during the procedure. The patient is placed in the lateral position; the shoulder to be examined is upward. A spinal needle is positioned 2 cm caudal and approximately 2 cm medial to the junction of the spine of the scapula and the lateral aspect of the acromion (Fig. 1). During placement of the needle, gentle traction is placed on the limb. The humeral head is grasped between the thumb and the index finger and manipulated. The needle is then positioned at the joint line and is slid over the top of the slightly inferiorly positioned humeral head. Saline is infused, and usually 50 ml can be instilled if joint contracture is not present. An incision is made next to the spinal needle, and the arthroscope obturator with its contained trochanter is introduced. The needle is then removed.

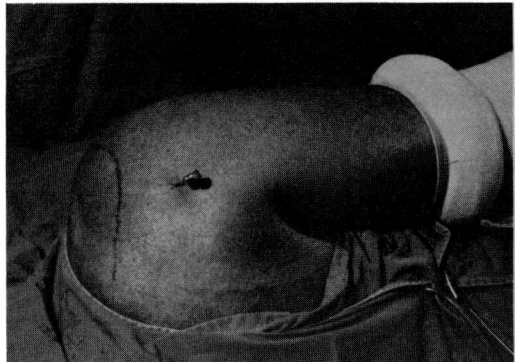

Figure 1 Posterior aspect of shoulder prepared and draped for arthroscopy. The spinal needle is positioned, saline is infused, and the portal incision is made adjacent to the needle.

Earlier, a small needlescope was used, but as experience was gained, a larger scope was introduced. The 4 mm arthroscope seems best for this procedure, as it is small enough to maneuver easily within the joint but large enough to allow maneuverability through the muscle planes without the need for reintroducing the scope in different directions, as had been necessary for the needlescope. Often, through-and-through irrigation is not needed, as irrigation can be satisfactorily obtained through the obturator. When additional irrigation is necessary because of difficulty with vision or for an arthroscopic surgical procedure, the needle should be introduced anteriorly just lateral and superior to the coracoid so that it enters the joint through the upper portion of the subscapularis or just above the subscapularis tendon. This portal is also useful if one wishes to insert a surgical instrument.

A standard order of evaluation is followed (Table 1). At the conclusion of the procedure, the joint is irrigated, the fluid is evacuated, and a single vertical mattress suture is placed, closing each portal.

TABLE 1 Sequence for Arthroscopic Evaluation of Shoulder Joint

1. Identify humeral head and biceps tendon
2. Follow biceps tendon to glenoid
3. Retrace along biceps to rotator tendons
4. Move posteriorly to inspect synovial reflection of humeral head, posterior synovial recess, inferior synovial recess, and posterior labrum
5. Return to central position to inspect cartilage surfaces
6. Advance forward to inspect glenohumeral ligaments and anterior labrum

RESULTS

Shoulder Instability

Three questions should be answered. Is instability still present and, if so, in what direction or directions? Is there evidence of continuing cartilage damage? Having answered these questions, what treatment is necessary, and especially if surgical treatment is necessary, which surgical approach would be better? As seen in Table 2, retrospective analysis in 28 cases established that routine history, physical examination, and roentgenograms were diagnostic in 10. The arthrogram did not add any information of diagnostic importance. In 12 shoulders, the arthroscopic evaluation offered some aid in selecting the path of treatment. In eight of the 12, no significant intra-articular changes were observed and, in addition to the other data, arthroscopic evaluation suggested that continuing conservative treatment measures would be adequate. In the four others, moderate cartilage changes were identified, suggesting the need for further treatment to control the instability and to delay the continuing loss of cartilage. In six other shoulders, arthroscopy revealed local labral injury and confirmed a diagnosis of instability that had been made secure at the time of examination under anesthesia. In only three shoulders was the diagnosis made at arthroscopy. In one of these, a large labral tear was identified anteriorly, and in two, the results of examination were normal, which with earlier diagnostic measures confirmed the suspicion that treatment was not necessary. Thus, for atypical instability problems, arthroscopy was crucial in three cases, was optional or helpful in 18, and was unnecessary in seven (Table 3).

Shoulder Impingement Syndrome

The rotator cuff was normal or inflamed on arthroscopic evaluation in 15 shoulders. There was an undersurface partial thickness rotator cuff tear in five, some fraying of the undersurface of the tendons in two, and a degenerated fibrillated biceps tendon in one. In these eight patients, arthroscopy was helpful in that it indicated no need for incision into the rotator cuff at surgery to inspect either the undersurface of the rotator cuff or the biceps tendon. However, a specific significant benefit was appreciated only for the eight shoulders in which a pathologic change was identified. For the other 15 shoulders, the procedure was helpful and optional but not necessary. Only one patient in this group and one patient in the entire series had an abnormal biceps tendon identified at arthroscopy. It should be recalled that the intra-articular portion of the biceps tendon is not usually involved by disease and that the extra-articular portion in the bicipital groove is most frequently affected. One would not expect to consistently identify this area of involvement at arthroscopic examination.

Glenohumeral Arthritis

Arthroscopy was helpful for the eight shoulders with degenerative glenohumeral arthritis and the one shoulder with arthritis secondary to pigmented villonodular synovitis. In four shoulders, the humeral head had lost cartilage on its central aspect, a finding that was not apparent by physical examination or on the roentgenogram. In the care of these patients, future surgical options were considered. In four other shoulders, the articular surface and synovial changes were minor, and a continued conservative treatment was recommended. In one shoulder, the arthrogram showed synovial irregularity that indicated a nonspecific inflammatory arthritis and not degenerative arthritic changes. At arthroscopy, this was confirmed, and synovial biopsy was interpreted as representing rheumatoid arthritis.

Rotator Cuff Tears

Art arthroscopy, rotator cuff tearing was identified in all seven shoulders. However, rotator cuff tearing was diagnosed by history, physical examination, routine roentgenograms, and shoulder arthrograms. The tear size was also effectively estimated by these measures. However, neither the above measures nor arthroscopy could effectively assess the quality or mobility of the tissue. This assessment is very important in predicting the outcome of surgical repair of a rotator cuff tear.

TABLE 2 Evaluation Crucial for Diagnosis of Shoulder Problems in 74 Cases

Diagnostic Category	History, Physical Exam, Routine X-ray	Joint Aspiration Arthrogram	Exam Under Anesthesia	Arthroscopy
Instability	10	—	15	3
Impingement	—	15	—	8
Arthritis	—	1	—	8
Cuff tear	—	7	—	—
Intra-articular fracture	—	—	—	2
Infection	—	2	—	—
Periarthritis	—	2	—	1
Total	10	27	15	22

Intra-articular Fractures

Both men with glenoid fractures whose displacement could not be ascertained by multiple routine roentgenographic views had their fractures identified with certainty at arthroscopic evaluation. In one patient, multiple fracture lines were identified without significant displacement, and surgery was avoided. In the other patient, a large articular surface fragment occupying the posterior one-third of the glenoid was seen to be slightly displaced but more importantly rotated approximately 40° such that open reduction and fixation was believed to be necessary and could be readily accomplished after identification of the intra-articular pathology. Although arthroscopy was very useful in these patients, the availability of computed tomography (CT) obviates the need for arthroscopy in most, if not all, patients with complex glenoid fractures.

TABLE 3 Value of Shoulder Arthroscopy in 74 Cases

Diagnosis	Important	Optional	Unnecessary
Instability	3	18	7
Impingement	8	15	—
Arthritis	9	—	—
Cuff tear	—	—	7
Intra-articular fracture	2	—	—
Infection	1	—	1
Periarthritis	1	—	2
Total	24 (32%)	33 (45%)	17 (23%)

Infection

The patient with acute Staphylococcus aureus septic arthritis who had had a proximal humeral prosthesis in place had the organism identified by aspiration at arthroscopy. It was possible to effectively irrigate all of the joint recesses and to identify that the synovial changes represented inflammation only and no significant synovial necrosis or extensive debris formation was present. Suction-irrigation tubes were placed, and this along with intravenously administered antibiotics resulted in resolution of infection, which has not recurred over a 1-year period. The second patient, with the subacute to chronic infectious process, had aspiration at arthroscopy, irrigation, and placement of suction-irrigation tubes. Significant synovial changes and debris formation also were identified, and a synovectomy was done. However, the infection recurred at 4 months and required open surgical treatment.

Periarthritis

In one patient with periarthritis, capsular scarring was noted and moderate glenohumeral arthritis was defined, affording a frank discussion with the patient about his disease and opening new potential lines for curative treatment. In the second patient, nonspecific synovitis was identified at arthroscopy, and in the third patient, a contracted joint volume without other abnormalities was seen. However, for these latter two patients, these changes were identified on the arthrogram. Arthroscopy offered no new knowledge.

DISCUSSION

Arthroscopy is useful in evaluating shoulder diseases, just as it is in evaluating other joints. However, the degree of its usefulness for various disease entities varies. Examination with the patient under general anesthesia is the most important measure for patients with glenohumeral instability. Arthroscopy is helpful in defining the intra-articular pathology, specifically the size and location of the labral and capsular damage, but it is only adjunctive in shoulders with instability. Arthroscopy in the evaluation of supraspinatus tendinitis is optional. It does identify undersurface rotator cuff tearing and will obviate the need for incision into the rotator cuff at surgery, if this is contemplated. However, a well-done shoulder arthrogram and careful examination of the exterior surface of the rotator cuff at acromioplasty should allow one to identify significant undersurface rotator cuff tearing, obviating the need for routine arthroscopy in this condition. When full-thickness rotator cuff tears are present and confirmed by arthrography, arthroscopy does not add any information that would alter the physician's discussion with the patient about his treatment options or change the patient's treatment.

Arthroscopy will help in staging the arthritic disease. If simpler measures will stage the arthritis, however, arthroscopy should not be done. In intra-articular fractures of the glenohumeral joint, if more conventional means, such as standard roentgenograms, cannot define the extent of fracture fragment displacement, arthroscopy can. However, since this series was undertaken, the use of CT has become more practical, and now when comminuted glenoid fractures are seen, CT almost always defines fracture fragment displacement, and arthroscopy is no longer necessary.

In patients with acute infection, arthroscopy offers a sure means of obtaining bacteriologic samples, carefully irrigating the joint, and placing suction-irrigation tubes to assure continuous lavage of the synovial cavity. In the presence of subacute or chronic infections though, it may not be possible to fully evacuate the infectious material and tissue via arthroscopy, and perhaps open measures are better in the treatment of nonacute joint infections.

In periarthritis, intrinsic joint disease must be excluded as a cause of the continuing shoulder pain and stiffness. The arthrogram will usually allow this. Once intrinsic shoulder disease has been excluded, treatment for the shoulder with periarthritis usually consists of physiotherapy, analgesics, and perhaps manipulation. These measures have proved to be extremely successful in the resolution of periarthritis of the shoulder. Surgical measures, including arthroscopic evaluation and surgery, should not be strongly considered.

SUMMARY

Seventy-four arthroscopic examinations of the shoulder were done between December 1979 and June 1982. These were done to evaluate glenohumeral instability in 28 shoulders, to assess the joint and tendons prior to acromioplasty for chronic tendinitis in 23, to diagnose or stage arthritic disease in 9, to define rotator cuff tearing in 7, to assess long-standing periarthritis in 3, to treat infection in 2, and to visualize articular fracture displacement in 2. Arthroscopy seemed to be important in 24 cases (32%), optional in 33 (45%), and unnecessary in 17 (23%). Examination of the shoulder with the patient under general anesthesia was more useful than arthroscopy itself in the patients with shoulder instability. In chronic tendinitis, arthrograms usually defined the pathologic change, but on occasion, undersurface rotator cuff tears were identified, leading to more specific treatment. Arthroscopy was valuable in staging intra-articular arthritic disease, in evaluating articular fractures, and in diagnosing and treating acute infections. However, arthroscopy may not be appropriate for treating chronic joint infections and is of no practical value in assessing rotator cuff tears or periarthritis.

REFERENCES

1. Andrews JR, Wilkes JS, Blackburn TA. Arthroscopic surgery in throwing athletes with glenoid labrum tears (abstract). Orthop Trans 1982; 6:203.
2. Bateman JE. The Shoulder and Neck. 2nd ed. Philadelphia: WB Saunders, 1978:170–176.
3. Burman MS. Arthroscopy or the direct visualization of joints: an experimental cadaver study. J Bone Joint Surg 1931; 13:669–695.

4. Caspari RB. Shoulder arthroscopy: a review of the present state of the art. Contemp Orthop 1982; 4:523–531.
5. Conti V. Arthroscopy in rehabilitation. Orthop Clin North Am 1979; 10:709–711.
6. Ha'eri GB, Maitland A. Arthroscopic findings in the frozen shoulder. J Rheumatol 1981; 8:149–152.
7. Johnson LL. Diagnostic and surgical arthroscopy, the knee and other joints. 2nd ed. St. Louis: CV Mosby, 1981; 376–389.
8. Watanabe M. Arthroscopy: the present state. Orthop Clin North Am 1979; 10:505–522.
9. Watanabe M, Takeda S, Ikeuchi H. Atlas of arthroscopy. 3rd ed. New York: Springer-Verlag, 1979; 134–150.
10. Wiley AM, Older MWJ. Shoulder arthroscopy: investigations with a fibrooptic instrument. Am J Sports Med 1980; 8:31–38.

TRAUMA

ASPECTS OF PROGNOSTIC FACTORS IN COMMINUTED AND DISLOCATED PROXIMAL HUMERAL FRACTURES

OLLE HÄGG M.D. and B. LUNDBERG, M.D.

The comminuted proximal humeral fracture is associated with great therapeutic problems. Several reports, where treatment has been either closed[8,29] or open, with varying methods of osteosynthesis,[1,12,21,23] have presented disappointing results. Neer[20] has shown that especially the IV-part fracture has a great tendency to develop avascular necrosis of the head fragment. He therefore, as others[11,29] do, recommends joint replacement as a primary procedure.

In the present report we have investigated the functional results after operative treatment with respect to an alternative primary joint replacement. We also evaluate the results of our mainly adopted procedure (open reduction with adaptation of fracture fragments combined with temporary transfixation with Kirschner wires). The investigation also seeks other factors of importance in the development of avascular necrosis.

MATERIALS AND METHODS

Thirty-three cases involving III and IV-part fractures with and without a dislocation were treated between 1971 and 1981. All patients were studied regarding early postoperative complications and postoperative x-ray anatomy. At the follow-up ten patients were not available. The follow-up time was from 1 to 10 years. The 23 cases included in the final study are:

III-part fracture	5	
IV-part fracture	6	
III-part fracture dislocation	3	(anterior)
IV-part fracture dislocation	9	(6 anterior, 3 posterior)

The mean age was 56 years, minimum 28 and maximum 75 years.

The treatment was open reduction in 20 cases. In 11 of these 1 to 3 Kirschner wires were used for temporary transfixation of the head fragment to the glenoid and to the humeral shaft (of these, ten were IV-part fractures or fracture dislocations) (Fig. 1a-c). In four cases a complementary tubercular fixation was utilized. The Rushpin technique was used in two cases (III-part fractures), staples in two cases of IV-part fractures, of which one also had tubercular fixation. AO-screw was used in one case (III-part fracture), merely osteosuture in one case (IV-part fracture), open reduction without internal fixation in two cases (III-part fracture dislocation). The majority of the fractures thus have been openly reduced, temporarily transarticularly fixated and the tubercular fragments have usually been only adapted without specific osteosyntheses. All but four cases (abduction frame 2–4 weeks) had the arm in the adducted position for 2–3 weeks. The Kirschner wires were then removed except in one case where they, by mistake, were left for 6 weeks and physiotherapy started with the wires still in place. Fourteen cases were treated within 24 hours, six within a week, one case after 10 days, one after 14 days and one after a month.

Associated injuries existed in four cases: One lesion of the brachial plexus (IV-part fracture dislocation), one fracture of the distal radius on the same side (III-part fracture dislocation), one cleavage fracture of the glenoide (III-part fracture dislocation) and one cerebrovascular lesion with propioceptive dysfunction in the fractured arm (IV-part fracture dislocation).

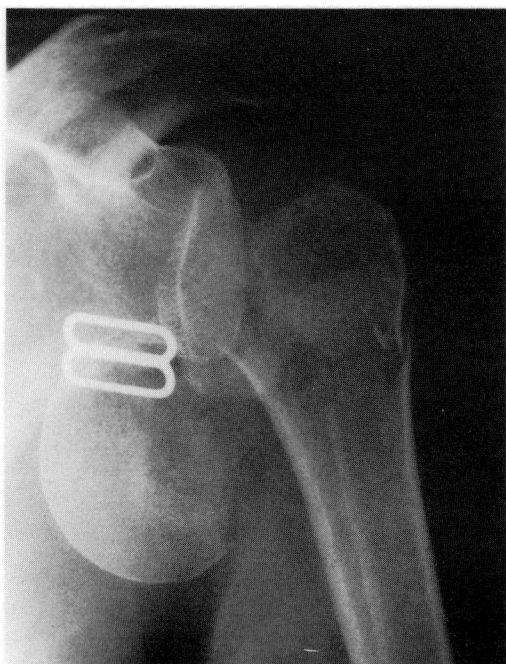

Figure 1a IV-part fracture-dislocation (anterior) in a woman aged 75.

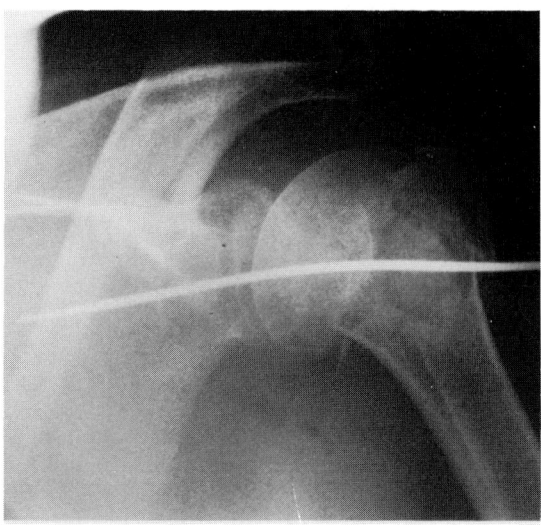

Figure 1b After open reduction and transfixation with Kirschner wire.

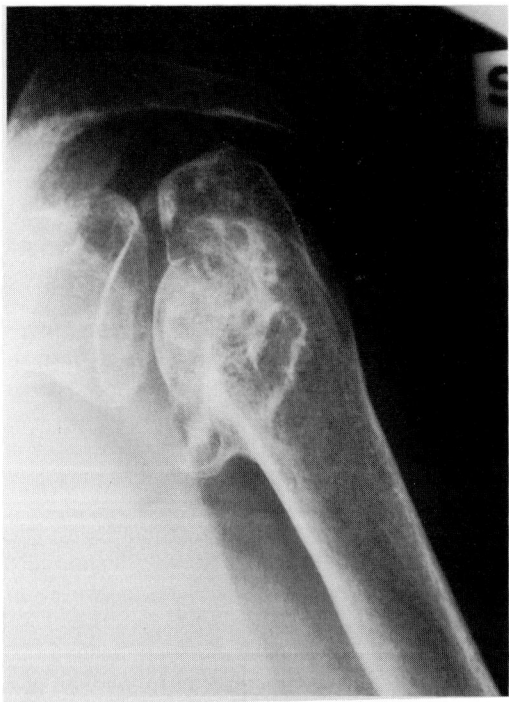

Figure 1c 21 months later—avascular necrosis of humeral head.

Results

In the evaluation of the results we have used two methods and compared them. One is the criteria established by Neer (maximum 100 points, excellent ≥ 90 points, satisfactory ≥ 80, unsatisfactory ≥ 70 and failure ≤ 70 points). The other method was originally practiced by Santee[25] and later by Knight and Mayne.[12] This method includes measuring of four movements:

1. Humeroscapular abduction, good if more than 60 degrees.
2. External rotation with arm in maximum abduction, good if the forearm reaches the plane of the body.
3. External rotation in the adducted position, good if more than 20 degrees.
4. Internal rotation in the abducted position, good if the forearm reaches 40 degrees below the horizontal plane.

It also includes estimation of strength and assessment of pain (none, minimal, moderate or disabling).

Postoperative complications in all 33 cases were three cases of deep infection, two of these requiring joint revision, two cases of superficial wound infection, which healed with antibiotics and two cases of secretion at the Kirschner wire entrance, which healed after extraction. The overall results at the follow-up, evaluated according to Santee were 52 percent excellent or satisfactory,

TABLE 1 Results of Evaluation Criteria According to Neer and Santee

	Excellent	Satisfactory	Unsatisfactory	Failure
Santee	5	7	7	4
Neer	2	6	3	12

TABLE 2 Results in Relation to Fracture Type (Evaluation According to Neer)

	Excellent	Satisfactory	Unsatisfactory	Failure
III-part fracture	0	2	2	1
IV-part fracture	0	1	1	4
III-part fracture dislocation	0	2	0	1
IV-part fracture dislocation	2	1	0	6

and evaluated according to Neer 35 percent excellent or satisfactory (Tab. 1). The IV-part lesions showed the worst prognosis. Dislocation of the head fragment, however, did not seem to affect the prognosis (Tab. 2).

Total avascular necrosis of the head fragment appeared in seven cases (all belonging to the IV-part group), one case of partial necrosis (III-part fracture), one pseudarthrosis (IV-part fracture) and one case of osteoarthritis (IV-part fracture dislocation). All were failures except the case of partial necrosis, which was unsatisfactory (Tab. 3). In Table 3 there is also a comparison between good x-ray anatomy and malunion (defined as ≤ 6 points) at the follow-up, considering final result, pain and movement. Table 3 shows that the necrotic head fragment results in a failure, not because of pain but because of restricted motion. The results also indicate a relation between malunion and restricted function.

Twelve persons were employed at the time of trauma. Five of these showed avascular necrosis at follow-up. The mean time of sick registration was in the whole series 5.7 months, for those with avascular necrosis 7.2 months and for those without avascular necrosis 4.6 months. One patient required a disability pension, one had to change occupation. The remaining ten including the five cases of avascular necrosis, could resume their ordinary occupation.

Only one patient had sought assistance because of shoulder disability, the case of osteoarthritis. He had a Neer prostheses implanted. All patients with avascular necrosis were offered joint replacement at the follow-up examination, but they all declined.

In the 15 IV-part fractures with and without dislocation we have tried to evaluate the importance of tubercular fixation, postoperative x-ray anatomy (Fig. 2) and operative delay (Tab. 4).

TABLE 3 Overall Results and Functional Restriction in Relation to Final Radiological Appearance

	Good X-ray	Malunion	Avascular Necrosis	Osteoarthritis Pseudarthrosis
Excellent	2	—	—	—
Satisfactory	5	1	—	—
Unsatisfactory	—	2	1	—
Failure	1	2	7	2
No or slight pain (≥30 p)	6	4	6	—
Pain	2	1	2	2
Abd/ext				
≥100	8	1	—	—
<100	—	4	8	2
Ext. rotation				
≥20	8	4	2	1
<20	—	1	6	1
Int. rotation				
≥30	8	1	5	2
<	—	4	3	—

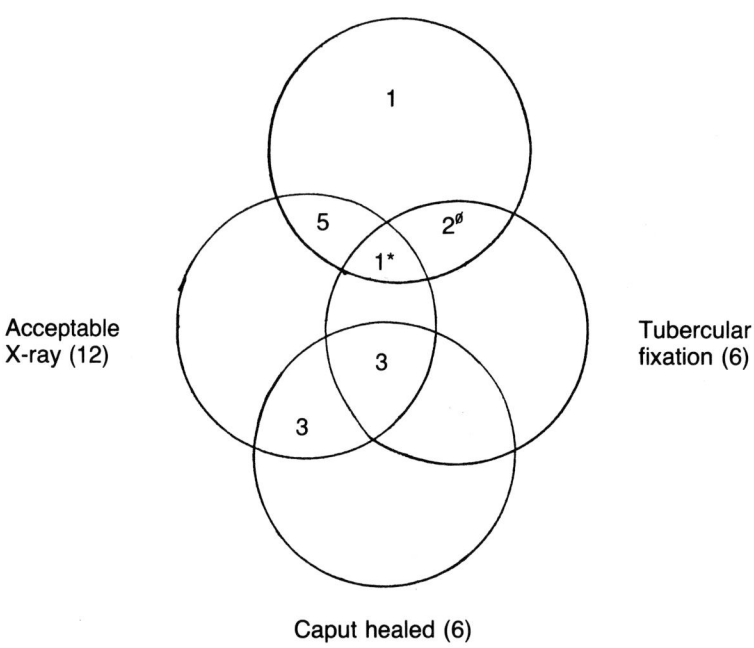

* Deep infection
∅ In both cases malplacement of tuberosities.

Figure 2 Survival of the head fragment in relation to postoperative x-ray and tubercular fixation in IV-part lesions (15 cases).

Acceptable postoperative x-ray is defined as a restoration to Neer's type 1 (minimal displacement), which means that no segment is displaced more than 1.0 cm or angulated more than 45 degrees (Fig. 3). An example of bad x-ray anatomy is shown in Figure 4. Two cases with tubercular fixation were technical failures (malplacement); they developed avascular necrosis. One case with the procedure had a deep infection resulting in avascular necrosis. The three cases with successful tubercular fixation and acceptable postoperative x-ray healed.

TABLE 4 Incidence of Avascular Necrosis in IV-Part Lesions in Relation to Operative Delay

	Avascular Necrosis	Healed
Op < 24 hours (6)	2	4
Op ≤ 1 week (4)	2	2
Op > 1 week (3)	3	—

DISCUSSION

Classification

Several different methods of fracture classification have been presented, often the surgeon's own modified system. Most authors apply anatomic divisions[7,8,9,13,16,18,24–28] but they are all different in some way. An etiological classification has been proposed,[4] and division into comminuted and noncomminuted fractures and fracture dislocation has been used.[12,17] This broad spectrum of classification makes all comparisons very unreliable or impossible. Fortunately the classification based on Codman's[3] original diagram and presented by Neer[20] has gained popularity and is adopted by several authors.[1,10,11,22,23,29] Apart from being easily reproducible, it also has a definite prognostic value as regards the survival of the head fragment. However, it is not always easy to make a distinction between III-part and IV-part fractures. The lesser tubercular fragment may be

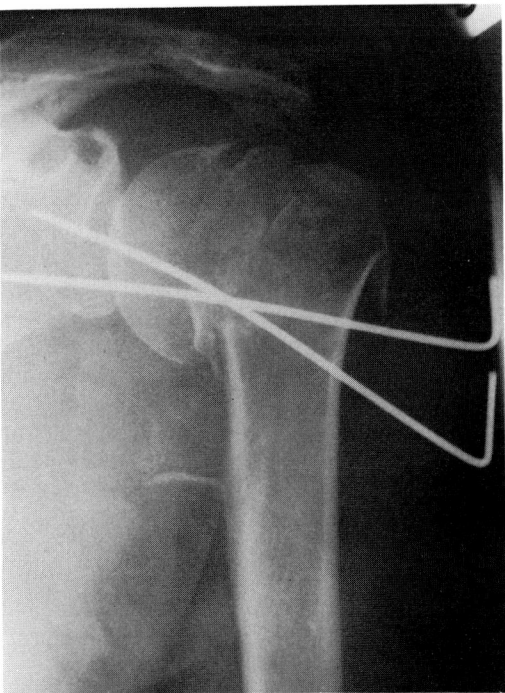

Figure 3 Acceptable postoperative x-ray in a IV-part fracture dislocation (posterior).

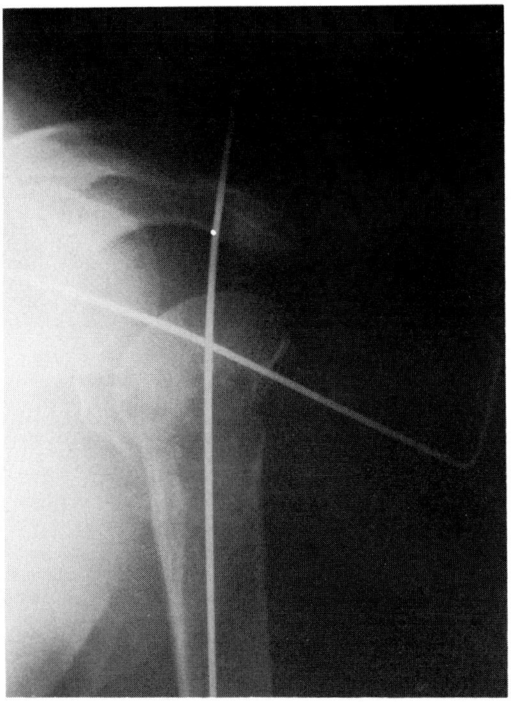

Figure 4 Bad postoperative x-ray in a IV-part fracture. Both tubercular fragments still displaced.

small and difficult to distinguish on x-ray. In our series there is one fracture allocated to the III-part group which might be a IV-part fracture. There are also two fractures actually having only 3 fragments but included in the IV-part group (Fig. 5). They are both fractures of the anatomic neck with displacement of the greater tuberosity but the lesser tuberosity attached to the humerus. In respect of the vascular state of the head fragment these fractures have the same prognosis as IV-part fractures and are therefore included in this group.

Treatment and Results

As with the fracture classification, there is also a great diversity of evaluation criteria, often undetailed.[4,7,13,17,23,30,31] In the interests of fair comparison we are restricted to works where both fracture classification and evaluation criteria are reproducible. This is the case where Neer's system is adopted.[10,20,29] A few other works, where fracture classification and evaluation criteria are different but clear[2,6,8,12,24,26] are also possible to compare.

In Table 5 we have tabulated the results of 9 different authors and our own results. It necessitated an approximation into III-part and IV-part lesions in works where different fracture classifications were adopted. By analysis of text and illustrations we consider it possible and reasonable with the following conversion:

III-part
  Supra-tubercular Non-comminuted (Knight/Mayne)
  Extra-capsular (Geneste)
  Vertical + Tuberosity (Duparc)
  Non-impacted Surgical Neck + Tuberosity (Razemon)
  Surgical Neck + Tuberosities (Baudin)

IV-part
  Supra-tubercular comminuted (Knight/Mayne)
  Intra-capsular (Geneste)
  Head + Tuberosity (Duparc)
  Non-impacted + Split Humeral Head (Razemon)
  Anatomic neck (Schultz)
  Comminuted Surgical Neck (Baudin)

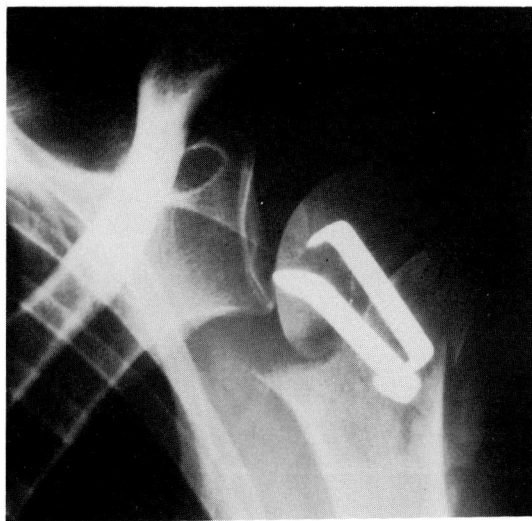

Figure 5 Fracture of anatomic neck and greater tuberosity—allocated to the IV-part group.

The investigations in Table 5 do not give any support to the thesis that open reduction is superior to closed treatment. With both methods III-part lesions have a better prognosis than IV-part lesions. When the results in Table 5 are compiled we find that III-part lesions treated by closed methods are satisfactory in 53 percent, by open reduction in 57 percent. Closed reduction in IV-part lesions gives satisfactory results in 34 percent and open reduction in 18 percent. In interpreting these figures one must be aware that the more displaced a fracture, the more one is prone to intervene surgically, thereby creating a bias in the distribution of therapeutic methods: more severely displaced fractures and therefore more severe injuries, in the operated group. On the other hand we find no prognostic difference between operated fractures and fracture dislocation of the same fracture group in Neer's, Knight/Mayne's and our own series. By definition, the degree of displacement between fracture dislocation and mere fracture is great. Still the results are equal. This seems to contradict the possibility that the operated group would contain more severe injuries and questions the aforementioned explanation of the different results in the two types of treatment.

Considering avascular necrosis, it is, as expected, most frequent in the IV-part group. If again the results in Table 5 are summed up, one finds the following:

III-part, closed treatment: 3–14% avascular necrosis
III-part, open treatment: 12–25% avascular necrosis
IV-part, closed treatment: 13–34% avascular necrosis
IV-part, open treatment: 41–59% avascular necrosis

The percentage is given as an interval, since some of the cases of avascular necrosis are of unknown fracture type or treatment group. There is a higher rate of avascular necrosis in the operated group. The reason could be that more severe injuries are operated on or it could be the negative effect of the surgical trauma. Svend-Hansen's[29] results of closed treatment are comparable to our own and Neer's operated cases. If anything, there is a tendency towards fewer cases of avascular necrosis in Svend-Hansen's series.

A further question is whether fracture dislocations need open reduction. Most authors in Table 5 consider it necessary, although Razemon and Baux,[24] Duparc[6] and Schuhl[26] recommended an attempt at closed reduction in all cases. Their works however include several failed attempts. Geneste et al[8] present 17 cases of fracture dislocation. They were all reduced by closed manipulation, sometimes using a percutaneous pin to hook the head fragment as described also by Dingley and Denham.[5] Remarkably, all cases were successfully reduced. Internal fixation was brought about by retrograde intramedullary Kirschner wiring from the olecranon fossa. The results are surprisingly good and only two cases of total and one case of partial avascular necrosis were encountered. The authors consider the advantage of their method was that it preserved what little vascularization remained and avoided further trauma to the soft tissues by surgery. Duparc's[6] series contains five cases treated by closed manipulation. All had the head fragment impacted upon the humeral shaft in the dislocated position. This may give a better condition for the survival of the head fragment. The operated cases were mainly stabilized with an AO-plate. Baudin's[2] fractures were reduced nonsurgically and fixated by retrograde intramedullary Kirschner wiring.

When comparing the different authors' results, two remarks are essential:

1. In the works of Razemon/Baux and Baudin the follow-up time was minimum 6 months.

TABLE 5 Results in 10 Comparable Series

		III-part[1]		IV-part[1]		
		Closed Reduction	Open Reduction	Closed Reduction	Open Reduction	
Neer	n:o	20	30	11	8	29 fract-disloc.
	a.n.	2	2	3	6	Prosthesis and head
	E/S	3	19	—	—	resections excluded
Haas	n:o		14		4	3 fract-disloc.
	a.n.			← 6* →		
	E/S		7		1	
Svend-Hansen	n:o	22		15		All fractures
	a.n.		← 4* →			
	E/S	11		5		
Razemon Baux	n:o	26	16	6	5	All fractures
	a.n.	← 1* →		← 1* →		
	E/S	20	10	4	1	
Baudin	n:o	8		7		All fractures
	a.n.	—		—		
	E/S	6		5		
Knight Mayne	n:o	8	14	6	4	18 fract-disloc.
	a.n.	1	7	3	2	Head resections excluded
	E/S	5	8	2	2	
Geneste	n:o	6		10		All fract-disloc.
	a.n.	—		3		
	E/S	6		7		
Duparc	n.o		4	5	7	All fract-disloc.
	a.n.		—	—	5	
	E/S		1	1	—	
Schuhl	n:o			9	7	All fract-disloc.
	a.n.			← 4* →		
	E/S			—	1	
Own series	n:o	2	6	1	14	12 fract-disloc.
	a.n.	—	1	—	7	
	E/S	1	3	—	4	

1. For explanation, see text
*. Fract type or treatment groups unknown
a.n. avascular necrosis
E/S. Excellent/satisfactory

In Baudin's series almost half the cases were examined between 6 and 12 months. This probably explains the very low frequency of avascular necrosis in this series, since it is well established that this development may be delayed up to two years. Geneste et al had two cases examined before one year. Actually, even a 1 year follow-up time is short in this respect, but it is an accepted limit.

2. The functional results differ partly because of different evaluation criteria. Neer, Sven-Hansen, Haas, Schuhl and we have applied Neer's criteria. The criteria used by the other authors in table 5 differ in one major aspect from Neer's criteria; namely the absence of radiological evaluation.

Since for example, avascular necrosis gives an automatic loss of 8–10 points in Neer's system, the result is always worse than other cases with the same functional state but good x-ray. This phenomenon probably accounts for the difference in results when our own series is evaluated with Santee's and Neer's methods (52 percent, 35 percent, respectively). One can suppose an equivalent difference in the other investigations as well. The functional results are thus actually better than those shown in Table 5. Interauthor comparisons must therefore be made with these remarks in mind. On the other hand it does not affect comparison between the two treatment groups, since the two systems are evenly distributed. However the rate of avascular necrosis in the total figures should probably be counted higher.

The main method of fixation in our series (percutaneous temporary transfixation) appears to give the same overall results as other techniques. It is a rather simple procedure requiring minimal dissection to achieve reduction. The achieved fracture position was maintained in all cases. Two cases of secretion at the cutaneous insertion of the Kirschner wire were seen; both healed without complications after extraction of the Kirschner wire.

Considering the details of operative technique, Neer has shown that III-part lesions treated with a successful technique and with good tubercular fixation are satisfactory in 86 per cent of cases. In our series we have tried to analyse the influence of time from injury to treatment, the quality of reduction and tubercular fixation in the IV-part lesions. As seen in Figure 2 and Table 4 it seems that early operation, good post operative x-ray and tubercular fixation reduce the risk of avascular necrosis. The problem with any technique is fixation of the head fragment to the humeral shaft. Also, when screws, pins or plates are used, the attachment in the minimal trabecular bone is difficult. A good contact between the trabecular bone of the head fragment and the shaft possibly reduces the risk of avascular necrosis. The results in Duparc's series support this hypothesis.

Immediate implantation of a prosthesis in IV-part lesions is proposed by Neer, since the prognosis is bad and the risk of avascular necrosis is high. His results are very good. 31 of 32 cases were satisfactory. Other reports have been more disappointing: Kraulis and Hunter[14] had nine failures in eleven prosthetic replacements (Neer-prosthesis). Marotte et al[16] consider their nine cases with Neer prosthesis satisfactory. However, the details of the results show that although strength was acceptable and the majority could reach the mouth and the top of the head, motion was quite restricted: on an average 120° in forward flexion and no one reached over 90° in abduction. This function is only somewhat better than what is shown in the cases of avascular necrosis in our series.

The patients in our series with avascular necrosis were all fairly satisfied with the shoulder function and the five previously working continued their ordinary occupation. At the follow-up examination they were all offered a prosthesis, but no one found it necessary. Furthermore, we had four IV-part lesions in which the head fragment survived, two were excellent, two satisfactory. We therefore doubt the necessity of emergency prosthetic replacement, and instead propose expectation and elective replacement in cases with a combination of disabling pain and restricted motion.

Conclusions

IV-part fractures and fracture dislocations carry a high risk of avascular necrosis of the head fragment, but the dislocation as such does not seem to increase the risk. Avascular necrosis results in failure, because of restricted motion and bad x-ray. Pain is insignificant. The patients are fairly satisfied and are often capable of continuing their ordinary occupation. Prosthetic replacement in all IV-part lesions is questioned. According to reviewed literature, closed reduction may be a preferable method of treating comminuted proximal humeral fractures. Surgery seems to require good reduction, tubercular fixation and early operation to be successful. It might then reduce the risk of avascular necrosis.

REFERENCES

1. Alberts KA, Engström CF. Fractures of the proximal humerus. Opuscula Medica 1979:24(4).
2. Baudin P. Intramedullary nailing of fractures of the proximal humerus. Thèse médecine, Bordeaux:1977.
3. Codman EA. The shoulder. Boston: Privately printed 1934.
4. Dehne E. Fractures at the upper end of the humerus. Surg Clin N Amer 1945; 25.
5. Dingley A, Denham R. fracture- dislocation of the humeral head. Bone Joint Surg 1973; 55A:1299–1300.
6. Duparc J, Largier A. Fracture- dislocations of the proximal humerus. Rev Chir Orthop 1976; 62:91–110.

7. Einarsson, F. Fractures of the upper end of the humerus. Acta Orthop Scand suppl. XXXII (1958).
8. Geneste R et al. Closed treatment of fracture-dislocations of the shoulder joint. Rev Chir Orth 1980; 66:383–386.
9. Heuget L et al. Bone cement in the treatment of certain fractures of the proximal humerus. Ann Chir 1973; 27:311–313.
10. Haas K. Displaced proximal humeral fractures operated by rushpin technique. Opuscula Medica 1978; 23 (4).
11. Heppenstall RB. Fractures of the proximal humerus. Orthop Clin N Amer 1975; 6:2.
12. Knight RA, and Mayne JA. Comminuted fractures and fracture-dislocations involving the articular surface of the humeral head. Bone Joint Surg 1957; 39A:.
13. Krakovic M et al. Indications and results of operation in proximal humeral fractures. Mschr Unfallheilk 1975; 78:326–332.
14. Kraulis J, Hunter G. The results of prosthetic replacement in fracture-dislocations of the upper end of the humerus. Injury 1976; 8:2.
15. Lundberg, BJ et al. Independent exercises versus physiotherapy in nondisplaced proximal humeral fractures. Scand J Rehab Med 1979; 11:133–136.
16. Marotte JH et al. Neer arthroplasty in complex fractures and fracture-dislocations of the shoulder joint. Chir 1978; 104:816–821.
17. Mills KLG. Severe injuries of the upper end of the humerus. Injury 1974; 6.
18. de Mourgues G et al. Fracture-dislocations of the shoulder joint. Rev Chir Orthop 1965; 51.
19. Neer CS. Fracture of the neck of the humerus with dislocation of the head fragment. Amer J Surg March 1953.
20. Neer CS. Displaced proximal humeral fractures part I and II. Bone Joint Surg 1970; 52A: 6.
21. Neviaser JS. Complicated fractures and dislocations about the shoulder joint. Bone Joint Surg 1962; 44A:5.
22. Paavolainen P, Björkenheim JM., Slätis P. Operative treatment of severe proximal humeral fractures. Acta Orthop Scand 1983; 54:374–379.
23. Pilgaard S, och Öster A. Four-segment fractures of the humeral neck. Acta Orthop Scand 1973; 44:124.
24. Razemon JP, Baux S. Fractures and fracture-dislocations of the proximal humerus. Rev Chir Orth 1965; 55:387–496.
25. Santee HE. Fractures about the upper end of the humerus. J Bone Joint Surg 1924.
26. Schuhl JF Fracture-dislocations of the proximal humerus. Thèse médecine, Lyon:1973.
27. Schwieger G, Ludolph E. Fractures of the shoulder joint. Unfallchir 1980; 6.
28. Sever JW. Fracture of the head of the humerus. N Engl J Med 1973; 24.
29. Svend-Hansen H. Displaced proximal humeral fractures. Acta Orthop Scand 1974; 45:359–364.
30. Weise K et al. Indications and operative technique in osteosynthesis of fracture-dislocations of the shoulder joint in adults. Langenbecks Arch Chir 1980; 351.
31. Vichard Ph, Bellanger P. Ascending bipolar nailing using elastic nails in the tratment of fractures of the upper end of the humerus. Nouv Presse Med 1978; 7.

TREATMENT OF COMPLEX FRACTURES OF THE PROXIMAL HUMERUS BY NEER HEMIARTHROPLASTY

J. E. DES MARCHAIS, M.D. and G. MORAIS, M.D.

Following an injury of the shoulder, according to Rockwood and Green,[1] 15 percent of the fractures of the upper end of the humerus involved displacement of major fragments. Even if these fractures were treated by open reduction, this procedure frequently resulted in a stiff shoulder.

This was the situation until 1970 when C. Neer published[2] his classification of these fractures according to the displacement of one or more of the four principal fragments, which are: the head of the humerus, the lesser tuberosity, the greater tuberosity and the diaphysis, each fragment having a tendency to be displaced by muscular insertions. Doctor Neer treats these fractures by early replacement of the head with an hemiprosthesis and careful reconstruction of the rotator cuff. Is this surgical procedure a good solution for these complex fractures of the proximal humerus?

In the literature,[3,4,5,6] the results of several small series were not encouraging, with the exception of those presented by Doctor Neer. We would like to present the experience of l'hôpital du Sacré-Coeur, Université de Montréal. We studied the fractures of groups 5 and 6 involving four displaced fragments.

METHOD

From 1971 to 1982, 43 Neer prostheses were inserted. Fourteen of these cases were not included: seven because of inadequate follow-up, five because of other factors which forced us to exclude them, one was lost to follow-up, and one died early from other causes. Therefore, 29 cases are included in our study, 12 men and 17 women. Their ages ranged from 33 to 84 years with a mean of 59 (See Fig. 1). The 29 cases involved four different surgeons; 20 patients were operated on by the same surgeon. A deltopectoral approach was used in all cases. Postoperative immobilization varied from one day to one month.

RESULTS

The follow-up varied from 16 months to 10 years for an average of 4.4 years (See Fig. 2). The only complication encountered was a partial paralysis of the deltoïd. There was no infection, no thromboembolic problem, no shoulder-hand syndrome, no diaphyseal fracture during or after surgery.

Evaluation

Neer's Protocol

Each patient was evaluated according to Neer's protocol. The evaluation is based on a total of 100 points:
  35 points for a painless shoulder
  30 for normal function
  25 for complete movement
  and 10 points for absence of anomaly on X-ray.
Using this scale, the resultant categories are:
  excellent (more than 89 points)
  satisfactory (80–89 points)
  unsatisfactory (70–79 points)
  failure (fewer than 70 points)
By using this evaluation, we have obtained the following results:
  13 excellent
  5 satisfactory
  6 unsatisfactory
  5 failures.
81 points is the average score for the whole group.

Pain

Assessing pain, 22 patients have no pain and seven little to moderate pain. One can conclude that the Neer prosthesis gives a relatively painless shoulder.

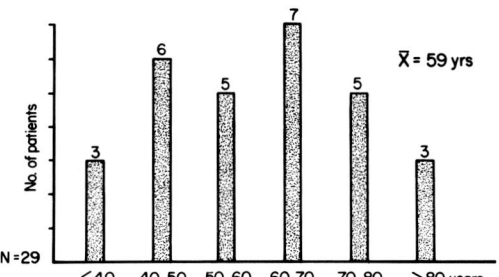

Figure 1 Age distribution of patient population.

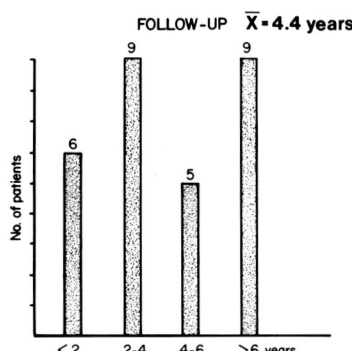

Figure 2 Distribution of the patients' follow-up.

Function and Movement

Considering function and movement, patients were divided into two groups:
- The first group of 18 patients with more than 80 points, have function of 27 and movement of 20 points.
- The second group of 11 patients with less than 80 points have function of 18 and movement of 11 points (See Table 1).

One sees that function is better than movement and that is because the patient can compensate for some stiffness of the shoulder. Despite a reduced abduction, the patient compensates by using anterior elevation and turning the body to bring the hand where he wants.

X-ray

Another criterion of evaluation is the X-ray study. Nineteen patients had a normal x-ray. In 10 patients, three had a score of more than 80 points despite some x-ray anomaly, such as calcification in the supra-spinatus muscle, which did not however affect the result in any way. The remaining seven patients had a score of less than 80 points with other anomalies, such as osteoarthrosis.

Biomechanics

In the evaluation of our results, we have also studied the biomechanics of the repaired rotator cuff. Using the studies of Freedman[7] and Poppen,[8] the center of rotation of the humeral head (while the patient is abducting his arm) should be on a perpendicular line, traced on the center of the axis of the glenoïd and meeting approximately the geometric center of the head of the humerus. We have confirmed this observation on the control shoulder of each of our patients.[9]

Correlation

Center of Rotation

The Neer prosthesis of those patients with good results has a center of rotation in normal position with the glenoid, showing a rotator cuff biomechanically functional. In the patients with poorer results, when the arm is abducted, the center of rotation of the prosthesis is moved upward. Let us now integrate this observation into the analysis of our results (see Table 2). In all 18 patients with a score of 80 points or more, the center of rotation of the prosthesis was normal. But nine of

TABLE 1 Evaluation of Function and Movement in Relation to Patient's Results

Results	Function/30	Movement/25
≥80 (N = 18)	27	20
<80 (N = 11)	18	11
average	24	17

TABLE 2 Evaluation of the Center of Rotation of the Prosthesis in Relation to Patient's Results

Results	Function/30	Movement/25	Center of Rotation
≥80 (N = 18)	27	20	Ⓝ
<80 (N = 11)	18	11	Ⓝ 2 ↑ ($\bar{X}$ = 9.3 mm) 9

the 11 patients, with a score of 79 points or less, had upward displacement of their center of rotation. This average displacement was 9.3 mm. The other two patients with a normal position of the center of rotation had a low score because one was immobilized too long after surgery, for one month, and the other was operated on three weeks after trauma.

Time

We then tried to correlate the results with the time between trauma and surgery, and with the length of post-operative immobilization. Table 3 shows that good results of 80 points or more, are obtained with early surgery and short postoperative immobilization. The difference between the two groups is highly significant.

Age

There was no correlation between the results and the age of the patient. A patient of 50 has a good result, and also a woman of 89 who obtained full passive abduction two weeks post-operatively and maintained it actively afterwards.

Conclusions

Complex fractures of the proximal humerus must be operated on early, before ankylosis sets in. Surgery should be done within seven days of the trauma. X-ray analysis has confirmed the importance of careful reconstruction of the rotator cuff in order to maintain the center of rotation of the prosthesis in good position relative to the glenoid. The study has also demonstrated that a short post-operative immobilization is imperative. On the third day, the patient must begin passive abduction exercises in order to obtain good results. When these conditions are met, Neer's hemiarthroplasty can give excellent results, and after a year, the strength will be sufficient to maintain the physical fitness of the patient.

TABLE 3 Statistical Analysis Correlating the Time Between Trauma and Surgery and Immobilization with the Patients' Results

Results	Time Trauma-Surgery	Immobilization
>80 (N = 18)	8 days	5.8 days
<80 (N = 11)	30 days	10 days

REFERENCES

1. Rockwood CA, Green DP. Fractures. Lippincott, 1975.
2. Neer CS. Displaced proximal humeral fractures (part I and II). J Bone and Joint Surg 1970; 52A:1077–1103.
3. Mills KLG. Severe injuries of the upper end of the humerus. Injury 1974; 6:13–21.
4. Duparc J, Largier A. Less luxations-fractures de l'extrémité supérieure de l'humérus. Rev Chir Orth 1976; 62:91–110.
5. Kraulis J, Hunter G. The results of prosthetic replacement in fracture dislocation of the upper end of the humerus. Injury 1976; 8:129–131.
6. Marotte JH, Lord G, Bancel P. L'arthroplastie de Neer dans les fractures et fractures-luxations complexes de l'épaule.
7. Freedman L, Munro R. Abduction of the arm in the scapular plane: scapular and gleno-humeral movements. J Bone and Joint Surg 1966; 48A:1503–1510.
8. Poppen MK, Walker PS. Normal and abnormal motion of the shoulder. J Bone and Joint Surg 1976; 58A:195–201.
9. Des Marchais JE, Benazet JP. Evaluation de l'hémi-arthroplastie de Neer dans le traitement des fractures de l'humérus. Can J Surg 1983; 26:469–471.

FRACTURES OF THE SCAPULA INVOLVING THE GLENOID FOSSA

ROLF IDEBERG, M.D.

Glenoid fractures are uncommon, comprising one-third of all scapular fractures.[2] In one year, 1975, only nine were treated at the University Hospital of Uppsala, Sweden, among 28 scapular fractures, compared to 380 other fractures and dislocations about the shoulder.

It is obvious that one single hospital cannot supply enough material for satisfying analysis. My research in 25 hospitals has provided 200 cases of glenoid fracture. A subdivision into five different types has been made, each requiring special consideration regarding mechanism and treatment. The results give rise to certain conclusions. Follow-up time varies from 1 to 22 years. Residual disability has been estimated in terms of pain and function.

TYPES OF GLENOID FRACTURE (FIG. 1)

There are five types of glenoid fracture.

Type 1 fracture involves avulsion of the anterior margin, sometimes as fracture dislocation, and is the most common fracture (130 cases). This is the only type of glenoid fracture caused by indirect trauma to the shoulder.

Type 2 fracture involves a transverse fracture through the glenoid fossa which separates the inferior part of the glenoid and neck as a triangular fragment, displaced together with the humeral head (6 cases). An oblique fracture of this type (seven cases) can dislocate the posteroinferior fragment, up to one-half of the articular surface, by rotation.

Type 3 fractures (17 cases) is often combined either with fracture of the acromion or the clavicle or with dislocation of the acromioclavicular joint or any combination of these. It runs obliquely from the glenoid and neck to about the middle of the cranial margin of the scapula. Incongruity arises with rotation of the big fragment including the coracoid process.

Type 4 fracture (23 cases) is horizontal, extending through the neck and blade, sometimes with severe displacement of the fragments and incongruity of the articular surface.

Type 5 fracture combines type 4 with a transverse fracture through the scapular neck or just its inferior half (20 cases).

Type 1 Fracture

Several years of recurrent dislocations may precede the sudden appearance of a fracture of the anterior glenoid margin (Fig. 2). This fracture, in association with dislocation, causes the fragment to be more displaced, and it can be seen together with a Hill-Sachs lesion or fragmentation of the greater tuberosity.[5] The size and shape of the fragment vary independently of dislocation and cannot be estimated without two interpretable x-ray pictures taken at right angles to each other. The transscapular view must show the contour of the glenoid free from the chest wall.[4]

Sixty-eight type 1 fractures occurred with dislocation and 62 without. Persistent subluxation is a serious complication of fracture dislocation and may, untreated, lead to severe osteoarthritis, as in three cases in this study.

Surgery for correction of subluxation was performed in four cases,[5] for unstable reduction in four cases, and for fixation of the fragment itself in three cases. All 11 were operated on within 14 days of the accident. The age of these patients varied from 30 to 81 years. The surgical results were classified as 6 good and 5 unsatisfactory. In two cases the unsatisfactory results were attributed to glenoid factors. The other three patients experienced recurrent dislocations until soft tissue surgery was successfully performed. The fragments in these cases were very small. The remaining 57 patients with fracture dislocation had uneventful recovery.

64 / Surgery of the Shoulder

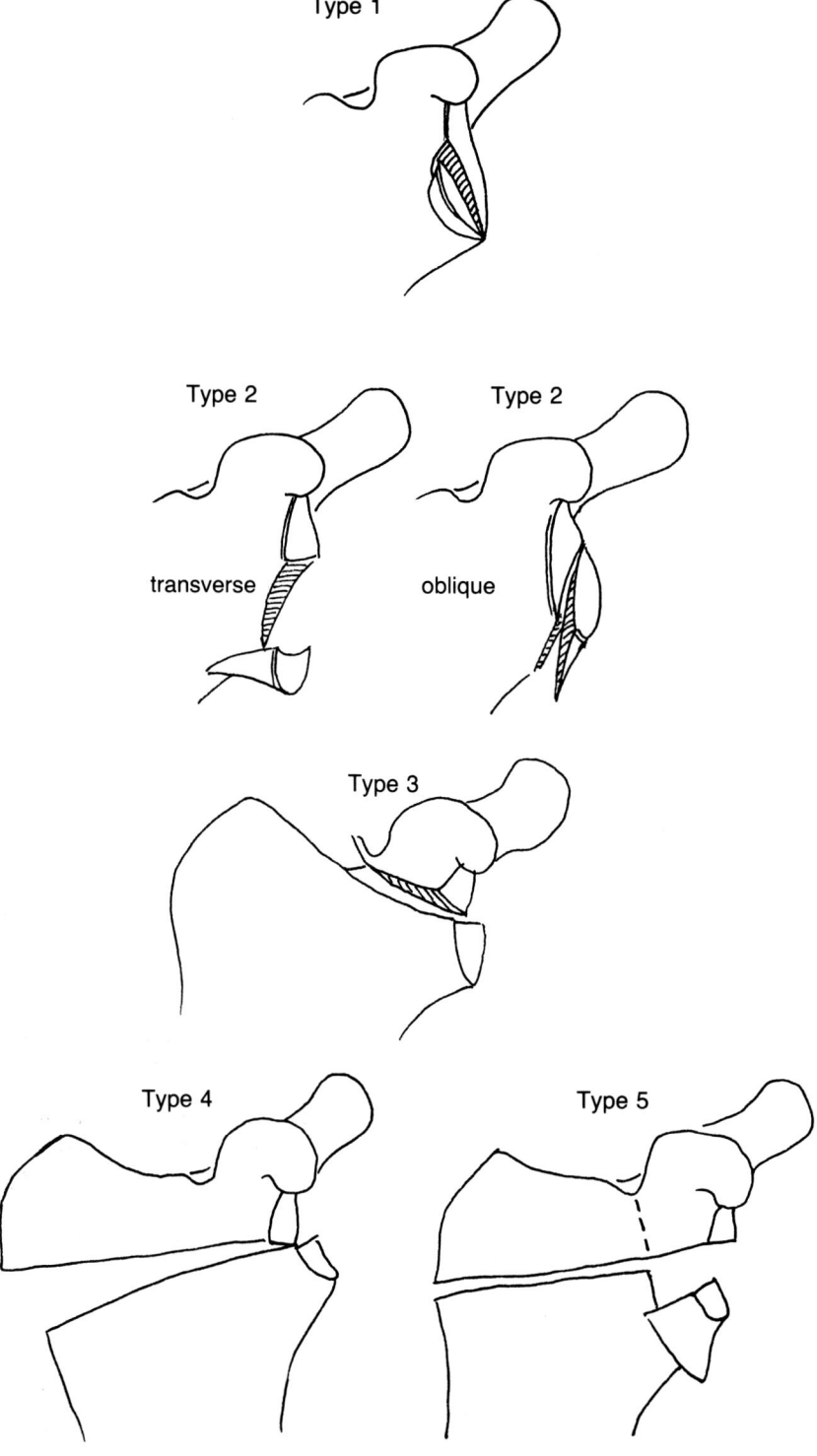

Figure 1 Glenoid fractures, 5 different types.

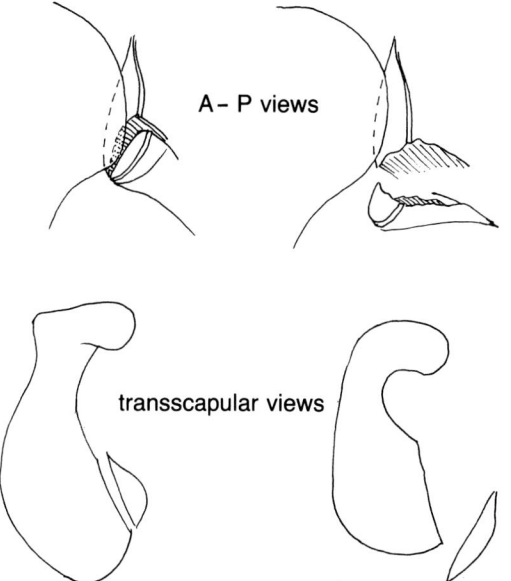

Figure 2 A–P views of the shoulder joint often show the fragment as an inferior part of the glenoid owing to anterior rotation of scapula. Correct transscapular views show the true site and size of fragment.

Fifty-nine of the 62 patients without dislocation were treated by conservative means. At follow-up the majority, including the three men who underwent operation, showed good to excellent results. A minority claimed mild disability, but not instability. Dislocation had not occurred in any of these patients.

The results of this study lead to the following conclusions:

1. Fracture dislocation may cause subluxation requiring surgery.
2. The size of the fragment in fracture type 1 is not prognostic.

Type 2 Fracture

The type 2 fracture results from trauma to the lateral aspect of the shoulder with significant violence.[1] Lacking its glenoid support, the humeral head slips inferiorly. In two untreated cases, the course was unsatisfactory, and in two other cases operation was not successful. Two patients had excellent results following stable fixation of the fragment.

In most cases in which the fracture line ran obliquely through the fossa, the fragment could be rotated inferiorly and surgery was not required despite major dislocation. The results were as good in the six patients treated conservatively as in the one patient who was operated on.

Type 3 Fracture

Severe trauma directed from above to the shoulder explains the concurrent lesions. Pseudarthrosis of the acromion and a destroyed acromioclavicular joint were responsible for the poor outcome in five of the 17 patients. Reduction of displacement was spontaneous in several cases and attributable to the surgery in one case. Slight incongruity did not influence the good result obtained in 12 patients.

Type 4 Fracture

There were 23 cases of type 4 fracture. Sixteen had good or excellent results, including two patients who were operated on. Seven had poor results, four because of complicating injuries in surrounding tissues, and three because of persistent irregularities in the glenoid surface.

Type 5 Fracture

Of the 20 cases of type 5 fracture, 13 had good to excellent results at follow-up, one having been operated on. Seven cases of this type had a poor outcome despite surgery in one of them.

Traffic accidents were the cause in most cases of direct violent trauma[6] to the scapula resulting in type 4 and type 5 fractures. Of the 43 patients, seven had other injuries so serious that surgery to the glenoid fracture was impossible or delayed, influencing the end result.

To summarize the results of these 200 glenoid fractures:

1. The fragment in type 1 is important only when associated with dislocation of the shoulder because of subsequent subluxation.
2. The size of the fragment does not affect the prognosis.
3. Loss of concavity of the glenoid fossa resulting in poor joint apposition must be rectified.
4. Disability after glenoid fractures may be of extra-articular origin.

REFERENCES

1. Aston JW, Gregory CF. Dislocation of the shoulder with significant fracture of the glenoid. J Bone and Joint Surg 1973; 55A:1531–1533.
2. Conradi P. Fractures of the scapula. Personal communication.
3. Ishizuki M. Avulsion fracture of the superior border of the scapula. J Bone Joint Surg 1981; 63A:820–822.
4. Pavlov H. Freiberger RH. Fractures and dislocations about the shoulder. Seminars in Roentgenology. 1978; Vol XIII. No 2:85–96.
5. Rockwood CA. Dislocations about the shoulder. In: Rockwood CA, Green DP, eds. Fractures. Vol 1. Philadelphia, JB Lippincott, 1975:656.
6. Wilber MC, Evans EB. Fractures of the scapula. J Bone Joint Surg 1977; 59A:358–362.

TREATMENT OF ACUTE COMPLETE DISLOCATION OF THE ACROMIOCLAVICULAR JOINT

FUMIO KATO, M.D., HIROMICHI HAYASHI, M.D., TEIJI MIYAZAKI, M.D.,
KUNINARI ITO, M.D., KATSUMASA TOMOTSUNE, M.D.,
and NAOFUMI SHIMIZU, M.D.

Over the past ten years we have treated 130 cases of acute complete dislocation of the acromioclavicular joint. Most of the injuries resulted from falls in "judo" which is compulsory for Japanese policemen. Judo is a dangerous contact sport as far as the shoulder is concerned. In Figure 1, a throw called "tomoe-nage," the player above is being thrown by the player below. Such a fall on the shoulder will surely put the joint in danger.

As background, we studied the incidence of injuries to the shoulder among 46,000 officers of the Tokyo Metropolitan Police. During a period of four years, from 1978 to 1981, there were 5078 injuries which occurred during their duty. Of these, injuries about the shoulder numbered 487 (9.6%). These 487 cases were classified as in Table 1. Injuries of the acromioclavicular joint, including dislocation, subluxation and sprain, numbered 242 or about 50 percent of the shoulder injuries. Following these were fracture of the clavicle, dislocation of the shoulder, rotator cuff tear, and contusion. These statistics show that the acromioclavicular joint is by far the most vulnerable part of the shoulder.

Materials and Methods

At Tokyo Metropolitan Police Hospital, we treated 130 acute complete dislocations of the acromioclavicular joint between 1971 and 1982. There was only one female patient, a young policewoman who was injured in the practice of "aikido", a kind of martial art. The right shoulder was involved in 72 patients, the left shoulder in 58. The age of patients at the time of injury ranged from 18 to 62 years, the majority being in the twenties and thirties. The causes of the injury were judo in 109 patients, other sports in 12 patients, and accidents in nine patients.

TREATMENT

We used three different types of treatment:
Group A: Open reduction with internal fixation was performed on 47 patients; the torn capsule and the acromioclavicular ligament were repaired, the coracoclavicular ligament was sutured when possible, and the joint was reduced and held in position with two Kirschner wires inserted across the joint.

Group B: Forty-one patients underwent closed reduction and percutaneous insertion of two Kirschner wires under fluoroscopic control.

Group C: Conservative treatment was used in 42 patients, involving strapping or Kenny-Howard's sling in most cases.

At the follow-up examination, which ranged from six months to ten years, roentgenographic as well as functional results, including the patient's sports ability, were evaluated.

RESULTS

Roentgenographic results were classified as reduction, subluxation and dislocation. These correspond with Tossy's grades 1, 2, and 3, respectively. The roentgenographic results in the three groups are summarized in Figure 2. In the group of open reduction with internal fixation, 60 percent of the joints were in a state of reduction, while 40 percent were in subluxation. This means that loss of reduction occurred in as many as 40 percent of these patients. In the group of closed reduction

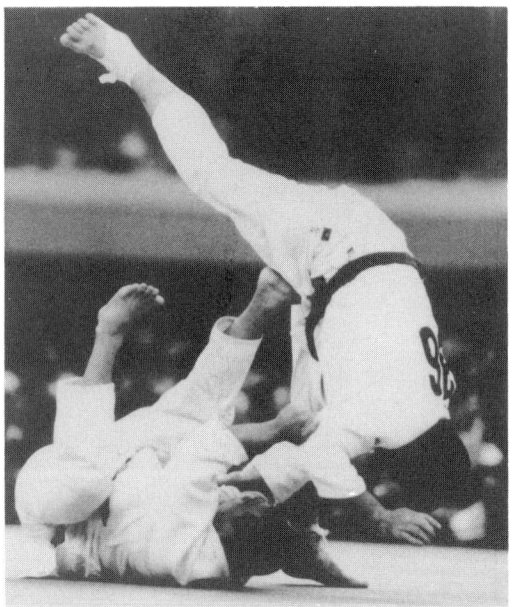

Figure 1 A fall in judo.

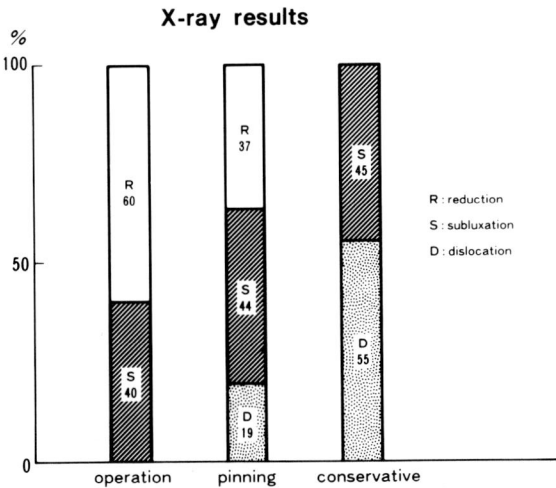

Figure 2 Roentgenographic results.

with percutaneous pinning, 37 percent were in reduction, 44 percent in subluxation, and 19 percent in dislocation. In the group with conservative treatment, no joint was in a state of reduction, 45 percent were in subluxation, while 55 percent remained dislocated. It is clear that open reduction with internal fixation gave the best result.

How to evaluate the functional result is important. Weitzman's classification includes pain, range of motion, and weakness as criteria.[5] There is no doubt that pain is a crucial factor. However, we have had no patient with limitation of motion or apparent weakness. Instead, we found that fatigue and loss of endurance were more frequent complaints. We also felt that recovery of sports ability was important, because this is essentially a sports injury. Accordingly, we included pain, fatigue, and sports ability in the criteria. The functional results were rated as excellent, good, fair, and poor as shown in Table 2.

The functional results in the three groups are summarized in Figure 3. In the ORIF group, excellent results were obtained in 34 percent of the cases, good results in 40 percent, and fair in 26 percent. With closed reduction and percutaneous pinning, excellent results were obtained in 19 percent, good in 44 percent, fair in 34 percent, and poor in 3 percent. In the conservatively treated group, excellent results were obtained in 14 percent, good in 36 percent, fair in 36 percent, and poor in 14 percent. If we regard "excellent" and "good" as satisfactory results, 74 percent of the ORIF group, 63 percent of the closed reduction-percutaneous pinning group, and 50 percent of the conservatively treated group were satisfactory.

TABLE 1 Injuries During Duty

(Tokyo Metropolitan Police 1978–1981)

Injury	No.
ACJ injuries	242 (49.7%)
Fracture of clavicle	86 (17.7%)
Dislocation of shoulder	57 (11.7%)
Rotator cuff tear	9 (1.8%)
Contusion	93 (19.1%)

Statistics from Tokyo Metropolitan Police

TABLE 2 Classification of Functional Results

Rating	Pain	Fatigue	Sports Ability
Excellent	none	none	full
Good	occasional pain on exertion	occasional	slightly reduced
Fair	occasional pain on routine motion	frequent	reduced
Poor	frequent	frequent	lost

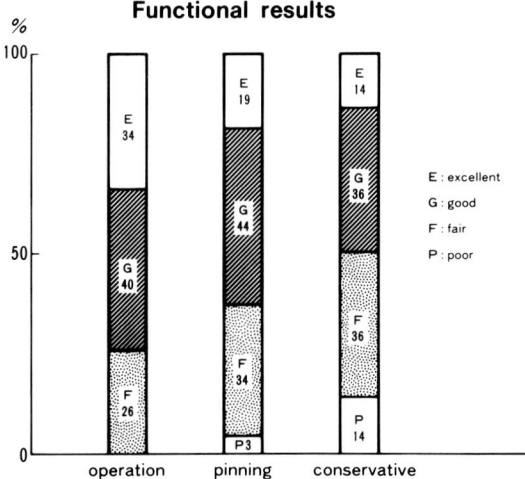

Figure 3 Functional results.

It was not a strictly prospective study. Rather, treatment was determined by factors such as availability of hospital beds or the patient's desire to avoid surgery. However, since the patient groups were similar in most respects, comparisons seemed justified.

From our data, we conclude that open reduction with internal fixation gave the best result, although we must realize that, even in this group, loss of reduction occurred in 40 percent of the patients and the functional results were not satisfactory in 26 percent.

Our criteria for evaluation of the functional results may be too strict. But most of the patients were young adults who had to return to vigorous physical activities involved in their occupation as well as in their athletic training. So, it seemed necessary to set a high standard of recovery for the results to be rated satisfactory.

DISCUSSION

When we started this study, we were not sure what was the best method of treatment for this injury. Opinions differed widely as to the method of choice.[1,2,3,4] It is true that the injury may leave little disability even if it is not treated at all. So, we tried to compare the results of three different types of treatment in a large number of patients.

REFERENCES

1. Bateman JE. The Shoulder and Neck. 2nd ed. Philadelphia: Saunders, 1978.
2. Jacobs B, and Wade PA. Acromioclavicular-joint injury. J Bone Joint Surg 1966; 48A:475–486.
3. Kessel L. Clinical Disorders of the Shoulder. New York: Churchill Livingstone, 1982.
4. Urist MR. The treatment of dislocations of the acromioclavicular joint. Am J Surg 1959; 98:423–431.
5. Weitzman G. Treatment of acute acromioclavicular joint dislocation by a modified Bosworth method. J Bone Joint Surg 1967; 49A:1167–1178.

A PROSPECTIVE STUDY OF THE TREATMENT OF ACROMIOCLAVICULAR DISLOCATION

G. C. BANNISTER, M.Ch., Orth.F.R.C.S., W. A. WALLACE, F.R.C.S.,
P. G. STABLEFORTH, M.B., B.S., F.R.C.S., and M. A. HUTSON, B.Chir., M.B.

It has long been known that a poor outcome could accrue from the conservative treatment of complete Grade III acromioclavicular dislocation. As long ago as 1861 attempts were being made to restore the anatomy of the joint.

The injury is, however, comparatively uncommon. It was not until 1946 that a single series of more than 40 cases was collected. In this study, Marshall Urist reviewed the literature and concluded that between 10 and 20 percent of cases had poor results. Closed reduction and bracing of the joint showed no significant improvement on this figure.

In 1954 Kennedy and Cameron from Western Ontario presented a series of 27 cases treated by coracoclavicular screw fixation. Excellent results were claimed in 87 percent of athletes under the age of 40.

This paper heralded an increasing tendency to operate on acromioclavicular dislocations. The standard reference works in Britain and North America recommend surgery and indeed postal survey of North American orthopaedic surgeons in 1974 revealed that 92 percent routinely operated on the injury. Referring to "the rather controversial decision not to operate in cases of complete acromioclavicular separation" the paper cited the case of a New York Jets quarterback who had been unsporting enough to return to first team duty in eight weeks whilst escaping the benefits of the knife.

Despite the literature, nonoperative management is generally employed in Britain. Orthopaedic practice owes much to the inherited conservatism of Robert Jones. Apocryphal tales abound of international rugby packs squaring up to each other with bilaterally unreduced acromioclavicular dislocations before scrumming down to conflict.

Academic fuel was added to the conservatives' fire when in the mid-70s James Glick left complete dislocations unreduced and, concentrating on early movement and weight-bearing, returned professional athletes to the sports field in an average of 3.5 weeks with 17 percent unsatisfactory results. A careful randomized prospective controlled trial from the U.S. Naval Medical Corps showed conservative treatment to have slightly better results over a variety of surgical procedures in complete acromioclavicular dislocation.

TRIAL DESIGN

It was in the presence of this controversy that in 1980 we decided that the only way to resolve the problem was to set up a randomized prospective controlled trial comparing what seemed to be the best of conservative and operative treatments. We calculated that 60 cases would be required and Bristol and Nottingham combined to produce this number.

The surgical procedure adopted was acromioclavicular arthrotomy and meniscectomy, reduction and insertion of an A.O. coracoclavicular cancellous screw. The coracoclavicular ligaments were not repaired. The deltoid was meticulously repaired. In the conservative regime, a broad arm sling was offered and patients treated with ultrasound until the pain subsided. Thereafter the shoulders were mobilized and strengthened with weights.

Follow-up was at 2, 6, 12 and 16 weeks and patients were tested for range of movement and shoulder pain and asked about pain. The 60 cases were randomly allocated to conservative or surgical treatment. Ninety percent of surgery was performed by or under the direct supervision of the first three authors.

The mean age of the patients was 30. There were 59 men and 1 woman, a nursery nurse, who sustained her injury in a martial arts contest.

The manner in which the injuries were sustained was from sport (mostly rugby), road traffic

TABLE 1 Results At 4 Months

	Conservative	Operative
Return to work (weeks)	5	11
Return to sport (weeks)	8	16
Return of full movement %	88	40
Satisfactory on Imatani score %	90	80

accidents (mostly motorcycles), and a variety of social and industrial mishaps, in that order. The mode of employment was manual in over 50 percent of the cases and, for this purpose, policemen were classified as clerical.

RESULTS (See Table 1)

Patients allotted to conservative treatment returned to work on average 5 weeks after injury— 6 weeks earlier than the operated group, who resumed at 11 weeks. The patient who took the longest time off was a scrap merchant treated by coracoclavicular screw fixation who took six months to get back to the job.

Those participating in sport returned on average 8 weeks after conservative treatment whereas after surgery it took twice as long. One conservatively treated rugby player returned to first team duty for the national club champions after 10 weeks on conservative treatment.

Four months from injury there was a full range of movement in 88 percent of conservatively

TABLE 2 Imatani Evaluation System for Acromioclavicular Dislocation

Points*	Pain
40	None
25	Slight, occasional
10	Moderate, tolerable, limits activities
0	Severe, constant, disabling
	Function (30 points)
20	Weakness
5	Use of shoulder
5	Vocational change
	Motion (30 points)
10	Abduction
10	Flexion
10	Adduction

*Excellent 90–100 points
 Good   80–89 points
 Fair   70–79 points
 Poor   <69 points

treated patients but only 40 percent of patients managed by the coracoclavicular screw. This was 10 weeks after removal of the screw and generally amounted to loss of the last 20° of abduction.

Return of power was tested by jerked shoulder flexion using a 5–lb weight and was achieved in a little under 90 percent in both groups. Only one patient in the entire series complained of disabling weakness.

Approximately 30 percent in both groups experienced continuing pain, usually being unable to sleep on the affected shoulder.

Cosmetic assessment revealed that the unreduced dislocation was best tolerated by heavily built patients whilst the best cosmetic scar came from a coronally orientated incision closed with a subcuticular suture.

Failures

Despite restricting operative procedures to the authors or residents under their supervision in 90 percent of cases, fixation failed in three cases. Whilst this should have been avoidable, 9 percent of Kennedy's series had technical problems and the occasional operator will encounter a similar experience.

Three patients conservatively treated required surgical intervention. A 24-year-old soccer goalkeeper had a painful subluxation and was unable to throw. A dynamic transfer of the coracoid relieved the pain but he was left with a weak shoulder and was still unable to throw.

A 29-year-old horse rider had gross weakness and deformity at 4 weeks from injury and requested surgery. Open reduction and internal fixation saw him back to full sporting activity at the sixth postoperative week.

A 22-year-old technician had good shoulder function at 4 weeks but his appearance was his Achilles heel; he demanded surgery. Open reduction and internal fixation saw full and early restoration of function and his shoulder to its rightful place.

CONCLUSION

Patients were assessed by the same independent scale used by Lieutenant Commander Imatani of the U.S. Naval Medical Corps to allow comparison of the 2 prospective controlled trials. See Table 2.

Ninety percent of conservatively treated pa-

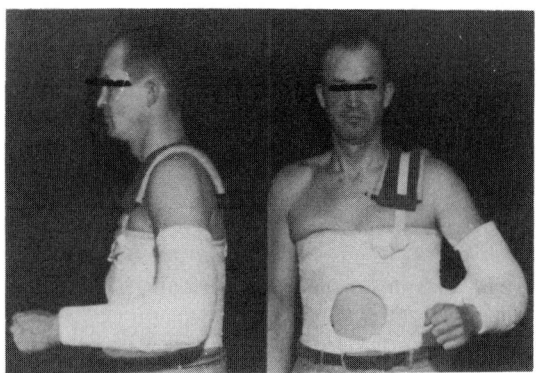

Figure 1 A popular body jacket used in the 1950's with downward pressure on the clavicle.

layer. A light dressing is applied, and a sling for a few days, after which the patient is allowed progressive use of his arm. Heavy lifting should be avoided for three weeks, after which forceful use and contact sports can be participated in as tolerated. Using this technique, patients have returned to professional hockey, football, tennis and basketball, with minimal loss of time.

In the 70's, an increasing number of surgeons noted that many patients with an unreduced complete dislocation of the acromioclavicular joint experienced very acceptable functional results without any form of treatment. The report by Glick et al[9] is significant. Although the deformity persisted, they had strong shoulders, no pain, and

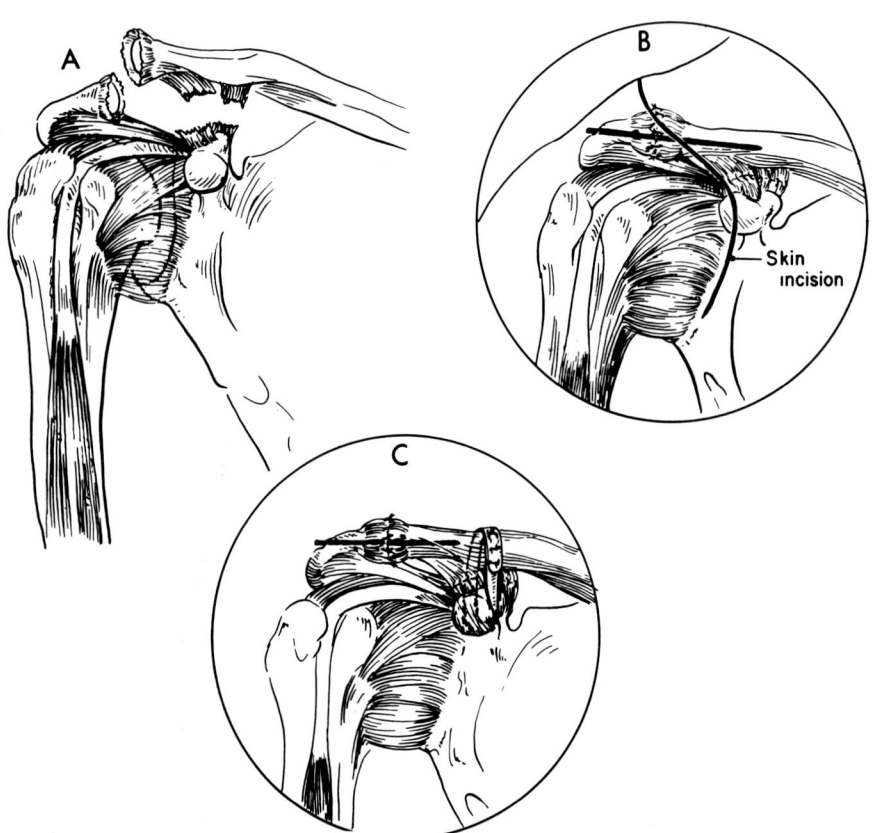

Figure 2 Transfixation of the acromioclavicular joint with 3–32″ Kirschner pin, reinforced by a strip of fascia lata around the clavicle and coracoid process. (Reprinted from The Shoulder in Trauma Management (Rowe), Yearbook Publishers, Chicago, 1974)

TABLE 1 Results At 4 Months

	Conservative	Operative
Return to work (weeks)	5	11
Return to sport (weeks)	8	16
Return of full movement %	88	40
Satisfactory on Imatani score %	90	80

accidents (mostly motorcycles), and a variety of social and industrial mishaps, in that order. The mode of employment was manual in over 50 percent of the cases and, for this purpose, policemen were classified as clerical.

RESULTS (See Table 1)

Patients allotted to conservative treatment returned to work on average 5 weeks after injury—6 weeks earlier than the operated group, who resumed at 11 weeks. The patient who took the longest time off was a scrap merchant treated by coracoclavicular screw fixation who took six months to get back to the job.

Those participating in sport returned on average 8 weeks after conservative treatment whereas after surgery it took twice as long. One conservatively treated rugby player returned to first team duty for the national club champions after 10 weeks on conservative treatment.

Four months from injury there was a full range of movement in 88 percent of conservatively

TABLE 2 Imatani Evaluation System for Acromioclavicular Dislocation

Points*	Pain
40	None
25	Slight, occasional
10	Moderate, tolerable, limits activities
0	Severe, constant, disabling
	Function (30 points)
20	Weakness
5	Use of shoulder
5	Vocational change
	Motion (30 points)
10	Abduction
10	Flexion
10	Adduction

*Excellent 90–100 points
Good 80–89 points
Fair 70–79 points
Poor <69 points

treated patients but only 40 percent of patients managed by the coracoclavicular screw. This was 10 weeks after removal of the screw and generally amounted to loss of the last 20° of abduction.

Return of power was tested by jerked shoulder flexion using a 5–lb weight and was achieved in a little under 90 percent in both groups. Only one patient in the entire series complained of disabling weakness.

Approximately 30 percent in both groups experienced continuing pain, usually being unable to sleep on the affected shoulder.

Cosmetic assessment revealed that the unreduced dislocation was best tolerated by heavily built patients whilst the best cosmetic scar came from a coronally orientated incision closed with a subcuticular suture.

Failures

Despite restricting operative procedures to the authors or residents under their supervision in 90 percent of cases, fixation failed in three cases. Whilst this should have been avoidable, 9 percent of Kennedy's series had technical problems and the occasional operator will encounter a similar experience.

Three patients conservatively treated required surgical intervention. A 24-year-old soccer goalkeeper had a painful subluxation and was unable to throw. A dynamic transfer of the coracoid relieved the pain but he was left with a weak shoulder and was still unable to throw.

A 29-year-old horse rider had gross weakness and deformity at 4 weeks from injury and requested surgery. Open reduction and internal fixation saw him back to full sporting activity at the sixth postoperative week.

A 22-year-old technician had good shoulder function at 4 weeks but his appearance was his Achilles heel; he demanded surgery. Open reduction and internal fixation saw full and early restoration of function and his shoulder to its rightful place.

CONCLUSION

Patients were assessed by the same independent scale used by Lieutenant Commander Imatani of the U.S. Naval Medical Corps to allow comparison of the 2 prospective controlled trials. See Table 2.

Ninety percent of conservatively treated patients were satisfactory compared with 80 percent of those allocated to surgery.

Early mobilization, then, gives comparable results to surgery but with lower morbidity. This is in itself of interest but a discerning student of the literature could have arrived at this conclusion from existing evidence. Urist, Kennedy and Glick using bracing, screws and nature, all achieved approximately 13 percent poor results.

The acromioclavicular dislocation is a benign injury generally overtreated but the facts remain that at least 10 percent of cases are unsatisfactory and a weak painful shoulder in a young manual worker who does not have the intellectual aptitude to change to clerical work is an economic and social disaster.

Before embarking on the project we were aware that reputable and eminent surgeons had advocated one or the other approach and were unlikely to be totally misguided in their views. Our aim was to try to identify a group that would fare poorly on conservative treatment but might benefit from surgery.

To do this we turned to the pathology of the injury. The general supposition is that a blow on the posterolateral aspect of the acromion drives it forward medially rupturing in sequence the acromioclavicular and coracoclavicular ligaments and the muscular attachments of the distal clavicle. In 1954, Horn of the Birmingham Accident Hospital explored the shoulders of 11 stokers who complained of weakness on shoveling after the injury. He found that the anterior deltoid was detached in all cases and the trapezius split.

It seemed that, if weakness here could be identified at presentation by an objective test, we would be able to spot the shoulder that was going to be at risk of giving way.

Accordingly, when patients attended the shoulder clinic, the tender areas around the shoulder were injected with local anesthetic. In addition to standard W.B. views, an additional x-ray was taken with the elbow flexed holding a 5-lb weight. This caused contraction of the anterior deltoid and 3 patterns emerged. In 20 percent, the acromioclavicular joint showed some attempt at spontaneous reduction; in 70 percent, it remained the same; and in the third group of 10 percent, the acromioclavicular distance widened.

In the group that widened, excellent results were obtained with surgery but the conservatively treated group had very poor cosmesis and 2 cases required surgery. These patients all had subcutaneously palpable clavicles.

The numbers do not allow parametric statistical analysis of this radiographic finding but do suggest that surgery has a very real contribution in the severest dislocations.

In summary, the Bristol–Nottingham trial has shown that the vast majority of acromioclavicular dislocations fare as well ultimately and recover more quickly when treated conservatively. A small group of 10 percent, with subcutaneous clavicles, may merit early surgical intervention.

REFERENCES

1. Glick JM, Milburn LJ, Haggerty JF, Nishimoto D. Dislocated acromioclavicular joint. Follow-up study of 35 unreduced acromioclavicular dislocations. Am J Sports Med 1977; 5:264–270.
2. Horn JS. The traumatic anatomy and treatment of acute acromioclavicular dislocation. J Bone Joint Surg 1954; 36B:194–201.
3. Imatani RJ, Hanlon JJ, Cady GW. Acute complete acromioclavicular separation. J Bone Joint Surg 1975; 57A 3:328–331.
4. Kennedy JC, Cameron H. Complete dislocation of the acromioclavicular joint. J Bone Joint Surg 1954; 36B 2:202–208.
5. Urist MR. Complete dislocation of the acromioclavicular joint. J Bone Joint Surg 1946; 24:4:813–837.

TRENDS IN TREATMENT OF COMPLETE ACROMIOCLAVICULAR DISLOCATIONS

CARTER R. ROWE, M.D.

There has been a slow but definite trend in the management of complete dislocations of the acromioclavicular joint over the past 30 years. In the 50's, although a small group of surgeons attempted to reduce and maintain reduction of dislocations of the acromioclavicular joint by an assortment of plaster casts with straps over the shoulder and downward pressure on the clavicle, these were uncomfortable and, as a rule, ineffective (Fig. 1). Reduction was often lost when the patient reclined in bed. Showers and baths were impossible. Consequently, open reduction and internal fixation were resorted to, in an effort to obtain a more efficient and acceptable reduction with less external apparatus. By the late 1950's, a number of operative techniques had been proposed. A popular one was transfixation of the clavicle by one or two smooth 3-32″ Kirschner pins, often with a strip of fascia passed over the clavicle and around the coracoid (Fig. 2). As the smooth pins frequently worked loose and protruded under, or through, the skin, heavier threaded pins were devised by Simmons.[18] As the fascial strips around the clavicle and coracoid seemed to encourage ectopic calcification, other methods were tried. Campos[6] separated the coracoacromial ligament from the acromion and passed it upward through the clavicle. Neviasser[15] in 1951 released the coracoacromial ligament from the coracoid, turned it upwards and reinforced the acromioclavicular joint superiorly. More recently, Weaver and Dunn[20] transferred the coracoacromial ligament upward into the medullary canal of the clavicle after an oblique osteotomy of the lateral 2 centimeters. There seemed to be no limit to the designs of innovative orthopaedic surgeons. Bosworth[4] in 1948 proposed the technique of securing the clavicle with a large screw which was passed through the clavicle to the coracoid process (Fig. 3). In some instances, when the patient became too active postoperatively, the screw was apt to pull out of the clavicle. This prompted Dewar[8] in 1965 and Bailey[2] in 1972 to turn the screw around, and transplant the coracoid process with its attached muscles upward into the clavicle (Fig. 4). In desperation, it seemed, Aldridge in 1965 proposed lashing the clavicle down to the coracoid with wire. Unfortunately, the wire frequently broke and had to be removed.

Efforts at closed reduction received a boost in 1967, when Allman[1] popularized the Kenny-Howard support which proved to be far more effective than the previous cumbersome methods of closed treatment (Fig. 5). The only drawback with the Kenny-Howard support was that it had to be tightened and adjusted daily by the surgeon or therapist for it to be most effective.

In the latter 1960's and early 1970's, a few surgeons noted the good results obtained by the Mumford[14] and Gurd[10] techniques of resecting the distal end of the clavicle in patients who had developed late degenerative changes of the joint secondary to trauma or other surgical techniques. We modified the technique as it was a simpler and less complicated procedure than open reduction with internal fixation. The method proposed by the author proved very successful (Fig. 6). It could be carried out at an elective time, did not require immobilization or external support, and eliminated the necessity of a second operation to remove the internal fixation devices. The results proved very satisfactory, allowing the athlete to return to competitive sports much earlier than with other surgical procedures. It is most important to point out, however, that a mistake is commonly made by removing too much clavicle. Usually 1 cm is adequate, so that there is no impingement against the acromion when the arm is placed in full elevation. If more space is needed, removing a small portion of the acromion is preferred to removing more clavicle. Care should be taken to narrow the clavicle a bit, to rongeur off the top angle smoothly, and to check the inferior margin of the clavicle to be certain no bony spicules are left. The periosteum, capsule, and muscles (the trapezius and deltoid) are then sutured securely together in one

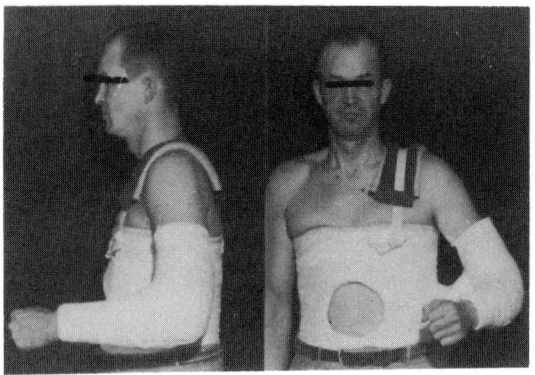

Figure 1 A popular body jacket used in the 1950's with downward pressure on the clavicle.

layer. A light dressing is applied, and a sling for a few days, after which the patient is allowed progressive use of his arm. Heavy lifting should be avoided for three weeks, after which forceful use and contact sports can be participated in as tolerated. Using this technique, patients have returned to professional hockey, football, tennis and basketball, with minimal loss of time.

In the 70's, an increasing number of surgeons noted that many patients with an unreduced complete dislocation of the acromioclavicular joint experienced very acceptable functional results without any form of treatment. The report by Glick et al[9] is significant. Although the deformity persisted, they had strong shoulders, no pain, and

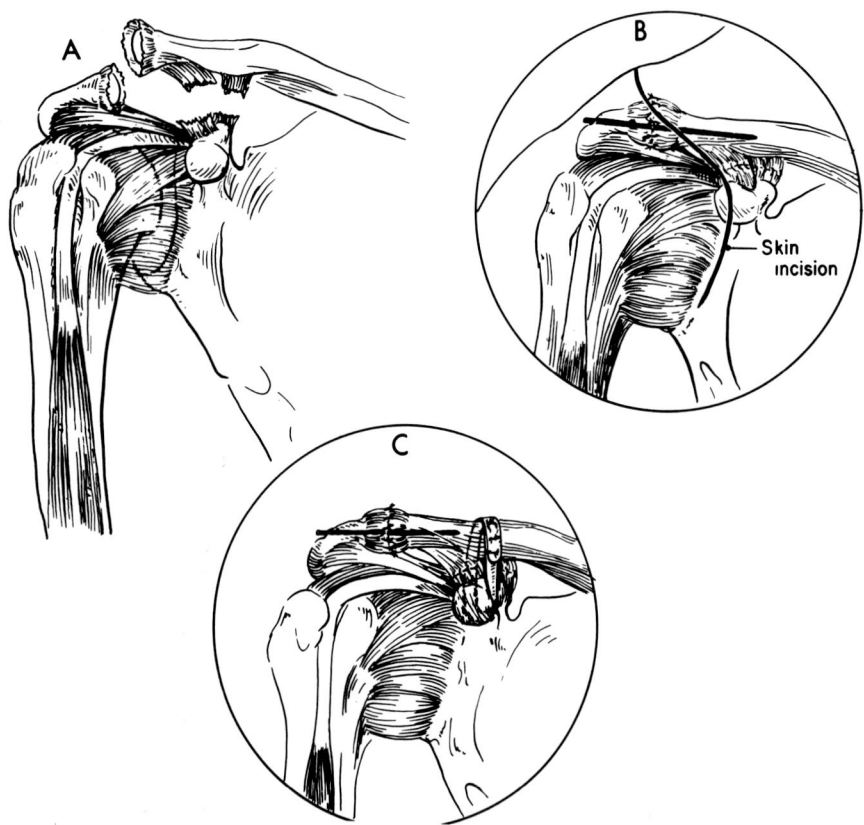

Figure 2 Transfixation of the acromioclavicular joint with 3–32″ Kirschner pin, reinforced by a strip of fascia lata around the clavicle and coracoid process. (Reprinted from The Shoulder in Trauma Management (Rowe), Yearbook Publishers, Chicago, 1974)

Trauma / 75

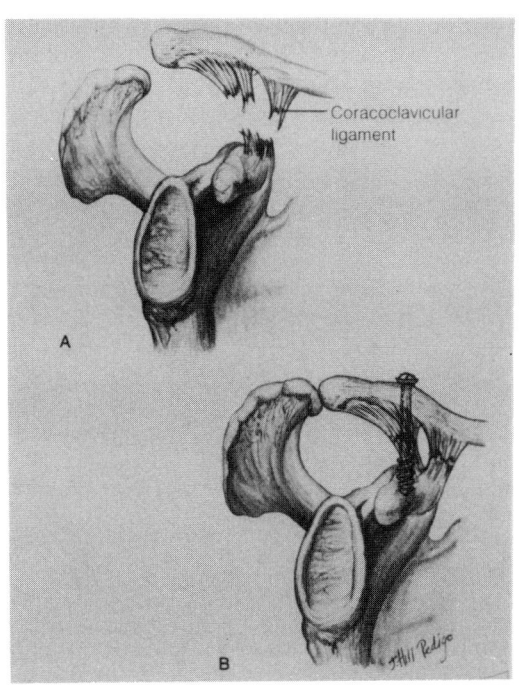

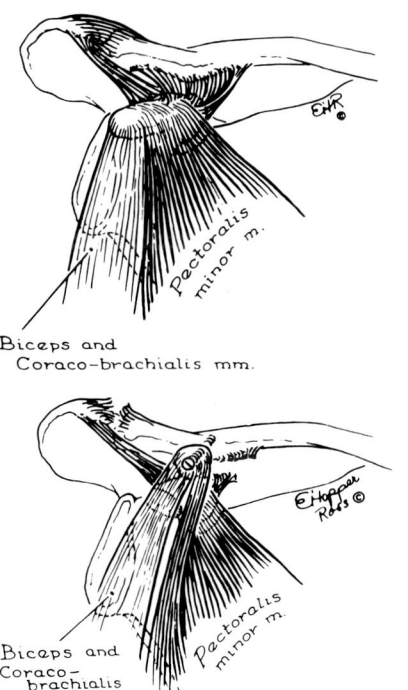

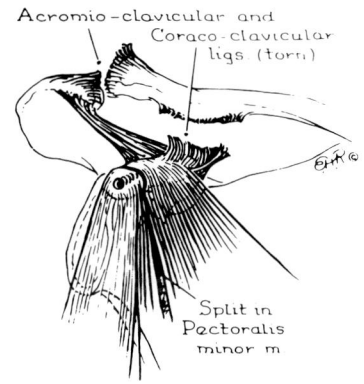

Figure 3 Bosworth method of screw fixation. Preoperative x-rays should be taken to exclude coracoid fracture. (Reprinted from Post, M. and Haskell, F: The Shoulder. With permission of Lea & Febiger, 1978, Philadelphia).

Figure 4 The Dewar and Barrington dynamic technique in which the coracoid process with its attached muscles is transferred to the clavicle for stability. (Reprinted from Dewar and Barrington: The Treatment of Chronic Acromioclavicular Dislocation. With permission of J Bone J Surg, 47B, 1965).

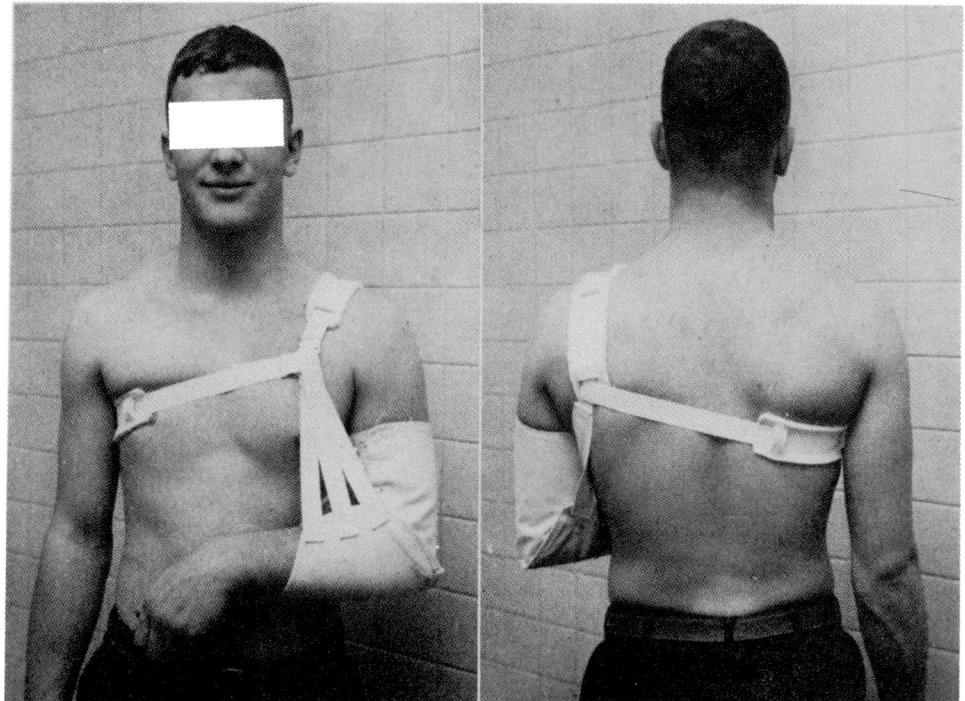

Figure 5 The Kenny Howard Sling Halter for closed treatment of acromioclavicular dislocation (Reprinted from Allman, F.: Fractures and ligamentous injuries of the clavicle and its articulations. J. Bone Joint Surg., 49A, 1967).

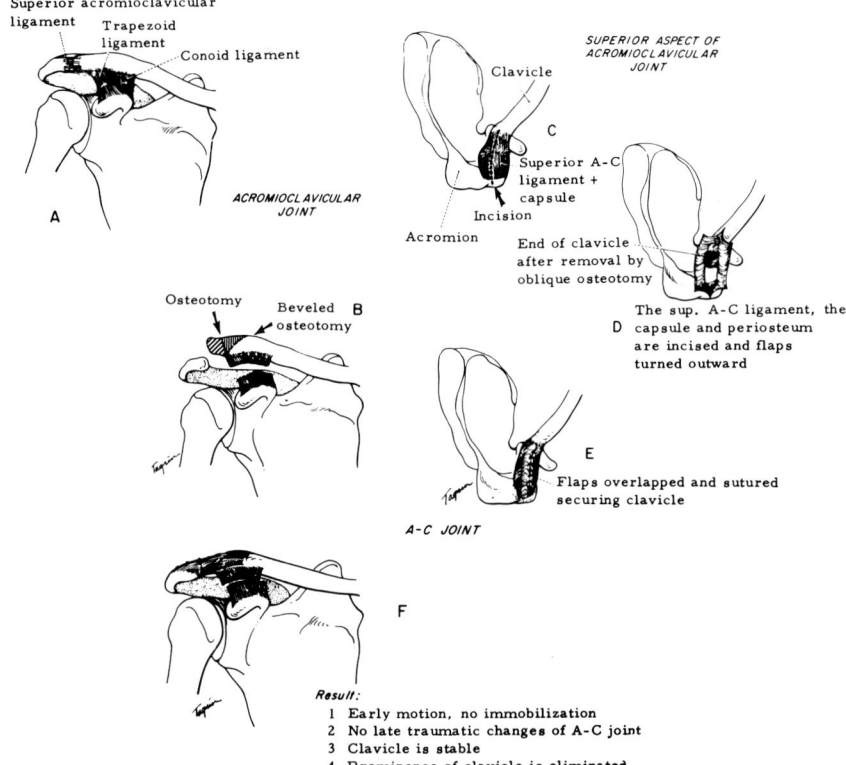

Figure 6 Rowe Modification of resection of distal end of clavicle for acute or chronic acromioclavicular dislocation. It is recommended that *not* more than 1 cm. of the end of the clavicle be removed, with enough clearance to avoid impingement with acromion. (Reprinted from Trauma Management, Shoulder Girdle Injuries, Rowe, C.R. Yearbook Medical Publishers, Inc., Chicago, Illinois, 1974).

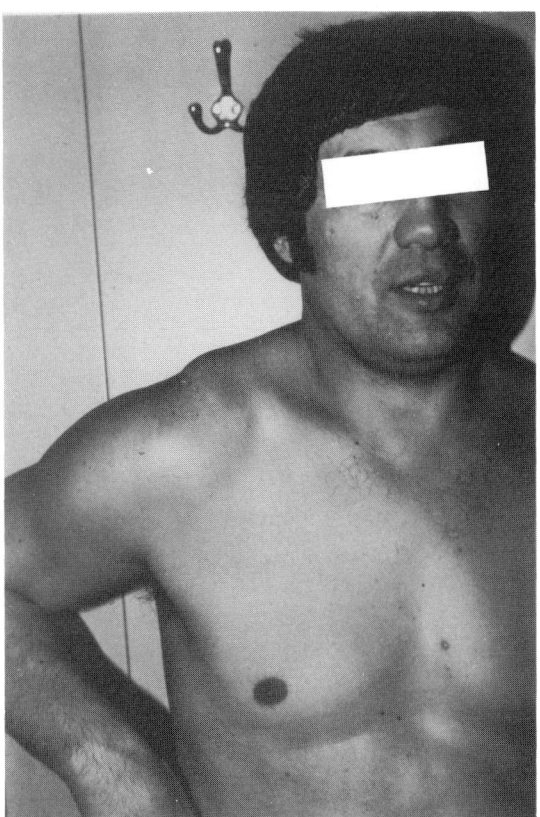

Figure 7 J.B. played professional hockey over a period of 20 years with an untreated complete acromioclavicular dislocation of his right shoulder. He had no complaints of his right shoulder.

in others), it did not disturb them. These patients included a number of professional athletes. Patient J.B. (Fig. 7) played over 20 years of professional hockey with complete dislocation of his right acromioclavicular joint, with full strength and power in his right shoulder and no pain. He is not conscious of his right shoulder deformity and is aware of it only when someone calls his attention to it. Patient G.B. (Fig. 8), a motorcycle racer were participating in all sports. Of interest, some of the deformities became less noticeable following return of muscle control and strength as noted by R.S. Bryan in 1975, "I have been surprised on occasion to see gross deformity almost disappear in time in patients who received no formal treatment, but did strenuous exercises of the shoulder muscles."

This stimulated me to look up the patients I had seen with complete acromioclavicular dislocation who had received no treatment other than a sling for a few days for comfort. On the grounds of these encouraging results, the patient was given the option of no treatment, along with closed or open treatment. Our experience with the patients who elected no treatment for their complete acromioclavicular dislocation has been worthy of note. Sixty percent reported no disturbing problem with their shoulder. They had full range of motion, strength and agility of their arm. Although the prominence persisted (less in some patients than

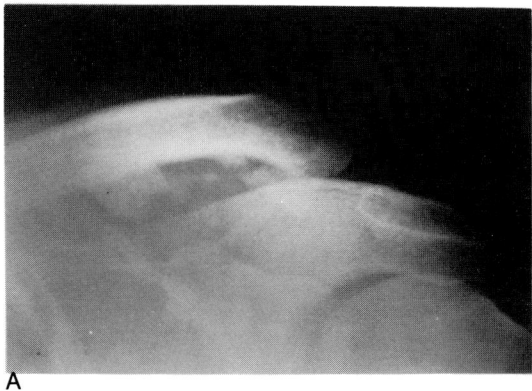

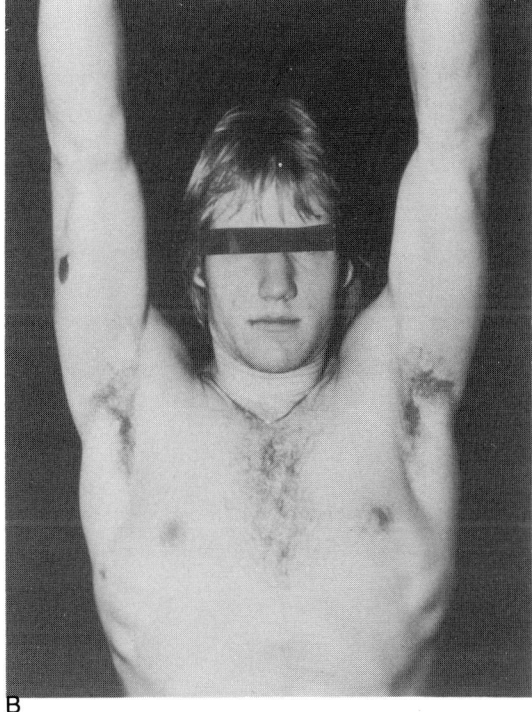

Figure 8 G.B. a motorcycle racer, one year after untreated dislocation of right acromioclavicular joint. Except for a few days rest, he lost no time from competitive motorcycle racing. (A) Complete superior dislocation of left clavicle. (B) Full range of painless motion.

seen here one year after complete dislocation of his left acromioclavicular joint. He received no treatment, lost only a few days from racing, lifts heavy equipment, has full range of motion, no pain, and no complaints about his left shoulder.

Twenty percent of the patients had minor complaints but wished to go along with their shoulders without surgery.

Twenty percent experienced disturbing symptoms and requested surgery. Resection of the distal clavicle relieved their discomfort and returned function in all except two thin female patients whose clavicle severely tented the skin. Open reduction with internal fixation was necessary in these two instances.

Thus, for the large majority of patients with complete dislocation of the acromioclavicular joint, my present advice to the patient is to apply ice, use a light sling for a few days and return to activities as soon as tolerated. Usually they have returned to light work within a week to ten days, to moderate work in three weeks, and to heavy work or contact sports in five to six weeks. Of course, treatment must be adjusted to specific situations and to the patient. With an occasional patient, as noted with the clavicle tenting the skin, open reduction and internal fixation is recommended. In chronic cases, if the patient does not care for the deformity, a modified acromioclavicular arthroplasty with removal of the distal centimeter of the clavicle is advised. This routine has eliminated the emergency treatment of acromioclavicular dislocations. It allows the patient to select the type of treatment which appeals to him. Two-thirds are happy with no treatment or closed treatment. Only one-third will possibly need operative treatment. I have found our overall results improved, that the patients are happier, and the management of a fresh, or an old, acromioclavicular dislocation is a much more pleasant experience than it has been in the past.

Perhaps we may close with the words of Codman,[7] "I personally have never found it necessary to operate on acromioclavicular dislocation, but in extreme cases, I should recommend Bunnell's operation."

REFERENCES

1. Allman FL, Jr. Fractures and ligamentous injuries of the clavicle and its articulation. J Bone Joint Surg 1967; 49A:774–784.
2. Bailey RW, O'Connor GA, Tilus PD, Baril JD. A dynamic repair for acute and chronic injuries of the acromioclavicular area. J Bone Joint Surg 1972; 54A:1802.
3. Bateman JE. Athletic injuries about the shoulder in throwing and body-contact sports. Clin Orthop 1962; 23:75–83.
4. Bosworth BM. Acromioclavicular separation. New method of repair. Surg Gynecol Obstet 1941; 73:866–871.
5. Bunnell S. Fascial graft for dislocation of acromio-clavicular joint. Surg Gynec Obst 1928; 46:563–564.
6. Campos OP. Acromioclavicular dislocation. Am J Surg 1939; 43:287–291.
7. Codman EA. The Shoulder. Todd Publishers, Boston (G. Muller & Co. Medical Publishers, Inc., Brooklyn, N.Y.) pg. 308, 1934.
8. Dewar FP, Barrington TW. The treatment of chronic acromioclavicular dislocation. J Bone Joint Surg 1965; 47B:32–35.
9. Glick JM, Milburn LL, Haggerty JF, Nishimoto D. Dislocated acromioclavicular joint: Follow-up study of 35 unreduced acromioclavicular dislocations. Am J Sports Med 1977; 5:264–270.
10. Gurd FB. The treatment of complete dislocation of the outer end of the clavicle. An hitherto undescribed operation. Ann Surg 1941; 113:1094–1098.
11. Imatani RJ, Hanlon JJ, Cady GW. J Bone Joint Surg. 1975; 57-A:328–332.
12. Jacobs B, Wade PA. Acromioclavicular joint injury. End result study. J Bone Joint Surg. 1968; 48A:475–486.
13. Moseley HF, Templeton J. Dislocation of acromioclavicular dislocation utilizing the coracoacromial ligament. J Bone Joint Surg. 1969; 51B:196.
14. Mumford EB. Acromioclavicular dislocation. J Bone Joint Surg 1941; 23:799–802.
15. Neviaser JS. Acromioclavicular dislocation treated by transference of the coracoacromial ligament. Bull Hosp Joint Dis 1951; 12:46–54.
16. Quigley TB. Injuries to the acromioclavicular and sternoclavicular joints sustained in athletics. Surg Clin N Am. 1963; 43:1551–1554.
17. Rowe R, Marble HC. Fractures and Other Injuries. Edited by E.F. Cave. Chicago: Year Book Publishers, 1958.
18. Simmons EH, Martin RF. Acute dislocation of the acromioclavicular joint. Can J Surg 1968; 11:473.
19. Urist MR. Complete dislocation of the acromioclavicular joint. The nature of the traumatic lesion and effective methods of treatment with an analysis of 41 cases. J Bone Joint Surg 1946; 28:813–837.
20. Weaver JK, Dunn HK. Treatment of acromioclavicular injuries, especially complete acromioclavicular separation. J Bone Joint Surg 1972; 54A:1187.

SPORTS INJURIES— SHOULDER STABILIZATION

CHRONIC SHOULDER PAIN IN THE ATHLETE

ROBERT E. LEACH, M.D. and DAVID SEGAL, M.D.

The shoulder joint appears to be second only to the knee joint as a cause of chronic disability in the athlete. Dislocations of the shoulder joint and the acromioclavicular joint are a common cause of acute disability, and recurrent dislocations of the shoulder are another cause of both acute and chronic disability. The most common cause of chronic disability is tendinitis of the rotator cuff and late attritional tears of the supraspinatus.[2]

Different sports put stresses on different anatomical areas in the shoulder. Contact sports such as football, hockey and wrestling are more likely to cause shoulder dislocations or AC separations. We see the changes of chronic tendinitis and rotator cuff damage in sports such as tennis, swimming, baseball and more rarely in bowling or at the quarterback position in football. These sports that demand the arm going overhead repetitively cause chronic stress on the rotator cuff, particularly the supraspinatus portion of that cuff. The term "impingement syndrome"[7] has been coined to indicate the usual symptom complex causing disability. As the arm is elevated, the rotator cuff, particularly its anterior and superior portions and the intervening bursa, is brought up against the anterior edge of the acromion, the coracoacromial ligament and possibly the undersurface of the distal end of the clavicle. This impingement repeated many times causes inflammation of the rotator cuff and of the subdeltoid bursa. As pointed out by the studies of Rathbun and Macnab,[9] there is a relatively avascular area in the rotator cuff approximately one centimeter from its attachment to the greater tuberosity. This area of relative avascularity predisposes to damage in that area or, at least, to the inability to repair damage in the rotator cuff.

The damage to the rotator cuff has been divided into three stages by Neer[7,8] and by Hawkins and Kennedy.[3] In stage 1, there is edema and hemorrhage in the rotator cuff; these patients should respond well to conservative treatment. In stage 2, there is reactive hyperemia and thickening of the cuff and the bursa; some of these patients may require surgery to have complete relief from symptoms. In stage 3, there is degeneration of the rotator cuff and, in some instances, small tears which may lead to complete tears of the rotator cuff (Fig. 1). Some of these changes may be age-related or related to the amount of activity of the individual athlete.

The athlete who is having chronic pain in the area of the rotator cuff usually describes an activity in which the arm is elevated from 80 to 120 degrees and repetitively internally rotated in that particular arc. If the arm is placed in that position by the examiner and some force applied to it, almost invariably the patient will have pain localized near the anterior superior aspect of the shoulder. Depending upon how long the symptoms have been present, there may or may not be visible atrophy of the supraspinatus and infraspinatus muscles. There will frequently be weakness of the supraspinatus muscle which can be tested with the arm at 90 degrees of abduction, 20 degrees of forward flexion and internal rotation (Fig. 2).

Such patients deserve a determined and organized conservative treatment regimen before we consider any surgical procedure. We start by having the athlete decrease the activity which is causing him or her pain. In many instances the athlete cannot or will not completely give up that activity, but it can be modified by, for instance, changing a swimming stroke or throwing motion, or by decreasing the number of repetitions done per day. We advise pendulum exercises with the athlete leaning far forward at the waist holding a three-pound weight in an effort to maintain or regain a full range of motion and to restore the gliding mechanism between cuff and bursa, and bursa and the acromion process and coracoacromial arch. Oral anti-inflammatory agents are frequently helpful and are usually given over a 3-week period. To

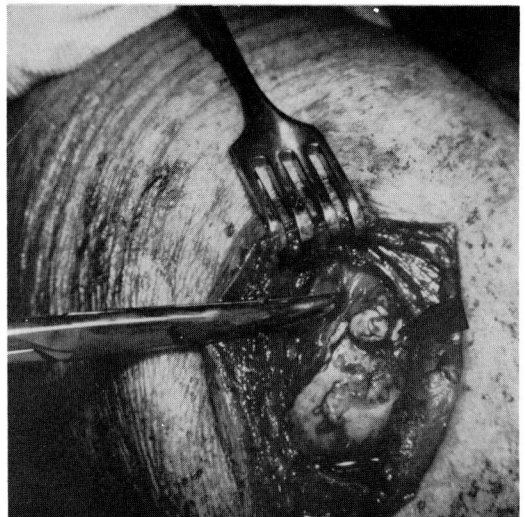

Figure 1 Arrow points to torn area of rotator cuff with Stage 3 changes.

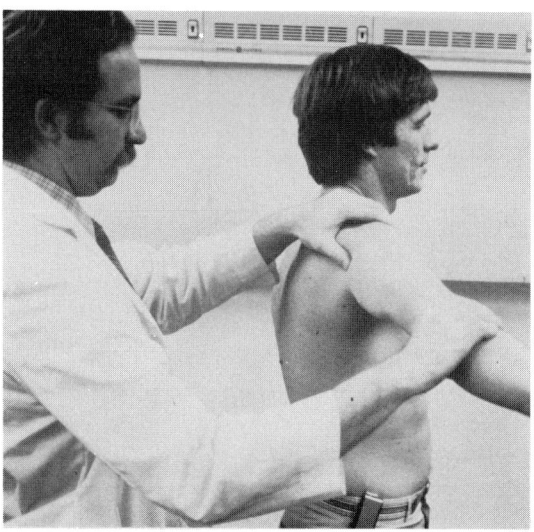

Figure 2 Testing for supraspinatus weakness.

this regimen, we add a strengthening program for the internal and external rotators of the shoulder with the exercises done with the arm at the side. We usually advise the patient to use surgical tubing or a bungee cord in performing internal and external rotation exercises with the arm at the side so that it is not in the position of elevation and internal rotation which causes pain. As the patient begins to improve with this program, we add stretching exercises to further regain the range of motion required. In throwing sports, the athlete needs external rotation beyond that which the normal person has or needs.

Most patients with an impingement syndrome will respond well to this program. If the patient does not respond, we inject a long-acting steroid preparation into the subdeltoid bursa with the intention of decreasing the local inflammatory process and following the rest of the conservative program previously outlined. Once we have injected a steroid we feel the patient should not, for a period of two weeks, do the usual activities of throwing, swimming, etc. This is because we are worried about the effect of the steroid on local healing and on the ground substance of the rotator cuff if there has been damage to it. In the course of several months we would be willing to inject a shoulder two times but do not feel that shoulders should be injected frequently or on a routine basis.

The question then arises as to what one does with the athlete who does not respond well to conservative measures. We will assume here that the patient does not have a major tear of the rotator cuff as we believe such tears should always be repaired in the athlete. What should be done depends to a large extent upon the particular activity of the patient, the amount of pain and what one assumes will be the pathological findings. The age of the patient is pertinent. In patients up to the age of 21 or 22 who have chronic pain secondary to an impingement syndrome and who do not respond to conservative treatment, we consider the possibility of resecting the coracoacromial ligament. We assume that these patients have stage 2 changes in the rotator cuff, i.e. that there is no actual degeneration of the cuff. At the time of resection of the coracoacromial ligament we feel the undersurface of the clavicle, and if there is a large osteophyte pointing inferiorly resect it or smooth it off. If the bursa is large, thickened and hyperemic we resect the bursa. In several instances, we have found large fibrin or "rice" bodies in the bursa (Fig. 3); it was felt that even with decompression, the bursa itself represented a potential source of encroachment upon the acromion process. The results of this surgery in younger patients, as noted by several authors,[4] are good and patients have gone back to full-time athletic activities. We have had several baseball pitchers in the collegiate and minor league ranks who have been able to return to effective pitching following this surgery. Each of them has had to go on a stringent rehabilitation program and regain normal strength of the internal and external rotators of the shoulder. Frequently

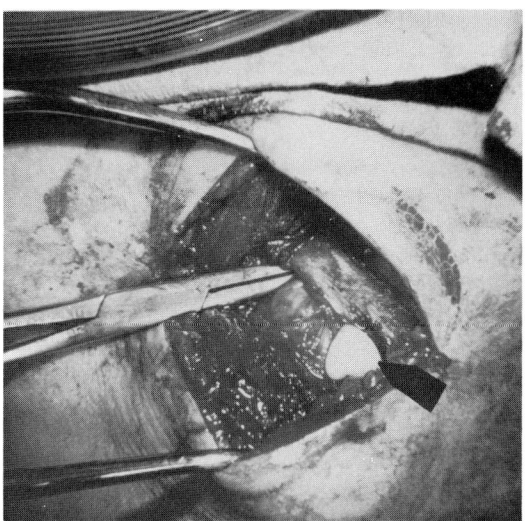

Figure 3 Hemostat under coracoacromial ligament; arrow points to rice body in enlarged bursa.

these patients are not aware of the strength loss which has happened over the long term and thus are unaware of their increasing disability.

Once the patient has gone beyond his early 20s or if there are any degenerative changes within the rotator cuff, we feel that resection of the coracoacromial ligament alone will not be effective and so move on to a more thorough decompression. The question is, how much constitutes enough decompression in these stage 3 shoulders? In the athlete, strength is a major consideration and anything which will significantly decrease strength, even if it decreases pain, cannot be viewed as effective.

Dr. George Hammond in 1969[1] published a long term study of almost 90 patients who had had complete acromionectomies. These patients were not athletes, but the results were excellent. In virtually all, there was excellent relief from pain and in most there was no noticeable weakness complained of by the patient. Since these were not athletes, they were not subjected to rigorous testing. He emphasized that total acromionectomy does relieve pain and that an air–tight repair of the deltoid muscle is important so that the patient loses neither shoulder function nor strength. This latter is critical to any removal of the acromion process.

Dr. Neer, in 1974,[7] reported a series of patients who had what he termed an anterior acromioplasty which entailed resection of the coracoacromial ligament and a beveling of the anterior portion of the acromion. He theorized that the vast majority of impingement syndrome cases are caused by impingement against the anterior aspect of the acromion and the coracoacromial arch. By leaving the acromion process intact, he provided the deltoid with the fulcrum which it normally has and did not have to worry about deltoid reattachment or sutures pulling free. Again, Dr. Neer's patients were not predominantly athletes, but the results were excellent in terms of pain relief. He felt it was likely that their deltoid strength was better than it would have been with an acromionectomy and the return of function, including strength, was quicker.

Subsequent to Dr. Neer's report, Leach and O'Connor[6] reported 16 partial acromionectomies which had been performed on athletes. In all cases, there had been stage 3 changes in the rotator cuff and, in a number of instances, small attritional tears of the cuff. The acromion process was resected back to the AC joint, the underside of the distal calvicle inspected, and osteophytes removed. The reattachment of the deltoid to a cuff of tissue consisting primarily of the acromioclavicular ligament was done easily, and the rehabilitation time, including strength gain, was much shorter than in the total acromionectomy patients of Dr. Hammond and others in the 1960s.

Inspection of the resected acromion in Leach's patients almost invariably showed a point of contact (which we called "the burnish point" for the polishing action) between the rotator cuff and the acromion which was quite anterior and near the acromioclavicular joint (Fig. 4). It would have been usually decompressed with a Neer anterior acromioplasty. In some instances the burnish point was larger and farther back from the anterior edge of the acromion, but never did it extend behind the acromioclavicular joint

We then decided to inividualize our treatment of patients with the impingement syndrome. In the majority, usually in the age range 25 to 40, we did a Neer anterior acromioplasty which also removed the coracoacromial ligament. We inspected the undersurface of the distal clavicle and removed any osteophytes found there. The bursa was inspected and, if it was thought to be markedly thickened and could mechanically interfere with recovery, we resected it. We inspected the rotator cuff and if there was a small tear of the cuff, in the younger patient, we repaired it and resected the anterior aspect of the acromion back to the acromioclavicular joint. If the cuff was intact we simply did the Neer anterior acromioplasty.

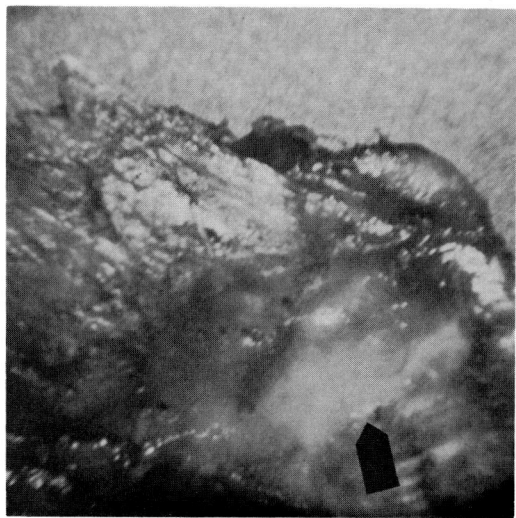

Figure 4 Arrow points to "burnish point" on undersurface of anterior acromion.

In patients over the age of 40, particularly those who have weakness of the supraspinatus muscle and in whom a small tear of the rotator cuff is likely, we perform a partial resection of the acromion back to the acromioclavicular joint. In some patients a small rotator cuff tear will have been proven by arthrogram or arthroscopy. In others, because of the length of time, weakness, and disability we assume there has been a small tear. One must be careful to preserve the undersurface of the deltoid muscle when it is being taken off the acromion. It must be skived off, carefully preserving the deep tendinous portion. Also, we must preserve the soft tissue on top of the acromion consisting of the periosteum and the acromioclavicular ligament as this is the tissue to which the deltoid muscle will be tightly sutured to allow the patient to regain strength postoperatively. We think that by removing the anterior portion of the acromion, particularly in those people who have small tears, that we have completely decompressed that area and our suture repair is protected.

The postoperative period is longer in patients with a partial acromionectomy. They are kept in a sling and swathe for seven days, then started on pendulum exercises for another seven days, and then gradually on active assistive and eventually active resistive exercises. It takes about three months for these patients to return to athletic activity and even then their strength, power and endurance is diminished. At six months they are usually doing well, with improvement up to a year. They must have a solid rehabilitation program which includes resistive exercises for all shoulder muscle groups.

In some instances in which the rotator cuff is very thin and resection of the tissue and repair would be difficult, we have done a partial acromionectomy and not repaired the cuff. We recognize the dangers in this but feel it may be preferable to resecting all the damaged tissue and trying to do a repair. This is a surgical judgment as we would obviously prefer to do a repair. This patient is unlikely to pursue athletic activities such as swimming and tennis, with tennis being a particular problem because of the violence of the serve and overhead shots. Swimming may be more easily done once the decompression has been accomplished. In the athletic person, a repair of the rotator cuff is always preferable and only under exceptional circumstances would we simply decompress the cuff. In the nonathlete, there may be more instances in which a partial decompression might be effective without trying to reconstruct a torn and thinned rotator cuff.

In patients who have an acute rupture of the rotator cuff through essentially healthy tissue, we do not do an acromioplasty or a partial acromionectomy. We do an acromial splitting incision, repair the cuff, and put the acromion process together. There seems no reason to do a decompression in such athletes. Anterior resection of the acromion process gives good visibility for a repair of the rotator cuff, but is not necessary in acute ruptures with no previous history of disease.

We have had no experience with solitary resection of the distal end of the clavicle as a treatment for patients with the impingement syndrome. It seems unlikely to us that the distal clavicle would be the major cause of the impingement syndrome with the consistent findings that we find in relation to the undersurface of the acromion and with the success of coracoacromial ligament resections. If there is disease of the acromioclavicular joint plus changes in the rotator cuff, partial resection of the acromion more completely decompresses the rotator cuff than would resection of the distal end of the clavicle.

REFERENCES

1. Hammond G. Complete acromionectomy in the treatment of chronic tendinitis of the shoulder. J Bone Joint Surg 1971; 53A:173–180.

2. Hammond G, Torgerson W, Dotter E, Leach RE. The Painful Shoulder. Instructional Course Lecture XXI. St. Louis: CV Mosby, 1971.
3. Hawkins RJ, Kennedy JC. Impingement syndrome in athletes. Am J Sports Med 1980; 8:151–158.
4. Jackson DW. Chronic rotator cuff impingement in the throwing athlete. Orthop Trans 1977; 1:24.
5. Kennedy JC, Willis RB. The effects of local steroid injections on tendons: A biomechanical and microscopic correlative study. Am J Sports Med 1976; 4:11–21.
6. Leach RE. O'Connor P, Jones RP. Acromionectomy for tendinitis of the shoulder in athletes. Physician Sports Med 1979; 7:96–107.
7. Neer CS. Anterior acromioplasty for the chronic impingement syndrome in the shoulder. J Bone Joint Surg 1972; 54A:41–50.
8. Neer CS, Welsh RP. The shoulder in sports. Orthop Clin North Am 1977; 8:583–591.
9. Rathbun JB, Macnab I. The microvascular pattern of the rotator cuff. J Bone Joint Surg 1970; 52B:540–553.

COMPUTER TOMOGRAPHY ON RECURRENT SHOULDER DISLOCATION

U. LAUMANN, M.D., and H. A. KRAMPS, M.D.

We investigated the use of CT scanning in the preoperative diagnosis of shoulder dislocation and obtained the results which follow.

Diagnosis of Hill-Sachs Lesion

Hill-Sachs lesion can be demonstrated in the transverse plane without any difficulty. By a second scan at 90° to the first one, its extension can be more exactly localized. Compared to conventional radiographs, smaller depressed fractures can be visualized very well on CT scan. If a Hill-Sachs lesion is demonstrable, there is no doubt about the direction of the dislocation (Fig. 1).

Determination of Capsular Extension

To determine the capsular extension, air insufflation of the joint is necessary. By transverse scans demonstration of both the ventral and the dorsal capsular extension is possible. The evidence of capsular extension is particularly important when operative treatment of recurrent dislocation has failed. The obliteration of the subcapsular recessus can be exactly diagnosed by CT (Fig. 2). Again, CT is superior to ordinary arthrography.

Clinical Assessment of Bankart Lesions and Fractures of the Glenoid Rim

The glenoid labrum is a hypodense structure and therefore cannot be demonstrated by CT without auxiliary means. If the articular cavity is filled with self-hardening Sulfix plastics, a well-defined negative impression of the labrum is obtained. By CT with additional pneumoarthrography, the glenoid labrum can be visualized. Its demonstration is particularly successful if the glenoid capsule is relaxed by internal and external rotation of the arm. Then the fibrous cartilage is demonstrated as a small bulge-like structure, showing lighter contrast, directly adjacent to the anterior and posterior margins of the glenoid fossa. If there is a Bankart lesion, this structure has been destroyed or dislocated (Fig. 3).

Accompanying shearings from the bony margin of the glenoid cavity can also be clearly demonstrated (Figs. 4, 5). Thus, CT is far superior to common radiography in diagnosing a Bankart lesion. Usually, a similarly good demonstration of the glenoid labrum can only be obtained by the much more expensive procedure of arthropneumotomography after McGlynn. Lastly, CT permits control of the position of the bony graft at the operative procedure according to Eden-Hybbinette, which is frequently carried out in Europe. CT makes possible a clear visualization of the positioning of the bone graft.

Evidence of Humeral Head Torsion and of the Angle of Inclination of the Glenoid Cavity

Saha and Weber showed that, in addition to the soft structures, torsion of the humeral head, divergent from the physiological norm, or a pathological angle of inclination of fossa glenoidalis causes recurrent shoulder dislocation. The diagnosis of humeral head torsion requires an additional scan through the humeral condyles. It must, however, be postulated that the humerus does not change its position during this examination. By means of a geometrical construction according to the procedure of Mukherjee-Sivaya, the retrotorsion of the humeral head can be determined (Fig. 6).

In 32 patients with recurrent shoulder dislocation we found values between 28 and 31 degrees, not significantly different from normal. The determination of the angle of inclination of the glenoid cavity is easily carried out. By construction of two auxiliary lines, the "spinal-axis" (articular central point—point of margo medialis scapulae) and the plane of inclination of the

Sports Injuries—Shoulder Stabilization / 85

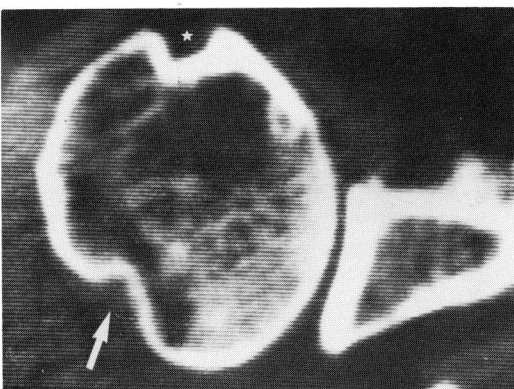

Figure 1 Posterior superior impacted fracture (Hill-Sachs lesion) plane S2, sulcus intertubercularis.

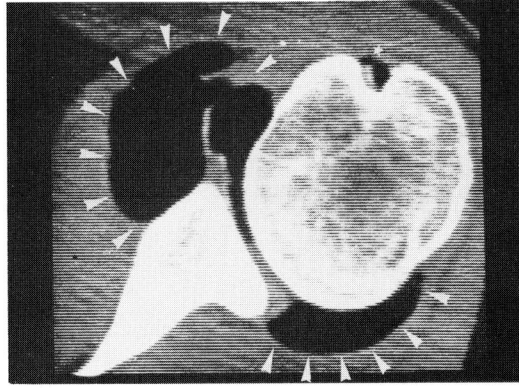

Figure 2 Anterior and posterior capsular extension (anteriorly, considerable widening of the capsule, the glenoid labrum has loosened). Diagnosis: recurrent shoulder subluxation; *sulcus intertubercularis.

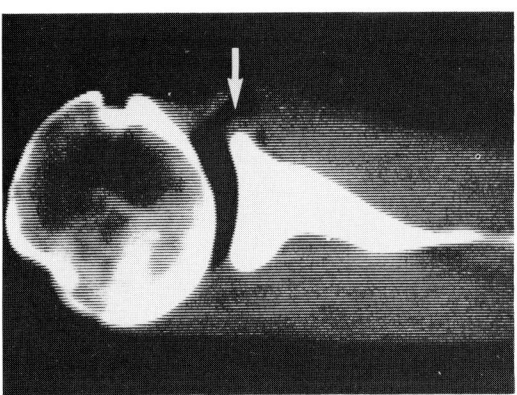

Figure 3 By internal rotation of the arm the hypodense structure of the anterior glenoid labrum is demonstrated.

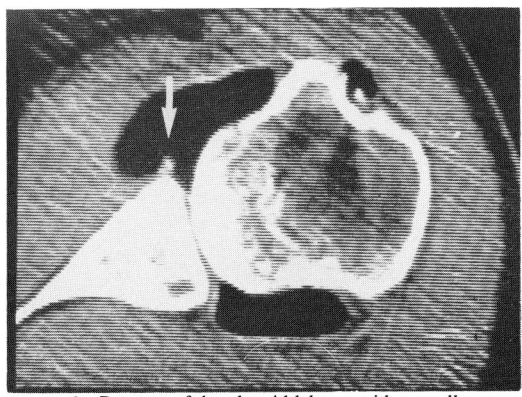

Figure 4 Rupture of the glenoid labrum with a small osseous lamella secondary to recurrent shoulder dislocation.

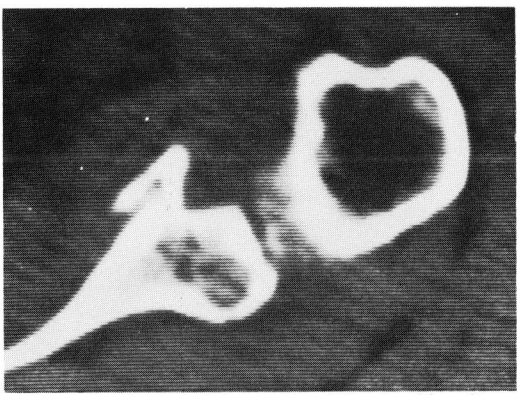

Figure 5 Fracture of the margin of the glenoid cavity.

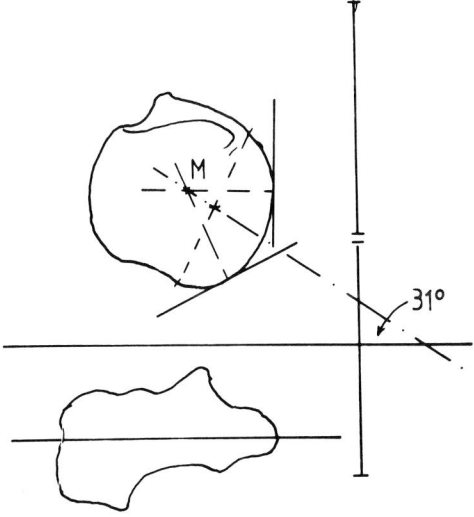

Figure 6 Determination of retrotorsion of the humeral head (Modification after Mukherjee-Sivaya)

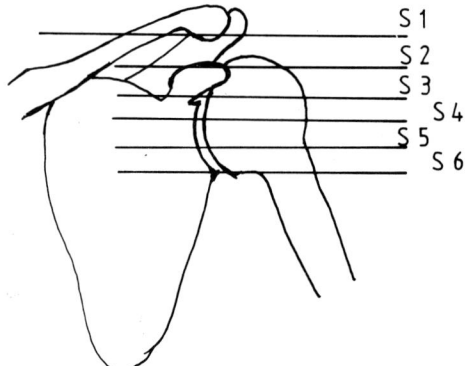

Figure 7 Series of transverse scans routinely carried out in our study.

glenoid cavity (angular points of the fossa glenoidalis), the retroversion of the fossa glenoidalis can be determined. Its complementary angle to 90 degrees amounted to a mean value of 7 degrees (4-11°) in our studies, and thus it was within a range of 2 to 12 degrees, as determined to be normal by Das and Ray, in all patients with recurrent shoulder dislocation.

Conclusion

CT diagnostics permit comprehensive assessment of all relevant structures in recurrent shoulder dislocation. With a series of 6 transverse scans and, if necessary, one additional scan through the area of the elbow condyles combined with an arthropneu, all information can be obtained by one procedure (Fig. 7). Since this procedure is still rather expensive and common radiodiagnostic methods are sufficient for preoperative planning in many cases of recurrent shoulder dislocation, we restrict CT diagnostics as yet to the following cases: failed operatively treated shoulder dislocation, in cases of doubt about the direction of the humeral head dislocation, and, if there are special questions of medicolegal concern.

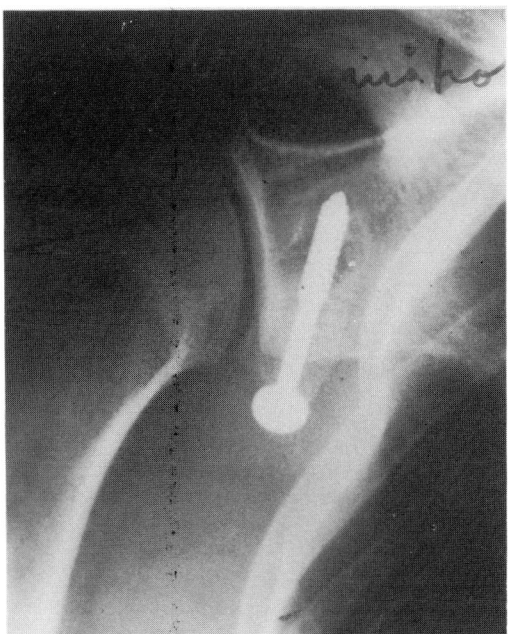 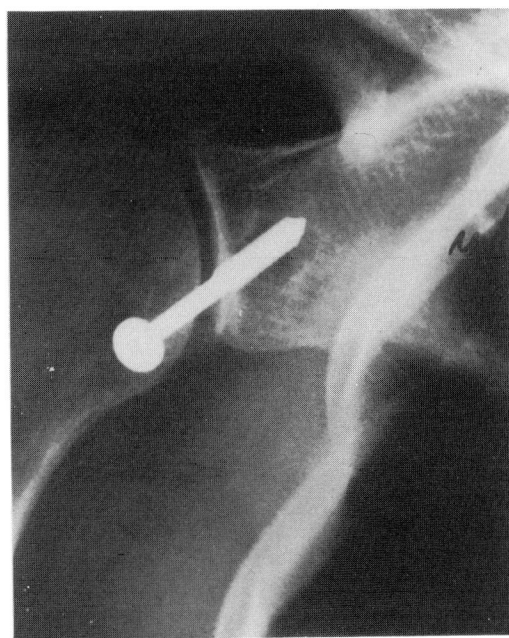

Figure 3 Radiograms at follow-up 2 years after a Bristow-Latarjet procedure. (a) A-P view with the arm in inward rotation; (b) The same view with the arm in outward rotation. The boneblock and screw have moved outward ("loose transplant"). Note cavity around the intrascapular part of the screw.

the anterior part of the joint is enough to cure some unstable shoulders.[19] One-third of our patients are operated upon not only with a longitudinal incision in the subscapularis tendon muscle, but also with a transverse incision engaging two-thirds or more of the tendon, which results in shortening and scar formation to this structure. How much importance does this have as regards the result? Some of these latter mechanisms may explain a successful result even after a procedure in which the transplant is severely migrated or in a position more than 1 cm medial to the glenoid rim.

Our follow-up time is at least 2 years. Patients with stable bone blocks should have a good prognosis even with a longer follow-up time but we cannot overlook the fact that late recurrences will appear especially in the group with loose transplants. Our radiologic technique[11] with four different projections is sufficient to confirm whether the transplant has healed with osseous or fibrous union or migrated. However, in a future study the stability of the transplant should also be considered in the fibrous union group. Figure 3 demonstrates that two exactly similar anteroposterior views can establish whether the transplant moves outwards when the arm is rotated.

Our results in the group of patients with dislocations caused by a trivial trauma (spontaneous) were not as favorable as in the traumatic group.[9] Even if this difference were not significant, it is possible that need for correct positioning and healing of the bone block increases with spontaneous dislocation. It is possible that reefing of the capsule should be included in the management of these cases. Hill et al[7] reported poorer results with the Bristow procedure in cases with subluxations but demonstrated no difference between spontaneous and traumatic dislocations regarding the results postoperatively. These results are at variance with those of DePalma.[3] Our opinion is that, when correctly performed, the Bristow-Latarjet procedure yields favorable results in spontaneous dislocations. Eight of our patients reported occasional subluxations which did not bother them. A longer follow-up period will reveal the true significance of these although we at present consider them unimportant.

Carter Rowe (personal communication, 1979) writes "unfortunately, the Bristow procedure is becoming very popular and many are being sent to me now who are recurring." Our opinion however is that "the orthopaedic surgeon who can not play the violin (Bankart) has to beat the drum (Bristow-Latarjet)."

REFERENCES

1. Bankart ASB. Recurrent or habitual dislocation of the shoulder joint. British Med J 1923; 2:1132–33.
2. Collins HR, Wilde AH. Shoulder instability in athletics. Orthop Clinic. N. Amer 1973; 4:759–774.
3. DePalma AF. Reflections on dislocation and recurrent instability of the shoulder. Proc Inaug Internat Conf Surgery of the shoulder. London, 1980. Shoulder surgery. Berlin, Heidelberg, New York; Springer-Verlag, 1982; 100–103.
4. Du Toit GT, Roux D. Recurrent dislocation of the shoulder. Twenty-four year study of Johannesburg Stapling operation. J Bone and Joint Surg 1955; 37-A:633.
5. Helfet AJ. Coracoid transplantation for recurring dislocation of the shoulder. J Bone and Joint Surg 1958; 40-B:198–202.
6. Hellum C, Rugtveit A. Luxatio humeri habitualis (abstract). Acta Orthop Scandinavica 1973; 44:127.
7. Hill A, Lombardo SJ, Kerlan RK, Jobe FW, Carter VS, Shields CL, Collins HR, Yocum LA. The modified Bristow-Helfet procedure for recurrent anterior shoulder subluxations and dislocations. Am J Sports Med 1981; 9:283–287.
8. Hovelius L, Åkermark C, Albrektsson B, Berg E, Körner L, Lundberg B, Wredmark T. The Bristow-Latarjet procedure for recurrent dislocation of the shoulder. A 2–5 year follow-up study on the results of 112 cases. Acta Orthop Scandinavica 1983; 54:284–290.
9. Hovelius L, Körner L, Lundberg B, Åkermark C, Herberts P, Wredmark T, Berg E. The coracoid transfer for recurrent dislocation of the shoulder: Technical aspects of the Bristow-Latarjet procedure. J Bone and Joint Surg 1983; 65A:926–934.
10. Hovelius L, Thorling J, Fredin H. Recurrent anterior dislocation of the shoulder. Results after the Bankart and Putti-Platt operations. J Bone Joint Surg 1979; 61A:566–569.
11. Lamm CR, Zachrisson BE, Körner L. Radiography of the shoulder after the Bristow repair. Acta Radiol 1982; 23:523–528.
12. Latarjet M. A propos du traitement des luxations récidivantes de l'epaule. Lyon Chir 1954; 49:994–997.
13. Lombardo SJ, Kerlan RK, Jobe FW, Carter VS, Blazina ME, Shields CL. The modified Bristow procedure for recurrent dislocation of the shoulder. J Bone and Joint Surg 1976; 58A:256–261.
14. May JV. A modified Bristow operation for anterior recurrent dislocation of the shoulder. J Bone and Joint Surg 1970; 52A:1010–1016.
15. Morrey BF, Janes JM. Recurrent anterior dislocation of the shoulder. J Bone and Joint surg 1976; 58A:252–261.
16. Osmond-Clarke H. Habitual dislocation of the shoulder. The Putti-Platt operation. J Bone and Joint Surg 1948; 30B:19–25.
17. Reider B, Inglis AE. The Bankart procedure modified by the use of prolene pull-out sutures. J Bone and Joint Surg 1982; 64A:628–629.
18. Rowe CR, Patel D, Southmayd WW. The Bankart procedure. A long-term end-result study. J Bone and Joint Surg 1978; 60A:1–16.
19. Watson-Jones R. Fractures and joint injuries. Vol 2. 4th ed. London: E. & S. Livingstone Ltd, 1955:492.

dard anterior approach showed very different results. Seven patients (30.4%) in this second group were dissatisfied with their cosmetic results owing to extensive keloid scar formation. Fourteen patients classified their results from good to moderate, whereas only two patients considered their results to be excellent.

Range of movement. Two patients explicitly stated that they had a limitation in the range of movement. The great majority of patients seemed to be unaware of any limitations. Objective assessment of shoulder movement told a different story. All patients had some limitation of external rotation, as well as forward elevation, although we found a considerable variation in the degree of limitation. The limitation of external rotation varied from 15°–35° (average 25°), whereas the limitation of forward elevation varied from 10°–25° (average 15°).

Muscular power was good in all patients but one. This patient had a deep wound infection, which ultimately led to severe atrophy of nearly all muscles of the shoulder region. One patient had temporary paralysis of the musculocutaneous nerve which disappeared after 6 months. At the time of follow-up the patient had regained full motor power.

Failures. As mentioned above one patient developed a deep wound infection, which finally resulted in redislocation and consequently in a severe loss of mobility and motor power in the shoulder. Although the infection has cleared up, the patient firmly declined any further treatment. One patient had a recurrence after four years (motor car accident). This patient underwent reoperation and is doing well at the moment. One case of temporary musculocutaneous paralysis owing to a technical error regained full motor power within 6 months.

CONCLUSION

In 1975 we were looking for a technically simple and reliable method of repairing recurrent anterior dislocation of the shoulder. Bankart's procedure combined with Putti-Platt's operation proved to be simple and reliable. The axillary approach, although technically more demanding, gives superior cosmetic results. Pull-out wires, modified after Sterling Bunnell, are an easy method for secure attachment of the lateral flap of the capsule just beyond the rim of the glenoid without leaving implants behind to be removed at a later date. Superficial wound infection at the point where the wires perforated the dorsal shoulder skin was never a problem. The one case of deep wound infection was probably due to a combination of technical errors and a bad choice of patient. This patient, a 64-year old farmer, had mild diabetes as well as undetected lymphatic leukemia. The other recurrence was precipitated by a severe motor car accident.

THE ANTEROINFERIOR VULNERABLE POINT OF THE GLENOID RIM

D. PATTE, M.D., J. BERNAGEAU, M.D., and P. BANCEL, M.D.

The anteroinferior rim of the glenoid, reinforced by the labrum, is the primary restraint of the shoulder joint for the humeral head, when the arm is in abduction and extension, in the "cocked" position. This is the weak spot in the stabilizing structures of the shoulder, lesions of which are generally underestimated, as they are poorly seen at arthrotomy and frequently obscured radiographically for lack of appropriate views. This area seems to us to be an important one to study in the diagnosis of so–called minor degrees of instability (subluxations or distorsions) which leave residual structural changes in this area, and because the anatomical defect should dictate the choice of reconstructive technique.

The use of a particular radiographic projection, the glenoid profile view[3] permits precise analysis of the anteroinferior border of the glenoid and the labrum as well as when used in conjunction with contrast arthrotomography.[2]

A permanent collaborative effort between the surgeons and radiologists during more than 15 years has permitted us to make several observations based on 40 patients with recurrent dislocation, 40 patients with minor instabilities which we call painful and unstable shoulders.[5,16,18] These correspond to the recurrent transient subluxations of C. Rowe[23] or the "Labral syndrome" of Trillat.[27]

THE ANTEROINFERIOR VULNERABLE POINT

The motor function and stability of the shoulder are inseparable, as represented by the dynamic, stabilizing, coaptive components of the shoulder girdle musculature, especially the rotator cuff.

The self–stabilizing muscular control functions in external rotations by tensioning the functional anterior sling.[26,14,28] This control, however, is only effective in the first half of abduction when the subscapularis covers the humeral head. To dislodge it in this position requires a high energy force of sufficient magnitude to produce a capsulo–periosteal detachment.

In the cocked arm position, the humeral head has less stability. The humeral head is progressively less covered by the subscapularis[6] and escapes its control. Under the action of gravity and the force of the other shoulder muscles which now sublux rather than stabilize, the humeral head escapes inferiorly and anteriorly (Fig. 1). The subscapularis itself in the last degrees of abduction also becomes a subluxation force.[10,25]

The remaining structures which tend to stabilize the humeral head are passive restraints including the capsule, the labrum, and the prominence of the anteroinferior glenoid rim reinforced by scapular rotation and elevation during shoulder abduction.

To the extent that a constitutional or acquired capsular laxity exists, the huge kinetic energy developed for example, in cocking the arm for a "smash" in tennis, exceeds the strength of the passive restraints subluxing the humeral head in the anteroinferior direction. This dynamic instability may be manifested clinically by a primary dislocation or by a painful syndrome wrongly interpreted and treated in vain as a tendinitis. If the diagnosis is delayed, one can demonstrate a clinical evolution of the painful shoulder toward greater instability, first marked by a simple "click" and later by a movement in internal rotation which seems to be a self–reduction of a subluxation.[1,4]

Our 40 records of painful shoulders can be divided into three groups. These groups have a different character if they are at the beginning of the syndrome or close to the surgical decision (Fig. 2).

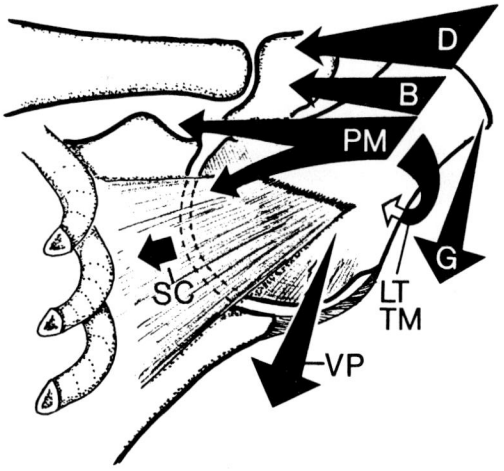

Figure 1 The humeral head escapes the self-stabilizing sling of the subscapularis.

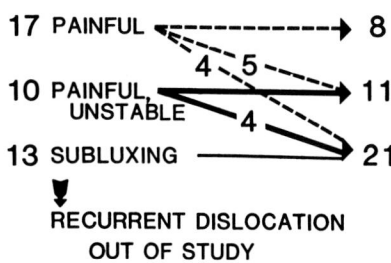

Figure 2 Clinical course.

Paralleling this clinical evolution, the lesions provide evidence of the passage of the humeral head out of its anatomical bounds. These lesions increase and become more complete in proportion to the frequency of the repeated episodes of instability which they facilitate. Initially, lesions of the labrum are seen as bony lesions of the glenoid rim and, finally, as detachment of the capsule and periostium. Therefore, early in the course, when the instability cannot be demonstrated clinically, the demonstration of these lesions of "passage" is most important for establishing the diagnosis.

RADIOGRAPHIC OBSERVATIONS

The lesions of the anteroinferior glenoid rim are even more frequently underestimated[4,13,15,21,24,28] than are Hill-Sachs lesions (which we are not considering in this study). The classical views (AP view and axillary lateral view), demonstrate only lesions extending beneath the inferior contour of the glenoid which are large enough to be seen on the axillary profile view, in which the whole anterior contour of the glenoid is superimposed on the area of the lesion.[13,21] With the scapula straightened (cocked arm position), the anteroinferior glenoid is projected forward in the shape of a prominent and easily recognizable triangle. This is the basis of the glenoid profile view. The technique is simple, the incident beam is 30° to 40° oblique from above. The image of a normal rim is superimposable on an anatomic drawing which verifies that the correct angle of incidence has been chosen (Fig. 3). The coracoid process must be close to the humeral head. If it is too far from the head as in the classic axillary view, the middle part of the anterior rim and not the inferior part is demonstrated.

Major fractures, demonstrating varying degrees of healing, involving one-third of the anteroinferior part of the glenoid are not rare in subluxations or recurrent dislocations. A beveled or worn appearance is easily recognizable when compared with the uninvolved side and is frequently seen in painful and unstable shoulders. Even a subtle lesion of this type is a sufficient basis for the diagnosis as we have shown in our comparison of the radiographic and operative findings in our 40 cases (Fig. 4). In two-thirds of our patients these lesions were only visible on the glenoid profile view even though sometimes the lesions could be

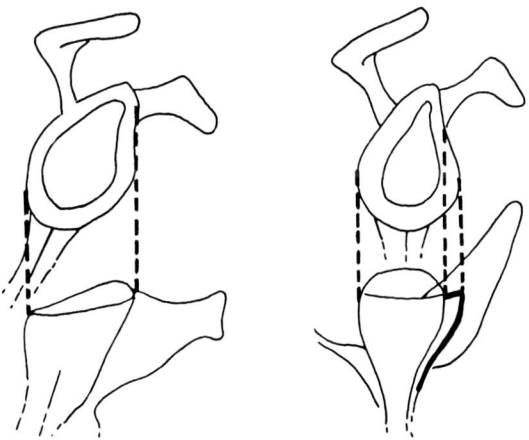

Figure 3 Steroid profile view—30° to 40° oblique from above.

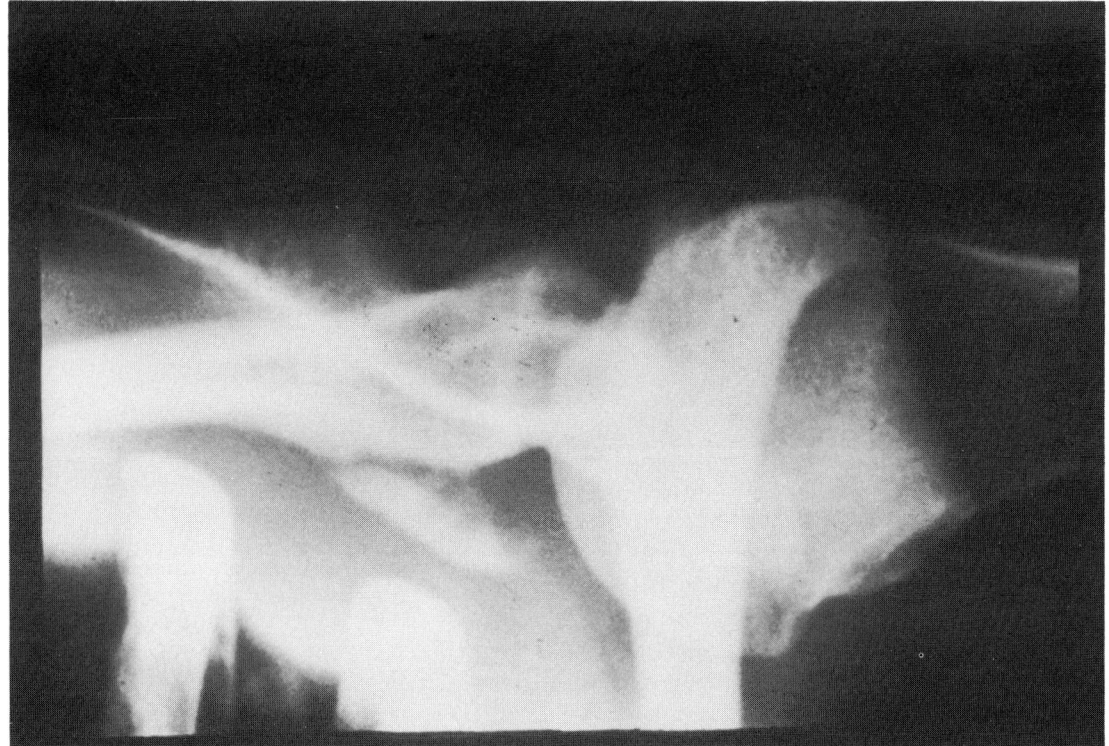

Figure 4 Glenoid profile view. Nonunited detached fragment of the anteroinferior glenoid rim.

suspected on the AP view by the loss of the inferior portion of the dense subchondral line.

With this radiographic view, we have demonstrated more lesions of the anterior glenoid rim than other authors.[17,18,20] This observation permits a better choice of procedure, in the operative treatment of recurrent dislocations. More than half of the lesions of the glenoid rim [23/40] were not suitable for a Bankart type repair.

It is in the diagnosis of the painful shoulder with inapparent instability that this study is the most important. In 58 percent of the painful syndromes and in 90 percent of the subluxations, this study permitted us to make the proper diagnosis.

If we add the Hill-Sachs lesions, alone or associated with glenoid rim lesions (17 out of 40 cases), we made 82.5 percent of formal diagnoses with a simple but rigorous radiographic protocol.[16] (Fig. 5).

Visualization of the Labrum

All the subluxations had bony lesions of the humeral head or the glenoid rim. Only seven of 13 painful shoulders with clinically inapparent instability had a totally negative standard radiographic protocol.

Different authors have emphasized the difficulties of diagnosis and the possibility of errors in such cases,[13,23,21] and seemed to be satisfied by an apprehension test for their operative decision.

We would rather try to visualize lesions of the labrum and have used contrast arthrotomography in the glenoid profile view, as opposed to arthroscopy which is a relatively new technique. Thus, as compared with a normal labrum, one can demonstrate displacement either by destruction or

40 PAINFUL UNSTABLE SHOULDERS

	BONEY LESIONS		
	HILL-SACH	GLENOID	TOTAL
8 PAINFUL	2	2	3
11 PAINFUL-UNSTABLE	7	9	9
21 SUBLUXATION	17	19	21
TOTAL-40	26	30*	33
			82.5%

* 2/3 ONLY VISIBLE ON GLENOID PROFILE VIEW

Figure 5

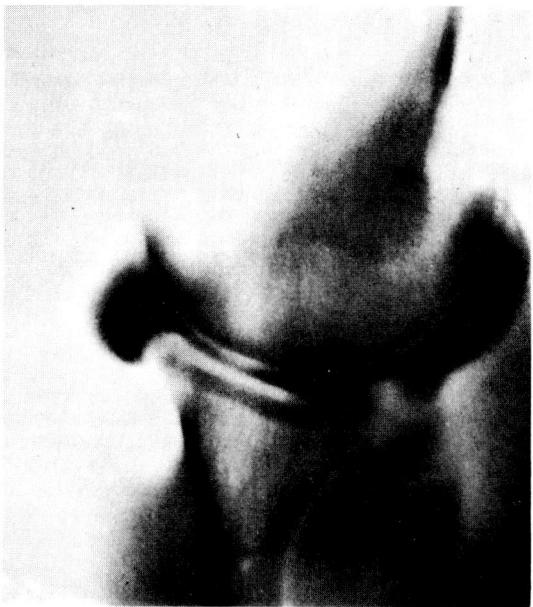

Figure 6 Contrast arthrotomography in the glenoid profile view. Complete avulsion of the labrum, which is still attached to the avulsed anterior capsule.

by detachment (Fig. 6). Destructive lesions as well as bucket handle tears of the labrum crossing the anterior joint space predict pathology with a high level of confidence. A comparison between arthrotomography and operative observations in 25 cases confirms no errors of interpretation.

On the other hand, a truncated appearance or a small or irregular labrum in normal position has to be interpreted with the same care as in the knee menisci. Two categories of diagnostic errors were made in these cases. At arthrotomy the lesions of the labrum were not constant, (31 lesions in 40 interventions for painful and unstable shoulders), and 3 times we found only simple capsular hyperlaxity.

When neither the radiographic protocol nor the arthrotomography can demonstrate a lesion, one should follow the patient to await the development of the anatomic lesions, or the evolution of clinical symptoms towards more instability. Surgical intervention should be contemplated only after formal confirmation of the diagnosis.

RECONSTRUCTION OF THE ANTEROINFERIOR BUTTRESS

It is important in the treatment of painful and unstable shoulders in athletes that full external rotation be preserved. To ensure this, an operative technique excluding any shortening of the subscapularis and providing for early postoperative mobilization is used. We trust neither the capsule nor the labrum, which we resect systematically, thus we have chosen the osseous buttress. A very complete buttress of the anteroinferior weak spot requires a triple locking technique with osseus, capsular and muscular restraint to subluxation (Fig. 7).

Osseus Locking

A buttress is carefully positioned far inferiorly and anteriorly at the level of the articular cartilage (without any step off) so that a wide retentive glenoid surface is rebuilt in its anteroinferior portion (as shown by the postoperative radiographic control).

The use of the coracoid buttress strongly screwed described by Latarget on 1954,[11] then by Helfet who had published a modified technique of Bristow procedure in 1958[8] resolved the problem of the bone graft and its union, things which had troubled Eden and Hybinette.[9] The position of their graft at the level of the articular cartilage was however the right one.

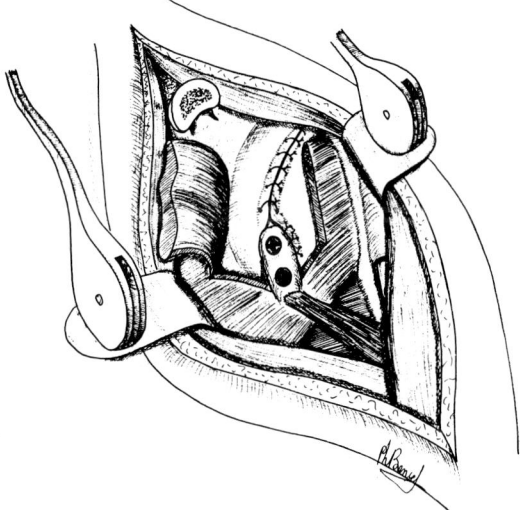

Figure 7 A very complete buttressing of the anteroinferior weak spot must be assured. We combine:
- a coracoid buttress placed far inferiorly
- a Bankart type repair between the anterior capsular "cul de sac" and the insertion of the short head of the biceps on the coracoid buttress
- an interwoven hammock constructed of the intact inferior half of the subscapularis and the short head of the biceps.

Capsular Locking

A Bankart repair is done between the anterior and inferior capsular cul de sac and the insertion of the short head of the biceps on the osseus buttress (transferred coracoid).

Sometimes if the capsule is of good quality we try to continue the Bankart repair higher, suturing the capsule to the remaining structures of the coracoacromial ligament on the external edge of the coracoid process.

Tendinomuscular Locking

This is essential from the point of view of dynamics. During the vertical section of the subscapularis, necessary for a wide arthrotomy, it is necessary to leave one-third of the inferior part of the muscle which will stay, therefore, behind the conjoined tendon. This portion will be maintained in position by the coracoid buttress. Using the Bristow idea, and improving the May[12] procedure, a very solid interwoven hammock constructed of the intact portion of the inferior subscapularis and the short head of the biceps is obtained, and can support the humeral head in the cocked arm position. This dynamic support seems to us to be fundamental; with the strength of the reconstruction thus assured, immediate postoperative rehabilitation can be used. This guarantees a return to normal external rotation, speed and power which is indispensible for the return to top–flight athletics—our only criterion of an acceptable result. We have had no recurrences in more than 100 cases.

In 30 shoulders in athletes with the dominant side operated (follow-up average 2 years), 23 had returned to their top level performance in the same sport. However, only 50 percent of very high risk competitors (such as javelin throwers, gymnasts, and martial arts competitors) who subject their shoulders to intense distorting forces returned to their preoperative form.

Conclusions

The potential of shoulder radiography seems to us to be undervalued. AP views with the humeral head in different positions, an axillary profile view, and mainly a glenoid profile view with or without an arthrotomography permits us to demonstrate the entire anteroinferior glenoid rim of which lesions are both common and significant.

Anterior instability of the shoulder is in fact an anteroinferior instability; this is the weak spot in the stabilizing structure of the shoulder. A rigorous radiographic protocol identifies accidents of instability, clinically unapparent and unknown, and points the way to effective surgical procedure for many incapacitating painful shoulders.

Furthermore, without this approach many of these shoulders would be ineffectively treated as only tendinitis.

REFERENCES

1. Bateman JE. The Shoulder and Neck. Vol. 1. Philadelphia, WB Saunders, 1978.
2. Bernageau J, Faguer B, Debeyre J. Etude arthropneumotomographique d'une luxation recidivante de l'epaule. Rev Rhum 1966; 33:135–137.
3. Bernageau J, Patte D, Debeyre J, Ferrane J. Interet du profil glenoidien dans les luxations recidivantes de l'epaule. Rev Chir Orthop 1976; 62:142–147.
4. Blazina ME, Satzman JS. Recurrent anterior subluxations of the shoulder in athletics. A distinct entity. In Proc Am Acad of Orthop Surgeons, J Bone Joint Surg 1969; 51-1:1037–1038.
5. Courroy JB. Les Epaules Douloureuses et Instables en Traumatologie sportive. Theses, Paris, 1979; 82.
6. Cyprien JM. La luxation recidivante de l'epaule. Theses 3649, Bale, Schwabe Ed. 1978.
7. Depalma AF. Surgery of the shoulder. Vol. 1. Philadelphia, JB Lippincott, 1973.
8. Helfet AJ. Coracoid transplantation for recurring dislocation of the shoulder. J Bone Joint Surg 1958; 40B-2:198–202.
9. Hybbinette S. De la transplantation d'un fragment osseux pour remedier aux luxations recidivantes de l'epaule. Acta Chir Scand 1934; 71:411.
10. Inmann VT, Saunders M, Abbott LC. Observation on the function of the shoulder joint. J Bone Joint Surg 1944; 26:1–30.
11. Latarget M. Technique de la butee coracoidienne preglenoidienne dans le traitement des luxations recidivantes de l'epaule. Lyon Chir 1958; 54-4:604–609.
12. May VR Jr. A modified Bristow operation for anterior recurrent dislocation of the shoulder. J Bone Joint Surg 1970; 52A-5:1010–1016.
13. Morton KS. The unstable shoulder: Recurring subluxation (in proceeding and reports of Gen. Orth. Assoc.). J Bone Joint Surg 1977; 59B-4:508.
14. Moseley HF, Overgaard B. Anterior capsular mechanism in recurrent anterior dislocation of the shoulder, J Bone Joint Surg 1962; 44B-4:913–927.
15. Neer II S, Welsh RP. The shoulder in sports. Orthop Clin of N Amer 1977; 8-3:583–591.
16. Patte D, Bernageau J, Rodineau J, Gardes JC. Epaules douloureuses et instables. Rev Chir Orthop 1980; 66:157–165.
17. Patte D, Debeyre J, Bernageau J. Die Bedeutung des vorderen Pfannenzardes bei rezidivieren den Schulter luxationen. Orthopade 1978; 7:194–198.

18. Patte D. Luxations recidivantes de l'epaule. E.M.C. Appareil Locomoteur 1980; 14037 C 20, 4.
19. Patte D, Debeyre J. Luxations recidivantes de l'epaule. E.M.C. Techniques chirurgicales, Orthopedie 1980; 44265.4.4.02.
20. Patte D. Instabilities anterieures de l'epaule. Cahier d'enseignement de la SOFCOT, Vol. 1, Exp. Scientif 1981; 15:55–66.
21. Protzman RR. Anterior instability of the shoulder. J Bone Joint Surg 1980; 62A-6:909–918.
22. Rodineau J, Krzentowski RL, Courroy JB. Une cause meconnue des douleurs de l'epaule: Les lesions du bourrelet et durebord glenoidien. Ann Med Phys 1978; 21:988–997.
23. Rowe CR, Narins B. Recurrent transient subluxation of the shoulder. J Bone Joint Surg 1981; 63A-6:863–861.
24. Rowe CR, Patel D, Southmayd WW. The Bankart procedure, a long-term result study. J Bone Joint Surg 1978; 60A:1–16.
25. Symeonides PP. The significance of the subcapularis muscle in the pathogenesis of recurrent dislocation of the shoulder. J Bone Joint Surg 1972; 54B:476–483.
26. Townley CO. The capsular mechanism in recurrent dislocations of the shoulder. J Bone Joint Surg 1950; 33A-2:370–380.
27. Trillat A, Dejour H, Roullet J. Luxation recidivante de l'epaule et syndrome du bourrelet glenoidien. Rev Chir Orthop 1965; 51-6:525–544.
28. Trillat A, Leclerc-Chelvet F. Luxation recidivante de l'epaule Vol. 1, Paris, Masson Ed, 1973.

GLENOID OSTEOTOMY FOR LOOSE SHOULDER

KATSUYA NOBUHARA, M.D. and HITOSHI IKEDA, M.D.

The shoulder complex is unique for the close interrelationship of three separate joint complexes working in unison to provide the greatest range of motion of any joint in the body yet preserving stability throughout this whole range.[1] There are varying degrees of mobility of the shoulder complex, with certain body types being predisposed to abnormal hypermobility. The idiopathic loose shoulder syndrome involves a multidirectional instability which can constitute a severe clinical problem. This is well demonstrated in Figure 1 where there is an anteroposterior instability of the humeral head and outward slipping of the arm in an elevated position.

The important feature of this condition is that this instability is strictly intracapsular. There is no breech of capsular integrity, unlike recurrent dislocation where the glenoid labrum has been stripped from the anterior aspect of the glenoid rim. The glenoid in this condition appears to be deficient, and the loosening would seem to be attributable to a dysplasia of the glenoid itself. It is for this reason that we have recommended glenoid osteotomy to patients disabled by the loose shoulder syndrome.

Clinical Material

Fifty-five patients with 76 involved shoulders were treated surgically. 21 patients had bilateral problems, there was a slightly higher incidence in females. The ages ranged from seven to 39 years with an average of 18, confirming that this is a problem among adolescents and young adults. Prior to surgery, a considerable observation period with conservative orthopaedic care was undertaken for an average of 2.5 years. Patients were commonly disabled by pain with activity, 86 percent being affected in this way. Instability was a common feature with 58 percent being severely limited by insecurity of shoulder function.

Objectively, major instability was evident in all patients, with easily demonstrable anteroposterior instability in 74 percent and marked apprehension and discomfort in 42 percent. In every instance, x-ray confirmation of instability was demonstrated with the arm elevated. An arthrogram showing an accumulation of contrast media in the upper portion of the humeral head (snow cap phenomenon) induced by downward traction of the upper limb carried out as a routine part of the arthrographic examination (Fig. 2).

Most importantly, all cases confirmed on axillary x-ray a deficiency of the posterior margin of the glenoid. (Fig. 3).

The range of motion of these involved shoulder joints was demonstrably greater than that found in normal subjects. The strength of muscle groups, however, was basically unaffected although there seemed to be a slight tendency for latissimus dorsi to be a little weaker than that of normal subjects.

SURGICAL PROCEDURE

With the patient positioned prone, a longitudinal incision 7 centimeters in length was made from the acromial angle toward the axilla. The posterior fibers of the deltoid and infraspinatus were separated to reveal the capsule. The capsule was frequently found to be quite slack and actually impinging in the posterior joint space. The capsule was opened vertically with a transverse extension made inferiorly towards the scapular neck to expose the inferior surface of the glenoid. Careful exposure of the inferior surface of the glenoid was essential to define the scapular neck. One to 1.5 centimeters from the glenoid margin, an osteotomy was made in the scapular neck and wedged open until loosening in the capsular structures was eliminated. The optimal position having been determined, an iliac crest bone graft was interposed to wedge the osteotomy open. Postoperatively, the

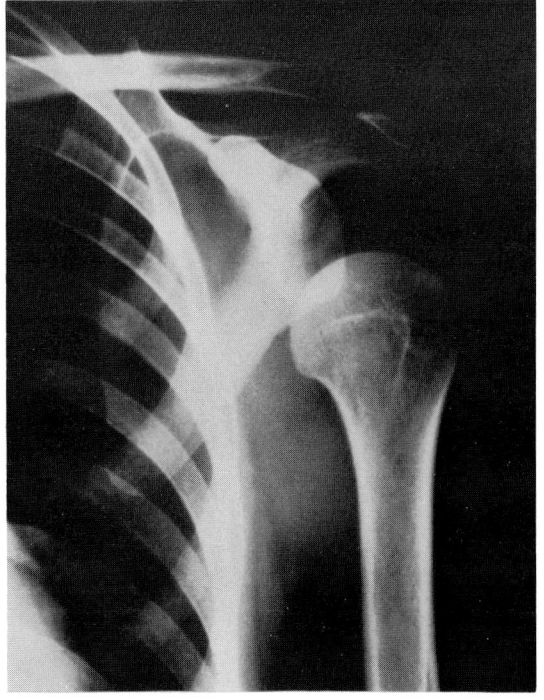 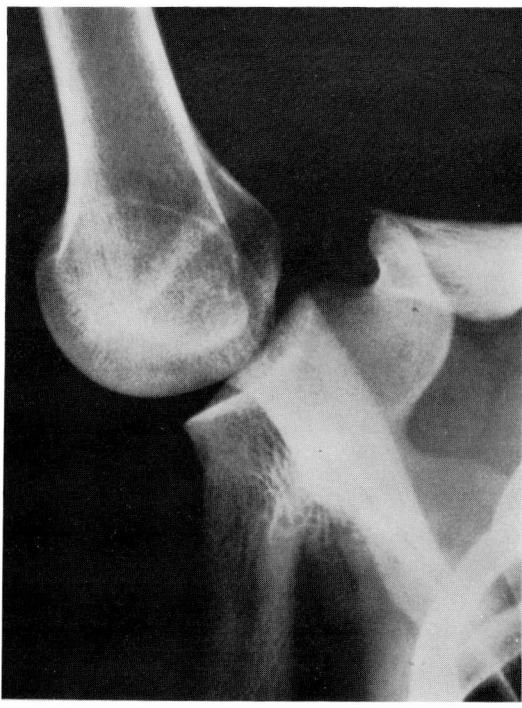

Figure 1 (a) Inferior subluxation, (b) Posterior subluxation

Zero^2 position was maintained with skin traction, before a body spica was applied maintaining an abducted position for two weeks before the shoulder was gradually allowed to return to the side of the body.

Fifty-six of the 76 patients have been reviewed more than one year following osteotomy. The average follow-up time was 2 years 8 months with the most common symptom noted being pain with activity in 26 instances. Some local discomfort was present in 27 percent, and in 32 percent a sense of instability with heavy lifting was noted. Clinical loosening was observed in only one instance; symptomatic instability was almost completely controlled.

X-ray examinations show effectively the control of the tendency to slip (Fig. 4). To quantitate the degree of slipping preoperatively and the control achieved postoperatively, x-ray studies were obtained in the elevated position. Two angles were measured, the angle between the straight line drawn from the inferior margin of the glenoid toward the center of the humeral head and the horizontal (alpha), and the angle between the straight line from the inferior margin of the glenoid to the superior margin of the glenoid, and the horizontal

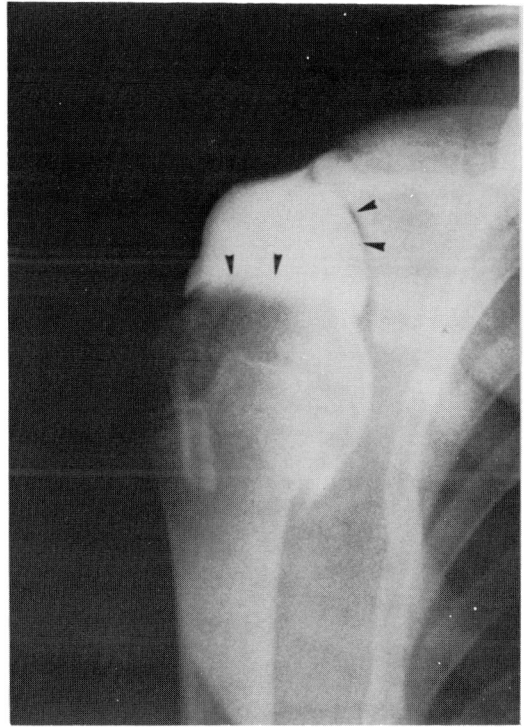

Figure 2 Snow cap phenomenon

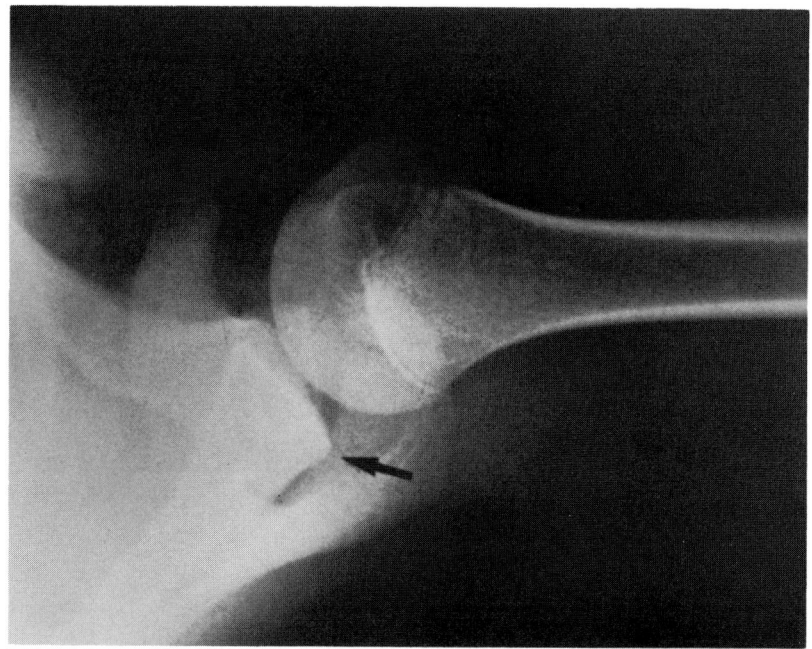

Figure 3 Posterior defect of the glenoid

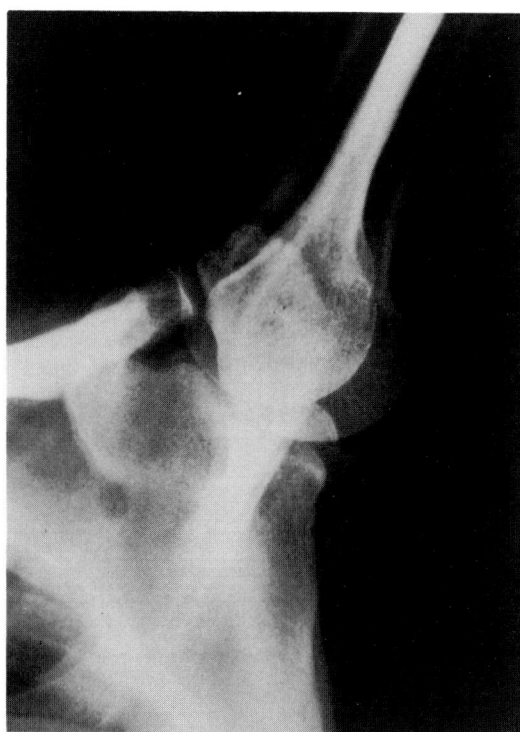

Figure 4 The effectiveness of osteotomy

(beta). Used in conjunction, a glenohumeral index could be determined, these angles being measured in pre- and postoperative patients as well as in 60 normal, healthy subjects between the age of 10 and 40 years.

Results indicate that the alpha and beta values were greater in preoperative patients than in the normal, indicating the slipping of the humeral head beyond the glenoid margin. It is interesting that the values for postoperative patients closely approximate those in normal subjects, suggesting that the humeral head regained its normal fulcrum as a consequence of the osteotomy.

The range of motion in postoperative subjects was certainly reduced from the previous preoperative hypermobile tendency. There was a significant difference in lateral elevation and external rotation between the preoperative group and the postoperative group, but the flexion range was within the normal values in both pre- and postoperative cases.

It was interesting to note that muscular strength was improved in many instances, particularly in the trapezius, the pectoralis major and the middle fibers of the deltoid. It is suggested that, with restoration of the normal fulcrum, a greater efficiency is possible for those muscles acting about the shoulder joint.

Complications encountered included anterior dislocation of the shoulder in two instances due to excessive anterior inclination of the glenoid. Breakdown of the graft occurred in one instance following a fall while one further patient suffered nerve damage from a compression syndrome in cast.

DISCUSSION

Glenoid osteotomy is an effective means of dealing with the problem of the loose shoulder syndrome with multiaxial instability. The benefits of glenoid osteotomy include:

1. Establishment of a new fulcrum for functioning of the shoulder musculature because of the increased inclination of the glenoid and the reestablishment of normal tensions within the rotator cuff.

2. Tendency of the humeral head to slip is controlled by the bony reconstitution of the posterior-inferior margin of the glenoid.

3. The slackness of the posterior joint capsule is completely controlled by a combination of osteotomy and capsulorrhaphy.

4. The reestablishment of the setting phase[3] of shoulder movement is enhanced by osteotomy and repositioning of the glenoid.

REFERENCES

1. Codman EA. The shoulder. Boston: Thomas Todd, 1934.
2. Saha AK. Zero position of the glenohumeral joint. Ann R Coll Surg 1958; 22:223–236.
3. Inman VT et al. Observations on the function of the shoulder joint. J Bone Joint Surg 1944; 26:1–30.

THE ROLE OF THE TENDON OF THE LONG HEAD OF THE BICEPS BRACHII IN ANTERIOR SUBLUXATION OF THE SHOULDER

PAUL M. GRAMMONT, M.D., RAINER P. MAYER, M.D., and JOCHEN R. LÖHR, M.D.

CLINICAL FINDINGS

In a 6-year period we observed six cases of conjoint luxation of the long biceps tendon with complete anterior dislocation of the shoulder. The first such case was a 50-year-old man who had sustained a high velocity fall. Anterior dislocation of the shoulder was diagnosed and treated by closed reduction under general anesthesia. The reduction proved to be difficult and unstable and the patient was therefore referred to our orthopedic clinic with symptoms of a frozen shoulder and residual sensitive paralysis of the ulnar nerve. On examination it became obvious that the shoulder had been left in anterosuperior luxation, and it was decided that the patient should go on to an open reduction of his shoulder.

The operation was performed by a delto–pectoral approach with the patient supine. Since the humeral head appeared to be displaced under the coracoid process and coracoid muscle group, the apophysis was detached in order to permit verification of the shoulder dislocation and the nerve injury. The brachial plexus was found to have an increased vascular injection, but no macroscopic lesion was found. The head of the humerus was then reduced by lateral rotation of the arm; it redislocated spontaneously, until, by superior approach to the joint along the subscapularis tendon, it became evident that the long biceps tendon had become entrapped into the joint. The intertubercular groove at the humeral head was found to be empty, the tendon being medially luxated with the transverse ligament torn; the tendon's path ran directly from the superior edge of the pectoralis major to its glenoid attachment.

Once the tendon was freed from the joint by traction, the humeral head was easily reduced, but could not be kept in place until the tendon had been repositioned into the intertubercular groove.

It was evident that the tendon, functioning like a bowstring, held the humeral head back and downwards, thus prohibiting recurrent anterior dislocation. In lateral rotation of the arm, the biceps tendon would give even more support; in medial rotation this would be diminished, allowing the head in extreme medial rotation to dislocate completely. In this case the tendon would jump over the medial tuberosity, and therefore become dislocated. To obviate this double luxation of both head and tendon, the biceps tendon was secured under the tuberosities in a deep groove, the bone bed being smoothed with bone wax.

The tendon was now stable in all rotational positions and would easily move vertically when the elbow was moved from full extension to full flexion. The coracoid process was then reaffixed with a screw and wound closure was facilitated in layers. A suction drain was implanted, to be removed after 48 hours. Active-passive ROM exercises were initiated immediately postoperatively and two months after the operation, the shoulder was found to be stable, painless, and with a good ROM, but strength appeared to be insufficient.

We have treated two other quite similar cases, one being a chronic recurrent dislocation in a 70-year-old farmer, the other an acute case in an active sportsman. In all three cases the tendon appeared to be the major obstacle in reducing the head; and reposition and fixation of the biceps tendon in a deep groove was the only way to attain a stable position of the head anteriorly.

DISCUSSION OF CLINICAL SYMPTOMS

Studies on the stability of the long head of the biceps brachii have rarely been reported with reference to the stability of the glenohumeral joint, especially from a clinical point of view. During the same six years of our report, we have treated 8 other cases of so-called isolated luxation of the biceps tendon; in all cases the major clinical sign was painful jumping of the tendon, always associated with a relative degree of instability and weakness of the shoulder, especially in the active sportsman. We believe that in these types of "singular luxation of the tendon" the humeral head is unstable to a minor degree.

Bera (Paris, 1910) described the general symptoms for biceps tendon luxation and elongation and emphasized a special sign of permanent luxation of this tendon. On physical examination, it appears abnormally long and can be palpated under the anterior head of the deltoid when the biceps is contracted. Gilcrest (1934) studied 100 cases with pathologic biceps tendons and described his own test: reproduction of the painful jump when the shoulder is passed from an elevated position into its normal functional position. Abbott and Saunders (1939) described six cases of surgery for acute luxation of the biceps tendon; their technique consisted of excision of the intra-articular part of the tendon and fixation of the distal portion in the intertubercular groove. We believe that this suppresses the painful jump, but provides weaker anterosuperior stability of the shoulder. Hitchcock and Bechtol (1948) undertook a large study on the anatomical structures emphasizing the importance of a flat chest and short forearm in the mechanism of luxation; they also demonstrated clearly how the medial wall of the sulcus intertubercularis determines the luxation tendency.

Each of these authors studied luxation of the biceps tendon separate from the functional motion of the shoulder joint. In our experience, the long head of the biceps has two main functions: (1) To guide the humeral head in abduction-lateral rotation movements. This type of movement is essential before throwing: the tendon of the long biceps obeys the rule of "progressive straightness" especially when the biceps is contracted, the elbow flexed and, e.g., a javelin kept in the hand. (2) To keep the humeral head low and retropositioned during the throwing movement. The predominant action of the lateral rotating muscles and the humeral elevation at the beginning of the cyclus aim at an anterosuperior instability; the long biceps tendon counteracts this mechanism. Sliding of the tendon in its groove is necessary during the movement; this explains the frequent tendinitis of the long biceps tendon in throwing sports.

The surgical technique used for all cases of tendon luxation, with or without associated humeral dislocation, was the deepening of the tendon's groove and its reduction of tendon in the groove, as well as suture of the transverse ligament. We feel that isolated suture of the ligament is insufficient in avoiding future dislocation.

RESULTS AND DISCUSSION

Deepening of the groove and reduction of the tendon were performed in three cases of "double luxation" and in five of eight cases for "single luxation." In each case, immediate postoperative active-passive motion exercises were initiated and ROM was excellent after two months. There was full stability immediately postoperative except in one case of secondary "labrum syndrome" in a 20-year-old woman. The joint was surgically opened and part of the labrum removed; the shoulder has since been stable. Pain was a constant finding (long head tendinitis) during the first three postoperative months; it was treated by chemical and physical means, never by local injections. After three months, all shoulders were virtually pain free. The strength of the shoulder, depending on stability and pain, was found to be good three months post surgery.

Of the remaining cases, one was treated with the Abbott technique and went on to a good result; two patients refused surgery and were treated by physiotherapy alone, without any improvement of the clinical signs. The diagnosis was made based on clinical findings since radiology is so far of limited use. It is difficult to make a diagnosis from an arthrogram with the long head of the biceps being medially displaced; it is similarly difficult in the case of a recurrently dislocating humeral head because the film has to be made exactly at the moment of the dislocation. Computerized tomography appears to be useful in obtaining a real measurement of the abnormality in the tendon groove.

As instability of the long head of the biceps tendon is rather frequent (probably more than 10%) some cases will need surgical treatment. The role of the tendon in the stability of the humeral head lies especially in the prevention of an anterior-superior displacement; further it avoids subacromial impingement or chronic rotator cuff tears. For these reasons the deepening of the intertubercular groove seems to provide a double stability, i.e. to the tendon as well as to the humeral head (although it does not prevent a postoperative tendinitis).

OUDARD-IWAHARA'S OPERATION FOR RECURRENT ANTERIOR DISLOCATION OF THE SHOULDER

RYUJI YAMAMOTO, M.D.

Some years ago, after reviewing the operative methods then available, the late Professor Jinnaka[1] of Kyushu University commented that what he needed was a new operation for recurrent dislocation of the shoulder which would be applicable to all cases, simple to perform, free of postoperative recurrence, and would preserve full joint mobility. This sounds naïve and optimistic today considering the various bony, ligamentous and muscular defects and dysfunctions found responsible for recurrent dislocations. He postulated an ideal, but did not elaborate a solution.

Oudard's operation as modified by Iwahara is basically an augmentation of the coracoid process, an extra-articular, simple procedure which is uniquely free of postoperative recurrence and complication. Oudard[2] first described it in 1924 as an operation consisting of augmentation of the coracoid process with bone grafting and tightening of the subscapularis muscle by plicating sutures (Fig. 1). The original method gave disappointing results in the early days because of frequent recurrences. Jinnaka[3] in 1939 proposed a modification in which he placed the grafted bone anterior to the humeral head. Plication of the subscapularis muscle was not included in this modified version. Iwahara[4] in 1954 further modified the method by embedding the graft in the coracoid process after splitting it longitudinally in the middle, thus eliminating the use of fixing devices for the graft. Plication of the subscapularis muscle was again omitted in this version. This is the operation I now regularly apply to cases with recurrent dislocation, with further minor modifications of my own.

OPERATIVE TECHNIQUE (Fig. 2)

A skin incision is made over the medial border of the deltoid muscle and extended toward the coracoid process reaching the lower edge of the clavicle. The fascia is incised along the cephalic vein and blunt dissection is carried out between the deltoid and the pectoralis major muscles down to the anterior aspect of the coracoid process. The coracoid process and the conjoined tendon of the coracobrachial and the short head of the biceps muscles are now brought into full view by dissecting away the soft tissues surrounding them. The coracoid process is divided longitudinally in the middle. While doing this, the osteotome is pointed to the clavicle rather than in an anteroposterior direction to avoid injuring the major vessels. The conjoined tendon is also divided in the middle for a distance of 3 cm or so in an extension of the split of the coracoid process.

A bone graft measuring $5 \times 1.5 \times 0.8$ cm, with periosteum attached, is taken from the iliac crest. I have found it helpful to trim the upper end of the graft from both sides so that it will fit snugly into the slit in the coracoid process. The graft is placed with the attached periosteum facing up and driven into the slit by gently tapping it. The tail of the graft is embedded in the muscle substance. The coracoid process and the conjoined tendon are closed over the graft with interrupted silk sutures.

The shoulder is immobilized in a Desault bandage for 3 weeks. Active movement is allowed at the fourth week while the arm is held in a sling, the latter being removed at the sixth postoperative week.

Results

Over the past 22 years I have operated on 88 patients with recurrent dislocation, amounting to a total of 90 joints in all. During the first half of this period, 1961 to 1975, Oudard-Iwahara's operation was my choice only for those patients who dislocated infrequently, five or six times a year or so. For those with more frequent episodes I

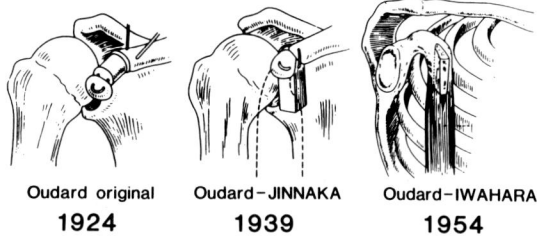

Figure 1 Stabilization of the shoulder by subcoracoid bone block.

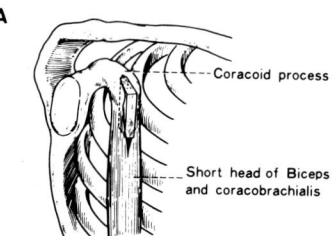

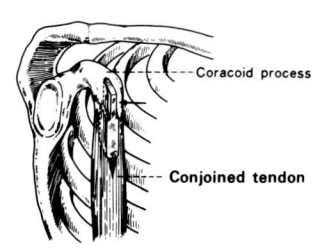

Figure 2 Technique.

would do either Bankart's or Bristow's procedure, or Eden-Hybbinette's operation for those with bony defects on the glenoid rim. A review at this point revealed that those who had undergone Oudard-Iwahara's operation fared much better in terms of the incidence of postoperative recurrence and complications than those who had been treated otherwise.

I started doing exclusively Oudard-Iwahara's operation on all the cases with recurrent dislocation regardless of its clinical and anatomical features, except for a few conditions to be discussed below. Table 1 summarizes the clinical features of the 76 patients in this series. A criterion for inclusion in the study was a reliable postoperative follow-up longer than one year. Males overwhelmingly outnumbered females with a ratio of four to one. It somewhat more frequently affected the dominant arm. Mean age of the initial episode of traumatic dislocation was 19 years. The patient came to operation at a mean age of 23, an average of 4.5 years having elapsed from the initial dislocation. Only 29 joints (37%) received adequate immobilization of the affected shoulder following closed reduction at the initial episode.

TABLE 1 Clinical Features of the Series

Total	76 patients, 78 joints	
Male	61 patients	
Female	15 patients	
Right shoulder	44 patients	
Left shoulder	30 patients	
Bilateral shoulder	2 patients	
Dominant side	44 joints	
Non-dominant	34 joints	
	Range	*Average*
Age < Initial dislocation	12–59	19
Age < Operation	13–62	23
Interval	1–23	4.5
Immobilization as the initial treatment	29 jts (37%)	

Postoperative recurrence was seen in five cases (6.4%) in the entire series (Table 2), three in 22 (13.6%) following Bankart's operation, one each following Bristow's (8.3%) and Oudard-Iwahara's (2.3%). This last patient dislocated one year after the operation when he was involved in a motorcycle accident. The dislocation was caused by the impact of the full weight of the motorcycle on his operated shoulder. He has never dislocated since then.

Limitation to range of movement, especially to external rotation, was the postoperative complication in 21 of 78 joints (27.0%) in the entire series while only in seven of 43 cases (16%) following Oudard-Iwahara's operation. It was observed in over 40 percent of the cases treated with other types of operation. Fate of the graft was studied carefully throughout the follow-up period by repeated roentgenography (Tab. 3, Fig. 3). In no case was the graft totally absorbed. Among the various changes the graft underwent as it stayed in the site, tapering at the distal end was found in 22 out of 43 cases (51.2%), thinning-out in its entire length in 14 cases (32.6%). The progress of these changes seemed to be arrested at two years postoperatively and the graft appeared about the same on the repeat x-ray thereafter.

Fracture of the grafted bone occurred in four cases (9.3%) and the graft was displaced from the coracoid process in three cases (6.9%). It was notable that none of these patients had recurrence of dislocation.

TABLE 2 Operative Results

Operative Technique	No. of Joints	Follow-up (Mean) In Years, Months	Recurrence	Limited ROM
Bankart	22	10, 4	3 (13.6%)	9 (40.9%)
Bristow modified	12	7, 1	1 (8.3%)	5 (41.5%)
Eden-Hybbinette	1	16, 0	0	
Oudard-Iwahara	43	5, 6	1 (2.3%)	7 (16.0%)
Total	78	6, 11	5 (6.4%)	21 (27.0%)

Case 1. (Fig. 4) A 35-year old female, on the nondominant side, 21 years postoperatively, no recurrence, full range of movement. The graft appears tapered, well fused and stable. She is currently engaged in active professional skiing.

Case 2. (Fig. 5) A 35-year old male, on his dominant side, 12 years after operation, no recurrence, full range of movement. The thinned out graft, shows clearly on the axial view. He is an active professional bowler.

Case 3. (Fig. 6) A 28-year old professional baseball player, with frequent dislocations. I implanted an extra-large graft measuring 7 cm in this case. Four years after the operation, the graft appears slightly tapered but stays in situ and intact. He has full range of movement and won the award for stealing the most bases during the 1982 season.

Case 4. (Fig. 7) A 30-year old housewife. The appearance of the graft on these films taken at two years and 7.5 years postoperatively is unchanged. Resorption apparently did not progress after two years.

DISCUSSION

Oudard-Iwahara's operation can claim two distinct advantages over other methods. Its simplicity and better results are evident. It is an entirely extra-articular procedure and spares the delicate joint structures from operative injuries. It is an improvement over its predecessors in eliminating the use of foreign material for fixation of the graft. Thus it is a simple and safe procedure. This presumably contributes to its second major advantage: postoperative limitation to range of movement occurred far less frequently following this operation than any other. Moreover, postoperative recurrence was an exception in this group, one in 43 cases. Even this solitary case was a result of a motorcycle accident and the patient has never dislocated since. This is without doubt a case of traumatic dislocation and not of postoperative recurrence.

There seem to be two separate mechanisms by which Oudard-Iwahara's operation effectively prevents recurrence. The augmented coracoid process

TABLE 3 Fate of the Graft

	No. of Cases	Percentage
No resorption	0	
Tapered	22 joints	51.2%
Thinned out	14 joints	32.6%
Fractured	4 joints	9.3%
Displaced	3 joints	6.9%

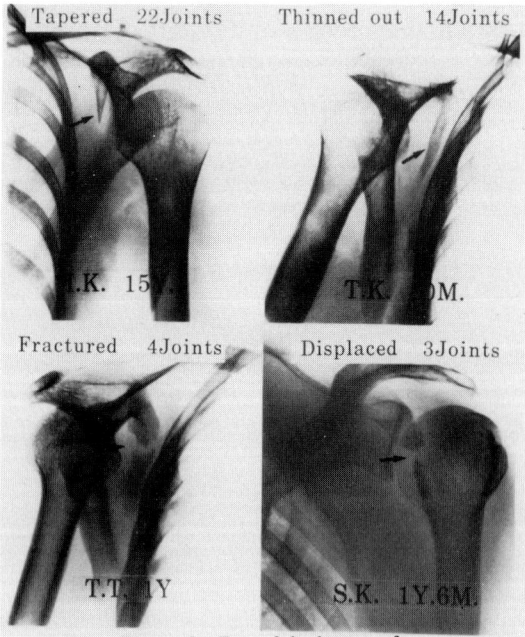

Figure 3 Fate of the bone graft.

Sports Injuries—Shoulder Stabilization / **109**

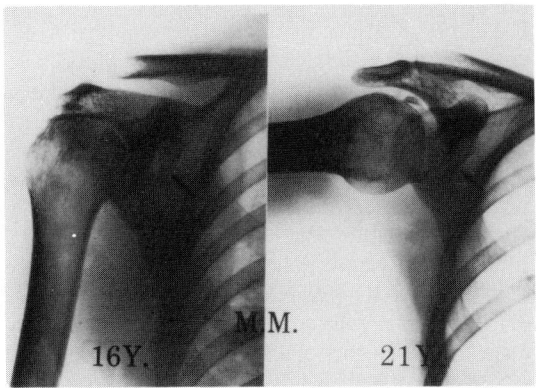

Figure 4 Graft well stabilized 21 years after operation.

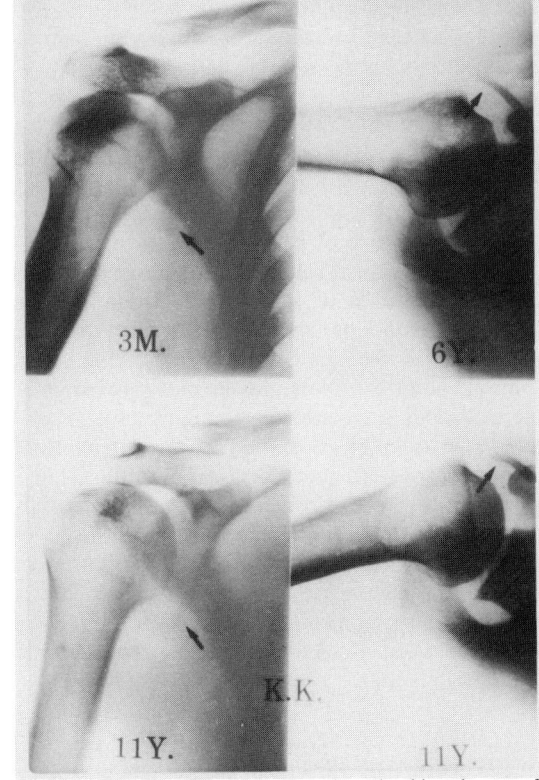

Figure 5 Twelve years after operation, the thinned-out graft is clearly seen in axial view.

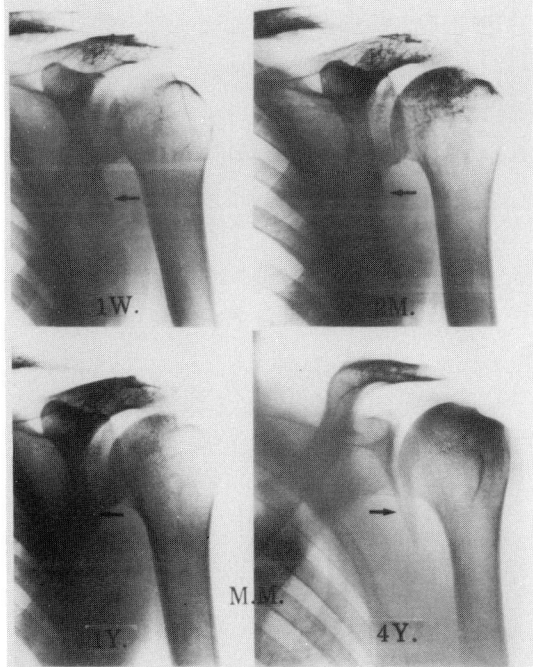

Figure 6 A large graft is tapered but intact 4 years after operation.

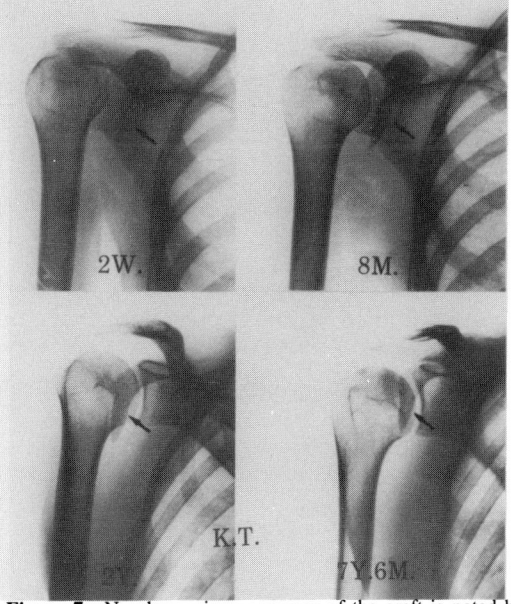

Figure 7 No change in appearance of the graft is noted between 2 and 7½ years after operation.

can act as a mechanical block preventing the humeral head from sliding over the anterior ridge of the glenoid fossa. In addition, or as an alternative, the graft sits on the subscapularis muscle and enhances the tone of this muscle by compression. It is conceivable that the enhanced tone and function of the subscapularis muscle brought about by the presence of the graft in the conjoined tendon play an important part in producing uniquely good results in this group of patients.

My only reservation in recommending this method for cases of recurrent dislocation is for those based on loose shoulder. I have not tried this operation as the sole procedure in these cases. Some type of capsulotendinous plasty is indicated here. In addition, certain congenital anomalies preclude the use of this operation. I[5] have encountered a patient with frequent dislocations following a rugby injury whose coracoid process was grossly hypoplastic. In addition, the short head of the biceps muscle originated from the soft tissues around, instead of from, the coracoid process in this case, making Oudard-Iwahara's operation out of the question. Bankart's procedure produced satisfactory results.

Summary

Oudard's operation originally consisted of augmentation of the coracoid process with bone grafting and plication of the subscapularis muscle. Later modifications of the method established the current Oudard-Iwahara's operation which is a simple, extra-articular bone-grafting to augment the coracoid process without subscapularis plication. My personal experience with the method in about 50 percent of the total 88 patients (90 joints) proved its efficacy in terms of prevention of recurrence and preservation of full joint mobility. Many patients have gone back to professional athletic activity. Its enhancing effect on the subscapularis muscle was considered the main mechanism by which this operation effectively prevents postoperative recurrences.

REFERENCES

1. Jinnaka S. Textbook of orthopedic surgery. Ed. 9. p. 335. Tokyo. Nanzando. 1966.
2. Oudard M. La luxation recidivante de l'epaule. Procede operatiore. J Chir 1923; 23:13–25.
3. Jinnaka S. Modification of Oudard's operation. Geka 1939; 3:1–5.
4. Iwahara T. Modification of Oudard's operation. Shujitsu 1954; 8:393–399.
5. Yamamoto R. Anomalous coracoid process as a cause of recurrent dislocation of the shoulder joint. The Journal of the Western Pacific Orthopedic Ass. 1974; Vol. 11, No. 2.

ANALYSIS OF FAILED REPAIR FOR SHOULDER INSTABILITY—A PRELIMINARY REPORT

TOM R. NORRIS, M.D. and LOUIS U. BIGLIANI, M.D.

To achieve a successful surgical repair of the glenohumeral joint, ideally one must be able to establish an accurate diagnosis, perform a repair based on the anatomical pathology, avoid hardware complications and conduct appropriate postoperative management. Errors in following these steps have resulted in surgery for the wrong diagnosis, to the wrong side of the shoulder, or repair of only one component of a multidirectional instability (Tab. 1). This has been an ongoing problem in orthopaedics. Sisk and Boyd stated: "It has been universally accepted that an operative procedure is the only sure way of curing a recurrent anterior dislocation of the shoulder while retaining its function. There all unanimity of opinion ceases." Reoperations may be required for arthritis resulting from a repair which was too tight, hardware complications, retained loose bodies, infection or neurovascular injury. Large Hill-Sachs defects, failure to repair labral detachments[11] or inadequate postoperative immobilization may result in residual subluxation or redislocation.

Anatomy

The shoulder has the greatest range of motion of any joint in the body. This is at the expense of bony stability. Unlike the acetabulum of the hip, the glenoid is rather flat and does not match the curvature of the humeral head.[3] At all times, only one-quarter to one-third of the head articulates with the glenoid. The stability of the glenohumeral joint is provided by the static support of the capsule and ligaments and reinforced by the dynamic action of the rotator cuff.[12] With the addition of the glenoid labrum, the arc of curvature approaches that of the humeral head.[18] The posterior labrum blends with the long head of the biceps, the posterior capsule and the glenoid periosteum. The anterior labrum, comprised primarily of the medial portion of the inferior glenohumeral ligament, is the strongest ligament in the shoulder. It provides an important barrier against anterior inferior subluxation, and is especially important when the arm is abducted and externally rotated.[20]

Clinical Evaluation

The differential diagnoses of shoulder instability include impingement lesions, arthritic lesions of the glenohumeral joint and acromioclavicular joint and a snapping scapula. In the absence of a complete dislocation, the patient may report episodes of locking, catching, slipping or even transient neurological symptoms extending down the arm.[17] Common findings of physical examination include anterior or posterior apprehension with stress testing,[14] a palpable subluxation or bounce, excessive external rotation or evidence of other loose joints. Common associated roentgenographic findings may include a Hill-Sachs posterior lateral humeral head defect,[4] loose bodies, and soft–tissue calcification on the anterior-inferior glenoid rim with anterior instability.[15] With posterior instability there may be a "reverse Hill-Sachs" head defect, bone reaction or soft tissue calcification adjacent to the glenoid rim or fracture of the posterior glenoid. Wear with loss of version in the posterior one-third to one-half of the glenoid may even occur. Upright traction films with 25-lb weights strapped to the forearms may demonstrate excessive inferior subluxation of the humeral head with inferior capsular laxity.[8] Double-contrast arthrotomograms and CAT scans to demonstrate glenoid labrum tears are difficult to interpret but helpful in specialized centers where the radiologists have developed the expertise.

Most important is a reassessment at the time of surgery. During the examination under anesthesia, the instability and its direction(s) can be confirmed. The C-arm fluoroscopic unit in the axial plane allows for visual confirmation of the palpable clicks, subluxations, or bounces. It is particularly helpful in avoiding surgery to the wrong side of the shoulder.[10]

TABLE 1 Causes of Failed Instability Repairs

Wrong Diagnosis	Ununited Bone Block
Wrong Side of Shoulder	Missed Loose Body
Multidirectional	Arthritis
Redislocate	too tight
Residual Subluxation	too loose
Labral Detachment Unrepaired	Neurovascular Injury
Hardware Complications	Infection
intra-articular	Inadequate Immobilization
or loose	

Materials

Between 1979 and 1983 we evaluated 42 patients with shoulder instability who had had 73 previous failed surgeries. These included 33 males and nine females ranging in age between 15 and 57 (mean = 31.5 years); 25 involved the right and 17 the left shoulder, one was bilateral. The dominant shoulder was affected in 25 patients.

Nine patients underwent 13 operations for the wrong diagnosis. These included operations for suspected impingement lesions, subluxing biceps, or acromioclavicular arthritis despite normal roentgenographs. It is often difficult to distinguish postoperatively between repairs that were carried out to the wrong side of the shoulder and repairs addressing only one component of multidirectional instability. In the latter, a repair to one side of the loose shoulder will displace it to the opposite side.[8] To the next examining physician it will appear that the repair was carried out to the wrong side.

There were four patients in this series who, in our opinion, had undergone operations to the wrong side of the shoulder. There were 3 patients who underwent 10 operations for multidirectional instability. An example is one patient who had had an anterior procedure resecting his glenoid labrum, a reexamination under anesthesia for instability, followed later by a posterior Putti-Platt for suspected instability. Postoperatively he was immobilized in wide abduction and forward flexion in an airplane splint. Obvious surgical errors included resection of the anterior labrum which increased his anterior and inferior instability and improper positioning following a posterior repair. A less obvious error was that the patient was not unstable posteriorly prior to his surgery to that side. Approaches to both sides subsequently were required for successful reconstruction.

Seventeen of the patients redislocated, 15 were symptomatic residual subluxers and six were found to be excessively tight.

The potential hazards of using metal in the shoulder region cannot be overemphasized.[7] Hardware complications played a role in 17 patients. In one a staple penetrated the joint and destroyed the articular surface (Figs. 1A, B). Residual inferior instability was still present two operations later. Loose or broken staples necessitated additional surgery in six.

Symptomatic nonunions (Fig. 2) of the coracoid with loosening of the screw occurred in 11 patients. Residual inferior subluxation below the Bristow repair (Fig. 3) in eight required special steps to recreate and dissect free the inferior capsule for a successful reconstruction. These were among the most difficult reoperations in the series since the scar extended from the skin down to the bone and imtimately involved the axillary nerve. Attempts to recreate the normal planes of anatomy are far more difficult than it would have been to

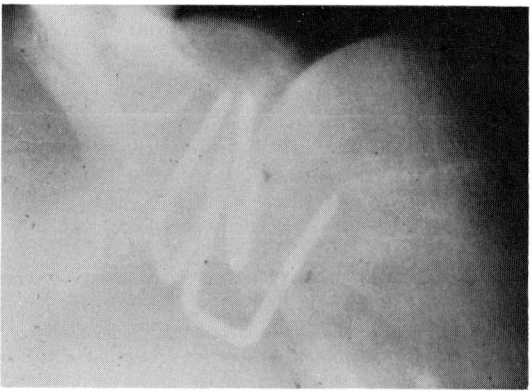

Figure 1A Joint penetration with staples.

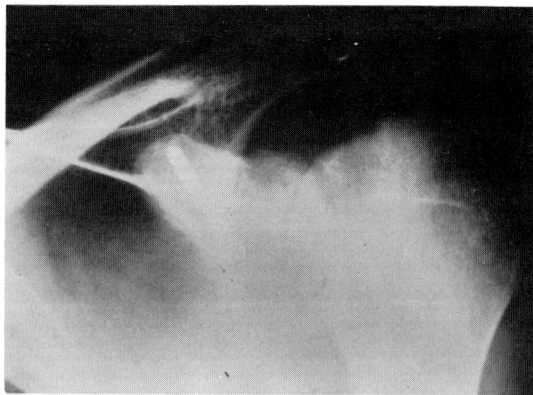

Figure 1B Loss of articular cartilage

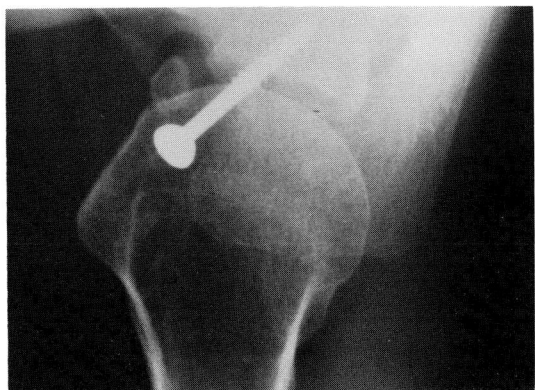

Figure 2 Symptomatic coracoid nonunion with impingement of the head of the screw on the humeral articular surface. Marked restriction of motion required lengthening of anterior structures at the time of screw removal with an excellent final result.

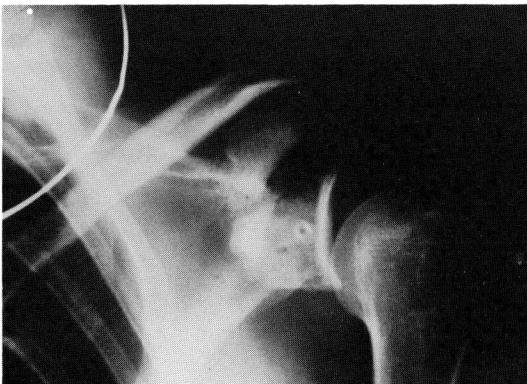

Figure 3 Removal of the loose screw did not alleviate the pain of residual inferior glenohumeral subluxation. An inferior capsular shift did. Surgery in this scar is tedious.

reattach the avulsed glenoid labrum which had often been overlooked.

In a second group there were three patients who were excessively tight following the Bristow transfers. These were associated with secondary arthritis with large subcortical cysts and, in two, loss of the normal joint space (Fig. 4). All required lengthening of the capsule and subscapularis either by a coronal plane Z-plasty or by elevating the subscapularis insertion, beginning with the soft tissue from the lateral side of the biceps groove. A total shoulder replacement was required in one.

Other complications included ligation of the musculocutaneous nerve with permanent loss of biceps function, laceration of the axillary nerve due to a poorly placed incision, a deep postoperative wound infection and a postoperative wound hematoma requiring reoperation with residual instability following the reoperation.

Eighteen were thought to have ugly scars. As noted in the reoperations for failed Bristow procedures, these scars extend from the skin down to the bone involving all structures.

Arthritis occurred in 13 patients. It was thought to be secondary to metal complications in five, recurrent dislocations in three, and repairs which were too tight in another five (Fig. 5A). Excessive tightness of a repair may cause displacement to the opposite side (see Fig. 5B).

ANALYSIS OF FAILED REPAIRS

Failed repairs occurred in all categories of surgical procedures for glenohumeral instability.

Attempts to alter bony stability with Bristow or other bone block procedures were unsuccessful in 12. A glenoid osteotomy for posterior instability failed in one. Tendon shortening such as the Magnuson-Stack or Putti-Platt was unsuccessful in 17

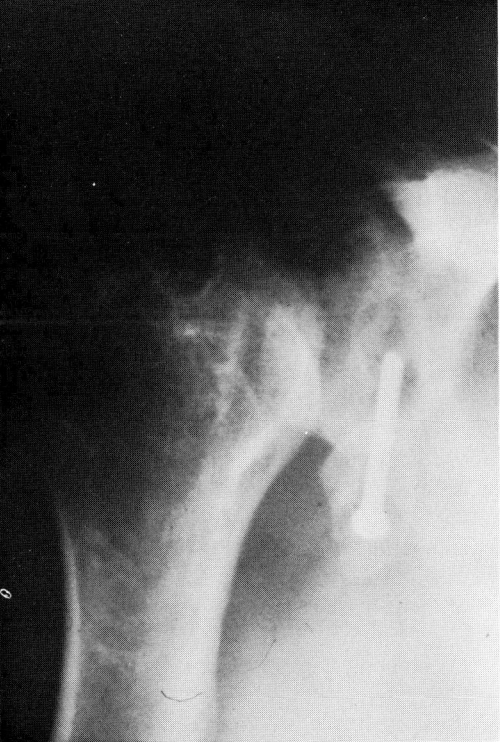

Figure 4 Symptomatic coracoid nonunion. Arthritis with subcortical cysts and fibrillation of cartilage from a tenodesis operation that was too tight.

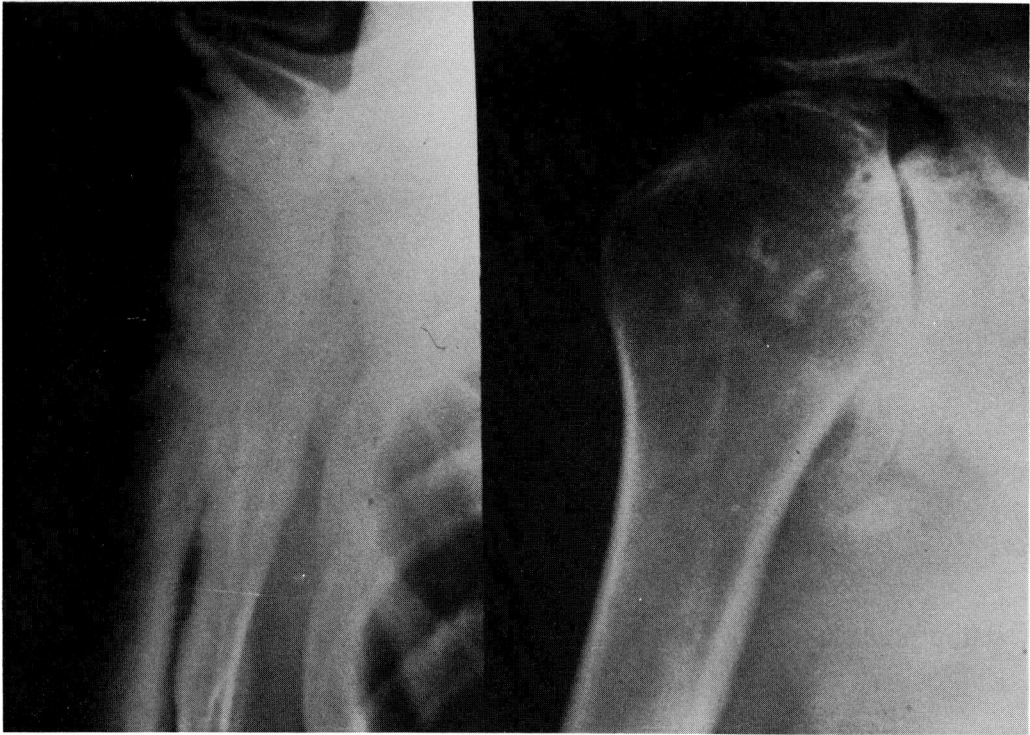

Figure 5A Posterior displacement with wear on both the humeral head and posterior glenoid from an anterior repair that was too tight or to the wrong side.

and capsular reefing procedures as in the Bankart, Dutoit, simple reefings, and capsular shift procedures failed in 15. The one Nicola suspensory operation evaluated in the series was likewise unsuccessful. Fifteen failures were attributed to unrepaired labral detachments or surgical excision, either by arthroscopy or during an open procedure. Residual inferior subluxations below a standard transverse repair occurred both in patients who were too loose in the direction of repair and also in those with marked limitation of motion on the side of repair. Placing a standard transverse repair such as a Putti-Platt or Magnuson-Stack does not adequately deal with the inferior capsular laxity.[8] Likewise, those subluxing below Bristow repair occurred with either a loose or detached capsule.[5]

Combining Bankart[16] capsular reattachment procedures with Putti-Platt or Magnuson-Stack[6] tendon shortening procedures rendered the shoulder tight and displaced it to the opposite side in four loose-jointed individuals. Improper or inadequate immobilization was a significant factor in three patients, causing redislocations. In one, no immobilization was used. In the second, the patient was improperly immobilized in internal rotation for two weeks following a posterior repair and in the third, the patient was immobilized in an airplane splint with the arm forward following a posterior capsular shift. Two other patients redislocated into large posterior lateral humeral head defects.

One advance in our understanding of instability is that we now appreciate it to be a vector of anterior and/or posterior and inferior capsular laxities (Fig. 6). Previous tendon shortening operations frequently repaired only the anterior or posterior portion of the vector leaving a significant residual inferior component.[8,13] Multidirectional instability is more common than previously appreciated. It may result from stretching of the capsule on the opposite side of a dislocation at the time of an acute injury, from generalized ligamentous laxity on a congenital basis, or from repetitive stretching with vigorous overhead sports, such as butterfly and backstroke swimming.

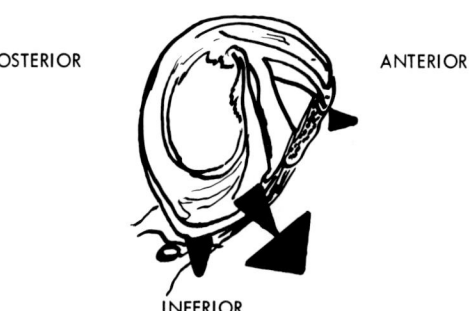

Figure 6 Shoulder instability may be a combination of vectors. Treatment of only one component is not sufficient for optimal results.

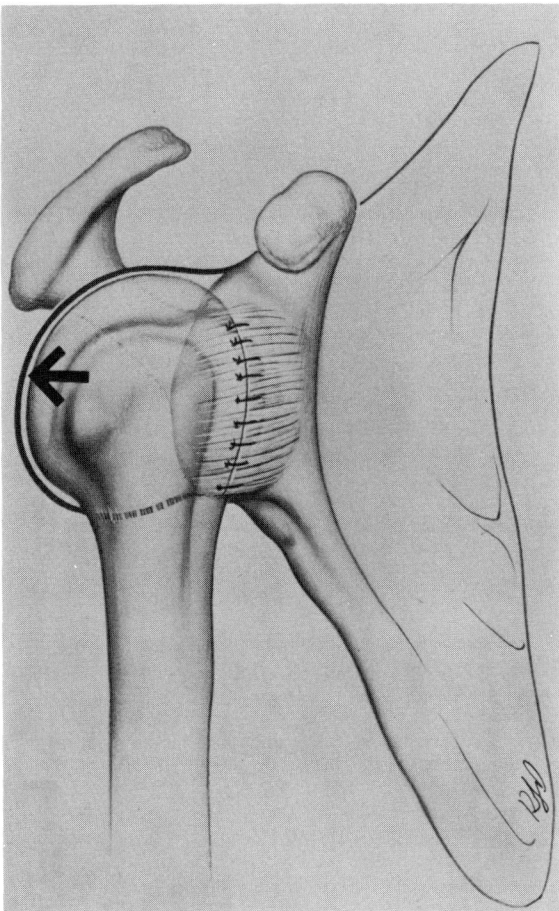

Figure 5B Tight repair causes displacement to the opposite side.

Operative Experience

Thirty patients with 50 previous failed surgeries underwent operative procedures to correct the anatomical pathology and to restore stability and function. In these patients, the operative approach for capsular shift was employed except for those requiring tendon lengthening or total shoulder replacement.

Our approach includes reassessment of the patient's stability with an examination under anesthesia. This is followed by an operative approach on the side of the greatest instability. The principles of reconstruction involve restoration of normal anatomy. These would include repair of labral detachments, reinforcement of the capsule and ligaments with partial thickness of the overlying tendon and restoration of the appropriate ligament tension anteriorly, posteriorly and inferiorly. If previous surgery has caused muscle and scar contracture then lengthening of the tendon and freeing of the muscle from the underlying capsule to regain a functional range of motion is necessary. Conforming surfaces with a humeral head or total shoulder replacement are used when necessary. Arthritis can occur from recurrent dislocations or repairs which have been too tight. Loss of glenoid version may be treated with bone graft and in situations where a total shoulder is necessary the bone graft is readily available from the resected humeral head.[9]

The methods of repair include an anterior capsular shift in 14 and a posterior capsular shift in nine. Seven required reattachment of the labrum and one a repair of the split between the inferior and middle glenohumeral ligaments reduced the abnormal laxity. Humeral head or total shoulder replacements were necessary in four.

CONCLUSIONS

From our analysis of this series, we would stress the importance of making an *accurate* diagnosis. Inability to do so resulted in unsuccessful surgery in one-third of these patients. Especially helpful is the examination under anesthesia and again during surgery prior to opening the rotator cuff. Use of the C-arm fluoroscopic unit for an axial exam under anesthesia can confirm the diagnosis, direction(s), and magnitude of relative displacement, thereby eliminating surgery to the wrong side of the shoulder or for only one component of multidirectional instability.

Avoidable hardware complications occurred in 40 percent of the patients in the series. The additional risk of using metal which may penetrate the joint or loosen and migrate to nearby structures should be carefully weighed. We favor reserving bone block procedures for glenoid deficiency or large humeral head defects.

Physiological repairs include reattachment of the glenoid labrum and plication of capsular laxity without shortening the rotator muscles. This can provide excellent stability, return of strength, and range of motion.

The postoperative immobilization position and duration are likewise important to allow for adequate healing of a capsular repair. The emphasis is placed on active rather than passive motion after the sling or cast is discarded.

The deranged anatomy makes repairs following previous failed surgery more lengthy and difficult, but worthwhile. Those following a failed Bristow procedure are especially difficult due to the amazing amount of scar and obliteration of anatomical planes. Freeing up the subscapularis and capsule from the coracoid muscles and preserving the axillary and musculocutaneous nerves provide a special challenge. Subsequent reattachment of the glenoid labrum and attention to the inferior capsule avoid many of the pitfalls seen in this series.

When these principles are followed, the patient can work confidently for near normal motion with good strength and stability.

REFERENCES

1. Artz T, Huffer JM. A major complication of the modified Bristow procedure for recurrent dislocation of the shoulder. J Trauma 1973; 13:564.
2. Bankart ASB. The pathology and treatment of recurrent dislocation of the shoulder joint. Brit J Surg. 1939; 26:23–29.
3. Grant JCB. Grant's Atlas of Anatomy. 6th ed. Baltimore: Williams and Wilkins, 1972.
4. Hill HA, Sachs MD. The grooved defect of the humeral head Radiol. 1940; 35:690–700.
5. Hovelius L, Korner L, Lundberg B, Akermark C, Herberts P, Wredmark T, Berg E. The coracoid transfer for recurrent dislocation of the shoulder. J Bone Joint Surg. 1983; 65A:926–934.
6. Magnuson PB, Stack JK. Bilateral habitual dislocation of the shoulders in twins, a familial tendency. JAMA 1940; 144:2103.
7. Matsen A, Zuckerman JD. Anterior glenohumeral instability. In: Symposium on Injuries to the Shoulder in the Athlete. 1983; Vol. 2, No. 2:330–332.
8. Neer CS II, Foster CR. Inferior capsular shift for involuntary inferior and multidirectional instability of the shoulder—a preliminary report. J Bone Joint Surg. 1980; 62A:897–908.
9. Neer CS II, Watson KC, Stanton FJ. Recent experience in total shoulder replacement. J Bone Joint Surg. 1982; 64A:319.
10. Norris TR. C-arm fluoroscopic evaluation under anesthesia for glenohumeral subluxations. Presented at 2nd Internat Conf Surgery of the Shoulder, May 29, 1983.
11. Perthes G. Uber Operationen bei Habitueller Schulterluxationen. Deutsche Zeitschr Chir. 1906; 85:199–277.
12. Poppen NK, Walker PS. Normal and abnormal motion of the shoulder. J Bone Joint Surg., 1976; 58A:195.
13. Protzman RR. Anterior instability of the shoulder. J Bone Joint Surg. 1980; 62A:909–918.
14. Rockwood CA Jr. Dislocations about the shoulder. In: Rockwood CA Jr, Green DP, eds. Fractures. Philadelphia: JB Lippincott, 1975; 1:677–680.
15. Rokous JR, Feagin JA, Abbott HG. Modified axillary roentgenogram. A useful adjunct in the diagnosis of recurrent instability of the shoulder. Clin Orthop 1972; 82:84–86.
16. Rowe CR, Patel D, Southmayd WW. The Bankart procedure: A long-term, end-result study. J Bone Joint Surg. 1978; 60A:1–16.
17. Rowe CR, Zarins B. Recurrent transient subluxation of the shoulder. J Bone Joint Surg. 1981; 63A:863–872.
18. Saha AK. Mechanism of elevation of glenohumeral joint. Its application in rehabilitation of flail shoulder in upper brachial plexus injuries and poliomyelitis and in replacement of the upper humerus by prosthesis. Acta Orthop Scand. 1973; 44:668.
19. Sisk DT, Boyd HB. Management of the recurrent anterior dislocation of the shoulder. Clin Orthop Rel Res. 1974; 103.
20. Turkel SJ, Panio MW, Marshall JL, et al. Stabilizing mechanisms preventing anterior dislocation of the glenohumeral joint. J Bone Joint Surg. 1981; 63A:1208.

MISSED POSTERIOR DISLOCATIONS OF THE SHOULDER

R. J. HAWKINS and C.S. NEER, II, M.D.

Although there has been emphasis in recent years regarding the importance of an early diagnosis for locked posterior dislocation, the majority continue to be missed by the initial physician. This report describes the method of diagnosis, the determination of the size of the defects in the humeral head and glenoid, and the treatment of a series of such missed lesions. The lesion considered is a missed posterior dislocation of the glenohumeral joint with an impression fracture of the articular surface of the humeral head as described by McLaughlin.[1] Associated displaced fractures after the classification of Neer are not included in this series.[2]

The following case illustration points out many of the features relevant to a missed posterior dislocation of the shoulder. A 45-year old male was involved in a motor vehicle accident with multiple injuries. X-rays of the shoulder demonstrated what was reported as a seemingly undisplaced fracture of the humeral neck. The patient was treated symptomatically in a sling with early physiotherapy. Eight weeks later, there had been little progress in overcoming the significant internal rotation deformity and functionally the arm was of little use to the patient for hygienic care about the face and head. Pain however, was minimal. At this stage, an axillary view demonstrated the missed posterior dislocation of the shoulder and the always present characteristic impression fracture of the humeral head.

MATERIALS

This series consists of 45 shoulders in 41 patients, four bilateral, of whom 29 patients were treated at the New York Orthopaedic Columbia Presbyterian Medical Center and 12 patients were treated at the teaching hospitals at The University of Western Ontario, London, Canada. Follow-up was conducted by the senior authors. There were thirty-two males, and nine females. The average age was 49.2 years with a range from 17 to 80 years. Twenty-eight of the cases involved the right extremity, which was dominant.

Mechanism of Injury

The mechanism of injury in the 45 patients was as follows:

Motor vehicle accidents	15
Seizures	17 (alcoholic—6, idiopathic—11)
Electro shock	7
Hypermobility of the joint	1
Unknown	5

Interval from Injury to Diagnosis

The average interval from injury to diagnosis was one year, however, those at the top end of the curve skewed the results. Twenty-five of the 41 patients were diagnosed in less than six months. The tabulation is as follows:

one to six weeks	13 patients
six weeks to six months	12 patients
six months to twelve months	3 patients
one year to two years	5 patients
two years to ten years	5 patients
Unknown	7 patients

METHOD OF DIAGNOSIS

History

These patients had certain features in common. Following a motor vehicle accident, seizure or electroshock therapy, a painful shoulder was x-rayed and the diagnosis missed. Associated undisplaced fractures about the shoulder and associated injuries were common. Despite physiotherapy, external rotation did not improve in these patients. They were often referred from the physiotherapist because of impeded progress in rehabilitation, many with the diagnosis of a "frozen shoulder." The chief complaint of these patients was a functional disability related to inability to comb their hair, and wash their face, because of the "stiffness." Although pain was frequently present, it was not debilitating, and was not a factor precipitating referral. In fact, in most cases pain was only mild.

Physical Examination

On physical examination there were certain pertinent clues that allowed the diagnosis to be established. On inspection, the humeral head was prominent posteriorly, and the acromion was squared off anteriorly. The coracoid was likewise prominent anteriorly. When visualizing the shoulder from the lateral view, there was malalignment of the humeral shaft under the acromion, in that it was in a more posterior position. Forward elevation and internal rotation were limited to varying degrees, although frequently functional. There was a marked limitation of external rotation; this was a consistent finding. Patients could not rotate to neutral and in fact had internal rotation deformities averaging 40 degrees. This was the key physical sign.

Radiological Examination

In most cases, the shoulder was x-rayed initially and still the dislocation was missed. The routine AP and lateral thoracic views taken in many radiological departments are inadequate to consistently recognize this dislocation. Associated undisplaced fractures and other injuries frequently misled the initial examiner. An AP at right angles to the scapula and a lateral in the scapular plane are more helpful to determine the dislocation; however even these x-rays can mislead the unwary. Only on suspecting the diagnosis or routinely obtaining the axillary view is the diagnosis confirmed. None of the patients in this series had an immediate axillary view. All diagnoses were finally established with the key radiological investigation; an axillary view. Associated fractures of the proximal humerus excluding the characteristic impression fracture, were present in 50 percent of the cases. These were undisplaced fractures.

The axillary view determines the presence of the characteristic impression defect and usually allows estimation of its size and of the amount of remaining articular surface. Laminograms (tomograms) were used and were helpful to further delineate the size of the defect and the status of the remaining humeral head articular surface. Recently, the CAT scan has helped further elucidate glenoid and head changes and may be more helpful in the future as a tool for investigation.

TREATMENT

Many patients had undergone treatment prior to referral. Many of these treatments went on to further modifications. The initial treatments of the missed posterior dislocation and their results once the diagnosis had been established are as follows:

Spontaneous reduction—1 patient
Attempted closed reduction—13 patients (6 successful)
Sub-scapular transfer—9 patients (5 failed because the defect was too large, going on to hemi- or total arthroplasty)
Tuberosity transfer—4 patients (all successful results)
Hemiarthroplasty—9 patients (3 have been revised to total shoulder, all are successful)
Total glenohumeral replacement—10 patients (1 still dislocated posteriorly, the remainder are satisfactory)
Bone grafts—2 patients (1 anterior and 1 posterior which went on to total glenohumeral replacement)
Excisional arthroplasty—1 patient (a poor functional result)
No treatment other than physiotherapy—8 patients (all with a poor functional result).

The group of patients that had no treatment other than physiotherapy had significant difficulty and disability in utilizing the hand above and about the head level. All had a marked internal rotation deformity, although pain was not a significant complaint.

The average follow-up in this review is 5.5 years. Thirty of the patients had longer than two years follow-up. The final follow-up results are as above.

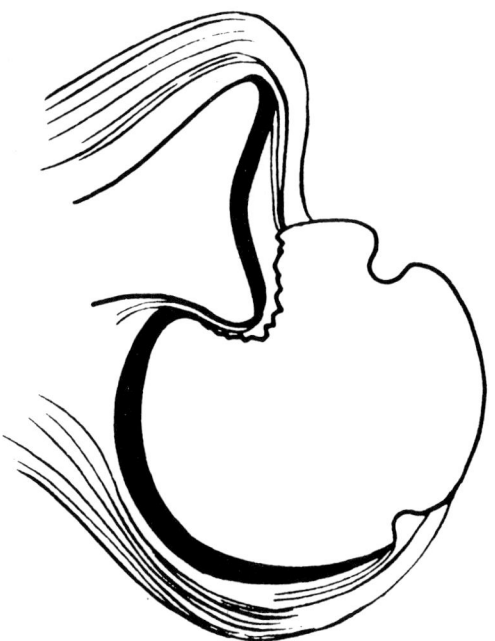

Figure 1 Diagramatic illustration of a missed posterior dislocation demonstrating the posterior glenoid rim located within the impression of the humeral head.

DISCUSSION

The method of closed reduction consists of flexion, adduction, and traction with direct pressure from behind to push the humeral head into the socket. Following successful closed reduction, the shoulder should be assessed for stability and immobilized with the arm at the side slightly externally rotated for four to six weeks.

Patients with a smaller impression defect may have less of an internal rotation deformity, and have less of a functional disability, and may choose to accept that disability. Patients with large and longstanding impression defects, if active, require surgical intervention.

Tuberosity transfer seems to provide a more favorable result than the McLaughlin subscapular muscle transfer. Following tuberosity transfer or subscapularis tendon transfer, the shoulder should be immobilized in approximately 20 to 30 degrees of external rotation in a spica for four to six weeks.

Hemiarthroplasties provided satisfactory results when appropriate technique and rehabilitation were followed. The prosthesis should not be inserted in the usual 35 to 40 degrees of retroversion from the coronal plane, but in neutral version to the coronal plane. Too much retroversion may result in recurrence of the dislocation. The version of the prosthesis can control the tendency to subluxation and if successful no postoperative immobilization is necessary and exercises may be

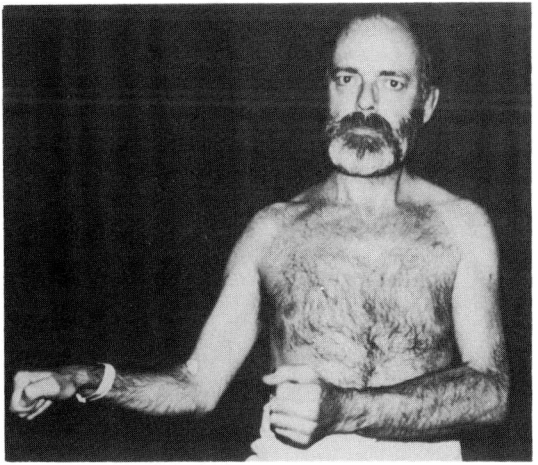

Figure 2 This gentleman has a missed posterior dislocation of his left shoulder and he has a 50° internal rotation deformity. The left arm demonstrates the full extent to which external rotation is possible.

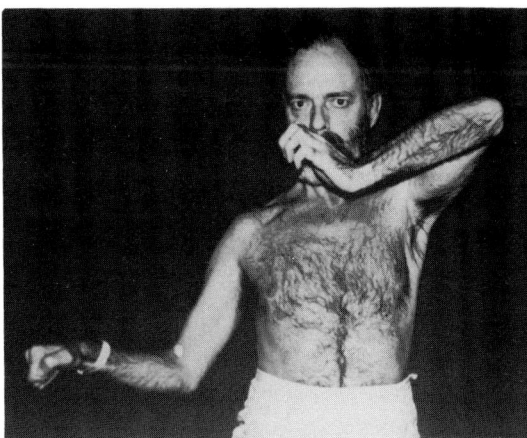

Figure 3 Because of the internal rotation deformity, patients with missed posterior dislocations find it extremely difficult to function for hygienic purposes about the head and neck.

commenced immediately. If, however, the shoulder is unstable, it should be positioned in 20 to 30 degrees of external rotation in a shoulder spica for four to six weeks. Plication of the posterior capsule may be added to increase stability. In the presence of glenoid deficiency or glenoid defects, bone grafting may be required in conjuction with total shoulder arthroplasty. Unfortunately, any pathology of significance on the glenoid side will require total shoulder arthropathy as part of the reconstruction. Again appropriate version will ensure stability.

The surgical approach for tuberosity transfers, subscapularis transfer and hemiarthroplasty is most easily performed from the front. Care should be taken when attempting to salvage the humeral head, not to lever on it while performing reduction. Leverage can be obtained by placing the instrument in the impression defect. Appropriate soft tissue releases will allow reduction without too much trauma.

The usual trauma series consists of an AP at right angles to the scapula, and a lateral in the scapula plane. It should be emphasized that if an axillary view is part of the routine trauma series, this diagnosis will not be missed. The axillary view can be obtained with minimum movement of the patient's arm and this can be performed in the presence of the examing physician. As little as 20 degrees abduction of the arm will allow an adequate axillary view. The cone is placed at the hip and the beam is directed upward with the plate above the shoulder.

Summary

A missed posterior dislocation is a diagnostic trap for the unwary physician and surgeon. Failure to diagnose this condition is related to its rarity but more importantly, to failure to interpret the available physical signs and take the appropriate x-rays. A history of seizure or associated shoulder fractures, particularly in the presence of multiple trauma must alert the surgeon to the diagnosis. Marked limitation of external rotation or more accurately an internal rotation deformity is the key physical sign to establish the diagnosis, particularly late. An axillary view is mandatory in all trauma studies of the shoulder, particularly in patients complaining of shoulder pain following epilepsy, electrocution, ethanol intoxication, and patients involved in motor vehicle accidents.

The size of the impression defect of the humeral head may be determined by a) An axillary view; b) Tomograms; c) CAT scan.

The present policy regarding treatment based on this series is as follows:

- Less than six weeks with a 20% defect—closed reduction may be attempted with the humerus held externally rotated 20 to 30° in a spica for six weeks.
- Greater than six weeks to 20 to 40% impression defect—requires an open reduction preferably with lesser tuberosity transfer with the arm held at the side and externally rotated 20 to 30° for four to six weeks.
- Greater than 50% head defect and/or a dislocation present for less than six months with a normal glenoid—suggest the use of a hemi-arthroplasty.
- Greater than 50% head defect and/or dislocation for greater than six months with a deficient glenoid—we would recommend a total glenohumeral replacement. (If the dislocation has been longstanding, then the remaining articular surface and/or glenoid would likely be destroyed requiring total glenohumeral replacement.)

In conclusion, with appropriate attention to the history and a careful physical examination, especially with the use of an axillary view in all traumatic injuries to the shoulders, "missed posterior dislocation" as a diagnosis will disappear.

REFERENCES

1. McLaughlin HL. Posterior dislocation of the shoulder. J Bone Joint Surg 1952; 34A:584.
2. Neer CS. Displaced proximal humeral fractures, Part I, Classification and evaluation. J Bone Joint Surg 1970; 52A:1077.

ROTATOR CUFF

THE SUBACROMIAL BURSA: A CLINICOPATHOLOGICAL STUDY

HANS K. UHTHOFF, M.D., F.R.C.S.(C), KIRITI SARKAR, M.D., and D. IAN HAMMOND, M.D.

A bursa allows a highly mobile part of skin or a musculotendinous structure to glide smoothly against a bony prominence. Because of its position, it is conceivable that the bursa is susceptible to friction–induced injuries, resulting in bursitis. Among deep bursae, the subacromial bursa has most often been suspected of being inflamed, and "bursitis" is a commonly applied diagnosis in painful shoulder syndromes. This seems partly justified, because injection of antiphlogistic agents directly into the subacromial bursa often gives dramatic relief from pain.

It is becoming generally recognized however, that a primary disease of the subacromial bursa may be a rarity,[1] and the term "bursitis" is often used even when a primary disease of a contiguous structure is evident.[6] Subacromial bursitis is most likely to be secondary either to a neighboring tendinopathy or to diseases of other adjacent structures. Although the source of "bursitis" is being clarified, there is very little information not only on the incidence of subacromial bursal inflammation in rotator cuff tendinopathies, but on the structural changes in the bursa occurring in relation to those conditions as well.

The purpose of the present study, in the beginning, was to examine morphologically, random samples of the subacromial bursa obtained during surgical interventions on rotator cuff tendinopathies. We realized, however, that the "normal" bursa itself may be subject to age-related wear-and-tear changes due to its strategic location. Therefore, we examined subacromial bursae from post mortem cases ranging in age from infancy to persons in the ninth decade for whom no shoulder diseases were recorded in the chart. Recently, we have added preoperative subacromial bursograms to our investigations of patients with rotator cuff tendinopathies to determine if the radiologic appearance of the bursa correlates with the morphology of surgically obtained bursal tissue.

Our study indicates that reactions of the subacromial bursa are almost always secondary in nature.

MATERIALS AND METHODS

Surgical Cases

Specimens of subacromial bursae were randomly obtained during surgery from 14 cases of calcifying tendinitis, seven cases of rotator cuff tear, five cases of tight coracoacromial ligament, three cases of acromioclavicular osteoarthritis and 1 case of rheumatoid arthritis.

Post Mortem Specimens

To obtain subacromial bursae from post mortem cases, the usual Y-shaped incision was slightly extended over the shoulders. The glenohumeral joint was exposed, and the supraspinatus tendon extending from the bony insertion to the musculotendinous junction was removed along with the overlying subacromial bursa. No attempt was made to collect samples for electron microscopy as the autopsies were performed eight hours or longer after death. Methods for processing specimens for light microscopy are described below.

Bursogram

With the patient supine a 22-gauge, 7.6 cm spinal needle was inserted into the shoulder under local anesthesia. The needle tip was directed a few millimeters inferior to the anterior edge of the acromion, slightly lateral to the midpoint of its inferior surface. The needle was advanced under fluoroscopic control, and as it reached the bursal sac, the patient complained of a slight but sharp pain. An amount of 3–5 ml of a water soluble iodinated contrast material (Hypaque M-60%, Winthrop) was then injected. A gentle abduction of the arm helped to distribute the medium throughout the bursa.

Morphology

For morphological examinations, a small portion of surgically removed biopsy samples was processed for electron microscopy, and the rest for light microscopy. For electron microscopy, tiny pieces of tissues were fixed: first in one—half strength Karnovsky's fixative for 24 hours and then in 1% osmium tetroxide for one hour, both at 4°C. Fixed pieces of tissues were dehydrated in graded ethyl alcohol and finally in propylene oxide. They were embedded in epon. Thick sections for preliminary light microscopic observations were stained with toluidine blue, while the thin sections for electron microscopic photography were stained with uranyl acetate and lead citrate.

For light microscopy, tissues were fixed in 10% neutral buffered formalin. Sections of paraffin-embedded tissue were stained routinely with hematoxylin and eosin, toluidine blue and trichromes, and selectively by von Kossa's method to detect calcification.

RESULTS

Post Mortem Bursae

As subacromial bursae from post mortem cases were obtained to serve as controls, our assumption was that the adjacent supraspinatus tendon would show no other changes but those related to aging, such as thinning and fibrillation of fascicles. We were surprised, however, to find that a majority of tendons from the third decade onward showed significant changes at their bony insertions, although there was no clinical history of enthesopathy. The blue line was irregularly split and it often showed calcific excrescences in older persons. Thinning and fibrillation worsened with age, and were most conspicuous at the region where tendon fiber proper merged with Sharpey's fibers. Small incomplete tears at the tendon attachment near the articular surface were seen in some cases of older age groups. Two cases in the eighth decade showed large calcific deposits adjoining the Sharpey's fibers, apparently in the region of old complete tears.

How these changes in the supraspinatus tendon would have affected the overlying bursa could not be ascertained. The structural changes undergone by the bursa from infancy to adulthood were readily discernible. At no time, was there a distinguishable cleavage line between the bursa and the tendon. The connective tissue of the bursal wall was continuous with that of the peritenon, and it was impossible to demarcate the former from the latter. This zone of connective tissue was minimal during infancy. At that age, the straightened inner lining of the bursa, consisting of a single layer of cells, was closely approximated to the tendinous tissue (Fig. 1). With age, the connective tissue layer gradually increased in thickness, containing a varying mixture of vascularized fibrofatty tissue. Concurrently, the bursal lining developed pseudostratification of two or more layers of cells. These developments were already identified by the third decade. It was difficult to determine whether advancing age or an underlying supraspinatus tendinopathy altered the basic architecture of the bursa.

Bursograms

The preliminary results of bursography revealed the subacromial bursa to be a shallow, semicrescent structure with smooth margins, lying be-

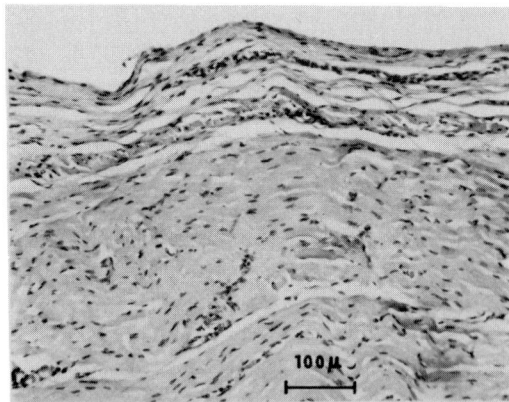

Figure 1 The base of subacromial bursa overlying supraspinatus tendon from a one-year-old male shows that the inner lining is composed of a flattened layer of cells. The bursal wall is indistinguishable from the peritendinous connective tissue. Hematoxylin and eosin.

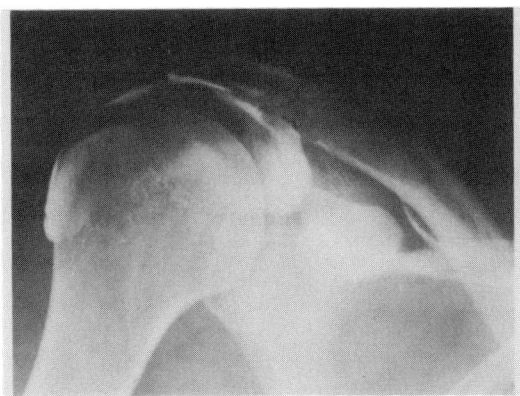

Figure 2 Bursogram shows normal large capacity of a smoothly outlined subacromial subdeltoid bursa.

tween the acromion and deltoid muscle above, and the superior margin of the rotator cuff below (Fig. 2). The lateral extent of the bursa was variable, depending upon the presence or absence of communication between the subacromial and subdeltoid portions of the bursa. Usually these two compartments formed one space. The bursogram showed characteristic changes in cases of complete rotator cuff tear when the contrast material flowed immediately from the bursa into the glenohumeral joint. In patients with impingement syndrome, bursograms demonstrated the obliteration of the mid-portion of the bursa between the greater tuberosity of the humerus and the coracoacromial arch as the arm was progressively abducted, with the concomitant distension of the bursa lateral to the obliterated zone (Fig. 3). In some cases, the bursa appeared contracted and irregular (Fig. 4), but our investigations are still inconclusive as to whether this indicates faulty technique or reduced bursal cavity.

Surgical Biopsies

Biopsies of subacromial bursa obtained during surgery could be broadly divided into two categories according to their morphology: tissues showing no signs of degeneration and tissues containing degenerative changes. In the first group were the biopsies from cases of calcifying tendinitis, tight coracoacromial ligament and rotator cuff tear. Histologically, the general disposition of the bursal structure from this group was closely similar to that in the "normal" post mortem specimens (Fig. 5), although some bursae appeared more cellular, and vascular proliferation and en-

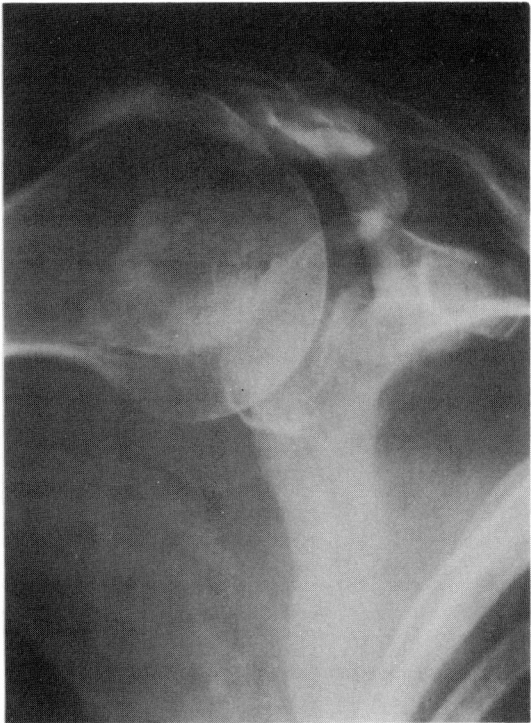

Figure 3 With the arm abducted, the subacromial bursa is compressed between the greater tuberosity of the humerus and acromion, indicating impingement.

gorgement were not uncommon (Fig. 6). Calcific deposits in the bursa did not necessarily elicit an inflammatory reaction (Fig. 7). On the other hand, macrophages, but only a few polymorphonuclear leukocytes, were present when the calcific deposits were being actively resorbed (Fig. 8).

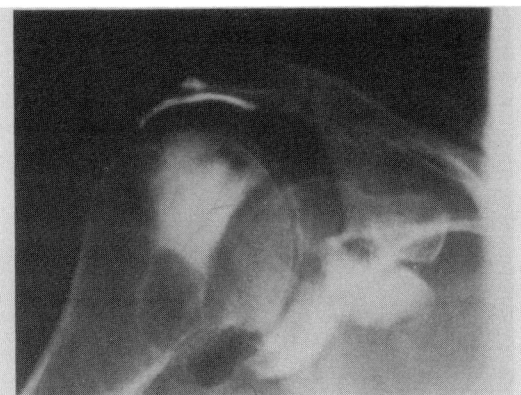

Figure 4 Bursogram shows a contracted and irregularly outlined subacromial bursa.

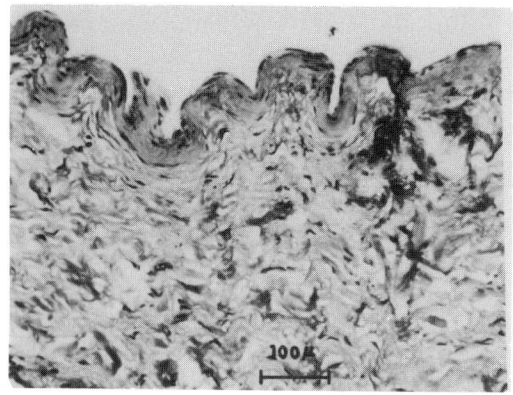

Figure 5 In a patient with tight coracoacromial ligament, the bursal lining appears as a compact band of connective tissue containing cells in pseudostratification. Hematoxylin and eosin.

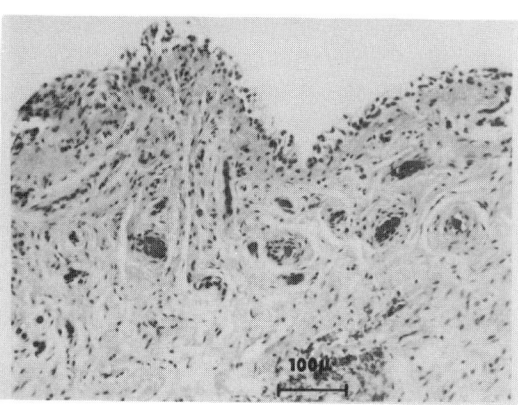

Figure 6 The bursa from a case of rotator cuff tear shows proliferation of lining cells and vascular congestion in the wall. Hematoxylin and eosin.

Ultrastructurally, the cells in the bursa corresponded to A and B types of synovial cells. Type A cells resembled macrophages with surface prolongations and intracytoplasmic vacuoles, while Type B cells resembling fibroblasts had well developed rough endoplasmic reticulum. Many cells, however, contained a combination of the features of both cell types. Proliferation of endothelial cells was common, and most of the vascular channels showed the presence of pericytes. The bursal cells as well as the endothelial cells contained an abundant number of intermediate filaments in the cytoplasm.

The second group of tissues that contained cells with degenerative changes included cases of acromioclavicular osteoarthritis and rheumatoid arthritis. During surgery, these bursae appeared thick and reddened with a rough surface. In a case of acromioclavicular osteoarthritis, the bursal cavity was denuded of the living cell layer. The undulated cavitary surface with villous protuberances alternating with deep clefts was covered by a fibrinous layer. Ultrastructurally, cellular fragments were dispersed in the interstitium surrounded by fibrin. Many cells were vacuolated, and lipidic droplets were frequent in the cytoplasm. Details of the ultrastructural findings have already been reported.[5]

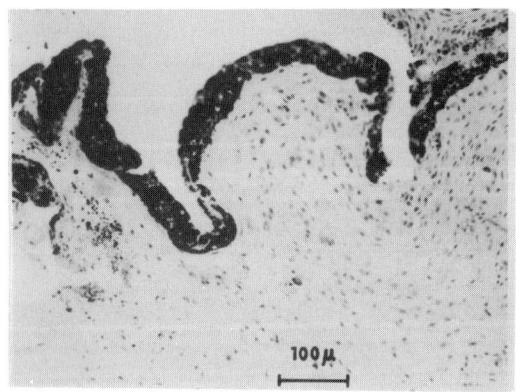

Figure 7 In a case of calcifying tendinitis, calcification of the bursa appears in a bandlike fashion along the lining. There is no evidence of inflammation in the adjacent wall. von Kossa.

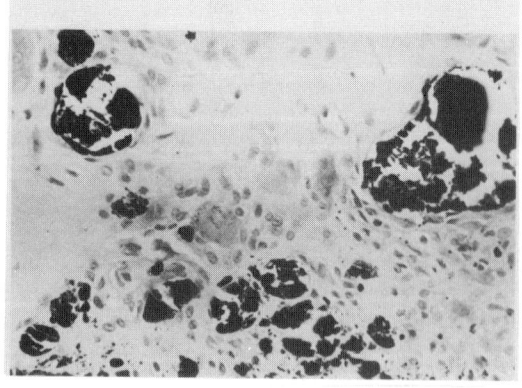

Figure 8 Numerous calcific deposits in the bursal wall are in the process of resorption. Multinucleated cells and most of the mononucleated cells are macrophagic in nature. von Kossa.

DISCUSSION

The subacromial bursa is continuous with the subdeltoid bursa in most individuals, thus constituting the largest deep bursa in the body. The diagnostic significance of preoperative bursograms has been established.[3,7] A filling defect in the bursa between the greater tuberosity of the humerus and the acromion when the arm is abducted, is clearly indicative of compression giving rise to impingement syndrome. A reduced filling of the bursa can be attributed to several causes: an absence of communication with the subdeltoid bursa, an edematous wall preventing normal distensibility, an obliterating cavity because of fibrosis, and, of course, a faulty technique.

The histological appearance of a normal bursa is generally described as a single layer of cells overlying a zone of connective tissue containing vascular channels.[4] In the present study, the examination of adult subacromial bursae that were obtained as post mortem specimens, rarely showed a uniform morphology. It appeared reasonable to conclude that a fair degree of variability might be expected not only in the lining layer but in the relative distribution of fibrofatty tissue and in the vascular component as well. The cells in the bursa are known to have the same features as those from the synovium. We noted in our study that the characteristic Type A cells were more likely to constitute the lining layer while the Type B cells and intermediate cells were predominant in the bursal wall. We would like to reiterate, however, that the delineation of the bursal wall was vague as it tended to merge with the peritenon of the supraspinatus tendon.

This apparent continuity between the walls of the tendon and the bursa leads us to believe that in the presence of clinically detectable tendinopathies, any structural alterations in the bursa suggesting bursitis are likely due to that underlying tendon disease. Recently, we have proposed a classification for rotator cuff tendinopathies that distinguishes between primary and secondary conditions in order to elucidate pathogenetic mechanisms, clinical behaviours and modalities of treatment of tendon-related painful shoulder syndromes.[8] Among the primary conditions, in which the disease process begins in the tendon, we include traumatic avulsion, calcifying tendinitis and rotator cuff tear. Most of the secondary tendinopathies, especially in the case of supraspinatus tendon, are induced by abnormalities in the contiguous structures. For example, a tight coracoacromial ligament or osteophytes from the acromioclavicular joint may be responsible for painful tendinitis. Rotator cuff tendons may also be secondarily involved in generalized systemic diseases such as rheumatoid arthritis and gout.

Both primary and secondary rotator cuff tendinopathies may affect the subacromial bursa. In the present study the bursal changes could be categorized in general descriptive terms as proliferative or degenerative. A true inflammation of the subacromial bursa, characterized either by effusion in the bursal sac or by a substantial degree of infiltration by polymorphonuclear leukocytes into the wall, was never seen, even when calcification was present. A small population of polymorphonuclears, in the range of 2.3 percent, could be found among a considerable number of macrophages during the resorption of calcific deposits.

Lack of inflammation of the subacromial bursa has been reported by other investigators.[2] In our experience, granulomatous diseases such as rheumatoid arthritis when affecting bursae secondarily, can either produce characteristic granulomas or give rise to an intense chronic inflammation with plasma cells and lymphocytes.

From a clinical point of view then, an acute subacromial bursitis must be a rarity, if it exists at all. An effort, therefore, should be made to avoid a diagnosis of acute bursitis in painful shoulder syndromes, even when a remarkable symptomatic relief is obtained through steroid injections into the bursa. Nonspecific changes in the subacromial bursa, with or without cell degeneration, are quite common, but the essential pathogenetic mechanism appears to originate in the contiguous structures, be they tendon, ligament or joint.

REFERENCES

1. Bland JH, Merrit JA, Boushey DR. The painful shoulder. Sem Arth Rheum 1977; 7:21–47.
2. Canoso JJ. Bursae, tendons and ligaments. Clin Rheum Dis 1981; 7:189–221.
3. Lie S, Mast WA. Subacromial bursography. Technique and clinical application. Radiol 1982; 144:626–630.
4. Reubens-Duval A. L'hygroma. Révisions histologiques. Rev Rheum Mal Ostéoartic 1972; 39:183–187.
5. Sarkar K, Uhthoff HK. Ultrastructure of the subacromial bursa in painful shoulder syndromes. Vichows Arch 1983; A 400:107–117.
6. Simon WH. Soft tissue disorders of the shoulder. Frozen shoulder, calcific tendinitis, and bicipital tendinitis. Orthop Clin N Am 1975; 6:521–539.
7. Strizak AM, Danzig L, Jackson DW, Greenway G, Resnick D, Staple T. Subacromial bursography. An anatomical and clinical study. J Bone Joint Surg 1982; 64A:196–201.
8. Uhthoff HK, Sarkar K, Hammond DI, Legault L. Die Pathologie der Rotatorenmanschette. Orthop Praxis (in press).

DIAGNOSIS OF ROTATOR CUFF TEARS BY DOUBLE CONTRAST ARTHROTOMOGRAPHY: RELIABILITY STUDY

JACQUES-E. DesMARCHAIS, M.D. and JEAN VEZINA, M.D.

Chronic shoulder pain in patients around fifty years old is sometimes due to a rotator cuff tear. To confirm the diagnosis, the surgeon may request a routine arthrography with iodine only. If this examination shows the opaque substance within the subdeltoid bursa from an injection into the joint cavity, then this is the sign "par excellence" of a rotator cuff tear. Should the surgeon then suggest to the patient a surgical repair of the torn cuff? In order to answer this question, one would like to know the extent of the tear. This could be very useful in anticipating surgical difficulties, and in forecasting results. At Sacré-Coeur Hospital, Montréal University, we studied the degree of reliability of double contrast arthrotomography in the diagnosis of rotator cuff tears.

METHODS

First, let us suggest hypothetically that it is possible to measure the extent of the tear prior to surgical intervention.

A short beveled needle is inserted anteriorly into the joint and obliquely oriented 15 to 25 degrees toward the socket, centering it on the humeral head. Double contrast arthrography uses only 3 ml of iodine injected intra-articularly along with 10 cc of air. The x-ray tube is then angulated caudad 10 to 20 degrees, in order to separate the acromion from the infraspinatus. A kidney-shaped filter made of plastic has been developed to equalize radiological densities and to better delineate soft tissues. The filter is placed behind the shoulder. The patient is in a sitting position holding a weight in his hand; this helps to increase the acromio humeral space. Exposures are taken in two series in order to study the sagittal and coronal planes. Whenever a tear is shown or suspected on these initial films on double contrast arthrography, then tomographic cuts, using a horizontal beam, are made at 5-mm intervals. This technique permits better visualization of the tendon, the tear and the surrounding bony structures. We can also measure the extent of the gap between the two ends of the torn tendon.

A second series of tomographic cuts helps to determine the extent of the tear in the sagittal plane. The x-ray tube is oriented along the flat axis of the scapula thus allowing a true lateral view of the shoulder. To be successful, this technique requires the collaboration of skillful technicians. Depending on the size of the tear, the humeral head will be more or less uncovered by the rotator cuff. A second series of tomographic films in the sagittal plane gives additional valuable information but is more difficult to interpret.

Thus, we see that with double contrast arthrotomography we can measure the extent of the tear in the cuff both in the coronal and sagittal planes.

RELIABILITY STUDY

In the second part of this study, we will show that double contrast arthrotomography is a reliable means of investigation. During the last three years, more than 400 cases of double contrast arthrography of the shoulder have been done in our hospital. The radiological examination was completed by tomography whenever a rotator cuff tear was suspected. We were able to compare the size of the tear as measured in the O.R. and as measured on the arthrography, in the 46 patients who had surgery. There were 39 men and 7 women with a mean age of 54 years.

Even though there was a 4.4 months time

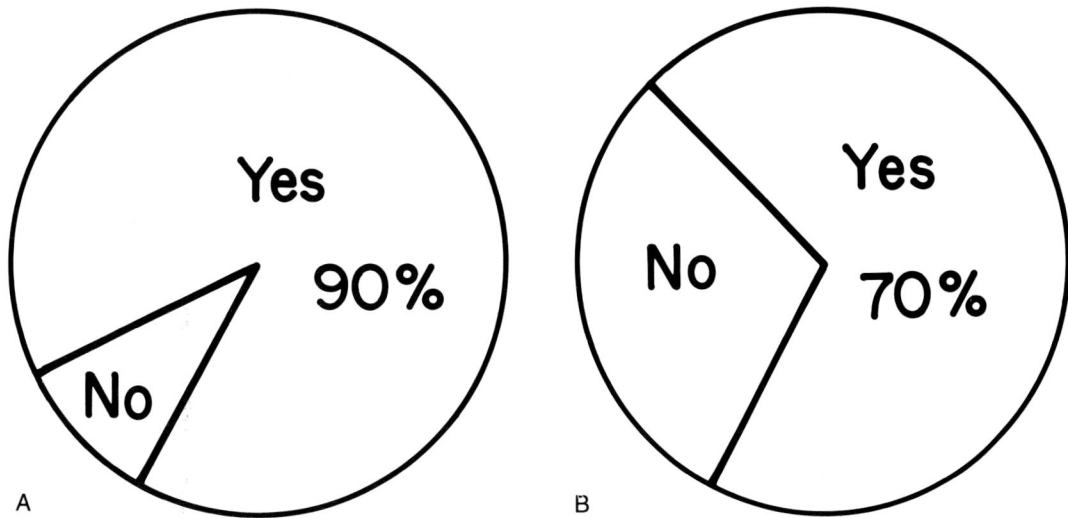

Figure 1 Reliability factors comparing surgical and radiologic findings. A, Coronal plane arthrogram. B, Sagittal plane arthrogram.

lapse between the two measurements, the reliability index did not seem to be related to this factor. We accepted a difference up to 5 mm between radiological and per-operative measurements as being due to radiological magnification.

From this study, we learned that arthrographic measurements were reliable in both planes in 30 of the 46 patients, that is, 65 percent. During these three years, we observed a gradual improvement in reliability from 56 percent to 67 percent. Let's take a close look at the reliability in each plane separately. Radiological and surgical evaluation in the coronal plane revealed that in 41 cases the two evaluations yielded identical results, thus giving a reliability of 90 percent (Fig. 1A). Of the five nonidentical cases, three were underestimated on the tomographs by 1.6 cm on average and two cases overestimated by 1.3 cm. Technically, it is easier to make good tomographic cuts in the coronal plane. Moreover, the tendon retracts beyond the superior edge of the glenoid, thus limiting the maximum size of tear to 4.5 cm and facilitating measurement in this plane.

Radiological and surgical evaluation in the sagittal plane revealed that in 32 cases the two evaluations yielded identical results thus giving a reliability of 70 percent (Fig. 1B). Of the 14 nonidentical cases, 11 were underestimated by 2.5 cm on average, and 3 overestimated by 1.8 cm. In the sagittal plane, technical difficulties in making tomographic films with good resolution make interpretation very difficult. Sometimes the radiologist must rely on the information learned from the coronal plane in order to estimate the tear in the sagittal plane. Also, the tear may be much larger, reaching 10 to 12 cm. Moreover, in complex tears when the edge is not clear, the radiologist calculates his measurements on the underside of the tendon (where the air has diffused), whereas the surgeon looks at the tear from above the tendon. All these factors may cause discrepancies between the radiological and surgical measurements. Finally, tears where the tendon is thin may compromise the reliability of the radiological diagnosis.

Therefore, our study shows four types of tears as measured at surgery both in the coronal and the sagittal planes (Fig. 2). In type 1, the tear is very small and the tendon is usually of near normal thickness. In type II, the tear enlarges up to 14 square cm. The tendon shows signs of wear and sometimes the humeral head starts to sublux towards the acromion. In type III, the tear extends mostly in the sagittal plane, the size of the tear being between 15 and 30 square cm. In complex tears, the head is also subluxed. In type IV, the tear is huge, the head is completely uncovered and so subluxed that an acromiohumeral arthrosis has developed.

A table of these various parameters indicates that the reliability of tomographic measurement varies with these 4 types of tears (Fig. 3). Despite the limited number of cases for types III and IV, the percentage of reliability decreases as the tear size increases.

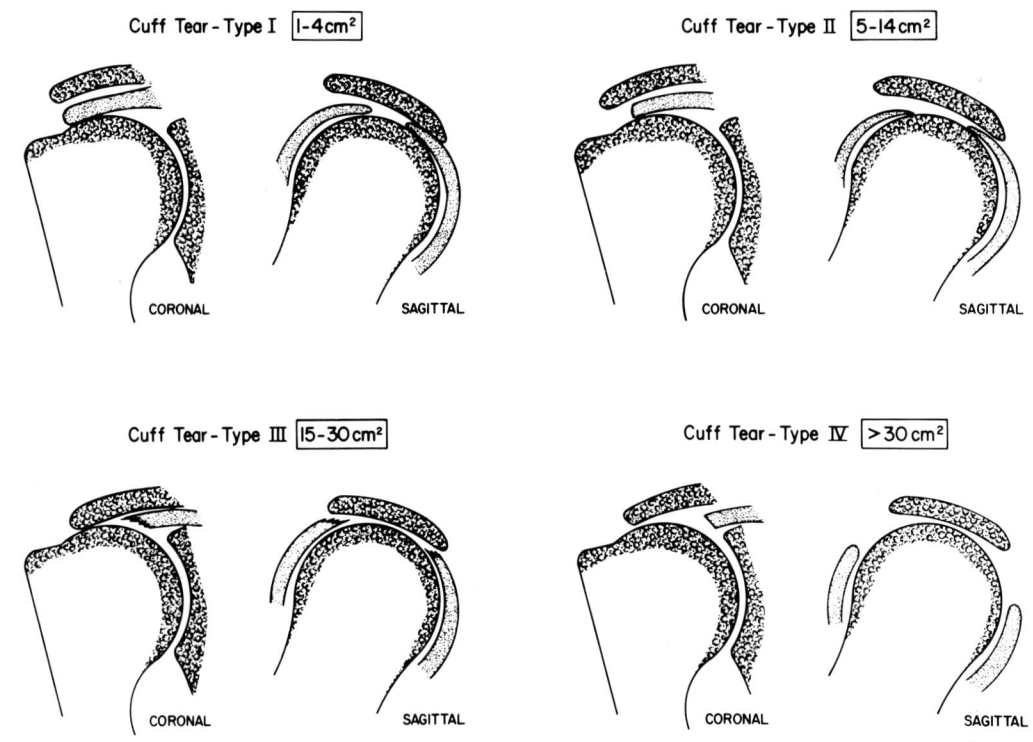

Figure 2 Four types of cuff tear shown by arthrotomography.

Type	Size (cm²)	Number of cases	
I	0-4	(5/20)	25%
II	5-14	(6/16)	38%
III	15-30	(4/7)	57%
IV	>30	(1/3)	—

Figure 3 Reliability of tomographic measurement decreases with increase in tear size.

Conclusions

We have demonstrated that double-contrast arthrotomography outlines the extent of rotator cuff tears with 90 percent reliability in the coronal plane and 70 percent reliability in the sagittal plane. From this study we conclude that double-contrast arthrotomography is a demanding but useful technique. It helps determine to a high degree of accuracy, particularly in the coronal plane, the extent of a rotator cuff tear allowing the surgeon to plan his surgical procedure.

THE SIGNIFICANCE OF DISTALLY POINTING ACROMIOCLAVICULAR OSTEOPHYTES IN RUPTURES OF THE SUPRASPINATUS TENDON

CLAES J. PETERSSON, M.D. and CARL FREDRIK GENTZ, M.D.

The acromioclavicular joint is intimately related to the supraspinatus muscle and tendon traversing its superior surface with very limited free space between. Degeneration of the acromioclavicular joint is an age-related process (DePalma,[1] Petersson[7]). Marginal lipping with osteophyte formation becomes increasingly frequent with increasing changes of the joint cartilages (Petersson[7]) (Fig. 1 a,b). Distally pointing osteophytes at the acromioclavicular joint reduce the subacromial sliding space of the supraspinatus tendon and might be potentially hazardous to the tendon by compressing it in abduction of the arm (Fig. 2). The significance of distally pointing acromioclavicular osteophytes in ruptures of the supraspinatus tendon was evaluated by two different methods.

MATERIAL AND METHODS

Radiologic Investigation

Forty-seven shoulder images of 47 patients with arthrographically verified supraspinatus tendon ruptures were reviewed (Tab. 1). The images were standard anteroposterior projections of the shoulder joint with the inferior border of the acromioclavicular joint clearly outlined. Distally pointing osteophytes at the acromioclavicular joint were measured using a ruler, and osteophytes greater than 2 mm were registered (Fig. 3, 4). In a control study, 50 shoulder images of 50 patients, 24 men and 26 women, aged 64 ± 12 years (mean ± SD) were reviewed. Most of these patients were trauma cases and none had a history of shoulder distress. Osteophytes of the undersurface of the acromioclavicular joint greater than 2 mm were registered. All images, both in the supraspinatus tendon rupture group and in the control group were obtained with the patient supine, with the same film-focus distance, and about the same position of the central beam. Therefore, the capability of exposing acromioclavicular osteophytes was comparable in the images of the two groups.

Anatomic Investigation

One hundred and seventy shoulder joints of 85 cadavers, 45 men and 40 women aged 69 ± 14 years (mean ± SD) were dissected. The cadavers were randomly selected at the Department of Pathology at the Malmö General Hospital. Four had a history of shoulder complaint and two of these had supraspinatus tendon lesions. The supraspinatus tendons were examined and ruptures—partial as well as full thickness—were registered. The acromioclavicular joints were scrutinized. Osteophytes of the undersurface of the joint were measured and osteophytes greater than 2 mm were registered.

Results

Distally pointing osteophytes of the acromioclavicular joint appeared in 24 images of patients with supraspinatus tendon ruptures and in seven images of the control group. This difference is significant ($p < 0.001$, chi-square test). In the rupture group, the osteophytes were registered on the clavicular side of the acromioclavicular joint in 15 shoulders and on the acromial side in eight shoulders, whereas osteophytes appeared on both sides of the joint in one shoulder only. In the control group five osteophytes were registered on the clavicular side and two on the acromial side of the acromioclavicular joint. The average size of the

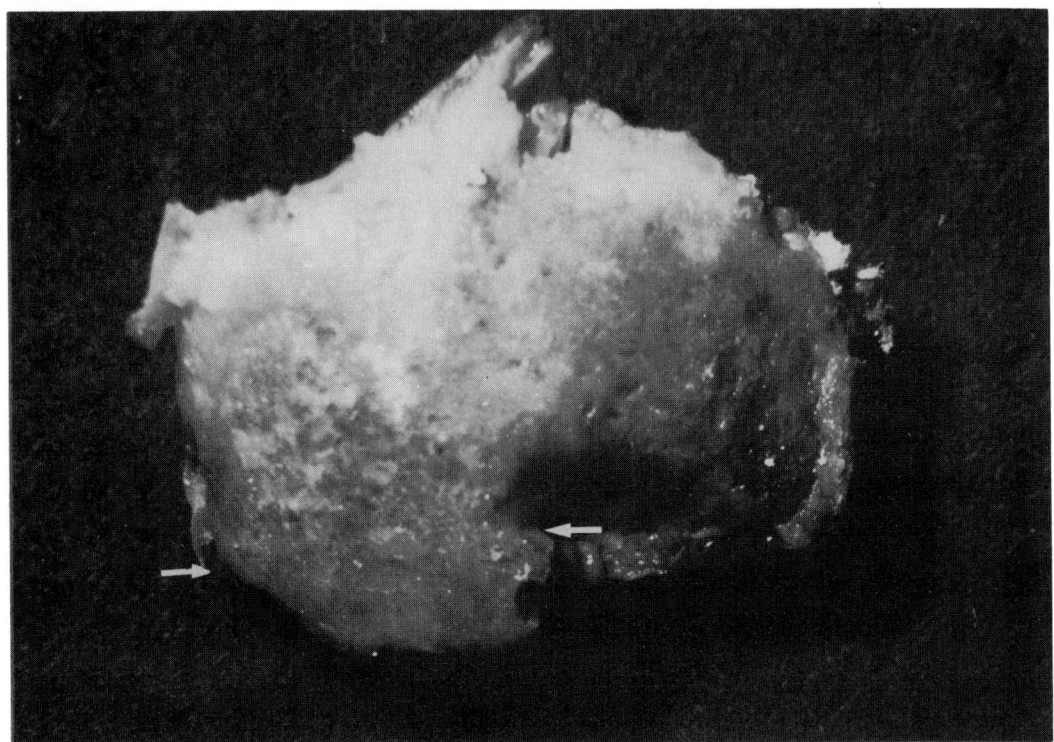

Figure 1a The right clavicular end of a 74-year-old man. Severe cartilage destruction and a large, distally pointing osteophyte indicated by arrows.

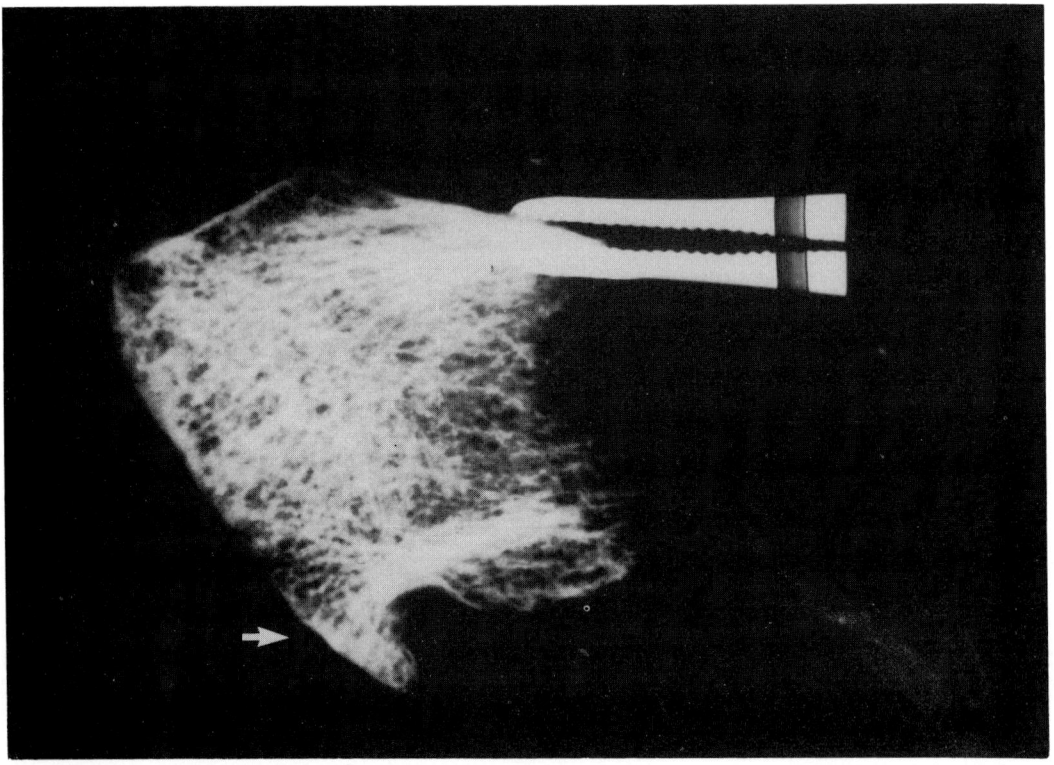

Figure 1b Lateral view of the same clavicular end on fine grain x-ray film. The osteophyte indicated by an arrow.

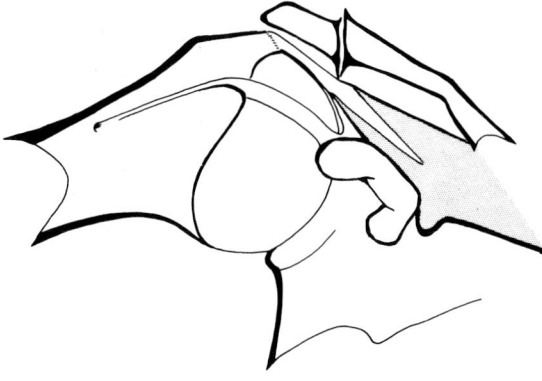

Figure 2 Schematic view of the supraspinatus tendon being compressed by distally pointing osteophytes at the acromioclavicular joint, when the arm is abducted.

	No.	Average Age ± SD	Ruptured Side	
			Right	Left
Men	29	61 ± 8 yrs	18	11
Women	18	63 ± 7 yrs	12	6

TABLE 1 Sex and Side Distribution of 47 Arthrographically Confirmed Ruptures of the Supraspinatus Tendon

distally pointing acromioclavicular osteophytes was 3.4 ± 1.4 mm (mean ± SD) in the rupture series and 2.7 ± 0.95 mm in the control series.

In the dissection study macroscopically normal supraspinatus tendons were found in 116 shoulders. Partial ruptures with penetrating degeneration of the supraspinatus tendon appeared in 32 shoulders (19%) and full-thickness ruptures were encountered in 22 shoulders (13%) (Tab. 2). Distally pointing osteophytes of the acromioclavicular joint were registered in 40 shoulders (24%). The osteophytes appeared in 29 shoulders with partial or full—thickness ruptures and in 11 shoulders with normal supraspinatus tendons. This difference is significant ($p < 0.001$, chi-square test). In 20 shoulders the osteophytes were found only on the clavicular side of the acromioclavicular joint, in five they were present on the acromial side and in 15 shoulders, distally pointing osteophytes were encountered on both sides of the acromioclavicular joint.

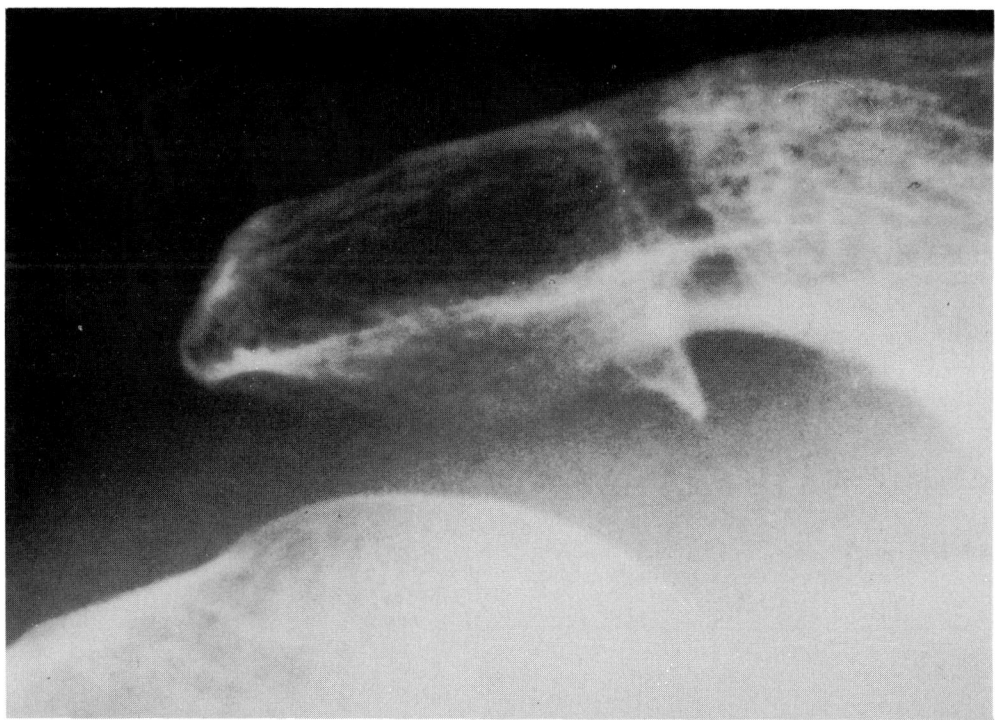

Figure 3 Radiogram of the right acromioclavicular joint of a 64-year-old woman with a large distally pointing osteophyte at the acromial side of the joint.

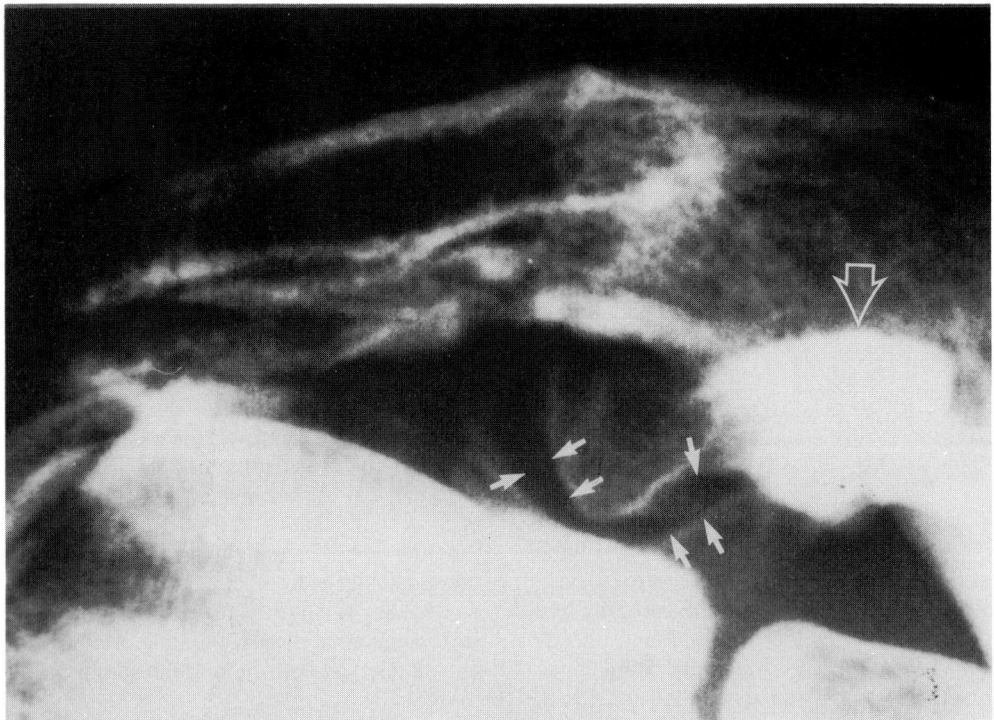

Figure 4 Arthrogram of the right shoulder of a 60-year-old man. The supraspinatus tendon, indicated by small arrows, is distally compressed by a large osteophyte at the clavicular end of the acromioclavicular joint. Contrast is escaping through a tendon rupture (open arrow).

DISCUSSION

Meyer[4] proposed attrition of the aponeurosis against the undersurface of the acromion as the main cause of supraspinatus tendon ruptures. Neer[6] found that impingement of the tendinous portion of the rotator cuff by the coracoacromial ligament and the anterior third of the acromion was responsible for a characteristic syndrome of shoulder disability. In a dissection study carried out in conjunction with surgical procedures, he found proliferative bone spurs and ridges on the anterior lip of the acromion. In several instances he also encountered bone spurs on the undersurface of the acromioclavicular joint. Kessel[2] and Watson[10] found lesions of the supraspinatus tendon associated with degeneration of the acromioclavicular joint in one-third of their patients.

The results of the present investigation very strongly suggest an association between distally pointing osteophytes of the acromioclavicular joint and ruptures of the supraspinatus tendon. The most plausible pathomechanism is that the osteophytes impinge on the supraspinatus tendon and press it against the humeral head when the arm is raised, especially in abduction. The continued impingement might, in addition to mechanical attrition, cause critical ischemia and subnutrition in the hypovascularized area of the supraspinatus tendon described by several investigators.[3,5,8,9] In consequence the tendon degenerates and eventually ruptures.

Conclusions

There exists a significant relationship between distally pointing osteophytes of the acromiocla-

TABLE 2 Age, Sex and Side Distribution of 54 Partial and Full-Thickness Supraspinatus Tendon Ruptures in 32 Cadavers

	No.	Average Age ± SD	Right	Left	Bilateral
Men	17	75 ± 8	3	2	24
Women	15	78 ± 11	5	0	20

vicular joint and supraspinatus tendon ruptures. Radiological examination of the shoulder in patients with rotator cuff symptoms should include an anteroposterior projection of the acromioclavicular joint with the undersurface of the joint clearly outlined. In rotator cuff surgery the acromioclavicular joint should be scrutinized and resected when distally pointing osteophytes are present.

REFERENCES

1. DePalma AF. Degenerative changes in the sternoclavicular and acromioclavicular joints in various decades. Springfield, CC Thomas, 1957.
2. Kessel L, Watson M. The painful arc syndrome. J Bone Joint Surg 1977; 59B:166–172.
3. Macnab I. Die pathologische Grundlage der sogennanten Rotatorenmanschetten-Tendinitis. Orthopäde 1981; 10:191–195.
4. Meyer AW. Further evidences of attrition in the human body. Am J Anat 1924; 34:241–267.
5. Moseley HF, Goldie I. The arterial pattern of the rotator cuff of the shoulder. J Bone Joint Surg 1963; 54A:780–789.
6. Neer II C. Anterior acromioplasty for the chronic impingement syndrome in the shoulder. J Bone Joint Surg 1972; 54A:41–50.
7. Petersson CJ. Degeneration of the acromioclavicular joint. A morphological study. Acta Orthop Scand 1983; 54:434–438.
8. Rathbun JB, Macnab I. The microvascular pattern of the rotator cuff. J Bone Joint Surg 1970; 52B:540–553.
9. Rothman RH, Parke WW. The vascular anatomy of the rotator cuff. Clin Orthop 1965; 41:176–186.
10. Watson M. The refractory painful arc syndrome. J Bone Joint Surg 1978; 60B:544–546.

CONTACT AREAS OF THE "SUBACROMIAL" JOINT

RICHARD J. NASCA, M.D., E. GEORGE SALTER, Ph.D., and CRAIG E. WEIL, M.D.

Painful shoulder arc, impingement syndromes and rotator cuff tears are common disorders which affect a significant number of people. Reduced volume within the coracoacromial arch and the unyielding nature of the coracoacromial ligament are considered to be causative factors.[15] Neer[13] implicates the anterior one-third of the acromion process, the coracoacromial ligament and at times, the acromioclavicular joint, as the anatomical culprits in impingement. Bigliani et al[1] observed that an unfused acromial epiphysis may be associated with an impingement lesion or a rotator cuff tear.

Stimulated by our clinical experience with disruptions of the rotator cuff, we were desirous of further defining the physical relationship of the cuff tendons to the acromion process. Impaling of the cuff tendons against the acromion process occurs with falls on the outstretched, flexed and abducted upper limb. In this manner, the undersurface of the acromion may act as a fulcrum through which shearing force is transmitted.

The purpose of our investigation was to delineate the area of surface contact between the cuff tendons and acromion process using a dye technique with the shoulder positioned in varying degrees of abduction.

METHODS AND MATERIALS

During the years 1981 and 1982, sixty cadaver shoulders were examined. Observations were made on the presence or absence of a rotator cuff tear, and areas of degeneration. The anatomical course of the coracoacromial ligament was studied. The inferior surface of the acromion process was inspected for osteophytes and other anatomic variations. The space between the acromion and the humeral head was measured. Acromioclavicular joints were evaluated for degenerative changes. Anatomic variations were noted on the courses and insertions of the tendons comprising the rotator cuff.

The deltoid muscle was released from its origin in order to provide exposure of the subacromial bursa, the acromioclavicular joint and the cuff tendons. Brilliant green dye was used to stain the inferior acromial surface (Fig. 1). The shoulder was then compressed manually as the humerus was abducted to an angle of 45 degrees in relationship to the sagittal plane of the body (Fig. 2). As abduction progressed, contact was made between the acromion and the rotator cuff tendons and the tendons became stained. These contact areas were triangular in shape; the sides of the triangle were measured with a caliper. Contact areas were then produced in 90 degrees of abduction (Fig. 3). To prevent inadvertent stain of the cuff tendons while applying the dye, a plastic shield was used as a barrier. Subsequently, an osteotomy of the acromion process was done in order to disclose and fully measure the contact area which was more extensive at 90 degrees abduction.

Anterior-posterior, lateral, oblique and superior-inferior radiographs of 12 of the acromion processes, with and without attached clavicles, were done after acromionectomy and soft tissue removal. The angle of inferior inclination of the anterior portion of the acromial edge was determined by constructing a line through the mid-portion of the acromion and another line parallel to its inferior surface (Fig. 4).

Statistical analysis of the contact area data was done by the Biostatistics Department at the University of Alabama in Birmingham.

The area of a triangle with three unequal sides such as occurred in our observations is computed as follows:

A, B and C will be designated as the three sides of the triangle. S is equal to the sum of the sides, A + B + C, divided by two. Therefore, the area is equal to the square root of S ×

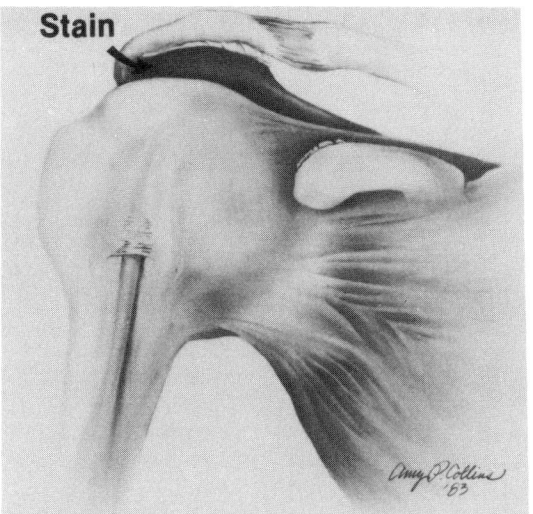

Figure 1 Exposed cadaver shoulder. Stain applied to undersurface of acromion process. Note resected coracoacromial ligament.

$(S - A) \times (S - B) \times (S - C)$. Computer analysis using the above formula was done.

RESULTS

In the 60 cadaver shoulders, eight rotator cuff tendon tears were observed. These varied in size from four centimeters to two millimeters in diameter. Usually, these involved the full thickness of the cuff tendons. A corresponding "irregular area" with osteophytes and bony excrescences was noted on the anterior-inferior aspect of the ipsilateral acromion process. These pathological changes in each instance corresponded to the contact area on the acromion process indicating the probable cause and effect relationship between the area of cuff defect and the anterior-inferior leading edge of the acromion. Occasionally, the anterior-inferior edge of the acromion appeared to have a curved, facet-like structure which reduced the space between the acromion and the cuff tendons (Fig. 5).

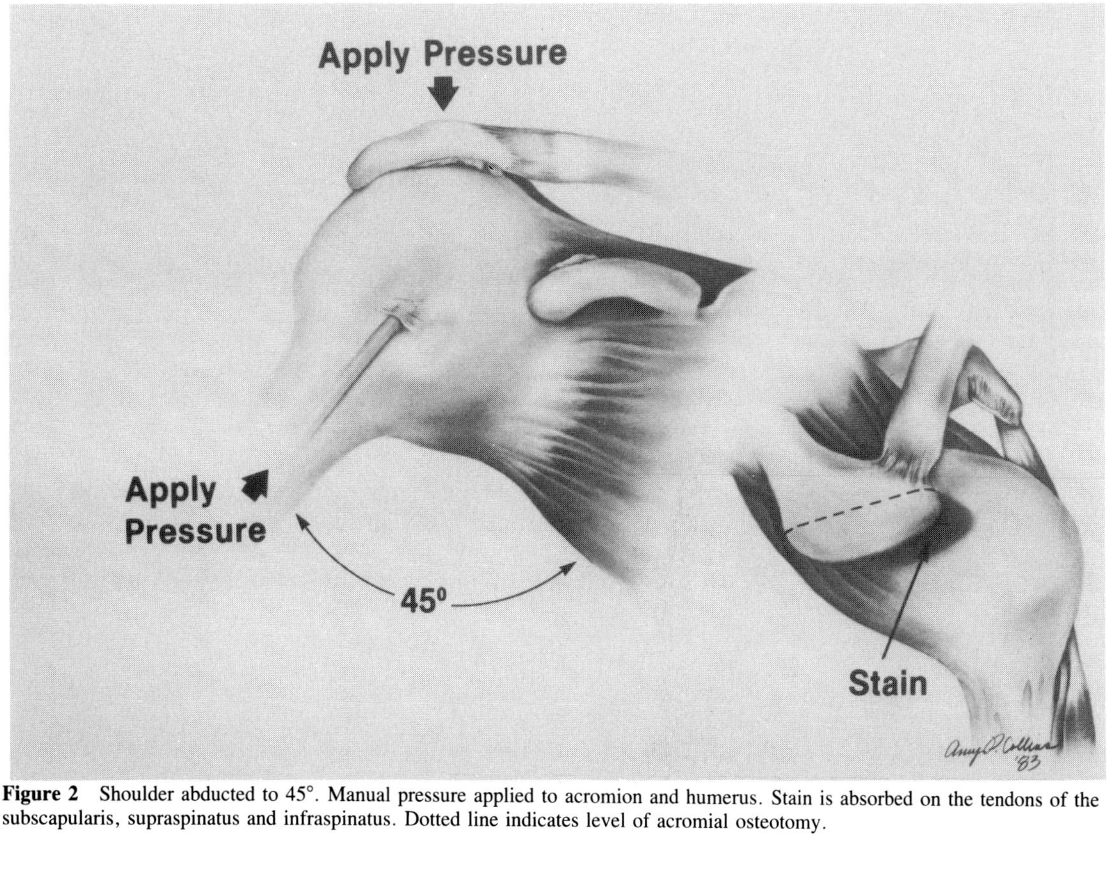

Figure 2 Shoulder abducted to 45°. Manual pressure applied to acromion and humerus. Stain is absorbed on the tendons of the subscapularis, supraspinatus and infraspinatus. Dotted line indicates level of acromial osteotomy.

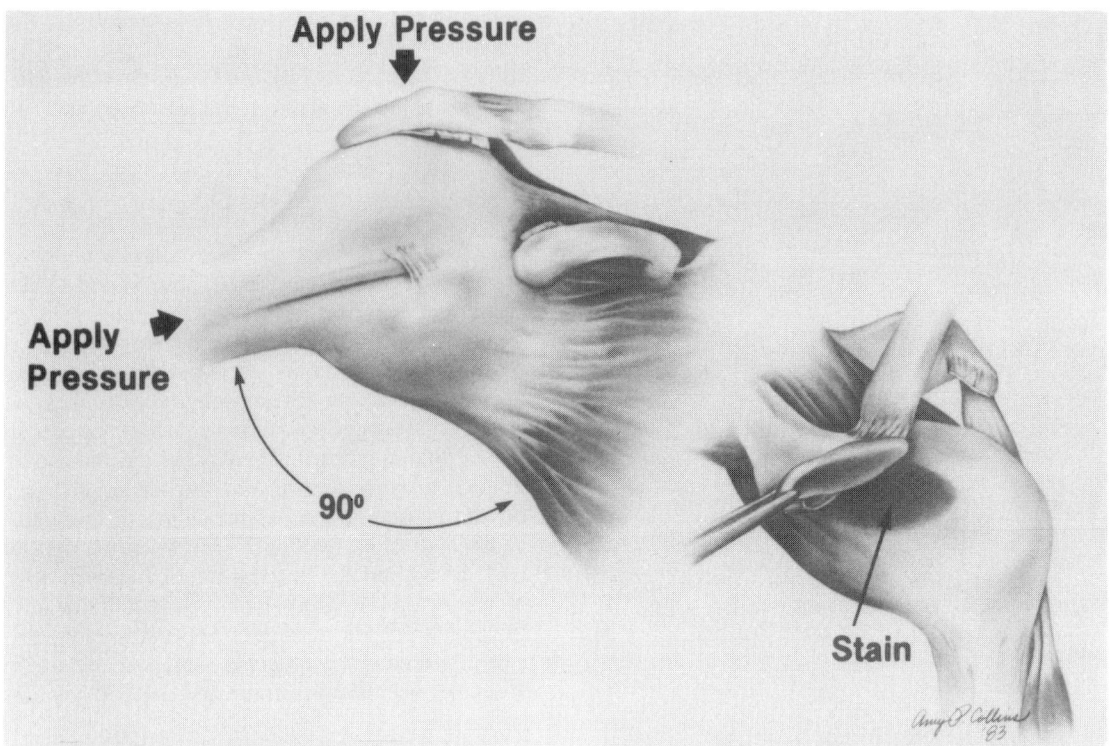

Figure 3 Contact area produced at 90° abduction. Acromial osteotomy completed uncovering the stained rotator cuff tendons.

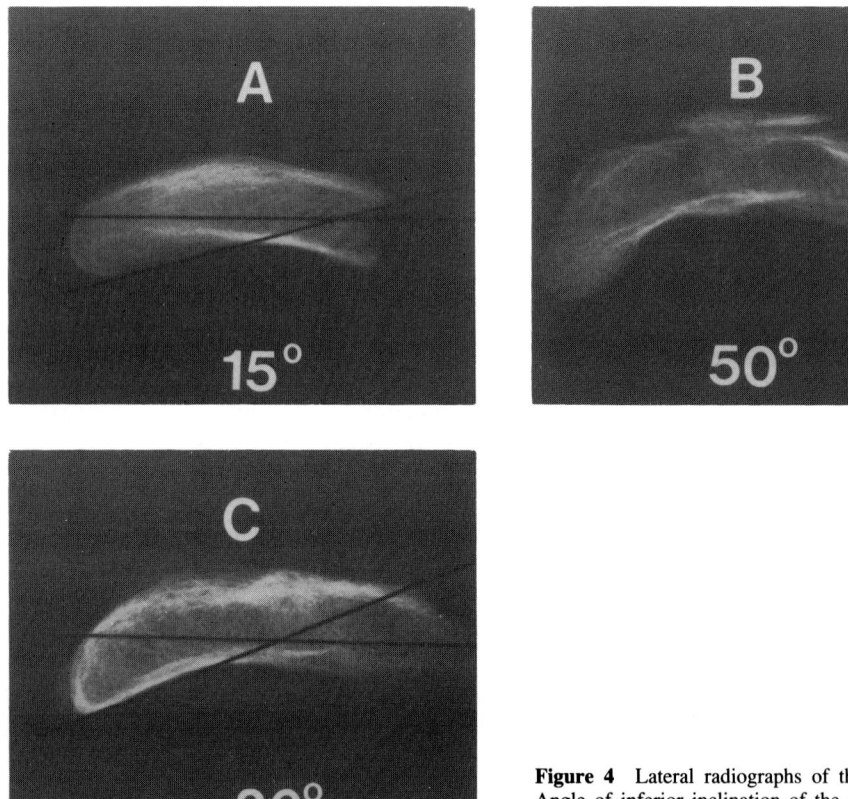

Figure 4 Lateral radiographs of three acromion processes. Angle of inferior inclination of the anterior edge constructed as shown in A and C. Note high angle of 50° in specimen B.

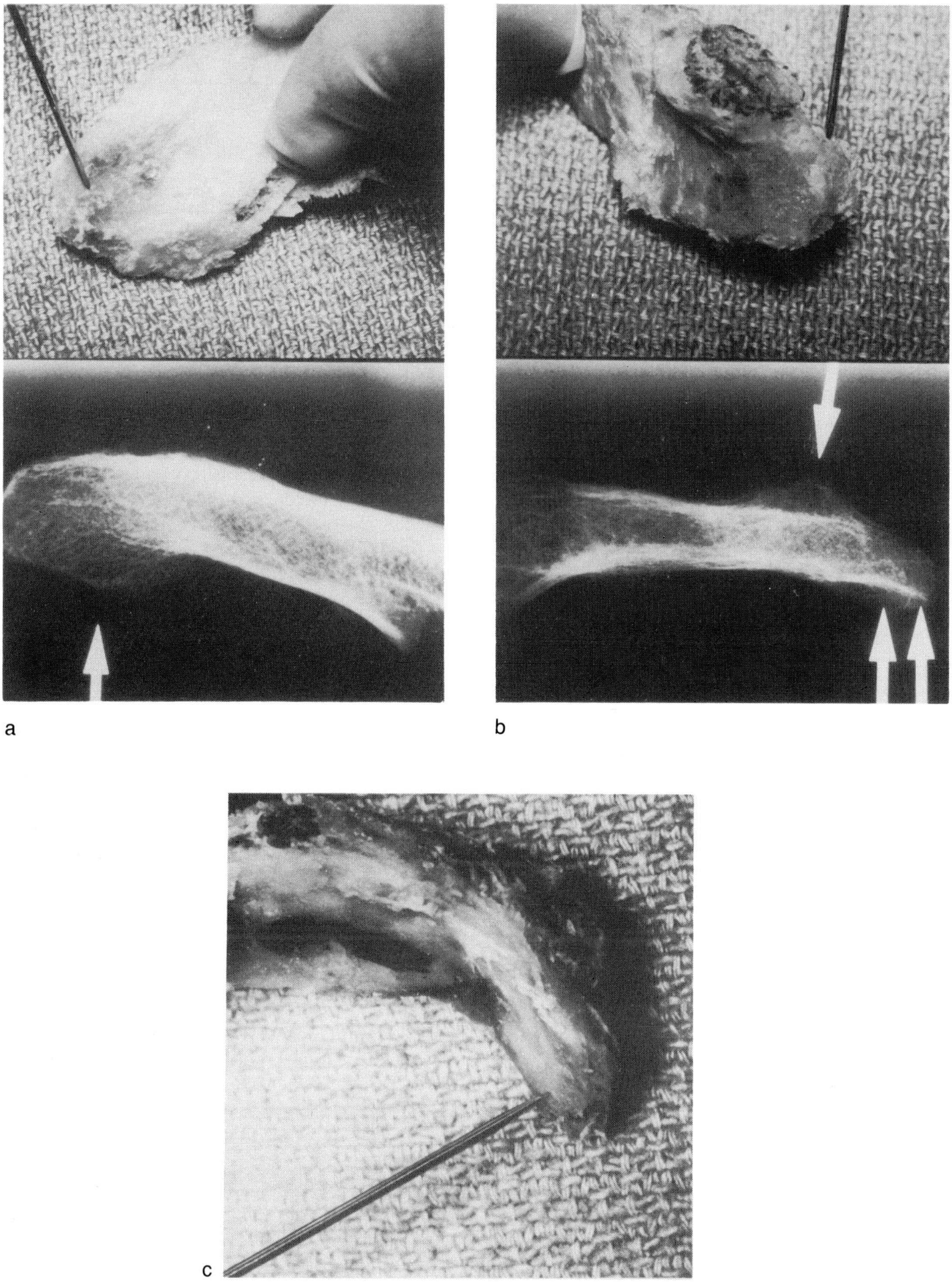

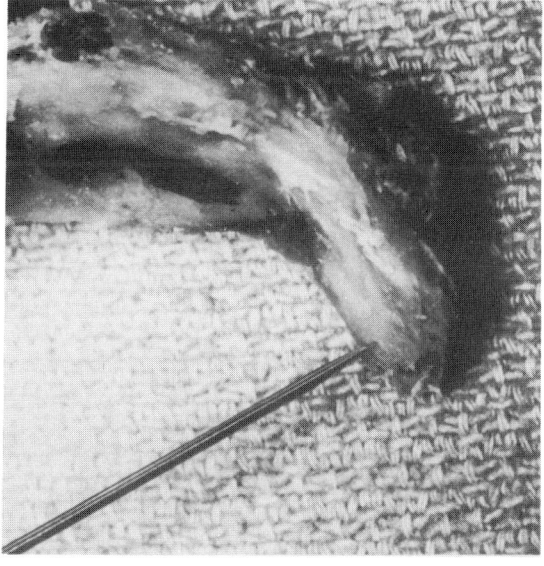

Figure 5 (a) Gross photograph and lateral radiograph of acromion process. Note arthritic change on inferior acromial surface (pointer), and inferior acromial osteophyte (arrow). (b) Gross photograph and lateral radiograph of acromion process. Note large osteophyte on acromial side of A-C joint (single arrow), and eburnated osteophytic area inferior surface (double arrow). (c) Gross photograph of acromion process with hook-like facet structure along its anterior-inferior edge (pointer).

The angle of inferior inclination of the acromial edge was measured on the radiographs of twelve specimens. An angle of 15 degrees to 30 degrees was considered normal. Angles of 50 degrees were noted in two specimens. These high angle acromion processes reduce subacromial space. Thus, the direction, orientation and size of the acromion process may be yet another causative factor in impingement and cuff tears. Compromise of the subacromial space will also result from arthritic changes on the inferior aspect of the acromioclavicular joint.

The coracoacromial ligament originated from the entire undersurface of the acromion process, with the exception of the anterior-inferior leading edge. It is difficult to appreciate how this ligament can reduce the space between the acromion process and the cuff tendons since it is so closely applied to the acromion process. In addition, this structure is broad, flexible and yielding. The coracoacromial ligament may act like a meniscus buffering the cuff tendons from the undersurface of the acromion process except in the crucial uncovered area at the anterior-inferior edge.

Degenerative changes in the acromioclavicular joint were noted in only four of 60 shoulders. The distance between the undersurface of the acromion and the humeral head with the upper limb by the side was measured in 15 shoulders and ranged between three and eight millimeters. Due to the stiffness of the shoulders studied and the fact that the deltoid muscle was released from its origin, this measurement may be spurious. In a few specimens it was noted that the muscle fibers of the supraspinatus and infraspinatus, rather than their tendons, inserted almost directly into the greater tuberosity. The tendon of the teres minor inserted consistently posterior and inferior to the greater tuberosity.

Dye was consistently absorbed on the tendons of the subscapularis, supraspinatus, and partly on the infraspinatus at 45 degrees abduction. A consistently larger area of contact was observed at 90 degrees abduction. All four of the cuff tendons were stained at 90 degrees of abduction.

Contact areas using the brilliant–green method as described were completed in 48 shoulders. The calculated area of contact was 4.77 square centimeters in 34 shoulders at 45 degrees abduction (P = 0.001). The calculated area at 90 degrees abduction was 7.08 square centimeters. In 14 shoulders, consistent 3-side measurements were not obtained and therefore not analyzed.

A 2-sided T-test was used to compare the mean measurements in Table 1. When the height of the same side was compared at 45 degrees and 90 degrees, all differences were statistically significant (P = 0.001).

TABLE 1 Mean Variability of Side Measurements of Contact Areas at 45 Degrees and 90 Degrees Abduction

Side	45 Degrees	90 Degrees
1	3.42 cm	4.09 cm
2	3.22 cm	3.98 cm
3	3.42 cm	4.15 cm

The course of the long head of the biceps tendon into the shoulder joint was traced upon opening the rotator cuff. This tendon was confluent with, and took origin from, the glenoid labrum rather than having an isolated origin from the supraglenoid tubercle as is depicted in anatomy texts. Little change in the gross appearance and continuity of the biceps tendon was noted, even with the coexistence of cuff tears.

DISCUSSION

Goodfellow and Bullough[6] used manual compression and a dye technique to map contact areas in 50 cadaver hips. Greenwald and Haynes[7] measured contact and weight-bearing areas in mechanically loaded and unloaded hip joints in 51 adult specimens using a dye technique. Using barium sulphate coating and AP and lateral radiographs on compressed knee joints, tibial-femoral contact areas were defined by Kettelkamp and Jacobs.[9] To our knowledge, these techniques have not been applied to the shoulder joint.

Fibrillation, lamination and thinning of the cuff fibers near their site of insertion into the tuberosities during the fifth decade in postmortem studies on 50 individuals were observed by DePalma.[4] In nine specimens, complete tears which communicated with the subacromial bursa were noted. He also noted evidence of contact between the greater tuberosity and the inferior aspect of the acromion process.

Cotton and Rideout[3] studied 106 necropsy subjects by anatomical and radiographic techniques. Radiographic abnormalities were found in 68 shoulders. Full-thickness tears of the cuff with the head of the humerus articulating with the acromion process were seen in seven specimens.

Olsson[14] carried out clinical and anatomical studies on 106 shoulder joints. He discussed the concept of the "superohumeral joint," ie. the coracoacromial arch as the socket and the top of the humeral head with the cuff as its ball.

Laumann's[10] anatomical studies on the shoulder resulted in his dividing the subacromial space into three separate segments: ventral, medial and dorsal. The subacromial space was narrowest in the medial and ventral segments.

Brewer[2] studied the greater tuberosity with the attached supraspinatus tendon. He found osteitis and cystic degeneration, decreased vascularity, disruption of the tendon of the supraspinatus to bone at Sharpys fibers, and fragmentation of the tendon with loss of staining quality.

Moseley and Goldie,[12] Rothman and Parke,[18] and Rathbun and MacNab[17] studied the vasculature of the rotator cuff. These investigators noted the relative avascularity of the supraspinatus tendon near insertion and termed this the "critical zone." Rathbun and MacNab[17] noted increased microcirculation of the supraspinatus tendon with abduction of the shoulder which they ascribed to relaxation of tension in the tendon of the supraspinatus. Neer[13] deonstrated in eight cadaver specimens a characteristic ridge of spurs and excrescences on the undersurface of the anterior process of the acromion. Without exception, it was the anterior lip and undersurface of the acromion along its anterior third that was involved. Mechanical impingement was noted in 11 of 100 dissected scapulae.

DeSeze[5] considered the coracoacromial vault, rotator cuff and humeral head to be the second "articulation" of the shoulder joint. We have coined the term "subacromial joint" as a descriptive term for this second articulation.

Using dynamic electromyography, Inman, Saunders and Abbott[8] found that all four of the rotator cuff muscles were active during shoulder abduction, although they individually varied in their intensity of action throughout the arc of motion. According to Perry,[16] the resultant force for the total cuff musculature depresses the humeral head and pulls it somewhat medially. Major tears of the rotator cuff deny patients adequate shoulder control by distorting the architecture.

A radiographic study on 1,800 shoulder girdles was done by Leiberson.[11] He found 25 cases of os acromiale. Hook-like, facet projections at the anterior-inferior edge of the acromion which extend inferiorly into the subacromial space may be implicated in impingement problems when the cuff tendons make contact in the position of abduction and forward flexion. These acromial variants, rather than a yielding structure such as the coracoacromial ligament, may well be the culprits in causing impingement in young athletes. These acromial variations do not appear to be unfused accessory ossification centers as described by Bigliani et al.[1]

Deficiencies in this study include inherent stiffness of the cadaver shoulders and the need to take down the deltoid attachments to the acromion process, clavicle and spine of the scapula. It is hoped that this study can be refined by using fresh necropsies and employing arthroscopic techniques in conjunction with the staining procedures.

REFERENCES

1. Bigliani LU, Neer CS, Norris TR, Fischer J. The relationship between the unfused acromial epiphysis and subacromial impingement lesions. Exhibit AAOS, Anaheim, CA, March 1983.
2. Brewer BJ. Aging of the rotator cuff. Am J Sports Med 1979; 7:102–110.
3. Cotton RE, Rideout DF. Tears of the humeral rotator cuff: a radiological and pathological necropsy survey. J Bone Joint Surg 1964; 46B:314–328.
4. DePalma AF. Surgical anatomy of the rotator cuff and the natural history of degenerative periarthritis. Surg Clin North Am 1963; 43:1507–1520.
5. DeSeze S, Ryckewaert A, Caroit M. Les ruptures traumatiques de la coiffe des rotateurs. Rev Rheumatisme 1960; 27 II:443–453.
6. Goodfellow JW, Bullough PG. Studies on age changes in the human hip joint. J Bone Joint Surg 1968; 50B:222.
7. Greenwald AS, Haynes DW. Weight bearing areas in the human hip joint. J Bone Joint Surg 1972; 54B:157–163.
8. Inman VT, Saunders M, Abbott LC. Observations on the function of the shoulder joint. J Bone Joint Surg 1944; 26B:1–30.
9. Kettlekamp DB, Jacobs AN. Tibiofemoral contact area, determination and implications. J Bone Joint Surg 1972; 54A:349–356.
10. Laumann U. Decompression of the subacromial space: an anatomical study. In: Bailey I., Kessel L,. eds. Shoulder Surgery. Berlin: Springer-Verlag, 1982.
11. Leiberson E. Os acromiale: a contested anomaly. J Bone Joint Surg 1937; 19:683.
12. Moseley HF, Goldie I. The arterial patterns of the rotator cuff of the shoulder. J Bone Joint Surg 1963; 45B:780–789.
13. Neer CS. Anterior acromioplasty for the chronic impingement syndrome in the shoulder: a preliminary report. J Bone Joint Surg 1972; 54A:41–50.
14. Olsson O. Degenerative changes in the shoulder joint and their connection with shoulder pain: a morphological and clinical investigation with special attention to the cuff and biceps tendon. Acta Clin Scand (Supp 181), 1953.
15. Penny JN, Welsh RP. Shoulder impingement syndromes in the athletes and their surgical management. Am J Sports Med 1981; 9:11–15.
16. Perry J. Normal upper extremity kinesiology. Physical Therapy 1978; 53:265–278.
17. Rathbun JB, MacNab I. The microvascular pattern of the rotator cuff. J Bone Joint Surg 1970; 52B:540–553.
18. Rothman RH, Parke WW. The vascular anatomy of the rotator cuff. Clin Orthop 1965; 41:176–186.

THE IMPINGEMENT SYNDROME IN SPORTSMEN

MICHAEL WATSON, M.A., M.R.C.P., F.R.C.S.

The sportsman is disproportionately incapacitated by injuries. Apparently trivial injuries may ruin his recreation and may even prevent him from earning a living. Impingement in the shoulder is frequently expectantly treated in the sportsman on the assumption that all cases are benign and that they resolve quickly and spontaneously. This is not always so. This paper describes the surgical management of a large series of consecutive cases whose symptoms did not resolve with conservative management.

Materials and Methods

Two hundred and seven cases were culled from an upper-limb clinic and a sports-injuries clinic over a six-year period. May 1976 to April 1982. They were the failures of a much larger group of sportsmen with impingement syndrome who were treated by a variety of nonoperative means such as local steroid and local anesthetic, ultra-sound treatment, short-wave diathermy treatment and mobilisation. The average age was 32, but the range was wide, from 19 to 60. The male:female ratio was 11:1. The sports varied from table tennis to weight-lifting. The two most commonly represented sports were rugby football (72 cases) and swimming (18 cases).

The impingement syndrome was defined as a combination of full active and passive movement associated with pain during part of the excursion of the joint which was more severe near the mid-range of the excursion than near the extremes. All the patients had severe localized tenderness over part of the rotator cuff.

After inclusion in the series because the patient continued to suffer severe symptoms after adequate nonoperative treatment, an anatomical diagnosis was made by a combination of clinical and radiographic means described by Kessel and Watson.[1] Exploration was by the anterior route as decribed by Watson.[2] Briefly an anterior skin cleavage line incision was made over the acromioclavicular joint. The outer centimeter of the clavicle was excised and the coracoacromial ligament was removed. This gave a good view of the whole rotator cuff, allowed any decompression necessary and permitted a very rapid rehabilitation.

Findings

Impingement of an element of the rotator cuff against an element of the coracoacromial arch could be identified in each case. In some there were several impinging structures, but one was always more severe than the others, and this was considered the cause of the symptoms. The cuff was usually red and swollen at the site of impingement except at the center of the supraspinatus tendon, which was either unaffected or thinned and frayed. In a small number there was a hole less than one centimeter in diameter in the center of the frayed area.

There were 103 cases of impingement of the cuff on the deep surface of the acromioclavicular joint. In 34 cases the coracoacromial ligament was judged the chief culprit. Acromial abnormalities were the cause in 23 cases. In 23 the long head of the biceps tendon was to blame. In 16 cases enlarged tuberosities caused impingement and in eight cases the coracoid process appeared to be the chief culprit.

Acromioclavicular Abnormalities

The acromioclavicular joint abnormalities were either acquired from previous trauma or due to a localised congenital abnormality.

The single commonest cause of impingement in the whole series was post-traumatic degeneration of the acromioclavicular joint. The joint was incongruous due to fracture or dislocation in 91 cases. The contralateral acromioclavicular joint was painless and within normal radiological limits in each case. The affected joint was enlarged and tender. Infiltration of the joint with local anesthetic did not abolish the symptoms, excluding degeneration as the cause of the symptoms. In all cases both sides of the joint were enlarged by osteophytic new bone visible on the radiographs. In all cases the joint space was abnormal: in 79 it was narrow and in 12 it was distorted by permanent acquired upward or downward displacement of the outer end of the clavicle. In some this appeared to be associated with malunion of the outer third of the clavicle, but in the others no juxta-articular bony abnormality could be discerned, suggesting that the displacement and degeneration were due to unreduced subluxation or dislocation.

In 12 cases the joint was swollen and tender but there was no joint space narrowing. But there was osteophytic new bone. These cases appeared to have congenital abnormalities, for the opposite side was radiologically similar although asymptomatic. Most had reciprocally curved, sloping articular surfaces with over-riding of the outer end of the clavicle.

Exploration of the cases due to acromioclavicular abnormalities revealed a common pattern of affection. The capsule of the joint was thick and vascular. The peripheries of both the acromial and the clavicular surfaces of the joint were enlarged by irregular osteophytes. The articular cartilage was soft and frayed. The meniscus was never seen in its entirety, but a ragged rim was sometimes seen in the roof of the joint space. The coracoacromial ligament was universally distorted by the overlying enlarged joint. It bulged down and compressed the rotator cuff beneath it.

Removal of the outer centimeter of the clavicle, of the osteophytic new bone on either side of the joint and of the coracoacromial ligament decompressed the cuff. The region of the cuff most severely affected varied. In 59 there was diffuse redness and swelling of the anterior part of the cuff. In 74 only the subscapularis was thus affected. In 11 the supraspinatus was thinner and softer than usual. In nine the fraying process appeared to involve the tendon of the long head of the biceps too, which was soft and yellow. Four of the supraspinatus-only affections had small degenerate holes in the tendon. These were closed with tough absorbable synthetic sutures.

Coracoacromial Ligament

In 34 cases the chief obstruction to cuff excursion was an enlarged stiffened coracoacromial ligament. The ligament was approached through the bed of the apparently normal acromioclavicular joint. The affected ligament was thicker and wider than normal. In 11 cases it was stiffened by plaques of ossification in its origin and insertion. Excision of the ligament decompressed the cuff and revealed similar findings to those seen in acromioclavicular joint disease.

Acromion

The acromion seemed the chief culprit in 23 cases. Twelve had the characteristic hook described by Neer. This projected downwards from the anterior acromion into the path of the moving cuff. If was dealt with by anterior acromioplasty as described by Neer.[3] In eight a large osteophyte jutted down and caused an almost identical syndrome. Three cases had incongruity of the subacromial joint caused by malunion. Two of these were the result of previous explorations. They were dealt with by acromioplasty: the downward projections were removed with an osteotome orientated horizontally so as to preserve the acromial origin of the deltoid muscle.

Long Head of Biceps Tendon

In another 23 cases exploration revealed that the long head of the biceps tendon caused most of the trouble. In 18 the tendon looped passively during abduction of the shoulder and bulged up between the supraspinatus and the subscapularis tendons. It appeared that the normally tough fibrous sheet between the two was unusually weak, and that the tendon advanced along the line of least resistance until it became trapped momentarily beneath the acromion. The looping phenomenon was abolished by reinforcing the fibrous hiatus with a nylon suture.

In four cases the long head of the biceps tendon had ruptured and the proximal stump had become enlarged. The stump intermittently locked the shoulder joint on passive movement. The proximal stump was excised back to the glenoid in each case.

In one case the tendon was extremely thick due to hypertrophy. It impinged on the deep surface of the coracoacromial ligament in abduction. The tendon was excised from the shoulder joint and the distal stump was attached to the transverse ligament with a nylon suture.

Enlarged Tuberosities

Degenerative or congenital enlargement of one or both of the tuberosities appeared to be the cause of impingement in 16 cases. The greater tuberosity was the offender in 10 cases. In abduction the cuff was trapped between the tuberosity and the overlying structure, the arch formed by the acromion, the coracoacromial ligament and the coracoid process. The tuberosity was nibbled down via a split in the supraspinatus tendon in each case. The lesser tuberosity was hugely enlarged in one case and was dealt with similarly. In five cases both tuberosities were affected; they were treated similarly.

Coracoid Process

In eight patients impingement appeared to be due to congenital enlargement and misalignment of the coracoid process. The subscapularis muscle belly jammed deep to the coracoid process on internal rotation. The muscle was much closer to the undersurface of the process than usual and passive internal rotation caused the muscle to bulge tightly beneath the process and the attached short head of biceps and coracobrachialis. The impingement was relieved by detachment of the muscles and reattachment to the stump of the coracoacromial ligament. Three of the cases also had enlargement of the lesser tuberosity which was dealt with by nibbling down through a split in the tendon near its insertion.

Results

One year after operation the patients were assessed for this study. Full painless excursion and return to sport was considered "good". Residual pain less than before the operation with full excursion and return to sport was considered "better". Residual pain more than before the operation, any stiffness, and failure to return to sport were all classified as "worse".

It was not possible to differentiate the cases into good-prognosis and bad-prognosis groups with the exception of the enlarged tuberosities group. In this group four out of 16 were better than before the operation, but not good, and one was worse. In all the other groups about nine out of 10 were good after the operation (Table 1).

TABLE 1 Results of Cuff Decompression

Surgical Site	Good	Better	Worse
Acromioclavicular Joint	93	10	0
Coracoacromial Ligament	31	2	1
Acromion	20	3	3
Long Head Biceps Tendon	22	1	0
Tuberosities	11	4	1
Coracoid	8	0	0

Repair of small defects in the cuff did not appear to affect the outcome.

Discussion

Most sportsmen are extremely well motivated. This helps the surgeon in dealing with them for rehabilitation after shoulder surgery is most important and the patients cooperate keenly. It is likely, however, that comparable results in sedentary patients will not be obtained for postoperative rehabilitation will not be so enthusiastically performed.

The very high incidence of this condition and the frequency with which it is associated with chronic permanently displaced acromioclavicular joint injuries calls into question our usual regime in dealing with acute acromioclavicular injuries. It would be valuable to know if anatomical reduction and stabilisation of all such injuries led to a reduced incidence of late impingement.

It seems from the study that careful examination of the patient and of his radiographs makes possible an accurate anatomical diagnosis in cases of impingement syndrome in sportsmen. Further, it seems that decompression of the impinging structures is always feasible, and that a good return of function can be expected if care is taken to preserve the deltoid and its anchors in cases of severe refractory symptoms.

REFERENCES

1. Kessel, L, Watson M. The painful arc syndrome. J Bone Joint Surg 1977; 59B:166–172.
2. Watson M. Refractory painful arc syndrome. J Bone Joint Surg 1978; 544–546.
3. Neer CS II. Anterior acromioplasty for the chronic impingement syndrome in the shoulder. J Bone Joint Surg 1972; 54A:41–50.

DIAGNOSIS AND TREATMENT OF PARTIAL THICKNESS TEARS OF ROTATOR CUFF

SHIRO TABATA, M.D. and HIROSHI KIDA, M.D.

When we consider rotator cuff tears we tend to concentrate upon complete tears and neglect partial thickness tears. The diagnosis of partial tears is not easy and there has been no clear description either of decisive clinical symptoms or supplementary diagnostic procedures for this type of cuff tears, Furthermore, there are still many unresolved issues concerning appropriate surgical procedures and the extent of resection.

From 1976 to 1982, 70 shoulders of 66 patients with cuff tear were subjected to surgery, including 19 shoulders of 18 patients with partial tear. This paper reports on the results of a clinical study on the diagnosis and treatment of these partial thickness tears.

MATERIALS AND METHODS

Fifteen of the patients were men and three were women. One of the women had both shoulders damaged, bringing the total number of cases to 19. Ages ranged from 19 to 64; the average age was 48.2 years. This was lower than the average age of patients with complete tear which was 57 years.

In 15 shoulders, we were able to draw a clear history of the injury. Thirteen of the patients (72% of the total) were engaged in occupations requiring heavy manual labor. The period from the onset of symptoms to surgery ranged from three weeks to three years with the average period being 7.3 months.

Clinical Signs and Symptoms (Table 1)

The characteristic symptoms were night pain of sufficient severity to awaken the patient, and persistent pain with motion, particularly when dressing, undressing and reaching above the head. The clinical signs observed were tenderness at the greater tuberosity and at the anteroinferior part of the coracoacromial ligament, restriction of active movements, such as abduction internal and external rotation, a positive resistance test, muscle atrophy in the deltoid, supra and infraspinatus muscles, and stiffness.

The incidence of shoulder stiffness was higher in those shoulders with partial tears than in those with complete tears. Shoulder stiffness was found in 12 of the 19 shoulders (63%) with partial tear but in only 50 percent of the shoulders with complete tear. Ten of the 12 shoulders also exhibited adhesive and inflammatory changes in the subacromial bursa (SAB) when directly observed during surgery.

On the other hand, only one out of seven shoulders that displayed no changes of SAB showed joint stiffness. Muscular atrophy was seen in 15 of the 19 shoulders; 15 in the supraspinatus, 13 in the deltoid muscle, and 8 in the infraspinatus. Crepitus with a soft audible snap due to impingement at the coracoacromial arch when the upper extremity was raised against resistance was frequently noted.

Classification of Tears by Type and Site (Table 2)

Partial thickness tears of the rotator cuff can be classified into three types according to operative findings:

1. Deep surface tear: The shallow layer of the cuff was normal but the deep layer of the cuff on the articular surface at the point of cuff insertion or critical area showed partial avulsion and tears.

2. Superficial tear: The shallow layer of the cuff showed partial ablation, small tear, or erosion at the cuff insertion or critical area.

3. Horizontal split: Development of a cavity was seen between the shallow and deep layers due to detachment of the cuff as a result of its progressive degeneration.

There were deep surface tears in 12 shoulders, superficial tears in five shoulders and horizontal splits in two shoulders. Deep surface tears

144 / Surgery of the Shoulder

TABLE 1 Clinical Signs and Symptoms

Pain: Night pain	16
Motional pain	19
Tenderness:	18
Degree of Mobility	
(Abd): <90	7
90–149	6
150<	6
Resistance Test:	14
Stiffness:	12
Muscular Atrophy:	15

Bursal Lesion and Joint Stiffness

Bursal Lesion (S.A.B.)		Stiffness
⊕12	→	⊕10 / ⊖ 2
⊖ 7	→	⊕ 1 / ⊖ 6

can be recognized by palpation and by color injection test; superficial tears can be seen directly during surgery; horizontal split can be detected by digital palpation and buckling of the superficial layer. Deep surface tears were frequently found in younger patients with an average age of 41. Further trauma was considered to be a contributing factor.

Superficial tears were seen in patients with an average age of 58, and horizontal split in patients whose average age was 63. Partial tears of the cuff were seen in the supraspinatus and the subscapularis, but partial tears of subscapularis showed only deep surface tears.

Clinical Diagnosis and Indications for Surgery

We emphasized clinical symptoms when determining if surgery was necessary. Decisions were made based on overall judgement taking into consideration resistance to conservative treatment, the duration of the disease, and the patient's social circumstances including such factors as a possible early return to his or her former occupation.

The main clinical signs and symptoms were persistent pain (night pain, pain with movement), weakness and atrophy, and restricted movement. No characteristic change was observed in the plain x-ray. No extravasation into the SAB was seen in the arthrography of the partial tear because there was no communication between the articular cav-

TABLE 2 Classification and Region of Partial Thickness Tear

Classification	Region	Insertion	Critical Area
Deep Surface Age: average 41.5 yrs.	12 (SSP 8, SSC 4)		
Superficial Age: average 58.2 yrs.	5 (SSP 5)		
Horizontal Split Age: average 63.5 yrs.	2 (SSP 2)		

ity and the shallow layer of the cuff. It is said that a local contrast filled defect is usually seen in the deep layer of the cuff in the arthrography but this was observed in only three of 12 shoulders (Fig. 1). In superficial and horizontal tears, no characteristic findings were obtained either by arthrography or by bursography (Fig. 2).

Diagnosis During Surgery; Extent of Resection of the Damaged Cuff

When the region of a deep surface tear was subjected to careful palpation during surgery it felt thin and fluffy. The region was darkly dyed by color injection test[3] (Fig. 3). In a superficial tear, when the bursal floor was resected vertically, we saw that the shallow layer of the cuff had detached from the greater tuberosity and presented a very rough texture at the critical area.

As the shallow layer of the cuff was ablated, the entire damaged layer of the cuff could be resected and restored, though the deep layer still remained unhurt. The presence of horizontal split could nt be easily confirmed either by palpation or by color injection.

In horizontal split, the lesion expanded widely and the boundary between the lesion and the normal region was not clear, leading to extensive resection.

Results

The follow-up period for 19 shoulders in 18 patients ranged from four years to six months: the average was eight months. The results of postoperative assessment were generally satisfactory considering that cases with short follow-up periods were included. According to Wolfgang's criteria,[7] 15 were excellent, three were good, and one was fair. The patients who had postoperative joint stiffness tended also to suffer pain and resisted functional improvement during postoperative therapy. This fact did not influence the results of the follow-up investigation.

The three cases which were restored by the patch method required long periods for recovery of muscle power. A slight decrease in muscle power resulted in 2 out of these 3 cases. Sixteen patients returned to their former occupations. Three patients were operated upon again.

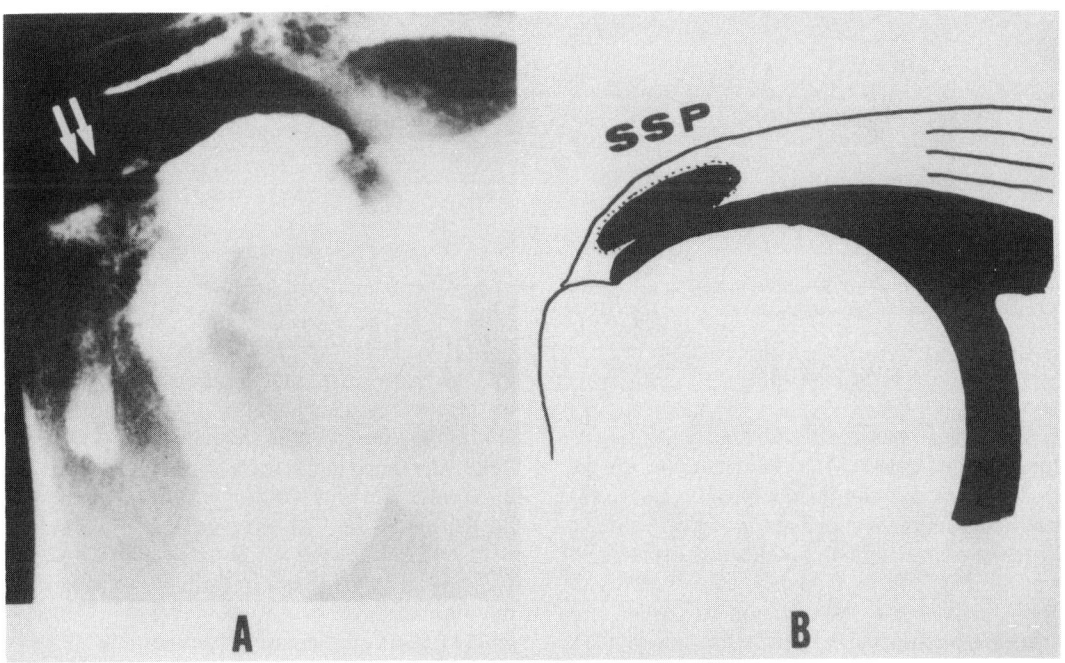

Figure 1 Deep surface tear in a 38-year old man.

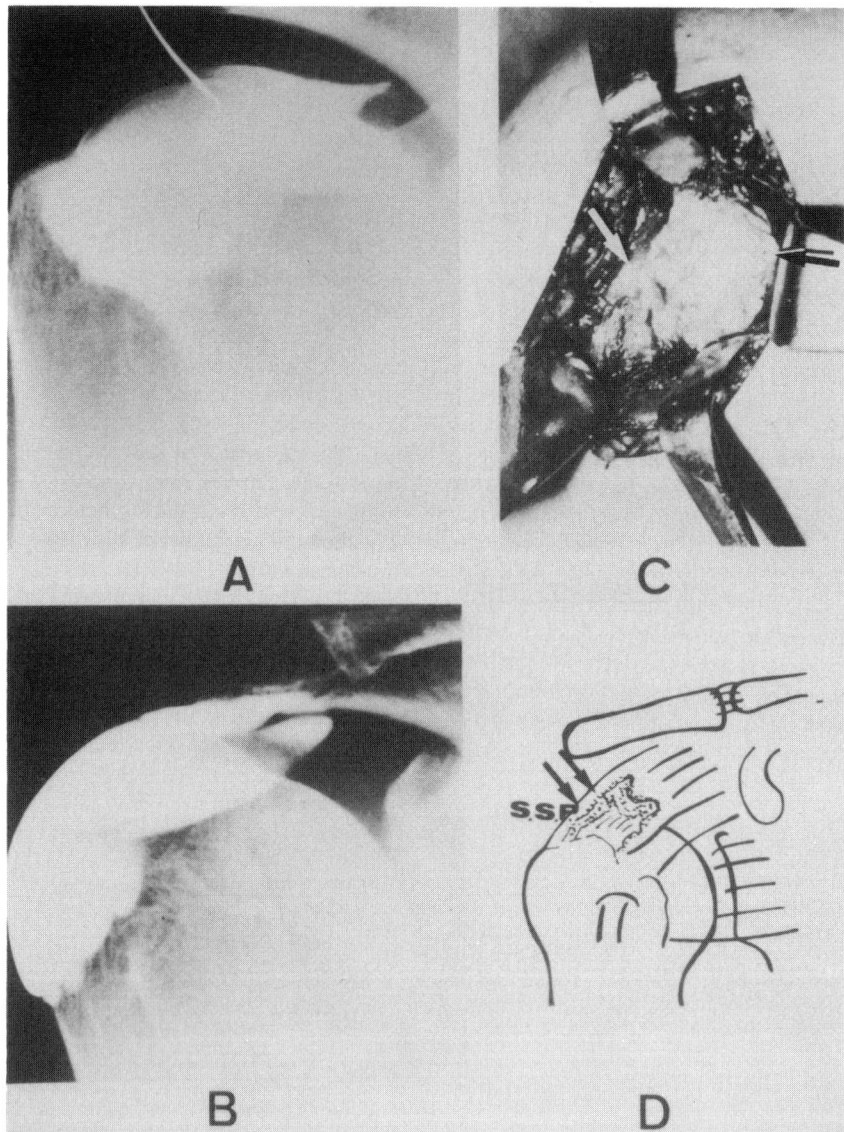

Figure 2 Superficial tear of the supraspinatus in a 46-year old man. A, B, no abnormal findings. C, D, the shallow layer of the supraspinatus showed rough scar and erosion.

DISCUSSION

Cuff injury has been classified according to shape, size and cause. We consider it convenient, both diagnostically and therapeutically, to classify partial tears roughly into three groups: full thickness tears, partial thickness tears, and rotator interval lesions. Since Codman,[1] the number of terms[4,7] used in the classification of partial tears has been numerous. The reclassification of these terms deep surface tears, superficial tears and horizontal split is shown (Tab. 3).

In many cases, deep surface tear is a result of serious trauma. Patients with deep surface tears tend to be younger than those patients with superficial and horizontal tears. Superficial tears and horizontal split may occur with minor trauma or no trauma at all. The average age of the patients with horizontal split tends to be high. However, these points are subject to further investigation as the number of cases investigated was small. Clinical symptoms are decisive factors in the diagnosis of partial tears. It is essential therefore that the patient be closely questioned about history of the

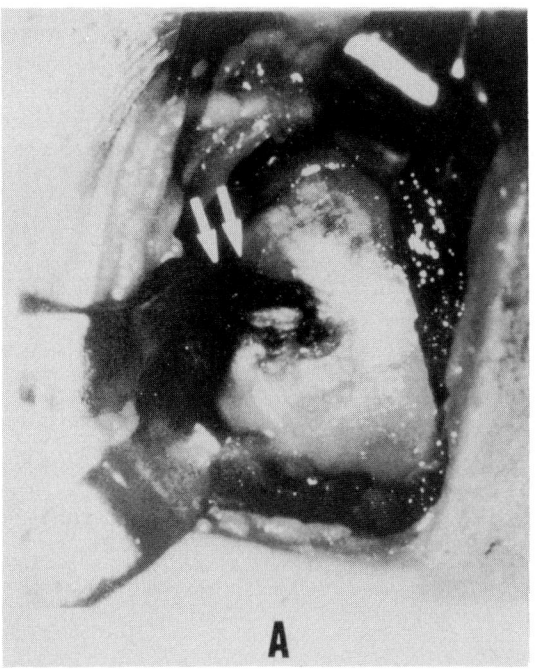 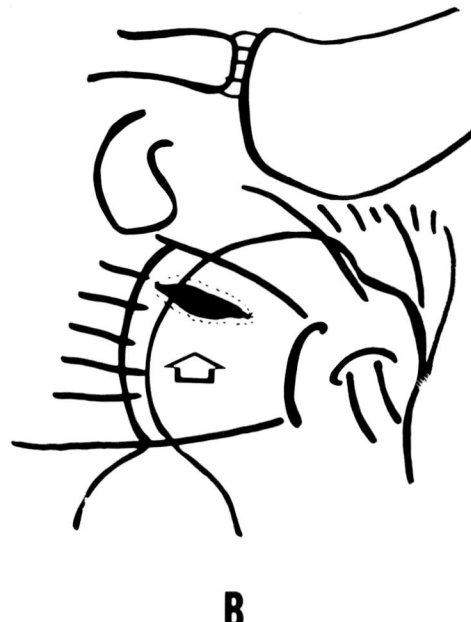

Figure 3 Deep surface tear of the subscapularis in a 50-year old man. Color injection test showed infiltration of the dye.

trauma, the localization of shoulder pain, ADL disorder, etc.

It is said that in the case of deep surface tears arthrograms reveal a shadow defect in the ulcer-like crater but in the case of subscapular tears, the shadow defect cannot be seen even by Y-view. We anticipate therefore that procedures will be developed to predict the presence of a tear by preoperative diagnosis. In the cases of superficial and horizontal tears, it is not possible to prove the shadow defect, but there were cases in which the flow of dye wasn't smooth and did not result in filling while it was infused. We should, therefore, pay attention to dynamic arthrography even if only for the purpose of obtaining a clue to cuff injury.

For superficial tears, diagnosis during surgery is easy; but for deep surface tears, palpation and a colour injection test are required. As it is difficult to predict preoperatively the presence of a partial tear of the subscapularis, it is necessary to perform careful palpation on the anterior medial surface of the cuff during surgery. It is not at all easy to confirm horizontal split even by careful palpation. Neviaser[11] confirmed the presence of tears by producing distortion resulting from pushing the shallow layer of the cuff toward the greater tuberosity with an instrument. We detected the presence of tears by digitally buckling the superficial layer of the cuff.

There are many papers[2,4] which admit the extreme difficulty of making a definitive diagnosis of partial tear, while finding conservative treatment remarkably effective.[2,4] Partial tears known to have been easily cured by conservative treatment include contusion of muscles, traumatic subacromial bursitis, tendinitis, etc. Therefore, when a partial tear is suspected but not confirmed,

TABLE 3 Classification of Rotator Cuff Tears

1. Full thickness tear (Complete tear)
2. Partial thickness tear (Incomplete tear)
   ① Deep surface tear
rim rent	(Codman)
concealed tear	(Bateman)
deep surface rupture } deep surface avulsion }	(Bosworth)
deep surface tear	(Neviaser)

   ② Superficial tear
Erosion on bursal side	(Codman)
upper surface split	(Bosworth)
superficial tear	(Bateman)

   ③ Horizontal split
   | parting of central fibers | (Codman) |
   | horizontal split | (Bosworth) |

3. Rotator interval lesion
   | small slit or rim rent | (Bateman) |
   | longitudinal rent | (Depalma) |

we make it a rule to put the patient in a sling or plaster cast for 2 to 3 weeks as a screening procedure. In view of our experience with patients who were reoperated, we believe that when deep surface or superficial tears are repaired, the entire layer including the normal region should be fully resected, even though the actual lesion is part of either the deep or the shallow layer.

The basic cause of horizontal split can be traced to the progressive degeneration of the cuff and because the lesion covers a wide area that lost elasticity, tight sutures are to be avoided. The measures we have taken with these patients included the application of the patch repair method which is considered adequate for tears covering a wide area especially in older patients who, because of their ADL conditions, are not required to be enlarged in strenuous physical activities.

Preoperative joint stiffness is often represented by adhesion or inflammatory change in SAB, for which the release of the coracoacromial or the coracohumeral ligament is required. Moreover, those same cases which are complicated by stiffness also tend to suffer pain during postoperative therapy which consequently tends to be prolonged.

REFERENCES

1. Codman EA. The shoulder, Thomas Todd, 1934.
2. Depalma AF. Surgery of the shoulder, JB Lippincott, 1973.
3. Fukuda H et al. Injury of the rotator cuff-colour injection test during surgery. J Jap Orthop Ass 1978; 52:1243–1244.
4. Neviaser JS. Ruptures of the rotator cuff. Clin Orthop 1954; 3:92–98.
5. Neviaser JS. Arthrography of the shoulder. Springfield: Charles C Thomas, 1975.
6. Wolfgang GL. Surgical repair of tears of the rotator cuff of the shoulder. J Bone Joint Surg 1974; 56-A:14–26.
7. Yamanaka Y et al. Pathohistological study on the supraspinatus tendon. The Shoulder Joint 1980; 4:83–86.

SURGICAL TREATMENT OF COMPLETE ROTATOR CUFF TEARS

RICHARD J. NASCA, M.D.

MATERIALS AND METHODS

This report reviews my experience with the surgical treatment of rotator cuff tears in 32 shoulders in 30 patients. These were consecutive cases done during a ten-year period, 1972 through 1982. The youngest patient was 32 years old; the oldest an 80-year-old male with a massive acute tear. The median age was 57 years. The majority of patients were males. Falls on the outstretched arm accounted for the mechanism of injury in 15 patients. Five patients injured their shoulder in automobile accidents. Seven patients were considered acute in that they were treated within six weeks of their initial injury; the remainder were considered chronic, being seen and treated six weeks to several years after injury. The right shoulder was more commonly involved than the left. Both patients with bilateral tears requested repair of the second shoulder soon after rehabilitating the first shoulder repair.

Clinical Presentation

Pain in the suprascapular region, base of the neck and deltoid tuberosity were common complaints. Night pain was very frequent and is quite typical of this problem. With the arm passively abducted and forward flexed 60 to 80 degrees, the pain was worse. Passive motion was maintained in spite of large tears in all but three patients. Weakness to resistive abduction was quite variable but appeared to be most consistent in acute tears. An audible or palpable click or clunk was often present when passively rotating the shoulder with the arm abducted and forward flexed. Atrophy of the supraspinatus and infraspinatus could be observed in thin patients. Occasionally, a defect in the cuff was palpable in slender patients with forward protruding shoulders and variable round back deformity.[1] Three patients continued to complain of pain after reduced anterior dislocations of the shoulder and were found to have associated rotator cuff tears and avulsions which required repair.

TREATMENT

Fifty percent of the patients had had one or more corticosteroid injections in or around the involved shoulder prior to our evaluation and treatment. Physical therapy consisting of active assistive range of motion, contrast applications of heat and cold, and ultrasound were commonly used. In those shoulders which received repeated injections of steroids, the cuff tendons were frayed, thin, friable and held sutures poorly. In four patients who received multiple steroid injections, primary tissue was so poor that excision and cadaver graft was necessary in order to achieve a repair.

Surgical Procedure

The patient is positioned in the semisitting position under general endotracheal anesthesia. The upper extremity is draped free so that the shoulder can be manipulated through a full range of motion during the procedure, especially extension. An arm holder assistant is helpful. The skin incision is made oblique to the anterior one-third of the acromion and continued down the deltopectoral interval; electrocautery is used to reduce blood loss. The anterior portion of the deltoid is subperiosteally detached from the clavicle and the acromion process, exposing the acromioclavicular joint and the anterior one-half of the acromion process. It is usually necessary to split the deltoid in line with its anterior fibers for 3 to 4 centimeters in order to provide access to the subdeltoid bursa. Often after getting to this point, joint fluid will be seen to leak through the torn cuff into the subdeltoid space. Traction applied to the arm with the elbow flexed helps to open up the subdeltoid space and makes exposure of the anterior edge of the acromion and the coracoacromial ligament much easier. The anterior and inferior edge of the acromion process is removed with its underlying coracoacromial ligament with an osteotome. The osteotomy of the acromion usually results in a wedge shaped piece of bone, 1.5 × 2.0 × 2.5 centimeters in size. If after the acromial osteotomy is done there is still impingement, additional acromion should be removed. The humeral head is protected during the acromioplasty. An arthroplasty of the acromioclavicular joint may also be necessary. This was done in three cases because of severe degenerative arthritis of the acromioclavicular joint. This consisted of removing the distal one centimeter of the clavicle in addition to the anterior-inferior portion of the acromion.

The greatest challenge in this type of surgery is dealing effectively with the torn retracted cuff tendons. The fresher the tear, the easier it is to repair and the less traction is required to bring the tendons back to their near normal anatomical loci of insertion. Chronic tears are characterized by significant retraction, fibrosis and attenuation of the cuff tendons. Tears vary greatly in size and location. Most of the tears occur between the leading edge of the supraspinatus and subscapularis tendons of insertion. Resection of a good portion of the thickened and proliferative subacromial bursa is necessary to provide good delineation of the tendons and their motors. These motors retract and adhere leaving a denuded head. An attempt is made to restore the resting length of the frayed retracted tendons by applying traction via sutures or clamps. If these maneuvers are successful, the tendon edges are trimmed in preparation for suture and reattachment to bone. If traction and mobilization is not successful, a graft may be necessary. This was done in seven cases. Interrupted nonabsorbable sutures are used to close the defect, starting furthest away from insertion. If present, the original tendons of insertion can be used to anchor the repair. However, it is usually necessary to prepare a channel in the bone just above the greater and lesser tuberosity but peripheral to the articular surface of the humeral head to anchor the tendons via drill holes. A watertight repair is the goal sought and is confirmed by injection of 5 to 10 cubic centimeters of saline into the joint through an intact portion of the cuff. Areas of leakage along the suture line usually can be repaired with additional interrupted sutures. The repair should not be tight with the arm against the chest wall.

In three cases (two were repeat surgeries), an abduction splint was used postoperatively. The deltoid muscle is resutured to itself and the fibers of origin are reattached to the periosteum and soft tissue overlying the remaining acromion process. If necessary, drill holes can be made in the acromion for reattachment with suture fixation; however, this is seldom necessary. A subcuticular closure is done and the patient is placed in a Velpeau type sling with pads in the axilla. Hospitalization is usually three to five days. If the biceps tendon is severely involved and attenuated, which has been rare in our cases, it can be removed from its supraglenoid attachment and sutured just distal to the intertubercular sulcus or tenodesed.

Postoperative Course

The commencement of active assistive motion usually depends on the size of the tear and the type of repair. In an uncomplicated repair, active assistive Codman's rotation exercises are started using the contralateral hand as the assistor at 14 to 21 days postoperatively. If a good deal of mobilization and traction is required, and drill hole fixation is used, it may be necessary to keep the arm at the side for four to six weeks. This regimen is also followed for graft cases. Patients are generally seen at two- to three-week intervals postoperatively or until the full Codman's routine is established. These exercises include circumduction, clockwise and counterclockwise, as well as forward and backward pendulum motion done at the side and across the frontal plane of the body with the torso flexed forward. Abduction of the shoulder without elevating the scapula is stressed. Doing these exercises in front of a mirror is helpful. Wall climbing in the coronal plane of the body is utilized. The patient is cautioned not to drop the arm from this abducted position because of fatigue, but to support it with the opposite member or hold it against the wall for support until control is regained. A broomstick is helpful in gaining abduction in multiple planes. Codman's exercises are augmented with a five-pound weight held in the hand as strength and range of motion increase. Four to six months is usually required to achieve the desired strength and mobility of the repaired shoulder in uncomplicated repairs. Some pain is not uncommon in the postoperative mobilization, similar to that noted in treating patients with adhesive capsulitis. Manipulation under anesthesia was not done in any of our cases. Deltoid strength and reversal of the atrophy of the rotator cuff muscles is noted at six months, although in two cases it took almost a year. Heavy lifting, golf, racquet sports and throwing are not recommended until reasonable range of motion and strength have returned. A smooth glenohumeralscapulothoracic rhythm without pain is the desired end point. Nearly full pivotal abduction is usually obtained, given time. Patients are encouraged to keep records of their progress; range of motion is recorded at each follow-up visit and shared with the patient who often becomes discouraged in the early months postoperatively. Patience and encouragement are necessary ingredients to a successful result in the cooperative and motivated patient.

ANALYSIS OF RESULTS

The final results were analyzed based on relief of pain, return of adequate range of motion and strength to the shoulder and patients' return to previous jobs and avocations. No attempt was made to quantitate these.

Acute Repair Group

Seven patients sustained acute injuries followed by repair within six weeks. One patient had avulsed the subscapularis from the lesser tuberosity and had an excellent result following repair. The other six patients had tears or avulsions involving the tendons attaching to the greater tuberosity. Results were excellent in this group. These patients with acute tears rehabilitated much faster and regained their range of motion with less difficulty than did those in the chronic repair group. Partial acromionectomy was done on four of the seven patients. In two patients, staples were used to secure the avulsed bone and tendon(s). One patient required staple removal. All patients but one (who was lost to follow-up) regained full range of motion. All returned to work except the one who failed to return for follow-up.

Chronic Repair Group

These patients underwent partial anterior-inferior acromionectomy and repair of their rotator cuff tears six weeks to several years after their original injury occurred. Results were good in this group of patients who required on the average six months to regain range of motion and strength in their shoulders. All but one patient had relief of pain.

Range of motion returned to normal or nearly normal in eleven patients. Five patients had greater than 110 degrees abduction and two patients had less than 90 degrees abduction. Fifteen of the 18 patients returned to work. Overall results were judged to be good to excellent in all but three patients.

Results of the Rotator Cuff Graft

Human homograft freeze-dried rotator cuff grafts obtained from the University of Miami Tissue Bank were utilized in seven patients. The average size of the graft in five of the seven patients was 5 to 6 centimeters in diameter. These were massive or global tears which could not be closed in any other fashion. An attempt was made to obtain a watertight repair. Five of the seven patients who underwent the cadaver grafts have been relieved of pain. However, the functional results are quite disappointing with the exception of two patients; one had full range of motion, the other greater than 110 degrees of abduction. Whether these grafts are actually functioning or not is difficult to say. There may be some problem with tension or the biomechanics of the reconstruction that is unknown to us. Only three of the seven patients returned to work.

It has been noted that if range of motion and strength are not improved by one year following the graft, they usually do not improve therafter. All patients requiring grafting had had several steroid injections in or about the shoulder. Steroid arthropathy with atrophy of the cuff tendons appears to be one of the unsolved problems related to this disease.

Complications

There were no infections. A suture granuloma which required excision and removal of the sutures used to carry out the repair, was done one month postoperatively. Two repairs have broken down and have been redone with cadaver grafts. There were no major anesthetic or medical complications in this group of patients, several of whom were in their 70s or 80s. Age appears not to be a significant factor in the decision to treat these patients surgically.

Discussion

Tears of the rotator cuff appear to be caused by trauma superimposed on poorly vascularized degenerating collagen. The anterior-inferior or leading edge of the acromion process may act as a cutting edge as force is transmitted through the upper end of the humerus as one falls on the outstretched arm or directly on the shoulder. Repeated corticosteroid injections in and around the cuff tendons lead to attrition, softening and fibrillation of the tendons[5] of the rotator cuff.

Night pain in and around the shoulder is a common complaint in those with cuff tears. Loss of motion is uncommon. Pain is reproduced at the point of impingement between the bare humeral head articular cartilage and the anterior-inferior undersurface of the acromion process.

Contrast arthrography remains the hallmark of diagnosis. It has also been helpful in evaluation of postoperative repairs. It is doubtful that a full thickness tear will heal without surgical intervention, considering the pull of the muscle motors on the tear(s) and the constant leakage of synovial fluid through the defect.

Repair of acute tears and tears with attached bony fragments (avulsions) are quite straightforward. The results of surgical repair in these types of tears are quite good. Small- to medium-size chronic tears whose remaining cuff tendons can be mobilized and repaired without tension also do very well. However, global or massive tears present major reconstructive problems since there is a paucity of good mobile tissue to use. Cadaver grafts have shown promise in the Neviasers' experience, but they are finding them difficult to obtain.[7] Tendon transfers and advancement of muscle tendon units offer additional ways to solve this problem. We have had no experience with advancement of the supraspinatus muscle to repair large cuff tears as originally described by DeBeyre, Patte and Elmelik[3] and advocated by Ha'eri and Wiley.[4] R. J. and T. J. Neviaser[8] have developed an alternative to biceps tendon graft and freeze-dried cadaver graft when the tendon defect is massive. They have used the tendons of the subscapularis and teres minor transferred superiorly and fixed to a trough made in a sulcus between the anatomic humeral neck and the tuberosities. They achieved 12 good-to-excellent results in 17 cases. We agree that a tension free, watertight repair utilizing tissue with good blood supply is essential for success. Neer's[6] technique of anterior-inferior oblique acromioplasty appears to give consistently good results in small- and medium-size chronic tears. These can usually be sutured by advancement of the retracted tendons using interrupted sutures or some variation of the Y-V plastic technique.

Use of an abduction shoulder spica or airplane-type abduction splint certainly relieves tension on the repair. Ideally, the final repair should be under little or no tension with the arm positioned next to the chest. The rehabilitation phase following repair appears to be of great importance and requires a motivated patient in order to achieve a good result. The patients who were judged to have excellent results in this series were highly motivated to obtain their full, or near full, range of motion and strength in the operated shoulder. Those considered to have a good result had occasional aching in the shoulder, greater than 110 degrees active abduction, and near normal strength in their deltoid and cuff muscles. Those patients with persistent pain, or less than 90 degrees active abduction, or loss of significant muscle power, were considered poor results.

Relief of night pain occurred early in the postoperative period. In three patients who complained of persistent pain in the early postoperative period, disruption of the repair occurred and further surgery was required. Anterior-inferior oblique acromioplasty rather than acromial osteotomy with screw fixation[2] appears a necessary step in successful management of a chronic tear. Subtotal or complete acromionectomy results in significant loss of the deltoid lever arm and deltoid muscle power.

Age is not a contraindication to repair providing the patient is medically fit for a general anesthetic and agrees to participate in the subsequent rehabilitation.

The deleterious effect of corticosteroid injections on collagen tensile strength and healing,[5] as well as articular cartilage integrity is considered a major factor in complicating the surgical repair. In a patient with a typical history and physical findings, early arthrography is advocated rather than steroid injection. If no tear is found, one can proceed with nonoperative therapy which may include bursal but not intratendinous or intra–articular injections of corticosteroids. Early recognition and repair of tears within the first six weeks after injury are usually technically easier and the results are better than those done after six weeks.

REFERENCES

1. Bateman JE. The Shoulder and Neck. 2nd ed. Philadelphia: WB Saunders, 1978
2. Bush LD. The torn shoulder capsule. J Bone Joint Surg 1975; 57A:256–259.
3. DeBeyre J, Patte D, Elmelik E. Repair of ruptures of the rotator cuff of the shoulder. J Bone Joint Surg 1965; 47B: 36–42.
4. Ha'Eri GB, Wiley AM. Advancement of the supraspinatus muscle in the repair of the ruptures. J Bone Joint Surg 1981; 63A:232–238.
5. Kennedy JC, Willis RB. The effects of local steroid injections on tendons. A biomechanical and microscopic correlative study. Am J Sports Med 1976; 4:11–21.
6. Neer CS. Anterior acromioplasty for the chronic impingement syndrome in the shoulder. J Bone Joint Surg 1972; 54A:41–50.
7. Neviaser JS, Neviaser RJ, Neviaser TJ. The repair of chronic massive ruptures of the rotator cuff of the shoulder by use of a freeze-dried rotator cuff. J Bone Joint Surg 1978; 60A:681–684.
8. Neviaser RJ, Neviaser TJ. Transfer of subscapularis and teres minor for massive defects of the rotator cuff. In: Bagley I, Kessel L, eds. Shoulder Surgery. Springer-Verlag, 1982: 60–63.

ADHESIVE CAPSULITIS OF THE SHOULDER

J. PATRICK MURNAGHAN, M.D.

Middle-aged patients presenting with spontaneous shoulder pain remain a diagnostic and therapeutic problem. The patients under study in this paper complain of a gradual onset of poorly localized shoulder pain which may radiate to the elbow, or occasionally to the outer aspect of the forearm. The pain tends to be worse at night. There is a progressive insidious decrease in the range of motion of the shoulder, most marked in forward elevation, external rotation, and abduction. The next phase is one of continuing aching discomfort in the shoulder, accentuated at the extremes of motion. In the final stages of this clinical symptom complex, pain decreases in step with a gradual relaxation of the restriction in the range of motion.

Is there such a separate clinical entity as primary adhesive capsulitis of the shoulder (ACS)? If so, it must be distinguished from other common clinical problems about the shoulder such as tendinitis or bursitis.

Duplay[4] described *"periarthrite scapulo-humerale"* to distinguish patients with a symptom complex similar to ACS from arthritis of the shoulder. A contracted shoulder capsule was recognized by Payr[14] and he aimed his treatment at the hydraulic distention of the capsule. Codman[2] coined the term "frozen shoulder," for a painful restriction in the range of motion of the shoulder. J. S. Neviaser[13] reported on the same clinical condition under the name of "adhesive capsulitis."

The pathology of an ACS seems to lie primarily in the capsule. The lack of true intra-articular adhesions has been confirmed by arthroscopy. Several pathological specimens have been made available by those advocating open surgical release. The capsule was found to be thickened, inelastic, and friable. In early cases, an acute inflammatory exudate is seen. Subsequently, there may be fibrosis and perivascular infiltration. Lundberg[11] identified alterations in the ground substance of the capsule, but could not state whether these changes were primary or secondary. Lundberg also recorded that the synovium for the most part appeared normal. The pathophysiology of primary adhesive capsulitis of the shoulder remains a controversial subject. Simmonds[16] and Macnab[12] have suggested an inflammatory response to cell death as the triggering factor. The cell death would occur on the basis of degeneration of the tendons of the rotator cuff. The auto-immune theory, though appealing, has not been borne out in recent preliminary reports of investigations by Kessel et al.[10]

A *forme-fruste* of shoulder-hand syndrome has also been suggested. The lack of response to sympathetic blocks makes the association between ACS and shoulder-hand syndrome somewhat tenuous. Bruckner and Nye,[1] in an interesting prospective series, examined 95 patients with subarachnoid hemorrhage. They demonstrated a 25 percent incidence of ACS, diagnosed by pain and decreased range of motion, in their patients. Bruckner and Nye identified prolonged immobilization as an etiological factor. In patients with impairment of consciousness, hemiparesis, or prolonged intravenous infusion in one arm, all had an increased incidence of the clinical syndrome of ACS when compared to controls.

The question has been raised whether there is a predisposed personality, as suggested by Coventry.[3] Tense, insecure, restless and vulnerable individuals were thought to be susceptible. Tyber[17] reported that Amitriptyline and Lithium were better than physiotherapy to manage the condition of ACS. Wright and Haq,[18] however, could find no evidence of a personality factor.

It has been suggested that ACS is possibly a self-limiting disease with no need for treatment. Robert Grey[5] followed 21 patients with 25 shoulders involved. Treatment was limited to reassurance and occasional analgesics. With his protocol, 24 of the 25 shoulders returned to normal within two years from the onset of symptoms. In contrast to this theory of self-limitation, Simmonds[16] found only six of 21 patients had normal function up to 6 years after diagnosis. Arthrography has perhaps given more tangible evidence for the diagnostic entity of adhesive capsulitis. The shoulder volume is uniformly decreased as low as 3 to 15 cc compared to a normal of 20 to 35 cc. Characteristically, there is a loss of the inferior capsular recess, as well as the subscapularis recess.

To this end, we tried to identify patients fitting into the symptom complex of primary idiopathic ACS. A small retrospective study was done on the patients seen in the Orthopaedic Clinic at the Ottawa Civic Hospital. Patients with the clinical diagnosis of primary idiopathic ACS with a minimum of two years follow-up from diagnosis were included. The study group included 29 patients. Seven patients were excluded on review of the old chart due to a change in the diagnosis over time. The exclusions included two patients with sudden catching shoulder pain, uncharacteristic of ACS. One patient was subsequently found to have polymyalgia rheumatica. Another patient had a third recurrence of similar pain in the same shoulder, which was felt to be atypical of primary ACS. A fracture of the proximal humerus eliminated another patient. The last patient continued to have tendinitis symptoms in keeping with a partial tear of the rotator cuff and was thus excluded. Thus, of the original group, 15 patients were available for follow-up. All were interviewed and examined. X-rays were not helpful. Two patients had involvement of the opposite shoulder, one during the period of the study, one before that period. Of the men, five patients had involvement of the nondominant side, and two of the dominant side. Four women had dominant side involvement. In four patients there was a history of minor trauma. One patient related the onset to a flare-up of cervical spondylosis. In all the others, there was no history of trauma or predisposing episode. The average age of this patient group was 62 years. All patients were asked to do autoassisted stretching exercises as described by Hughes and Neer.[8] The program involved both stretching exercises to increase range of motion and strengthening exercises within the range of motion.

At follow-up, 87 percent of the patients were pain free. The remaining patients had an aching discomfort, and had to be careful to avoid overusing the affected shoulder. A range of motion including 160° of forward elevation, and 45° of external rotation was achieved in 15 of the 16 shoulders.

No relationship could be established between the duration of symptoms before diagnosis and the time to return of a painless clinical status with a free range of motion. On an average, the duration of prediagnostic symptoms was five months. The duration of symptoms following diagnosis lasted on an average 9.3 months. The overall duration was 14 months.

Forty percent of the patients were better at six months; 90 percent of the patients were better at one year. All patients felt that soon after starting the exercises, they had improved their shoulder motion and the functional use of their shoulder. Return to a totally free range of motion of the shoulder without discomfort took many months in all patients. The group that exercised regularly unfortunately could not be distinguished from the study group over all.

In discussion of the above results, the shortcomings of our current methods of reporting shoulder motion are exemplified. A more useful representation of 3-dimensional shoulder movement is necessary.

The literature conflicts as to the treatment of ACS. Lloyd-Roberts,[9] comparing manipulation to a control group of patients, found that at 6 months, 44 percent of the control group had a good result, compared to 67 percent with manipulation. Reeves[15] confirmed that in a manipulation group, 66 percent were doing well at 6 months, but several had problems up to 2 years. Harmon,[6] in a 3 year follow-up, showed 66 percent of patients did well with exercises, achieving full painless range of motion, but over a longer period of time than those treated with manipulation. Hazelman[7] reported no difference in a prospective study comparing steroid injections, physiotherapy, and manipulation when patients were assessed as to pain relief and return of function.

Manipulation has been demonstrated to be effective in shortening the period of time during which the shoulder range of motion is extensively decreased. It does not, however, appear to shorten the overall course of the disease. The residual discomfort and stiffness of the shoulder tends to follow the same time course as those patients treated without manipulation.

In conclusion, primary ACS can be identified as a distinct clinical entity, which can be distinguished from other shoulder disorders by the history and physical examination. X-rays are usually normal. The pathogenesis remains unresolved, but it appears that a period of immobility and membership in a specific age group are two contributing factors to ACS.

It would appear that treatment should be directed to the stage of disease at which the patient presents. Where there is a restricted range of motion, autoassisted stretching exercises appear to be beneficial. Pain at the extremes of range of motion settles as motion is regained. This small study supports the theory that a more physiological stretching program can usually be successful, avoiding the need for manipulation under anesthesia. No definitive comment can be made as to whether in fact primary ACS is a self-limiting disease.

REFERENCES

1. Bruckner FE, Nye CJS. A prospective study of adhesive capsulitis of the shoulder in a high risk population. Quart J Med. 1981; 19:8:191–204.
2. Codman EA. The Shoulder. Boston, 1934.
3. Coventry MB. Problems of the painful shoulder. J Amer Med Ass. 1953; 151:177.
4. Duplay S. De la periarthrites scapulo-humerale et des raideurs de l'épaule qui en sont la consequence. Arch Gen Med. 1872; 20:513.
5. Gey RG. The natural history of "idiopathic" frozen shoulder. J Bone Joint Surg. 1978; 60A:564.
6. Harmon PH. Methods and results in the treatment of 2,580 painful shoulders. Amer J Surg. 1958; 95:527.
7. Hazelman BL. The painful stiff shoulder. Rheum Phys Med. 1972; 11:413–421.
8. Hughes MA, Neer CS II. Glenohumeral joint replacement and postoperative rehabilitation. Phys Ther. 1975; 55:85.
9. Lloyd-Roberts GC, French PR. Periarthritis of the shoulder. Brit Med J. 1959; 20:1569.
10. Kessel L, Bayley I. The frozen shoulder. Brit J Hosp Med. 1981; 25:334.
11. Lundberg BJ. The frozen shoulder. Acta Ortho Scand. 1969; 119.
12. Macnab I. Rotator cuff tendonitis. Ann Roy Coll Surg Eng. 1973; 53:271.
13. Neviaser JS. Adhesive capsulitis of the shoulder. J Bone Joint Surg. 1945; 27:211.
14. Payr E. Gelenk-"Sperreu" and "Anylosen." Behan Zbl Chir. 1931; 58:3, 2993.
15. Reeves B. Arthrographic changes in frozen and post-traumatic stiff shoulders. Proc Roy Soc Med. 1966; 59:827.
16. Simmonds FA. Shoulder pain, with particular reference to the "frozen" shoulder. J Bone Joint Surg. 1949; 31B:426.
17. Tyber MA. Treatment of the painful shoulder syndrome with amitriptyline and lithium carbonate. Can Med Assoc J. 1974; 111:137.
18. Wright V, Haq AM. Periarthritis of the shoulder. Ann Rheum Dis. 1976; 35:220.

ROTATOR CUFF TEARS IN THE YOUNG

V. PREM KUMAR, M.B.B.S., F.R.C.S.(Ed), OMAR BAYNE, M.D.,
R. PETER WELSH, M.B.Ch.B., F.R.C.S.(C),
and JAMES BATEMAN, M.D., F.R.C.S.(C)

Rotator cuff tears in the middle aged or elderly may present following trauma but equally as often present quite insidiously.[1,2,7,8,13] The reason for this, Macnab and Rathbun have suggested, may be an area of relative dysvascularity found at the insertion of the supraspinatus tendon acting as a point of focal weakness such that degenerative tears eventually occur at these sites. However, little has been written about rotator cuff tears in the young adult.[9,10] Avulsion of the greater tuberosity rather than cuff substance tears at the supraspinatus insertion may generally be expected with trauma, and degenerative tears are exceedingly rare.

This study was undertaken to emphasize that, while rare, true cuff tears do occur in young patients. A retrospective analysis to illustrate age and sex distribution, clinical presentation, investigative findings and results of treatment was carried out. A plan of management for cuff tears in the young was subsequently formulated.

MATERIALS AND METHODS

The records of 38 patients under age 40 years, who had rotator cuff repairs carried out at the Orthopaedic and Arthritic Hospital between 1970 and 1980 were reviewed.

Fourteen patients were lost to follow-up, leaving 24 patients with 25 surgically treated cuff tears for clinical assessment.

There were 18 males and six females with an age range of 15 to 37 years (average 30.5 years). The time of follow-up after surgery was 14 months to 11.2 years (average 6 years).

MANAGEMENT

Preoperative Assessment

Thirty-two of the 38 patients (87%) gave a clear history of antecedent trauma to the involved shoulder. Two patients had avulsion fractures of the greater tuberosity and two had associated anterior shoulder dislocations. There were an equal number of sports and industry related accidents. Six patients gave a history of chronic pain of insidious onset with only two of these giving a history of trauma to the shoulder. One patient who was an epileptic had had repeated falls on the involved shoulder while the other patient developed more intense shoulder pain and weakness after chiropractic manipulation for his "sore" shoulder (Table 1).

Prior to surgery, all patients had a trial of conservative management which ranged from three months to two years (average 8 months). This included nonsteroidal anti-inflammatory medication and physiotherapy with one-third of the group having up to three local steroid injections to the shoulder.

Eleven patients had had previous surgical procedures to the involved shoulder. Five in fact had undergone previous rotator cuff repair and five some form of soft tissue stabilization, three for recurrent subluxation and two for frank anterior shoulder dislocations. One patient had required an open reduction for an avulsion fracture of the greater tuberosity.

Intractable pain was the predominant presenting symptom in 11 cases, while pain with weakness was seen in 19. Three patients complained of weakness alone while one patient presented with a stiff and painless shoulder (Table 2).

Preoperatively, all patients had routine plain x-rays and an arthrogram of the involved shoulder. One patient underwent a diagnostic shoulder arthroscopy. A few patients with radicular symptoms and associated neck pain had electromyographic studies to rule out pathology in the cervical spine.

Surgical Technique

All tears repaired were full thickness tears. The tears were graded I to III using Bateman's

TABLE 1	
Type of Accident	No.
Sporting accidents	11
Industrial accidents	13
Road traffic accidents	5
Miscellaneous accidents	2
Spontaneous	6
	38

TABLE 2	
Symptoms	No.
Pain and weakness	19
Pain alone	11
Weakness	3
Stiffness	1
Miscellaneous symptoms	4
	38

criteria.[16] Repairs were carried out either by suture reapproximation or the use of fascia lata autographs. In the young individual, where the tear occurs in relatively healthy cuff tissue, a direct repair is more feasible than in the older patient where the quality of the cuff may necessitate fascial reinforcement. Decompression of the cuff by acromioplasty or acromioclavicular resection to protect the repaired area from subsequent impingement was performed in 29 instances.

Postoperative Care

The patients were immobilized postoperatively with the shoulder in 90 degrees of flexion and abduction and 15 degrees of external rotation with the arm supported on slings and springs when lying in bed, or a wedge support or Cantelever brace when ambulating. Physiotherapy, including isometric and isotonic exercises of the shoulder girdle musculature, was started as soon as the patient was comfortable. The use of the wedge support or Cantelever brace was discarded as soon as the patient was comfortable, approximately 3–6 weeks postoperatively. Physiotherapy to regain full strength and range of movement ranged from one month to four months (average 2.5 months).

Follow-up Assessment

Patients were assessed subjectively and objectively regarding pain, range of movement and strength in the involved shoulder, and graded according to our rating scale. These results were compared to the preoperative clinical findings.

RESULTS

Complications

There were three postoperative wound infections (7.8%), all growing Staphylococcus aureus. Two were superficial and healed without sequelae with the use of appropriate antibiotics. The other case, previously operated on for an avulsion fracture of the greater tuberosity, required removal of the hardware, debridement and appropriate antibiotic coverage to control the deep infection. There were no complications at the donor site following harvesting of the fascia lata grafts.

Pain Relief

Preoperative and postoperative pain was graded subjectively on a scale of 1 to 10, 1 being no pain and 10 being severe pain. Seventy-seven percent of the shoulders showed vast improvement over their preoperative condition, whereas 9 percent were unchanged. Fourteen percent experienced more pain postoperatively than they had prior to surgery.

Range of Motion

Preoperative forward flexion and abduction of the shoulder were compared to that present at the time of review and graded 25% to Full.

Fifty-seven percent of the shoulders had much improved abduction compared to thirty-five percent which had no improvement. Eight percent were made worse. Forty-four percent of the shoulders had much improved forward flexion compared to forty-three percent which remained the same. Thirteen percent showed decreased forward flexion.

Strength

Shoulder strength was graded as follows: 10 points for full strength and 1 point for complete paralysis. Seventy-one percent of the patients had much improvement over their preoperative condition. Twelve percent had decreased strength and 17 percent remained unchanged from their preoperative status.

DISCUSSION

Our study has shown that true rotator cuff tears do occur in the young and should be considered, especially following trauma to the shoulder. In our series, 84 percent of the shoulders had a history of severe trauma. Only two patients had associated avulsion fractures of the greater tuberosity and two had associated anterior shoulder dislocations. At surgery the majority of cuff tears were noted to be through relatively healthy, viable tissue rather than through degenerative tissue as is usually noted in the older age group.

Male predominance has always been stressed in the classical age distribution. Samilson and Binder[6] report a 7:1 male/female ratio in their analysis of 276 patients. A 3.5:1 ratio was the finding by Godsil and Linscheid[12] in their analysis of 59 patients with an average age of 60 years. Our study revealed a 2.7:1 male/female ratio in a population with an average age of 30 years. The pattern of more equal sex incidence reflects the greater likelihood of a traumatic tear in a young patient remaining symptomatic. In the older male patient with heavier recreational and occupational demands, the lesion is more likely to remain persistently troublesome than it is in the female although the true incidence of complete tears may closer approximate a more even ratio than previously reported.

Pain and weakness were the predominant symptoms in more than half the patients, with pain being the presenting complaint in almost 80 percent of this study population. Pain becomes a predominant symptom because of subacromial bursal inflammation and impingement. Weakness is not a predominant symptom even with a complete cuff tear because attachment to the tuberosity often remains secure, in many instances permitting full active motion. Weakness may be an initial symptom due to pain and inhibition but becomes superseded by pain as the main symptom the longer the delay following injury. The average time interval between injury and treatment in this series was 32 months with a range of 5 days to 10 years. Stiffness of the shoulder was a symptom in only one patient, the young patient showing a lesser tendency to shoulder stiffness than does the older individual with a shoulder injury or cuff tear.

EMG studies to exclude associated neural or brachial plexus injury in these patients have been emphasized.[2] In the three patients who had this investigation, one sustained an axonotmesis of the axillary nerve, another denervation of the levator scapulae and trapezius, while in the third case a normal study was demonstrated. We find this investigation useful but stress that a positive EMG finding should not contraindicate further studies to confirm a cuff tear.

While a history of injury, continuing pain and occasionally weakness of abduction may arouse suspicion of a cuff tear, an arthrogram is essential to confirm the presence of a full thickness cuff tear. Bateman[9] considers contrast studies the most accurate means of identifying cuff defects and recommends such investigation in all cases. Our review indicates that arthrogram may be unreliable for small complete tears (Grade I tears) in about half the cases. For grade II and III tears arthrograms were more reliable, confirming the diagnosis in 90 percent of cases. For dye to leak into the subacromial bursa not only must the cuff be torn but the bursal lining over the cuff as well. In small cuff tears, complete though they may be, a break of the bursal lining may not necessarily occur or may heal as any other endothelial lining, contributing to the negative arthrographic findings in the Grade I tears.

It is important to detect and repair a complete tear of the cuff as soon as possible. Delay results in further extension of the defect[13] and contracture of soft tissues which may require secondary reconstruction procedures. Delay also results in muscular atrophy[12] which interferes with rehabilitation. There is no place for the conservative treatment of cuff tears in the young.

In this study the average time interval between injury and treatment was 32 months. Our study confirms our assumption that the longer the delay, the more difficult the subsequent reconstruction. The average time interval for those shoulders requiring secondary reconstruction using fascia lata graft was 42 months as opposed to 22

TABLE 3

Grade of Tear		Numbers	A/C Decompression
Grade I Tears	Direct suture	17	13
	Fascia lata graft	6	3
Grade II Tears	Direct suture	2	2
	Fascia lata graft	5	4
Grade III Tears	Direct suture	1	0
	Fascia lata graft	7	7
	Total	38	29

months for those whose repair was effected by direct suture.

Acromioclavicular arthroplasty may be indicated in repairs in the elderly where tissue is necrotic and acromioclavicular osteoarthritis is an important associated pathology that may have contributed to the rupture in the first place. In the young this procedure should be less often indicated.

However, after repair of the cuff, the subacromial space is often reduced and passive abduction of the shoulder may result in impingement which is obviated by acromioplasty and excision of the coracoacromial ligament.

Other secondary procedures such as sacrifice of the long head of the biceps for reconstruction in the elderly are to be condemned in the young as this tendon has an important function in stabilizing the humeral head during resisted elbow flexion.

Long-term follow-up reports of a comparative group are lacking. Samilson and Binder[6] in 1975 reported 59 percent excellent to good results in full thickness cuff tears managed conservatively. However, with a selected group of full thickness tears treated by operation, they reported 84 percent excellent to good results. Young patients have not previously been studied as a separate group, and conservative treatment cannot be considered a viable treatment alternative because of the late morbidity of the neglected cuff tear leading in its extreme state to a rotator cuff arthropathy.

Conclusions

Rotator cuff tears may occur in the young adult, usually as a result of shoulder trauma. These show only a slight male preponderance compared to degenerative type tears which are much more common in the male.

Continuing pain after severe shoulder trauma is the most common symptom. Good strength and range of motion may be preserved in the presence of a complete cuff tear.

Arthrography is reliable for Grade II and III tears but is less helpful in identifying small or Grade I tears where bursal overgrowth may lead to false negative study.

The early diagnosis and treatment of cuff tears leads to a more favorable outcome—the longer the delay in treatment, the more difficult the reconstruction procedure.

REFERENCES

1. Rathbun JB, Macnab I. The microvascular pattern of the rotator cuff. J Bone and Joint Surg 1972; 52B:540.
2. Wolfgang GL. Rupture of the musculotendinous cuff of the shoulder. Clin Orth and Related Research 1978; No. 136:230–243.
3. Debeyre J, Palte D, and Emelik E. Repair of the rotator cuff with a note on advancement of the supraspinatus muscle. J Bone and Joint Surg 1965; 47B:36–42.
4. Hickel HVA. Rupture of the rotator cuff of the shoulder. Experience of surgical treatment. Acta Orthop. Scand 1968; 39:477–492.
5. McLaughlin HL, Asherman EG. Lesions of the musculotendinous cuff of the shoulder. IV. Some observations based upon the results of surgical repair. J Bone and Joint Surg 1951; 32A:76–86.
6. Samilson RL, Binder WF. Symptomatic full thickness tears of the rotator cuff. An analysis of 292 shoulders in 276 patients. Orth Clin of N Amer 1973, 2:449–466.
7. Codman EA. The shoulder. Boston, Thomas Todd Co., 1934.
8. McLaughlin HL. Lesions of the musculotendinous cuff of the shoulder. 1. The exposure and treatment of tears with retraction. J Bone and Joint Surg 1944; 26, 31.
9. Bateman JE. Cuff tears in athletes. Orth Clin of N Amer 1976; 4:721–745.
10. Neer CS, Welsh RP. The shoulder in sports. Orth Clin of N Amer 1977; 8:583–591.
11. Weiner DS, Macnab I. Superior migration of the humeral head. A radiological aid in the diagnosis of tears of the rotator cuff. J Bone and Joint Surg 1970; 52B:No. 3, 524–527.
12. Godsil RD, Linscheid RL. Intratendinous defects of the rotator cuff. Clin Orth and Related Research 1970; No. 69:181–188.
13. Nixon JE, DiStefano V. Ruptures of the rotator cuff. Orth Clin of N Amer 1975; Vol. 6:No. 2, 423–447.
14. Kessel L. Shoulder Surgery. Heidelburg, New York: Springer Berlin, 1982.
15. Rose SH et al. Epidemiologic features of humeral fractures. Clin Orth and Related Research 1982; No. 168, 24–30.
16. Bateman JE. The shoulder and neck. 2nd Edition, Saunders.

SURGICAL MANAGEMENT OF ROTATOR CUFF TEARS

R. J. HAWKINS, M.D.

The surgical management of rotator cuff tears has been a controversial issue for many years. Many strongly favor a nonoperative approach, whereas others believe that with appropriate patient selection reconstruction of rotator cuff tears can be rewarding. This report will consider the rationale for surgery, the surgical techniques, and attempt to offer a clearer concept regarding patient selection and expectation for surgery.

There is considerable terminology describing the variations in pathology that may be associated with rotator cuff tears. Tears may be described as degenerative, partial or complete thickness. They may represent an acute extension of a chronic process or may on rare occasions be acute. They may be described as small, medium, large or massive and, as massive tears, may be associated with changes in the glenohumeral joint (cuff arthropathy). They may have associated biceps involvement with biceps rupture. They are often associated with degenerative changes of the acromioclavicular joint. We must clearly understand the pathology involved before we can appropriately discuss surgical management, particularly as it relates to patient selection and expectation.

PATHOANATOMY

Neer has taught us that the functional arc of elevation of the shoulder is forward and not lateral, and that impingement occurs predominantly against the anterior inferior edge of the acromium and the coracoacromial ligament.[1] This is supported by pathology found at the time of surgery. Appreciation of this concept forms the basis for decompression, which therefore must almost always accompany rotator cuff reconstruction. Decompression is performed as an anterior acromioplasty along with resection of the coracoacromial ligament. Rathbun and Macnab injected microopaque into the subclavian artery to demonstrate the vascular compromise of the supraspinatus and biceps tendons.[2] This contributes to degeneration and subsequent rupture of these tendons and is important as it affects the healing process following cuff reconstruction.

The progression of pathology in the impingement process involves an initial tendonitis followed by wear and tear over the years with scarring of the subacromial bursa, resulting in degeneration, partial and finally complete thickness rotator cuff tears. The bursa is obviously involved; the biceps tendon which runs adjacent to the supraspinatus tendon frequently is involved with rupturing, and the acromioclavicular joint undergoes secondary degenerative changes. With time and progression the complete tear becomes larger, and may result in a massive rotator cuff tear and occasionally ends up as an end-stage cuff arthropathy with degenerative changes not only subacromially, but also in the glenohumeral joint.

The natural history of the impingement process is unknown. The frequency and rate at which patients progress from Neer Stage I tendonitis to scarring in Stage II and ruptures in Stage III are probably not very high. Once, however, a partial thickness or small cuff tear is established, then with ongoing impingement, the tear will likely enlarge with time. It would seem that the natural history of a cuff tear is one of progression and this is important in our surgical consideration. In considering the surgical approach to rotator cuff surgery, we must be aware of the pathoanatomy, particularly the presence of impingement, the staging of the disease as described by Neer,[3] and involvement of associated structures such as bursa, biceps, acromioclavicular and glenohumeral joints.

SURGICAL RATIONALE

Surgical considerations revolve around pain, function, and natural history. The important factors to consider in a decision to operate relate to analysis of the patient and the pathology. Activity level and physiological age would be influencing patient factors. Different patients have different expectations and demands and these must be honored. It would be important to know the severity of pain, how long it has been present, its response to conservative measures and the course it has taken in the preceding time. Weakness and its associated functional limitations must be assessed.

An analysis of pathology must consider the many variations as previously discussed. It would be important to know whether the process is acute or chronic, the size of a cuff defect, and the progression this pathology has taken over preceding months or years. It would also be important to know what associated pathology may be present, such as biceps ruptures or acromioclavicular degeneration.

The commonest and usually the primary indication for rotator cuff reconstruction is pain relief. Functional improvement may be a consideration and is very dependent on the patient's activity level. Another consideration is prophylactic prevention of progression of the disease process. The goals of cuff surgery are relief of pain, which is accomplished through decompression as well as through restoration of the rotator cuff; improvement in function, which is achieved primarily through the reconstruction of the rotator cuff but also through elimination of pain; and prevention of progression, which is achieved through decompression. The principles of cuff surgery are to preserve the deltoid by taking off as little as possible and reattaching as carefully as possible, to decompress through appropriate acromioplasty and ligament resection, and to reconstruct the rotator cuff as required.

SURGICAL TECHNIQUE

Historically the approaches to rotator cuff reconstruction have been described by such surgeons as Codman, McLaughlin, Neer, Debeyre and others. Codman originally described a sabre cut across the top of the shoulder, taking off considerable deltoid to achieve reconstruction.[4] McLaughlin described an anterosuperior approach and advocated decompression.[5] The transacromial approach has been popularized by Debeyre and employed by Kessel and allows an exposure of the rotator cuff but does not allow for decompression unless through a separate anterior approach.[6,7] The anterior acromioplasty approach through an anterior superior incision has been popularized by Neer and is our preference to approach cuff reconstruction.[1]

Common Tears

The majority of rotator cuff repairs are achieved through mobilizing and advancing the subscapularis from in front of, the infraspinatus from the back of and the supraspinatus from under the acromioclavicular joint, suturing these to a trough in bone at the junction of the anatomical neck and greater tuberosity (Fig. 2). A decompression is performed as described by Neer to help eliminate pain, protect the repair, and prevent progression (Fig. 1).

Some authors report that resection of the acromioclavicular joint acts as a decompression. We believe that a formal anterior acromioplasty is required in conjunction with cuff reconstruction. Resection of the coracoacromial ligament alone probably does not provide adequate decompression. Acromionectomy has been shown to be a debilitating procedure interfering with functional

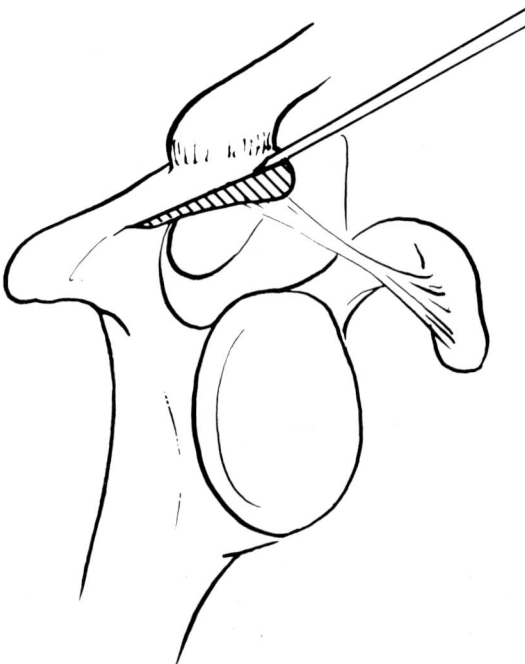

Figure 1 An anterior acromioplasty is routinely performed with rotator cuff repairs. The osteotomy cut commences at the anterosuperior border of the acromion and proceeds a distance of approximately 1½ cm to the undersurface of the apex of the acromion.

rehabilitation because of loss of fulcrum for the deltoid through difficulty in reattachment.

An anterior acromioplasty approach is performed with an incision bisecting the anterior acromium between the acromioclavicular joint and lateral border of the acromion. The deltoid is detached from the anterior acromion only and the anterior acromioplasty performed, resecting the anterior superior portion of the acromion back to the apex of the undersurface (Fig. 1). If the outer portion of the clavicle has prominent osteophytes on its undersurface, these may be osteotomized.

The surgical sequence may be as follows: excising and trimming, defining the defect, assessing tissue mobility, and a plan for closure either to a trough in bone, or side to side suture. Redundant excess tissue, particularly of the bursa, is excised and trimmed so that the edges of the cuff tear can be identified. The size of the cuff defect is then described as small (less than 1 cm), medium (1–3 cm), large (3–5 cm), and massive, encompassing the entire humeral head. The subscapularis is identified anteriorly, the supraspinatus medially, and the infraspinatus posteriorly. Stay sutures are positioned in these tissues and with careful dissection, adhesions are broken down both between the deltoid and underlying cuff and on the undersurface of the cuff, even dissecting tissue off the glenoid neck to achieve greater mobilization. The mobility of the tissue will determine how much dissection is required.

At this stage a plan for closure is devised. If it is a small tear, there may be a detached portion of cuff at the greater tuberosity and an end to end or side to side repair may be effected. Usually there is no detached portion of cuff at the area of the greater tuberosity, and although a side to side repair can be performed, there is no way of achieving fixation to bone without suture to a trough. A trough is then designed at the junction of the anatomical neck with a gentle slope and the tendons mobilized into the trough (Fig. 2). Sutures may be passed from the tendon through the trough to the outside of the greater tuberosity, back through the greater tuberosity into the trough and through the tendon again. In this manner the arm is abducted and the sutures tied, pushing the tendons into the trough (Fig. 3).

Large Tears

If the defect is large or massive, exposure can be increased by incising the deltoid in the direction of its fibers at the junction of its anterior and middle third, a distance of approximately 5 cm. A suture placed distally at this distance will prevent progression of the tear. The deltoid may be then opened like a book, allowing greater exposure. Further exposure may be achieved, particularly for mobilizing the supraspinatus by resecting the outer clavicle. We do not routinely resect the outer clavicle unless it is for greater exposure. Excision of the outer clavicle may also be entertained when there are significant degenerative changes with marked clinical findings and pain relief has been provided with a local injection directly into the acromioclavicular joint. We generally prefer to work on the undersurface of the outer clavicle, removing osteophytes rather than resecting the outer clavicle.

With large tears, plastic surgery principles such as pedicle advancement, rotation transposition, direct flaps or free grafts and other synthetic materials may be employed. We have found that the most advantageous way to repair a large rotator cuff defect is to transpose the subscapularis, leaving the underlying capsule in place, mobilizing this

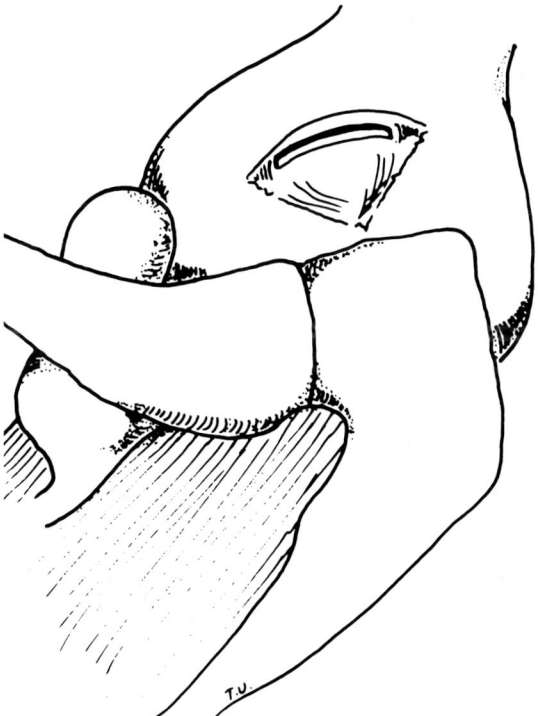

Figure 2 The triangular rotator cuff defect is demonstrated with a trough prepared in bone at the junction of the greater tuberosity and anatomical neck.

structure superiorly over the humeral head. In addition, by enlarging the usual incision to allow detachment of more deltoid laterally, the infraspinatus may be identified and advanced as a pedicle advancement from the infraspinatus fossa and brought to meet the subscapularis superiorly. These may then be sutured to a trough in bone (Fig. 3). The biceps tendon may be incorporated as a direct flap or may be detached and opened in half and reapplied as a free graft. Other synthetic materials may be used as free grafts. The use of synthetic materials is embryonic in its development and these are not commonly used in covering large cuff defects.

Another technique for large tears involves foreshortening the trough, moving it more up onto the humeral head as described by McLaughlin.[8] This would limit some elevation during rehabilitation.

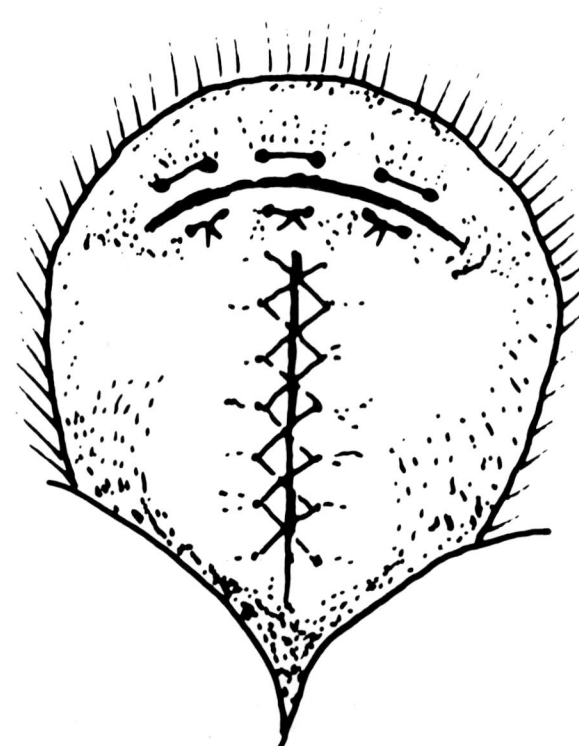

Figure 3 The rotator cuff defect is closed on the apex in shoelace fashion and then sutured to the trough in bone to effect a secure closure.

Postoperative Management

The postoperative management of patients following rotator cuff surgery must address the problem of when active exercises may be commenced. This depends upon the size of the tear and the security of the repair and must be tailored to each patient. Usually, however, at least six weeks should be allowed for healing before active exercises are commenced. In the majority of tears, which usually are small or medium in size, early assisted exercising, using the normal arm as a power, emphasizing elevation, external and internal rotation may be commenced immediately. At six weeks active exercises are added, followed quickly by resisted exercises to build up strength particularly of the anterior deltoid for forward elevation and the infraspinatus for external rotation. This is followed by an ongoing stretching and strengthening program for up to two years.

Elevation braces may be employed to protect the repair until it heals. If the reconstruction is for a large or massive defect, and excess tension is put on the reconstruction when the arm is brought down to the side, an elevation brace should be worn for four to six weeks. Depending on the security of the repair, assisted elevation and external rotation can usually be performed above the level of the brace since this will not compromise the repair. This also allows the patient to be more actively involved in the rehabilitation program early on. It is important to remember it takes six months following most rotator cuff reconstructions before active elevation of the arm is comfortably achieved.

Complications

Infection has been a complication encountered in rotator cuff reconstructions, particularly with large tears, probably because of the prolonged exposure and tight reconstructions. The shoulder is a contaminated area with the armpit, saliva running down from the mouth, and hair near the wound. With vigorous preoperative washing, appropriate draping and prophylactic antibiotics, this complication can be avoided. Deltoid retraction may be a complication but can be avoided by careful reattachment. The positioning of the stay suture in the deltoid at the lateral margin of the incision will prevent it from retracting underneath the skin during the surgery allowing easier closure. Reflex dystrophy can occur following cuff reconstruction and should be aggressively treated with stellate ganglion blocks and physiotherapy. Stiff shoulders require aggressive physiotherapy. Rerupture can occur, particularly with large defects. In fact, if a massive defect cannot be repaired, frequently decompression alone will offer a reasonable degree of pain relief. Operating on reruptures may not prove favorable unless the initial procedure did not include a decompression.

Special Considerations

Special considerations associated with surgery of the rotator cuff involve biceps rupture, associated dislocation in an older patient, and cuff arthropathy.

When a biceps rupture occurs, it is important to consider that the patient probably has underlying impingement and long term disability will be related to the cuff deficiency rather than the biceps rupture. An arthrogram will determine the status of the rotator cuff, and if surgery is performed, an anterior acromioplasty with exploration of the rotator cuff should be undertaken. Repair of the biceps may be added as indicated. However, biceps ruptures alone do not usually lead to late pain or a significant degree of functional weakness or disability. Ruptures of the biceps may occur in the absence of a cuff deficiency but are still usually associated with impingement. In such circumstances, these patients must be carefully followed if repair of the biceps is not undertaken, being alert for any subsequent development of a cuff tear. Muscle tendon rupture in a younger patient is a different pathological process and may require surgical repair.

Patients over the age of 50 years who have a first time dislocation usually have an associated rotator cuff tear and attention must be directed to this in their rehabilitation program.

The recently introduced concept of cuff arthropathy associated with longstanding cuff deficiencies implies degenerative changes not only in the subacromial area but also in the glenohumeral joint. Surgical management of such a problem can be challenging, requiring not only cuff reconstruction but also glenohumeral arthroplasty.

Conclusions

Most authors report improvement following rotator cuff repairs in over two-thirds of patients. However, the reports include all aspects of pathology and all aspects of pain, function, range of motion, and strength. We have alluded to the fact that there are many pathologies involved and patients have different demands and expectations as to pain and function and these must be considered individually to give us a better appreciation for patient selection and expectation.

Cofield at the Mayo Clinic has analyzed 43 patients with a seven year follow-up and with acute rotator cuff tears. These acute tears which were repaired at 0–3 weeks achieved better elevation than those that were repaired later. Wolfgang[11] analyzed 73 patients, presenting good early results at one year with 69 percent satisfactory, and in the same group of patients even better results at eight years with 75 percent satisfactory.

In our experience in well over 100 rotator cuff reconstructions we have been very pleasantly surprised at the pain relief afforded by the operation and at the functional improvement achieved by these patients. It is difficult to judge whether functional improvement is based strictly on reconstruction or on pain relief or both. It is our conclusion that small and medium sized rotator cuff reconstructions offer excellent functional improvement. Large and massive tears have variable functional improvement, but in most tears the pain relief is satisfactory. The functional success of the operation is related to the patient's preoperative loss of range of motion and its duration along with the size of the rotator cuff defect.

In active patients with acute tears we suggest an early decompressive operation and repair. In less active patients there may be a brief trial of physiotherapy and time. In inactive patients conservative management would be appropriate with decompression for pain relief. The indications for surgery in chronic tears would primarily be for pain relief, particularly in inactive patients. In active patients, repair may not only be for pain relief but also for functional improvement. Early surgery will prevent progression of the disease process and should be an important consideration.

The surgical approach to rotator cuff tears must be individualized. The spectrum of pathology is wide. Patient demands and expectations are varied. They are challenging, however, and provide great satisfaction with success.

REFERENCES

1. Neer CS. Anterior acromioplasty for the chronic impingement syndrome in the shoulder: A preliminary report. J Bone Joint Surg. 1972; 54A:41.
2. Rathbun JB, Mcnab I. The microvascular pattern of the rotator cuff. J Bone Joint Surg. 1970; 52B:540.
3. Neer CS, Welsh RP. The shoulder in sports. Orthop Clin N Am. 1977; 8:583.
4. Codman EA. The shoulder. Rupture of the supraspinatus tendon and other lesions in or about the subacromial bursa. 2nd ed. Boston: Thomas Todd, 1934.
5. McLaughlin MH. Rupture of the rotator cuff. J Bone Joint Surg. 1962; 44A:979.
6. Debeyre J, Patte D, Elmelik E. Repair of ruptures of the rotator cuff of the shoulder with a note on advancement of the supraspinatus muscle. J Bone Joint Surg. 1949; 47B:436.
7. Kessel L. Clinical disorders of the shoulder. London: Churchill Livingstone, 1982.
8. McLaughlin HL. Lesions of the musculotendinous cuff of the shoulder. J Bone Joint Surg. 1944; 26:31.
9. Neer CS, Bigliani LU, Hawkins RJ. Rupture of the long head of the biceps related to subacromial impingement. Orthop Trans. 1977; 1:111.
10. Hawkins RJ, Koppert GJ. The natural history following anterior dislocation of the shoulder in the older patient. Orthop Trans. 1981; 5:396.
11. Wolfgang GL. Surgical repair of tears of the rotator cuff of the shoulder. J Bone Joint Surg. 1974; 56A:14.

LONG TERM RESULTS OF SURGICAL REPAIR OF FULL THICKNESS ROTATOR CUFF TEARS

OMAR BAYNE, M.D., and JAMES E. BATEMAN, M.D., F.R.C.S.(C)

It is the purpose of this paper to review 452 consecutive complete rotator cuff tears treated surgically by one surgeon between 1970 and 1980 at the Orthopaedic and Arthritic Hospital and to report on the long-term results of 323 cuff repairs followed for an average of 7.7 years. It is our intention to draw conclusions from our results that may help to more clearly define or establish certain guidelines for the management of rotator cuff tears.

MATERIALS AND METHODS

The charts of 489 patients who had rotator cuff repair carried out between 1970 and 1980 were reviewed. Of these, 16 patients had partial cuff tears and were therefore not included in our study. Thirty-six patients were excluded because of inadequate preoperative records, leaving 437 patients with 452 complete cuff tears (15 bilateral).

There were 185 females and 252 males (ratio 1:1.4) with an average age of 57.8 years and 55.4 years respectively. Ages ranged from 15 to 84 years.

Preoperative Assessment

The predisposing cause of cuff tears ranged from severe direct trauma to the shoulder to minimal or nontraumatic. Sixty-one patients (15%) had compensable injuries. The right shoulder was involved in 284 (63% of cases) and the left in 168 (37%). Twenty-four patients (5.4%) had associated injuries about the shoulder: 13 had associated pure anterior shoulder dislocations and seven had anterior fracture dislocations. The remaining four patients had separation of the acromioclavicular joint.

Previous Shoulder Surgery

Eighty-five patients (27%) had had previous surgery to the involved shoulder done elsewhere. Thirty-eight (11.8%) had had previous rotator cuff repair. Twenty patients had had some form of soft tissue stabilization for recurrent shoulder dislocation. Twelve patients had had excision of the A/C ligament for impairment, 6 had had excision of the long head of biceps and 4 had had repair of calcium deposits.

Nonoperative Management

Ninety-four percent of patients had had a trial of conservative treatment prior to surgery ranging from two months to four years (average 11.4 months). This had included some form of nonsteroidal anti-inflammatory medication (95%), some form of physiotherapy (80%), chiropractic manipulation (20%); 109 patients (25%) had local steroid injection to the involved shoulder with 53 patients receiving three or more injections. Three percent had had acupuncture.

Ninety (20%) shoulders presented with intractable pain at rest or with activity. Of these, 2/3 had radiation of their shoulder pain down the anterior upper arm to the elbow. Two hundred and four shoulders (45%) had nocturnal pain only. One hundred and eighteen shoulders (26%) had pain only with activity. Forty shoulders (8.8%) presented with no pain.

One hundred and forty shoulders (31%) had a full range of active motion. One hundred and twenty-two shoulders (27%) had a painful arc between 90° and 120° of abduction. Ninety-nine shoulders (22%) had no glenohumeral motion (frozen shoulder).

Fifty-nine (13%) shoulders had full muscle power (5/5); 278 (62%) had a loss of at least one grade (4/5). Seventy-nine (17%) had no power against one finger resistance. Thirty-six (8%) had no power against gravity. One hundred and eighty-one (40%) shoulders had palpable crepitus and 352 (78%) had detectable muscle wasting involving mainly the spinatae, trapezius and deltoid muscles.

Roentgenographic Examination

Two hundred and forty (53%) shoulders were reported normal on plain x-ray evaluation, 127 (28%) had osteoarthritis involving the acromioclavicular joint, 22 (4.9%) had evidence of calcific tendinitis, 18 (4%) had an avulsion fracture of the greater tuberosity; 37 (8.1%) had evidence of snubbing of the humeral head against the acromion. Two patients showed evidence of a Hill-Sachs lesion and two had bipartate acromions.

Arthrogram

Preoperative arthrographic investigation was done in 417 (92.3%) shoulders. Arthrograms confirmed a tear in 385, (85.3%) of the shoulder. The percentage of accuracy was related to the grade of cuff tear. With grade 1 tear having an 82%, Grade 2 96% and Grades 3 and 4 100% accuracy rate verified at the time of surgery. Seven patients were noted to have dye extending from the subacromial bursa to the acromioclavicular joint. They were all noted to have chronic global cuff tears at surgery. Five patients were allergic to the contrast material and had their cuff tears diagnosed by shoulder arthroscopy.

Surgical Technique

The patient is placed in a semi-sitting position (at approximately 45°) with the head turned to the contralateral side; a towel is placed between the scapulae and the shoulder is allowed to hang over the edge of the table and draped free. The contralateral thigh is also prepared and draped for harvesting of fascia lata graft should the need arise. An anterior lateral utility shoulder incision is made extending two inches posterior to the acromion and three inches anterior, about two fingers breadth lateral to the deltopectoral groove. The anterior deltoid muscle is split along its fibers and subperiosteally dissected off the acromion, leaving a good cuff of tissue for reattachment. A routine acromioclavicular arthroplasty is carried out to aid in exposure of the cuff defect. If there are degenerative changes in the acromioclavicular joint, the outer ⅜ inch of the clavicle is excised. To maintain shoulder stability, a complete acromionectomy is avoided. Acromioclavicular arthroplasty, apart from improving the exposure of the cuff defect, also removes existing or potential impingement and decompresses the repair.

The fibrotic edges of the tear are debrided and the cuff mobilized as much as possible by digitally breaking down all adhesions and putting the shoulder through a full range of passive motion. For small, full thickness tears, a nonabsorbable synthetic suture is used to reapproximate the edges. For longer defects in which edge-to-edge approximation is impossible, fascia lata graft is used to bridge the defect using a darning technique. Occasionally a wedge of bone is removed from the humeral head and drill holes made to anchor the fascia. For large global tears with deficient cuff margins, several soft tissue procedures are carried out depending on the extent of the tear and the availability of usable local soft tissue structures.

Harvesting of Fascia Lata Graft

Fascia lata is obtained from the controlateral thigh using a standard fascial stripper. A transverse incision approximately 2 cm in length is made a hand's breadth above the fibular head. A strip of fascia measuring 2 × 8 inches is obtained. The free end of the fascia is first fed into the stripper which is then advanced proximally and the fascia is removed in one piece.

The fascia may then be divided into two equal strips and sutured onto two Gallie needles.

Postoperative Management

The postoperative management of rotator cuff repairs requires the help and supervision of skilled physiotherapists in order to obtain optimum benefits from the surgical repair. Immediately postoperatively the patient is immobilized in an abduction splint. In about 24 hours this is changed to slings and springs when lying or sitting in bed. Once the patient is ambulatory an abduction wedge or cantilever brace is provided which allows the shoulder to be immobilized in approximately 60° of abduction and forward flexion and 15° of external rotation. The brace is discarded as soon as the patient has adequate shoulder control and is able to abduct the shoulder against some manual resistance (approximately 6 weeks). Out-patient supervised physiotherapy is then continued until maximum function, range of motion and power are regained (average 6 months).

SURGICAL GRADING OF ROTATOR CUFF TEARS

Rotator cuff tears were graded according to our criteria into Grades 1 through 4 depending on the extent of the lesion. All tears reported in this series were full thickness tears.

Grade 1 (149/452 or 33%)

These were cuff tears of 1 cm or less measured in the longest diameter after debriding of the avascular edges which were always repaired by direct nonabsorbable interrupted sutures. The edges were easily approximated with the patient's hand at his side.

Grade 2 (127/452) or (28%)

These were cuff tears of 1 to 3 cm in diameter after debridement of the avascular edges; usually full approximation of the edges was possible with the shoulder abducted to 60°.
All grade 2 tears were reconstructable with fascia lata grafts without wedge resection of the humeral head.

Grade 3 (142/452 or 31%)

These were cuff tears of 5 cm or less in which the cuff margins approximated the shoulder at 60° only after wedge resection of the humeral head. Fascia lata grafts were routinely used in the darning technique. After wedge resection the fascial graft was secured in drill holes and woven in crisscross fashion to cover the defect.

Grade 4 (34/452 or 8%)

Those were global cuff tears in which there was little or no cuff left. A salvage procedure was carried out including sub scapularis transfer (9 shoulders), lateral transfer of the long head of the biceps tendon (10 shoulders), and coracoid transfer (12 shoulders).

COMPLICATIONS

There were neither intraoperative complications nor local complications relating to the fascia lata donor site. Eight patients (1.7%) developed postoperative wound infections. Six of these had superficial wound infections which cleared up after 7–14 days of systemic anti-biotics. The other two had deep wound infections which required sinus tract excision and debridement before the infection resolved. Five of the eight patients with postoperative wound infections had had previous shoulder surgery. All wounds grew Staphylococcus aureus except one superficial wound infection which grew staphylococcus epidermidis. Prophylactic antibiotics were not used in this series. Five shoulders (1.1%) developed ulnar nerve palsy as a result of pressure from the abduction wedge or cantilever brace. All were transient neuropathies except one which required an ulnar nerve transfer 10 months after the cuff repair. Two patients developed postoperative transient axillary nerve palsy associated with deltoid paralysis. One patient developed a deep vein thrombosis and was treated with anticoagulants. Two patients had acute upper gastrointestinal tract bleeds. Two had frozen shoulders that had to be manipulated 2 to 3 weeks postoperatively. One patient developed a nonfatal myocardial infarction and one, bronchial pneumonia. Six patients developed postoperative wound hematomas which resolved without sequelae.

CLINICAL ASSESSMENT AND CRITERIA

One hundred and seventeen patients returned for clinical reassessment; 139 responded to a written questionnaire; 60 responded to a telephone interview. Fifteen patients had died and 106 changed address and were lost to follow-up, leaving 316 patients with 323 cuff repairs (7 bilateral) for review.

The time of follow-up was 2.5 to 13 years (average 7.7 years). The patients reviewed according to grade of tears were as follows:

Grade 1 tears (81/147), grade 2 (96/127), grade 3 (116/142) and grade 4 (30/34). The patients were assessed subjectively and objectively with regard to pain relief, range of motion and return of shoulder function.

Excellent Result

An excellent result was obtained if there was no pain; abduction and forward flexion greater than 120° and the patient was able to return to his or her original job, sport or activity.

Good Result

A good result implied minimal pain without without activity, abduction and forward flexion between 90–120°. Minor modification of job, sport or activity.

Fair Result

Moderate pain requiring occasional analgesics, abduction or forward flexion less than 90°. Major modification of job, sport or activity.

Poor Result

No change from preoperative status or made worse by the surgery.

Results

Using the above criteria, there were 260/323 (80.5%) overall satisfactory results, (excellent and good) and 19.5% overall unsatisfactory results, (fair and poor). No patient was given a satisfactory result unless both the patient and the examining physician agreed.

Grade I tears as expected had 86.3% (70/81) satisfactory results.

Grade II tears had 81.25% (78/96) satisfactory results.

Grade III tears had 77.6% (90/116) satisfactory results.

Grade IV (global tears) 73.3% (22/30) satisfactory results. Taking all grades into account, 87.3% had complete pain relief, 76.7% had improved range of motion and 84.2% had improved power.

DISCUSSION

Sixty-three cuff repairs (19.5%) had an unsatisfactory result. Of these, 21 had compensable injuries. When these patients were compared to the general population, the overall satisfactory results showed that the general population did almost 50% better than the compensation group. There appeared to be no significant difference between grades 2 and 3 in reference to long-term results following surgery. However, there was a significant difference ($p < 0.005$) between grades 1 and 4 cuff tears in both the general population and the compensation group.

The mean time from onset of clinical symptoms to cuff repair was 20.6 months in the satisfactory group compared to 31.8 months in the unsatisfactory group. This confirms other reports that better results can be expected if the repair is carried out 6 months to one year after onset of symptoms.

Eighteen of 25 patients who received three steroid injections were reassessed following their repair. Only 50 percent of these had a satisfactory result. Twenty-one patients reviewed had had more than three injections and only 11.8 percent had satisfactory results. Almost all patients having fewer than three steroid injections had a satisfactory result.

Most patients who received three or more steroid injections were noted at the time of surgery to have developed a "steroid arthropathy" with reduction of the tensile strength of the cuff with associated soft, fragile bone, making cuff reconstruction and bone resection tenuous. It is therefore recommended that steroid injections used in the conservative management of cuff tears be restricted to one or two injections in order not to compromise the remaining cuff tissues should cuff reconstruction be attempted.

Complete pain relief was seen in 87.3% of cuff repairs. We felt that the prophylatic decompression of the repair by acromioclavicular arthroplasty assisted tremendously in pain relief especially during the early rehabilitation period when regaining range of shoulder motion is very important. Fourteen of the 22 patients with major complaints of pain had compensable injuries.

Improved shoulder motion was noted in 76.7 percent of cuff repairs. The majority of patients had no or minimal pain associated with their decreased range of motion. Thirty-five patients had limitations of abduction less than 90%. Two-thirds were noncompliant in adhering to the strict postoperative physiotherapy regimen. Six patients had deficient deltoid muscle as a result of previous shoulder surgery. Three had postoperative transient axillary nerve paralysis lasting between 3 and 6 months and one patient had a myocardial infarction immediately post operatively causing a delay in post operative physiotherapy.

Muscle weakness alone with no pain and a full range of glenohumeral motion was seen in 16% of shoulders following cuff repair.

RECONSTRUCTION OF CHRONIC TEARS OF THE ROTATOR CUFF

ROBERT J. NEVIASER, M.D. and THOMAS J. NEVIASER, M.D.

The problem of chronic tears of the rotator cuff remains a perplexing one to most orthopaedic surgeons. This is a result of inadequate exposure to surgery of the shoulder during their training as well as confusing literature on the subject. Nevertheless, lesions of the rotator cuff—from tendinitis to chronic tears—plus problems of instability make up the vast majority of shoulder disorders seen in orthopaedic practice. The intent of this discussion is to put into some order the chaos that exists concerning chronic tears of the rotator cuff.

DIAGNOSIS

There are two types of chronic rotator cuff tears. The more common of the two is the degenerative or attritional tear. Patients with such tears may present with or without history of an injury. The injury, if present, is often minor. The history dates back over a period of several months or even years and is one primarily of shoulder pain. Night pain is a prominent feature. One of the confusing and frequent findings is excellent motion, even approaching the normal range. On examination, however, weakness in external rotation can be detected, and there also will be pain with palm-down abduction.

The second type of chronic tear is traumatic. It is less common than the degenerative tear, but may prove to be a more difficult reconstructive problem. Traumatic tears are classified as chronic when the interval between injury and repair exceeds three weeks.[8,9] Often there is a significant history of injury with some loss of active motion, although this is not always the case. The patient complains of pain, weakness, and discomfort at night. Weakness in external rotation and abduction can be found. Both types of tears are found in patients over age forty but rarely in younger patients without a violent traumatic episode. The older the patient, the higher the index of suspicion.

TREATMENT

The initial treatment of the chronic traumatic tear is operative. The sooner one repairs the rotator cuff of a patient who has had a significant injury with subsequent pain and loss of motion, the more likely it is that the result will be successful.[1] The treatment of attritional tears with no significant injury can be nonoperative initially. Anti-inflammatory agents, either oral or local, can provide satisfactory relief. Gentle stretching exercises and avoiding the activity which produces the most pain can also ease the patient's complaints. There is a risk, however, that an injury could produce an acute extension of the already existing chronic tear, necessitating surgical repair. For patients with chronic degenerative tears who do not get relief from nonoperative measures, surgical reconstruction can be beneficial. The diagnosis, however, must be confirmed by arthrography.[11] Clinical assessment alone can result in missed diagnoses.

There are five procedures which have proved useful in the treatment of both types of tears. If the surgeon is sufficiently familiar with all five, closure of a rotator cuff defect should be possible in virtually every case.

Surgical Approach

The surgical approach is the same in all cases. Closure of the tear itself differs depending on the size of the defect and these differences revolve around the maneuvers done to obliterate the defect. All procedures are performed under general endotracheal anesthesia. The patient is in the sitting position with his head on a headrest so the shoulder extends above the edge of the table, allowing free access to its superior, anterior, and posterior aspects. The arm is draped free to permit appropriate positioning of the extremity. An anterior-superior approach is used. The incision begins at the posterior margin of the acromioclavicular joint and is extended across the superior surface of this joint in a straight line to a point just lateral and inferior to the coracoid process. This incision heals with an esthetically attractive result.

The deltoid is split at the level of the acromioclavicular joint in line with the skin incision. After the deltoid is separated bluntly from the underlying subacromial bursa, the acromioclavicular joint is incised from its inferior margin up to, but not including, the superior acromioclavicular ligament. The knife blade is then turned to lie parallel to the superior surface of the clavicle and the acromion. The deltoid and superior acromioclavicular ligament are dissected subperiosteally from the superior margins of the clavicle, the acromioclavicular joint, and the acromion. The deltoid is also dissected subperiosteally from the anterior margin of the acromion. This anterior and superior subperiosteal dissection of the deltoid from the acromion can be extended as far laterally and posteriorly as necessary to gain access to all components of the rotator cuff, even the teres minor. The outer 5 mm of the clavicle is excised with a power saw, eliminating one of the irritants of the rotator cuff and allowing increased exposure to the cuff itself.[2,7,13] The coracoacromial ligament is excised in its entirety, and an anterior-inferior oblique acromioplasty is performed.[4] This subacromial decompression is an important part of the reconstruction of any rotator cuff lesion.[12]

The subdeltoid bursa is incised in line with the deltoid splitting incision. It is dissected free from the underlying rotator cuff, tagged with a suture for the purpose of identification, and is routinely saved. After retracting the bursa, the surgeon can easily see the defect in the cuff. Traction downward on the arm opens the subacromial space, and by placing a retractor posterior to the humeral head and under the acromion, visualization of the entire cuff can be achieved.

The closure of this approach is accomplished by repairing the subacromial bursa with a running 3–0 plain catgut suture. The purpose of closure is to protect the suture line of the cuff and retain the gliding mechanism of the cuff under the deltoid. The deltoid is returned to its original position and the split in its fibers approximated with 0 nonabsorbable suture. There is no need to suture the deltoid to the acromion, since it has not been incised from its tendinous origin. Rather, it has been simply reflected subperiosteally, and the periosteal attachments of the deltoid remain intact. Thus the periosteum will heal to the underlying cortical surface and provide a secure origin for the deltoid.

Prior to closure reconstruction of the cuff itself must be done. As indicated earlier, there are five options available, depending on the size of the defect, the quality of the tissues, and their mobility. In all instances the rounded, scarred, friable edges of the cuff at the site of the tear must be resected. Enough of this friable tissue must be removed to leave a healthy, thick tendon edge capable of healing. If the friable margins are not removed, the repair cannot be expected to withstand any stress postoperatively and will inevitably rerupture.

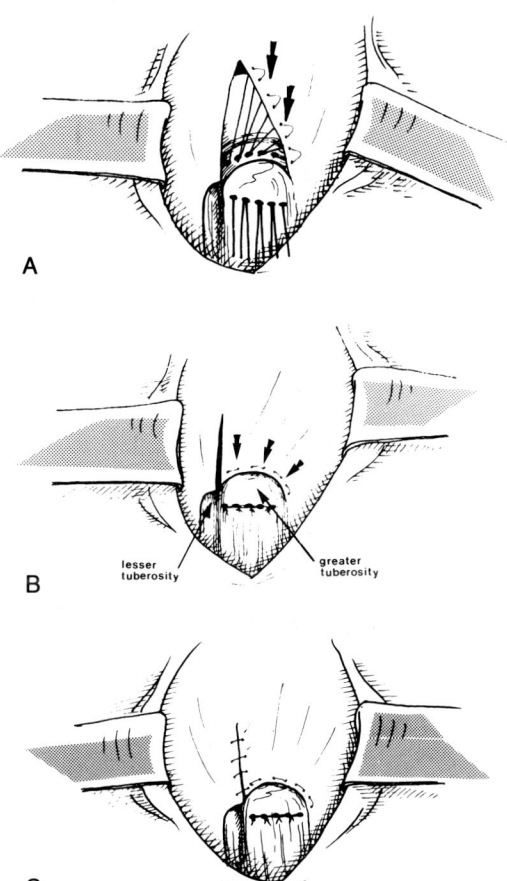

Figure 1 *A,* After resection of the unhealthy margins of the tear, one edge of the tendon is directed toward a trough cut at the anatomic neck of the humerus. *B,* After the tendon is secured to the trough, a single longitudinal limb remains. *C,* The residual longitudinal tear is closed by side-to-side opposition using interrupted, simple sutures.

Direct Closure

The first option is direct closure. This is frequently possible and, indeed, in most cases is the technique used. Traction sutures are placed in the edges of the tear and used to bring the tendon margins laterally. Blunt dissection along the tendons should allow increased mobility after the peritendinous adhesions have been released. This technique requires a great deal of patience and willingness to spend the time required for such a maneuver. Generally the anterior margin then can be brought to a cancellous trough of bone which should be made in the sulcus just medial to the greater tuberosity (Fig. 1A). The margins should be anchored to bone through drill holes which allow the sutures to be tied over a bridge of bone inferior to the apex of the greater tuberosity (Fig. 1B). This will leave a longitudinal tear which can be sutured side-to-side (Fig. 1C). Occasionally, it is possible to bring the entire free tendon edge to the trough.

Free Biceps Graft[5]

The next option, if mobilization of the tendons does not permit the free edges to be brought to the greater tuberosity and a small residual defect exists (Fig. 2A), is bridging by a free biceps graft. The intra-articular portion of the biceps is resected after fixing the tendon in the intratubercular groove by suturing it to the transverse humeral ligament. The free portion of the biceps tendon is then split in a book-like fashion, leaving a hinge on one side (Fig. 2B). The graft is placed so that the cut surface is exterior and the shiny surface is against the humeral head. The orientation of the graft depends on the orientation of the defect. The graft should be sutured to the free margins of the tendon on one side and to a trough of bone (made as previously described) on the other (Fig. 2C). Occasionally, reinforcing sutures may be necessary at the hinge of the graft.

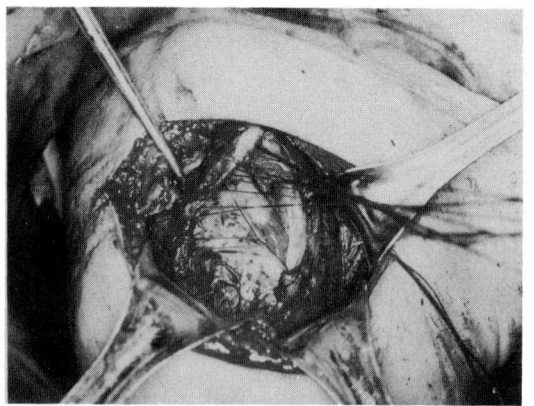

A

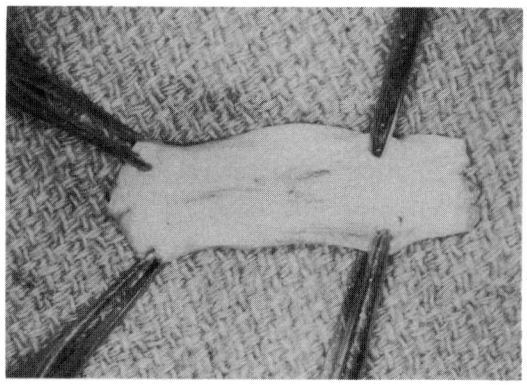

B

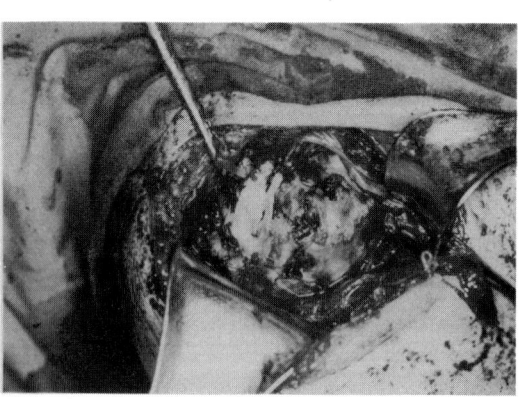

C

Figure 2 *A,* Traction is being applied through sutures and a defect is still present in the cuff. *B,* The intra-articular portion of the biceps tendon has been split in book-like fashion. (From Neviaser RJ. Tears of the rotator cuff. Orthop Clin N Am. 1980; 11:295–306). *C,* The biceps graft has bridged the defect in the cuff tendons. (From Neviaser RJ. Tears of the rotator cuff. Orthop Clin N Am. 1980; 11:295–306.)

McLaughlin Repair[3]

The remaining options are used for those defects which cannot be closed by direct suture or the free-biceps graft; they involve reconstruction of very large or massive tendinous defects. For surgeons who only attempt rotator cuff reconstruction occasionally, the easiest of these techniques is the McLaughlin repair. This involves creating a trough of cancellous bone in the humeral head at that point to which the tendons can be readily brought. If this is in the middle of the apex or dome of the humeral head, or further laterally, the depressing effect of the rotator cuff on the humeral head will be greater. If this trough is placed medial to the apex of the dome of the humeral head, the power of stabilization of the humeral head or of external rotation will be considerably weakened. The approach provides effective relief of pain, although, functionally, it is less satisfactory than other techniques. Once the cancellous trough has been created, drill holes are made from the middle of the trough to the lateral margin of the humerus below the greater tuberosity. Sutures placed through the cuff can be brought out through these holes and tied over bridges of bone to anchor them (Fig. 3).

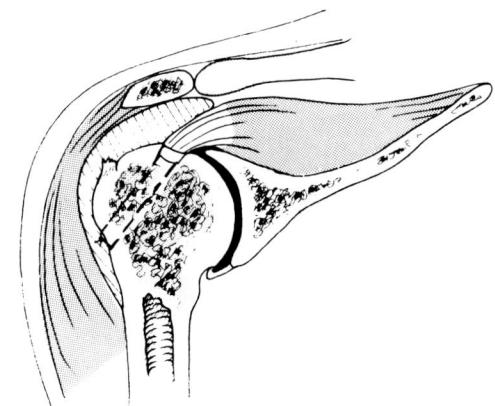

Figure 3 The technique which was described by McLaughlin consists of inserting the tendon into a cancellous trough made in the humeral head at whatever point it happens to reach.

Freeze-Dried Rotator Cuff Graft[6]

The next two options should be reserved for surgeons who are comfortable in operating on the shoulder—especially rotator cuff defects—and have developed some technical expertise. The first is the freeze-dried cadaver graft. It is used for

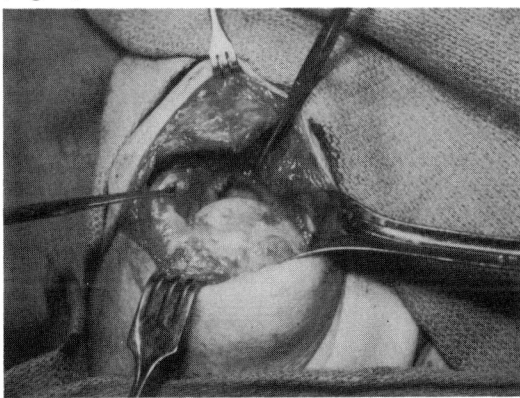

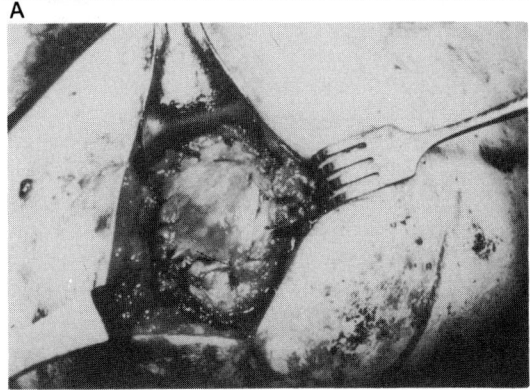

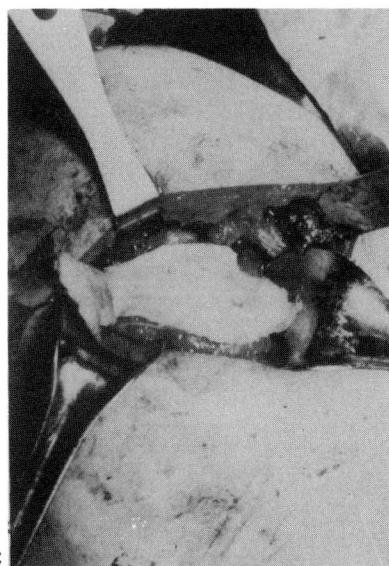

Figure 4 *A,* There is a massive chronic tear of the rotator cuff, which could not be closed by direct repair. (From Neviaser RJ. Tears of the rotator cuff. Orthop Clin N Am. 1980; 11:295–306). *B,* A reconstituted freeze-dried rotator cuff cadaver graft lies in the wound reflecting the size of the graft. (From Neviaser RJ. Tears of the rotator cuff. Orthop Clin N Am. 1980; 11:295–306). *C,* The graft has been sutured in place to bridge the massive defect. (From Neviaser RJ. Tears of the rotator cuff. Orthop Clin N Am. 1980; 11:295–306).

massive chronic tears (Fig. 4A). This graft should be harvested from a cadaver under forty-five years of age with no history of rotator cuff problems, systemic infection, or malignancy. The quality of the tissue is, therefore, generally quite good. The freeze-dried tissue can be reconstituted by simply soaking it in sterile saline for a period of thirty minutes (Fig. 4B). Once the graft has been reconstituted, it is trimmed to accommodate the margin of the free tendon edge and sutured securely with 0 nonabsorbable sutures to this tendon. The graft is then brought over the humeral head and trimmed to fit into a cancellous trough in the sulcus between the humeral head and the greater tuberosity (Fig. 4C). It is anchored to bone with drill holes as previously described. Massive defects can be readily closed by use of this graft.

Tendon Transfers[2,10]

The final option—tendon transfer—is reserved for the patient with a massive defect for which a freeze-dried graft is not available. The subscapularis can be utilized alone or in conjunction with the teres minor. When a decision has been made to utilize a tendon transfer, either tendon can be separated from the underlying capsule by starting medially near the musculotendinous junction and dissecting laterally toward its insertion. It is important to leave the underlying articular capsule undisturbed to provide support to the joint both anteriorly and posteriorly as well as a watertight closure. The tendon is separated as far laterally as possible and detached (Fig. 5A). Blunt dissection along the muscle belly will allow it to

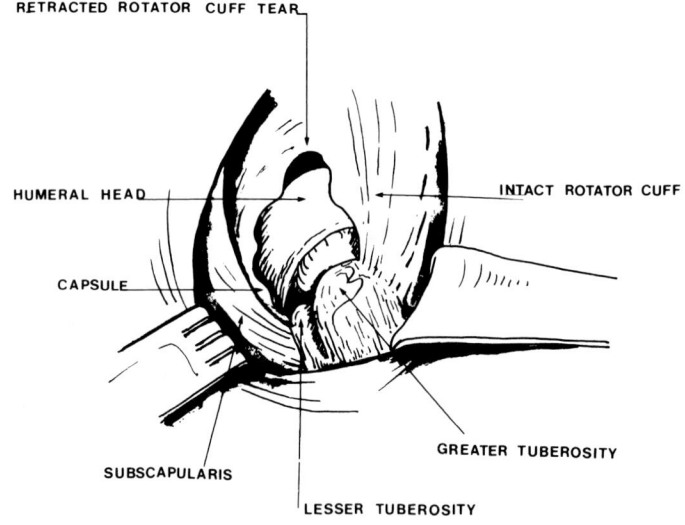

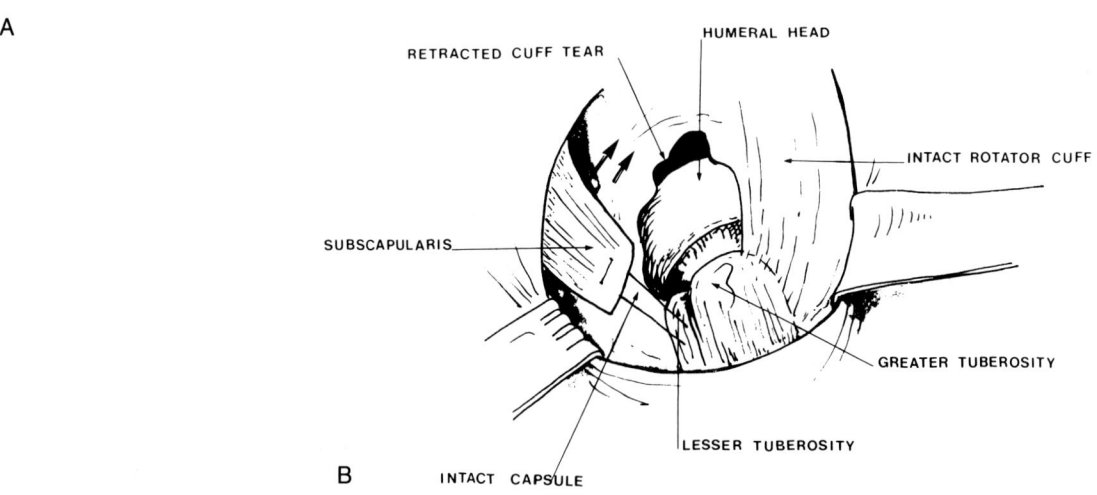

Figure 5 *A*, The subscapularis has been separated from the underlying capsule which is left intact. *B*, The subscapularis is detached as close to its insertion as possible and mobilized so that it can be shifted superiorly. The underlying anterior articular capsule remains undisturbed.

(Illustration and legend continued on the opposite page)

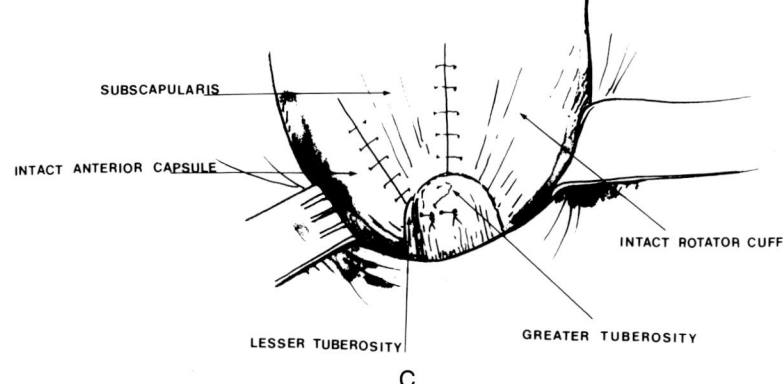

Figure 5 *(Continued)* C, The subscapularis has been moved superiorly. The edges of the tear have been resected. The subscapularis has been sutured to bone at the tuberosities. The superior edge of the subscapularis is sutured to the anterior edge of the remaining cuff and inferior edge of the subscapularis is sutured to the superior margin of the remaining undisturbed anterior articular capsule.

be mobilized sufficiently to swing it superiorly to close the defect (Fig. 5B). Once the subscapularis has been mobilized and transferred, and if it is large enough to fill the defect left after the unhealthy tendon edges have been resected, its lateral margin is sutured to the trough made in the anatomic neck just medial to the greater tuberosity. The transferred superior edge is sutured to the border of the intact cuff, and the inferior margin is sutured to the superior margin of the undisturbed remaining articular capsule anteriorly (Fig. 5C). If the teres minor is to be used as well, it is separated in the same fashion as described for the subscapularis (Fig. 6A). Both tendons are then mobilized sufficiently to allow them to be transferred superiorly (Fig. 6B). They are sutured together first, with their superior margins opposing one another to form a new broad common tendon. The lateral margin of this new common tendon is inserted into the trough as previously described (Fig. 6C). Final closure of the defect is then accomplished by suturing the inferior margin of the subscapularis to the superior margin of the undisturbed anterior capsule and the inferior margin of the transferred teres minor to the superior border of the undisturbed posterior capsule (Fig. 6D).

Aftercare

Postoperative care consists of immobilization in a sling and swathe immediately. Passive motion is permissible within the limits of the repair and is done for the first three to four weeks for those patients who have had a direct repair or a McLaughlin procedure. For patients who have had a biceps graft, a freeze-dried cadaver graft, or tendon transfers, passive exercises are continued for six weeks. At that point, in both instances, active rehabilitation is undertaken. This consists of routine exercises for the rotator cuff and stretching exercises to prevent joint contracture. Resistive exercises are not instituted until full active motion has returned. It generally takes a minimum of six months for full function to be restored.

CONCLUSION

The expected outcome for direct repair should be quite satisfactory. The published statistics for the various grafting or transfer procedures are still valid. As the surgeon's experience with the techniques increases, his success rate will increase also. Chronic tears of the rotator cuff are not an insoluble problem. Understanding the basic pathophysiology and pathomechanics is important. A subacromial decompression is an important part of any reconstructive procedure. Familiarity with all five of the available options should give the surgeon the ability to close and manage virtually all chronic rotator cuff tears.

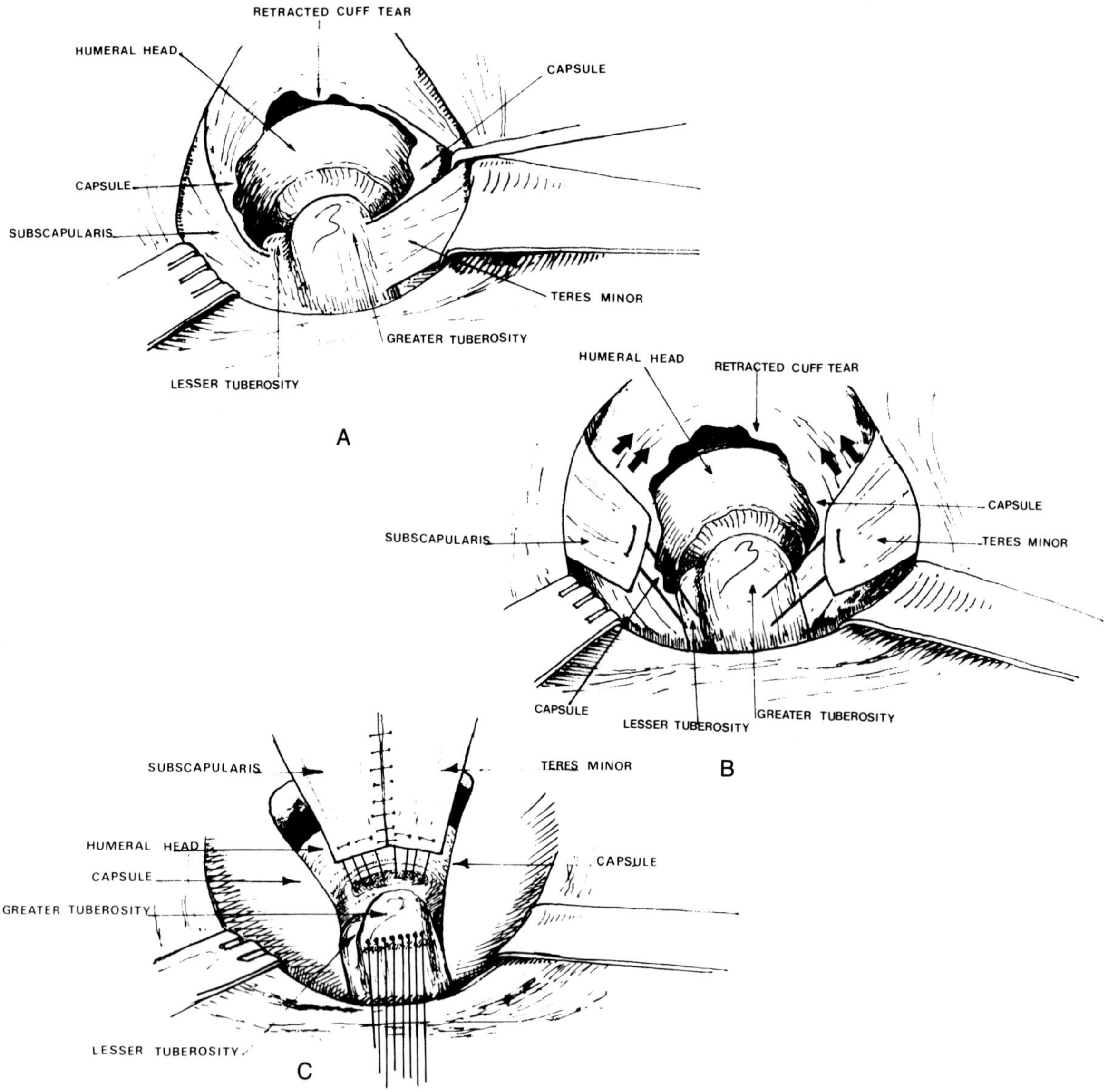

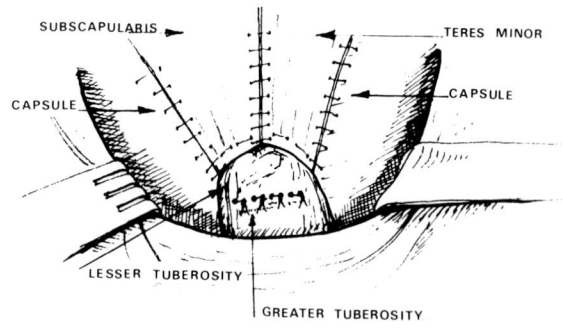

Figure 6 *A*, The subscapularis and the teres minor are separated from the underlying articular capsule which remains intact. *B*, The tendons are detached as close to their respective insertions as possible and mobilized sufficiently to allow their transfer superiorly. The anterior and posterior capsules are left undisturbed. *C*, The superior borders of the subscapularis and teres minor are trimmed to healthy tissue and then sutured together to form a new broader common tendon. This combined tendon is sutured to a cancellous trough in the anatomic neck. *D*, After securing the combined tendon into bone, the inferior border of the transferred subscapularis is sutured to the freshened superior margin of the undisturbed intact anterior articular capsule. An identical closure is performed posteriorly between the inferior edge of the transferred subscapularis and the freshened superior margin of the undisturbed posterior articular capsule.

REFERENCES

1. Bassett RW, Cofield RH. Acute tears of the rotator cuff. Clin Orthop Rel Res. 1983; 176:18–24.
2. Bateman JE. *The Shoulder and Neck*. 2nd ed. Philadelphia, WB Saunders Co, 1978
3. McLaughlin HL. Lesions of the musculotendinous cuff of the shoulder. I. The exposure and treatment of tears with retraction. J Bone Joint Surg. 1944; 26:31–51.
4. Neer CS, II. Anterior acromioplasty for the chronic impingement syndrome in the shoulder. J Bone Joint Surg. 1972; 54A:41–50.
5. Neviaser JS. Ruptures of the rotator cuff of the shoulder: new concepts in the diagnosis and operative treatment for chronic ruptures. Arch Surg 1971; 102:483–485.
6. Neviaser JS, Neviaser RJ, Neviaser TJ. The repair of chronic massive ruptures of the rotator cuff of the shoulder by the use of a freeze-dried rotator cuff. J Bone Joint Surg. 1978; 60A:681–684.
7. Neviaser RJ. Anatomic considerations and examination of the shoulder. Orthop Clin of N Am. 1980; 11:187–195.
8. Neviaser RJ. Tears of the rotator cuff. Orthop Clin of N Am. 1980; 11:295–306.
9. Neviaser RJ, Neviaser TJ. Lesions of the musculotendinous cuff of the shoulder. Part A: Tears of the rotator cuff. In AAOS Instructional Course Lectures, Vol. XXX. St. Louis; CV Mosby Co. 1981:239–250.
10. Neviaser RJ, Neviaser TJ. Transfer of the subscapularis and teres minor for massive defects of the rotator cuff. In Shoulder Surgery. Bayley JI, Kessel L, (eds). Berlin: Springer-Verlag, 1982:60–69.
11. Neviaser TJ. Arthrography of the shoulder. Orthop Clin of N Am. 1980; 11:205–271.
12. Packer NP, Calvert PT, Bayley JIL, Kessel L. Operative treatment of chronic ruptures of the rotator cuff of the shoulder. J Bone Joint Surg. 1983; 65B:171–175.
13. Watson M. The refractory painful arc syndrome. J Bone Joint Surg. 1978; 60B:544–546.

SHOULDER REHABILITATION AFTER ROTATOR CUFF SURGERY

MARILYN MODE, B.P.T.

It is essential that the physiotherapist see the shoulder surgery patient preoperatively so that she can perform a thorough assessment. The preoperative assessment should include subjective and objective findings such as the presence of pain, active and passive range of motion, patterns of movement, muscle strength, and, of course, function.

The effectiveness of physiotherapy depends to a large extent on meaningful two-way communication between the surgeon and the physiotherapist. This communication can make the difference between exceptional and ordinary physiotherapy. The physiotherapist must know the surgical approach and the structures it affects, the surgeon's estimate of the strength and stability and healing time for the repair, and the surgeon's expectations for the patient's functional improvement or result.

The physiotherapy department at the Orthopaedic and Arthritic Hospital divides patients who have had rotator cuff repairs into two main categories for postoperative management. In category I (Fig. 1) are those patients whose small tears have been repaired with synthetic sutures. In category II (Fig. 1) are patients who have had tears large enough to require another substance, such as fascia lata, to effect the repair.

We believe that the postoperative resting position of the shoulder is extremely important because it protects the repair, and is a starting point for exercise. Figure 2 illustrates the special pillow used to position the shoulder and which is placed under the patient in the recovery room. Note that the shoulder is in 90° abduction; that the elbow is off the bed to keep the shoulder in slight flexion and that the rotation is controlled by the attachment to the overhead pulley.

When the patient is in the sitting position (Fig. 2), the slings and springs hold the shoulder in 90° flexion and abduction and 15° external rotation. This balanced suspension allows the patient to experiment with gentle movement, and may be thought of as a forerunner to continuous passive motion.

Also illustrated in Figure 2 is the abduction wedge which maintains the resting position of the shoulder when the patient ambulates. It is used for patients in category I.

It is important to realize that the shoulder is maintained in this position at all times except when the patient is exercising or performing functional activities.

Category I

As a general rule, the patient in category I, whose small tear has been repaired by suture, has had a very stiff, painful shoulder preoperatively. Therefore, the immediate postoperative physiotherapy aims are to regain motion as soon as possible, and to relieve pain.

One of the ways in which we begin motion is by encouraging the patient to exercise his arm in the slings and springs (Fig. 3). This apparatus facilitates gentle bouncing and swinging motions. We believe that gentle motion stimulates the mechanoreceptors of the glenohumeral joint and therefore aids in reducing pain. We have also found that ice and transcutaneous nerve stimulation are very effective in relieving postoperative pain.

The patient progresses from gentle bouncing and swinging motions to assisted active and active exercises from the resting position upward through range. When the patient demonstrates strength and control from 90° up, exercises below the resting position are started.

We feel it is important to emphasize at the outset the difference between shoulder girdle motion or hunching and true glenohumeral motion (Fig. 4). To do this, we use proprioceptive and visual reinforcement techniques. In Figure 5, the physiotherapist stabilizes the scapula and assists the patient to gain flexion, adduction, external rotation at the glenohumeral joint. The mirror serves as visual feedback for the correct pattern of movement.

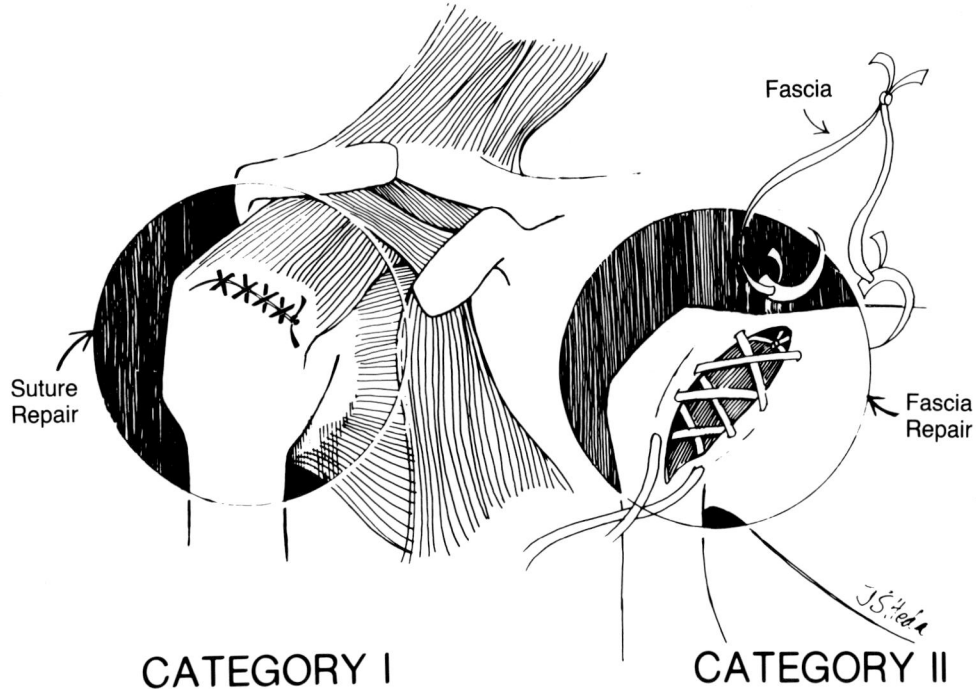

Figure 1 Rotator cuff tears are divided into two main categories.

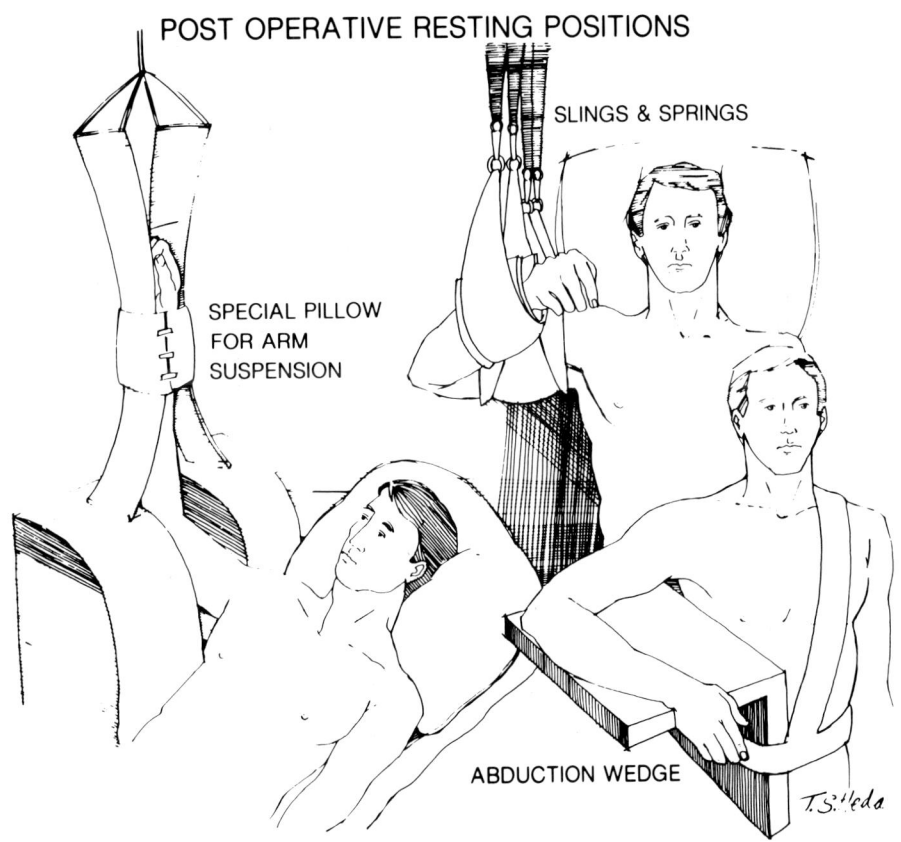

Figure 2 Postoperative resting position used in lying, sitting, and in standing.

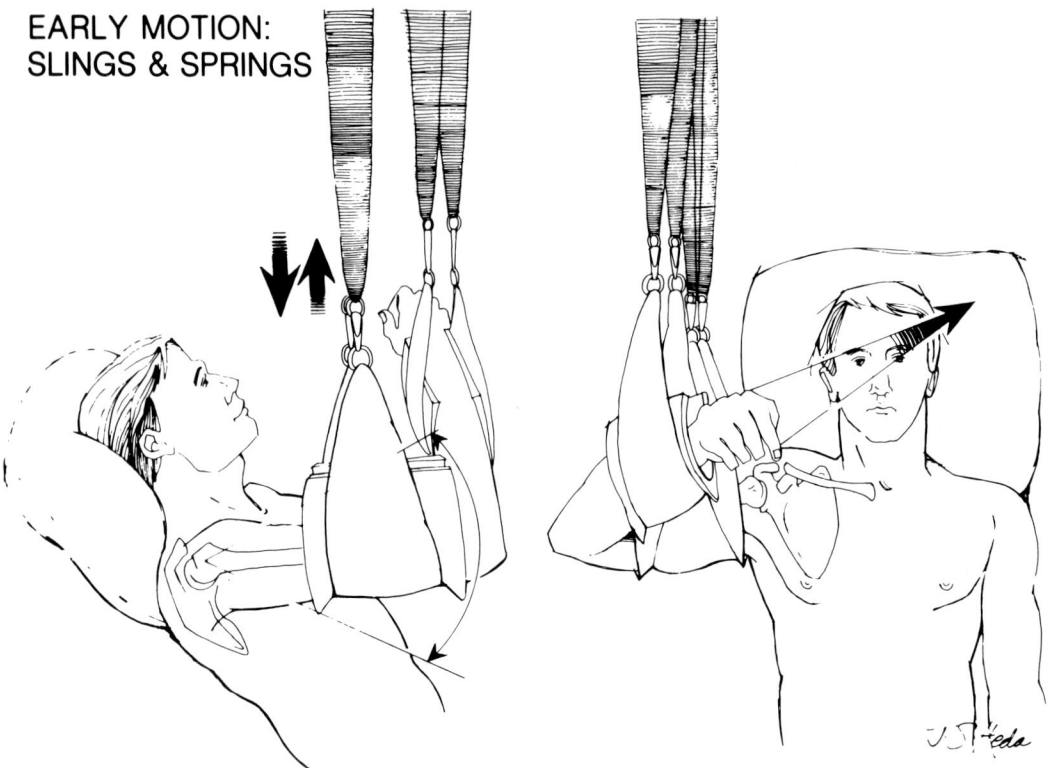

Figure 3 Early motion facilitated by the use of slings and springs.

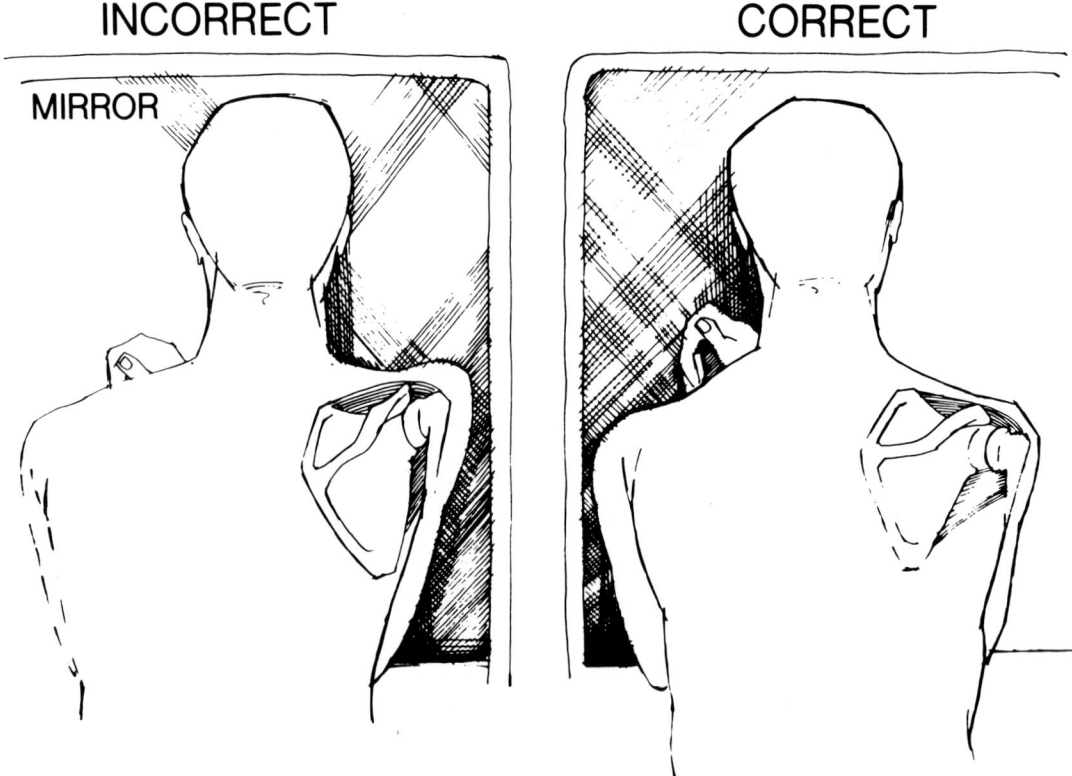

Figure 4 True glenohumeral motion is emphasized (as opposed to shoulder girdle or hunching motion).

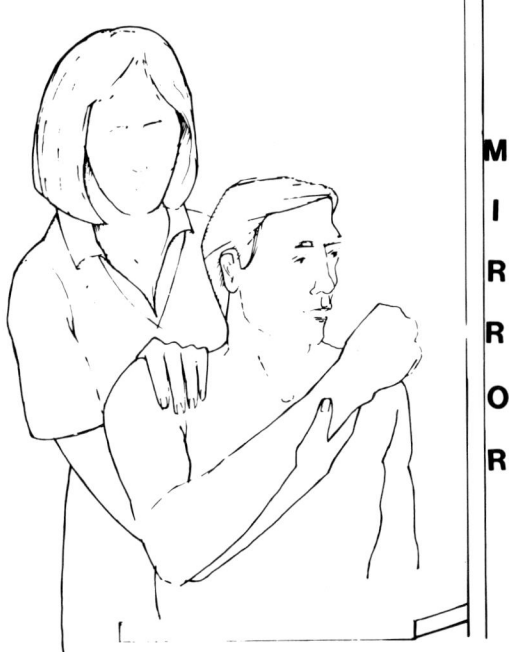

Figure 5 The physiotherapist stabilizes the scapula and assists the patient to gain flexion, adduction and external rotation at the glenohumeral joint.

Category II

Category II refers to patients who have had large tears repaired with fascia lata. The resting position is the same as that used for patients in category I, and the slings and springs are used in the same fashion (Figs. 2, 3).

Because of the extensive repair, protection is crucial for patients in category II. The cantilever brace (Fig. 6) is used to hold the shoulder in 90° flexion and abduction and 15° external rotation when the patient is not exercising. It is worn even for sleeping. Note the swivel joints at the shoulder and elbow which allow movement in the horizontal plane and the hinge joint in the axilla. The hinge joint is used to lower the brace at the appropriate time.

Category II patients, who have had a large tear preoperatively, usually have had full passive range of motion but have lacked strength. Therefore, the physiotherapist concentrates on increasing muscle strength. Isometric strengthening exercises starting at the resting position and then through the range above are emphasized. Because all functional activities involve groups of muscles working together in diagonal patterns, we teach

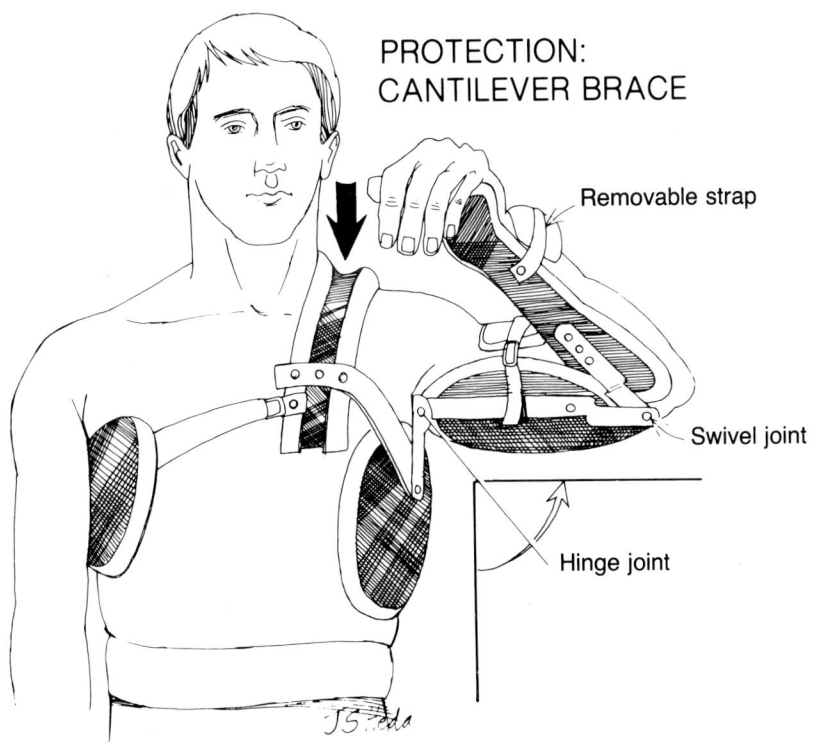

Figure 6 The cantilever brace is used to protect the Category II cuff repair.

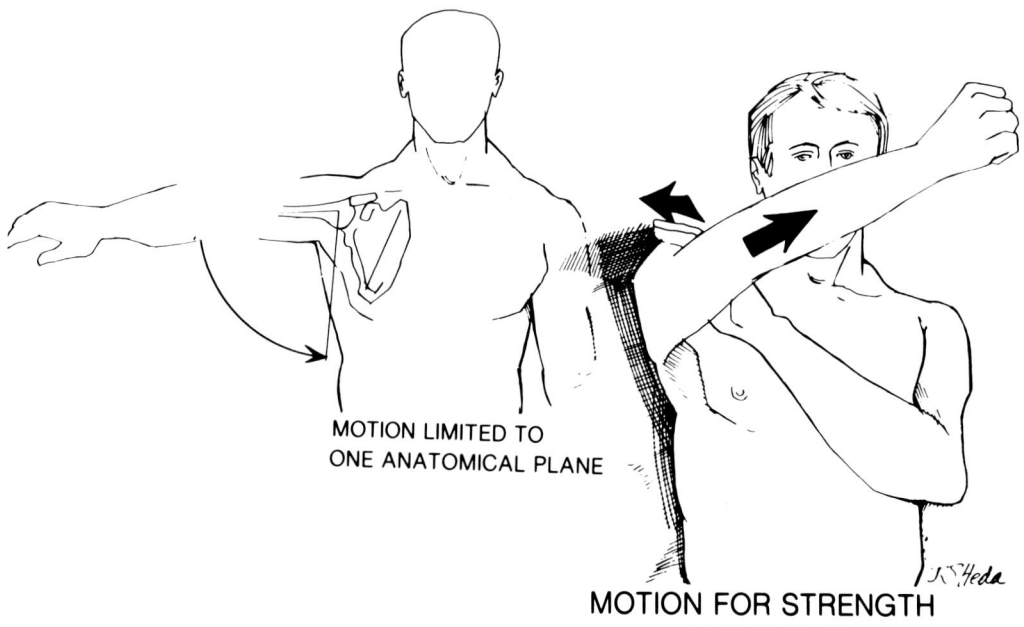

Figure 7 Exercises are performed in diagonal patterns used for functional activities not in the traditional anatomical planes.

the patient to exercise in diagonals as opposed to the traditional anatomical planes (Fig. 7).

In summary, although each patient is an individual with his own specific needs, we have found that for postoperative physiotherapy management, patients who have had rotator cuff repairs can be divided into two main categories as follows:

	Category I	*Category II*
Size of tear	Small	Large
Type of repair	Suture	Fascial
Common preop. status	Stiff painful shoulder	Weak muscles
Postop. emphasis	Early motion	Isometric strengthening exercises

Conclusions

As mentioned earlier, two-way communication between the surgeon and the physiotherapist is very important. The therapist must be aware of the surgeon's true expectations to that the patient does not receive conflicting messages. As the therapist is often the front-line answerer, it makes sense that she be informed.

It may be of interest to compare our method with another method known to most orthopaedic surgeons.

With respect to the suggestion that the other method may require fewer physiotherapists, fewer physiotherapists probably necessitate the expenditure of more time on the part of the surgeon.

	Orthopaedic & Arthritic Hospital Method	Other Method
Day 1	Active motion begins (in slings and springs see Figure 3).	Rest with arm at side in sling and swathe (O&A Hospital's resting position 90° abduction and flexion, 15° external rotation).
Day 3	Patient performs active exercises out of slings and springs (may be auto resisted).	Patient performs passive range of motion exercises to encourage range while avoiding excessive strain on the repaired muscles.
Six weeks post-op.	Fascial repair has been protected for 6 weeks. Brace and resting position now lowered gradually if the patient can abduct and flex against gravity and mild resistance	*Active* exercises are begun as anterior deltoid has healed.
Role of physiotherapist	*Re-educates* proper pattern of movement and muscle function. Responsible for *pacing* throughout the rehabilitation program. *Actively involved* in a hands-on fashion.	Patient is given a handout of written and illustrated instructions for exercises. The therapist is more of an *observer* and a *coach* or *resource person*.
Benefits	Fewer frozen shoulders	Fewer physiotherapists

REPAIR OF CHRONIC MASSIVE ROTATOR CUFF TEARS WITH SYNTHETIC FABRICS

JIRO OZAKI, M.D., SEI FUJIMOTO, M.D., and KENJI MASUHARA, M.D.

The surgical treatment of rotator cuff tear was first performed by Codman in 1909.[1] Since that time, the clinical manifestations of the lesion have been more clearly defined and treatment has progressed. However, not all methods hitherto described for the repair of chronic massive rotator cuff tears have been successful procedures.

We here describe a reliable surgical procedure for chronic massive rotator cuff tears using synthetic fabrics which has never been utilized by others until the present.

BIOMECHANICAL CONSIDERATIONS

According to Codman,[1] the supraspinatus muscle acts as a fulcrum to furnish the power for the deltoid muscle. On the other hand, Kapandji[5] described the supraspinatus as the "starter" muscle of abduction at the beginning of shoulder motion. Linge[6] concluded that the role of the supraspinatus muscle is only of a quantitative nature, and it has no specific function of its own. Thus, the action of the supraspinatus muscle has been a subject of controversy.

From the point of view of reconstruction of the shoulder joint with synthetic fabrics, we have developed the concept that the rotator cuff acts as a "tendinous glenoid" to compensate the small and shallow osseous glenoid. This concept was also described by Himeno in 1982. The diagram (Fig. 1) shows the function of the rotator cuff as a "tendinous glenoid." The articular surface of the glenoid is too small and too shallow to fit the humeral head. It is generally supported that the deltoid muscle is an abductor, but it cannot act as an abductor unless accompanied by the action of the rotator cuff. Figure 2 demonstrates that the deltoid alone tends to press the humeral head up to the acromion. In the case of massive rotator cuff tears, sliding fulcrum cannot be made on the glenoid. In normal abduction, the action of the rotator cuff as a "tendinous glenoid" tends to drive the humeral head towards the osseous glenoid. In other words, the action of the rotator cuff is to steer the humeral head on the glenoid and make the deltoid muscle work as the abductor effectively. Therefore, it is believed that the use of ideal synthetic fabrics to bridge the cuff defect leads to satisfactory functional results (Fig. 3).

Selection of Synthetic Fabrics

Synthetic fabrics as a substitute for the rotator cuff have not been used by others until the present time, but in the reconstruction of tissue defects, synthetic fabrics like Teflon fabric, Teflon felt, and Marlex mesh have been widely used in the field of thoracic and cardiovascular surgery.[12,13] They seemed to us ideal materials for a rotator cuff substitute, with the following requirements:
1. Quick coverage with satisfactory connective tissue proliferations.
2. Firm attachment with the recipient bed.
3. Less adhesion with the neighboring tissues.
4. Endurance to mechanical stress and ability to maintain their original tensile strength after implantation.
5. Convenience in cutting into desired size at operation, without fraying or unraveling.

In our experiments on rats using Teflon fabric, Teflon felt, and Marlex mesh, all of them proved to be satisfactory to replace the tendomuscular defect.

OPERATIVE TECHNIQUE

The patient lies on the operative table with the upper part of his body elevated 45° to 60° from the horizontal. The arm is placed so that it rests on the edge of the table. To permit easy manipulation of the extremity it is draped separately. A

NEW CONCEPTION as "TENDINOUS GLENOID"

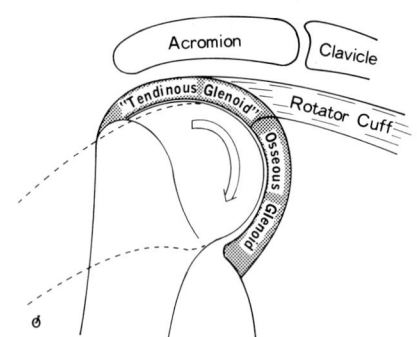

Figure 1 The rotator cuff acts as a "tendinous glenoid" to compensate the small and shallow osseous glenoid.

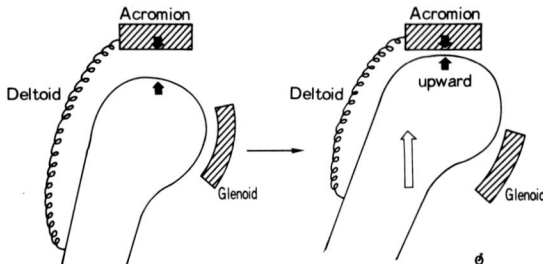

Figure 2 In the case of massive rotator cuff tears, the deltoid alone tends to press the humeral head up to the acromion.

sandbag is placed under the scapula. Finally, the table is tilted slightly away from the surgeon.

Transacromial Anterior Deltoid Approach

An S-shaped incision is started at a point a finger's breadth above the superior margin of the midlateral portion of the scapular spine, as shown in Figure 4a. It curves foreward over the acromion and extends to the anterior deltoid portion. The anterior portion of the deltoid is split downward from the acromion. The capsule of acromioclavicular joint is opened and the coracoacromial ligament is divided. An osteotomy of the acromion is done transversely and obliquely outward as shown in Figure 4b. When the osteotomised acromion is reflected anterolaterally, the humeral head can easily be exposed (Fig. 4c).

Repair of the Chronic Massive Rotator Cuff Tear

If the torn cuff edge retracted proximally and cannot be easily pulled out, and if a large defect

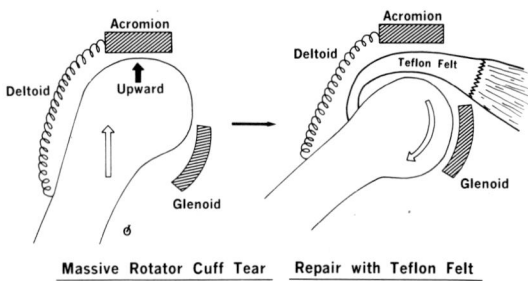

Figure 3 The use of ideal synthetic fabrics to bridge the cuff defect leads to satisfactory functional results.

over the humeral head remains, the use of synthetic fabrics should be indicated. The synthetic fabric, namely thick Teflon felt, is trimmed to the desired size with scissors. The proximal edge of the torn cuff is cut back to the healthy strong tendinous part exposed and the felt is firmly sutured with the cuff edge. It is pulled down laterally to be anchored around the tuberosities. It is essential that there be some tension on the graft when the sutures are tied, with the arm at the side. The edge of the graft can be firmly fixed near the tuberosities (Fig. 4d). If the biceps long tendon is displaced medially out of the groove, reduction of the tendon should be done after making the groove deeply and the intertubercular ligament is also repaired with Teflon fabric. The site of osteotomy of the acromion is reduced back and fixed with wires. The detached part of the deltoid muscle is sutured firmly to the periosteum on the superior surface of the acromion. An acromioclavicular arthroplasty is performed, on occasion following anterior acromioplasty.

Postoperative Management

Immediately after the surgery, the "zero-position" of the shoulder joint[10] should be maintained by skin traction while the patient rests in bed. After three days, a functional shoulder joint orthosis devised by us is applied to keep the same position on the scapular plane.[9] At the beginning of the second postoperative week, the upper limb in the orthosis extends at 100° abduction on the scapular plane and the patient is allowed to start gradual active-assisted abduction exercise of the arm. From the second to the fourth week after surgery, when the patient is able to perform active elevation in the range of 60° to 150°, the abduction angle of the orthosis can be decreased gradually to 30°.

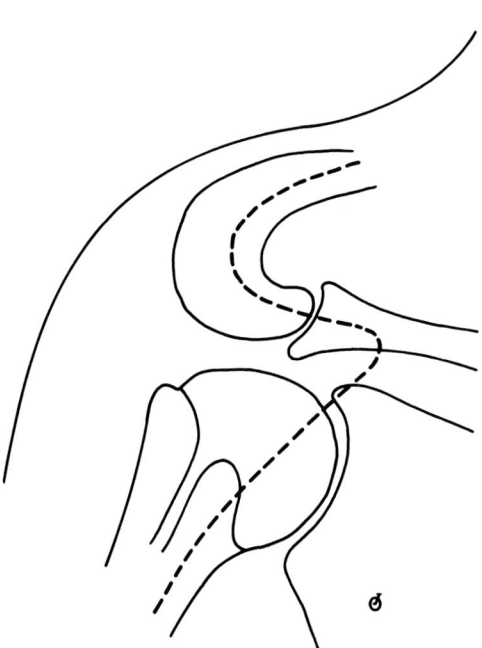

Figure 4a Skin incision.

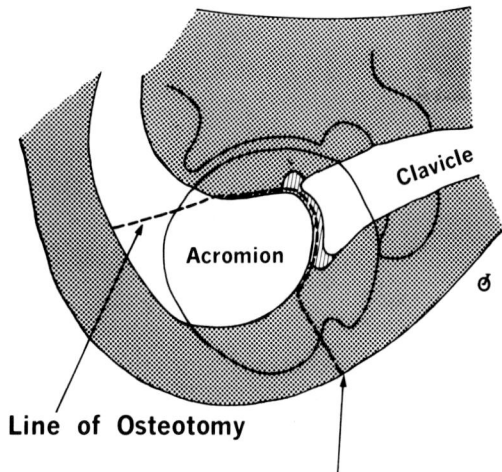

Line of Osteotomy

Anterior Portion of Deltoid is splitted and Capsule of A-C. Joint is opened.

Figure 4b Osteotomy of the acromion, separation of the acromioclavicular joint, and resection of the coracoacromial ligament. Although the anterior portion of the deltoid is split downward, the lateral and posterior portions of the deltoid should never be reflected from the acromion to keep the deltoid function as much as possible.

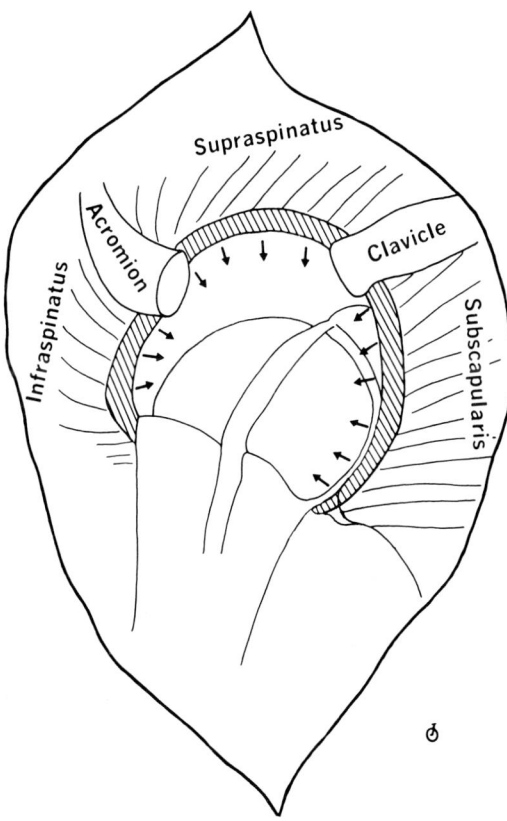

Figure 4c Exposure of the chronic massive rotator cuff tear.

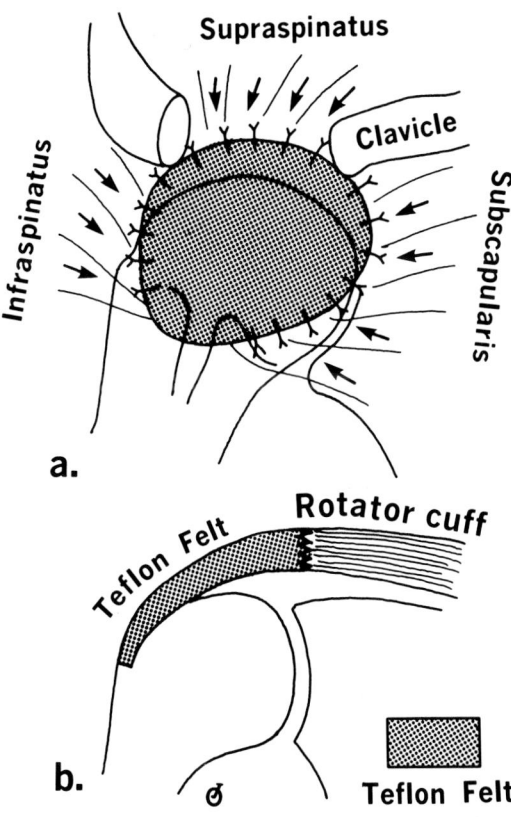

Figure 4d Synthetic fabrics graft in place. Some tension on the graft is essential when the sutures are tied. The graft edge can be firmly fixed near the tuberosities.

Mass movement exercise involving circular motion is indicated. Two to three months after surgery, the orthosis is removed. At this point, the patient is able to gain full range elevation (Fig. 5). And three to six months after surgery, the patient can recover his maximal range of motion.

CLINICAL DATA

In 170 patients operated on for repair of rotator cuff tears, 27 cases with chronic massive tear underwent synthetic fabrics implantations (Table 1). Patient age ranged from 47 to 79 years (average, 67.2 years) and duration between onset and operation was 1 month to 10 years (average, 2.9 years). The predominant complaints were dysfunction and pain in the involved shoulder. The extent of ruptured cuff was from 5 × 3 cm to 8 × 7 cm (average, 6.1 × 4.7 cm). In 27 patients, 6 were repaired with Teflon fabric, 6 with Teflon felt, and 15 with Marlex mesh.

TABLE 1 Summary of Cases

Total: 27 cases
Age: 47–79 years
   (average: 67.2 years)
Male: 20 cases, Female: 7 cases
Used synthetic fabrics
   Teflon fabric: 6 cases
   Teflon felt: 6 cases
   Marlex mesh: 15 cases
Duration between accident and operation
   1 month–10 years
   (average: 2.9 years)
Extent of ruptured cuff
   5 × 3 cm–8 × 7 cm
   (average: 6.1 × 4.7 cm)
Defect size of rotator cuff
   3 × 2–7 × 6 cm
   (average: 4.6 × 3.6 cm)
Condition of biceps long tendon
   Tear: 14 cases
   Dislocation: 2 cases
   Stenosis: 2 cases
Nerve injury: 4 cases

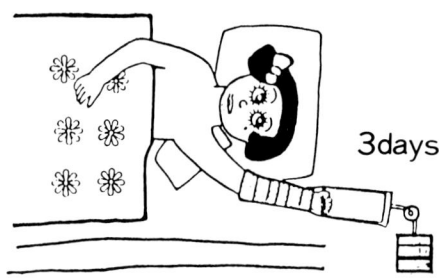

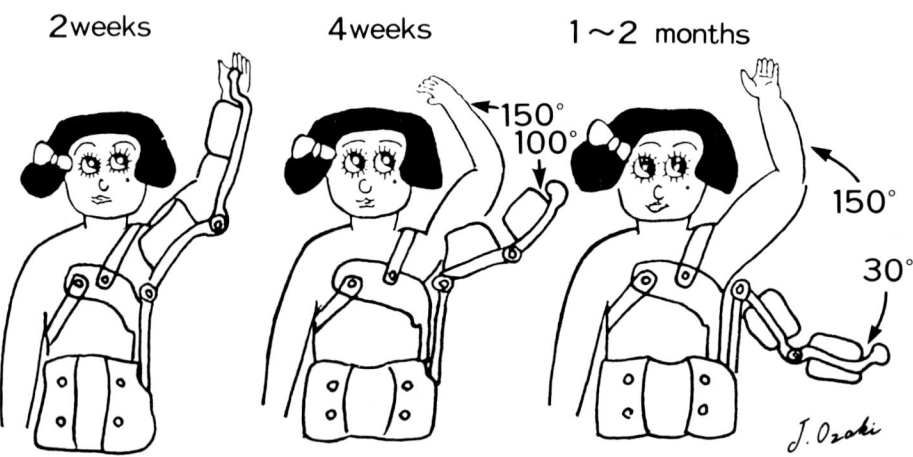

Figure 5 Postoperative management.

Results

The follow-up periods were 5 months to 3.5 years (average, 2.0 years), and there has been no sign of foreign body reaction in any case. The improvement of abduction was significant as shown in Table 2a. Before surgery, only two patients had a normal range of abduction, but with decreased muscle power. After surgery, however, 25 patients gained 120° to 160° of abduction. No patient's mobility was reduced by the operation. In two patients who had had coexistent axillary nerve injury, improvement of abduction was poor. In the remaining 25 patients, remarkable improvements in the range of motion were achieved. Relief of pain was generally remarkable (Table 2b); twenty-five patients out of 27 were completely free from pain, and only two patients who had had coexistent axillary nerve injury were less improved.

Case Reports

Some representative cases:

Case 1: A 54-year old man suffered a lateral blow on his left shoulder when he was lifting a large stone. He suddenly felt intense pain and became unable to abduct his arm. Although he consulted many doctors the disability and pain of his left shoulder were not relieved at all. Ten years later he came to our hospital for a comprehensive examination of his shoulder. On examination, his left shoulder joint showed typical signs of massive rotator cuff tear, such as atrophy of the supraspinatus and infraspinatus muscles, crepitus during the motion of abduction which occurred between the greater tuberosity and the acromion (Fig. 6a). The clinical diagnosis was confirmed by arthrography. At surgery, the roof of the subacromial bursa was thickened and when it was incised, strawcolored fluid was released. Since the torn rotator cuff edge had been retracted far under the acromion, it could not be seen (Fig. 6b). The bicipital long tendon had also been completely torn off the glenoid and retracted partly away. After osteotomy of the acromion, the supraspinatus, infraspinatus and subscapularis were caught with a tenaculum hardly. However, a large defect, 7 × 6 cm in size, was left. Teflon felt was used in this case to bridge the defect successfully (Fig. 6c). Three months after surgery, the patient could elevate his arm normally (Fig. 6d) with the pain completely relieved, and one more month later, he returned to his job.

Case 2: A 55-year old carpenter had a motor cycle accident 3 years ago. He has developed intense pain and disability of abduction in his right shoulder. Immediately after the injury, he consulted our clinic and was advised to have an operative treatment for the rotator cuff injury, but he refused. The pain subsided for approximately 3 years. Recently he came to our clinic again because of aggravation of symptoms. Clinical examination and arthrography confirmed the diagnosis of massive rotator cuff tear of his right shoulder joint. At operation, a transacromial anterior deltoid approach was made and the subacromial bursa was opened. The rotator cuff was torn massively and the bicipital long tendon had been displaced medially from the groove. The tendon was replaced to the groove with transverse humeral ligament repaired using Teflon fabric. A ruptured rotator cuff defect, 6 × 5 cm in size, was bridged with Teflon felt. The postoperative course was smooth and 3 months later, the pain was completely relieved and shoulder function was perfectly recovered.

TABLE 2a
Range of Abduction Before and After Operation

Range in degrees	Number of patients	
	Before op.	After op.
Normal	2	17
120-150	1	8
60-120	2	—
30-60	—	—
0-30	22	2*
Total	27	27

* who had had coexistent axillary injury

TABLE 2b
Pain Before and After Operation

Amount of pain	Number of patients	
	Before op.	After op.
None	2	25
Some	3	2*
Continual	14	—
Intolerable	8	—
Total	27	27

* who had had coexistent axillary nerve injury

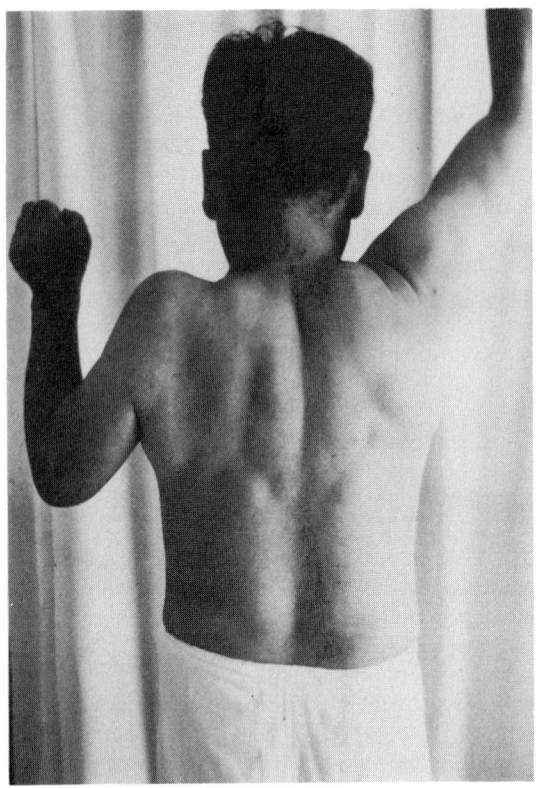

Figure 6a Case 1: Preoperative findings. Note that in attempting to abduct the arm he shrugs the shoulder. The normal scapulohumeral rhythm is completely disturbed.

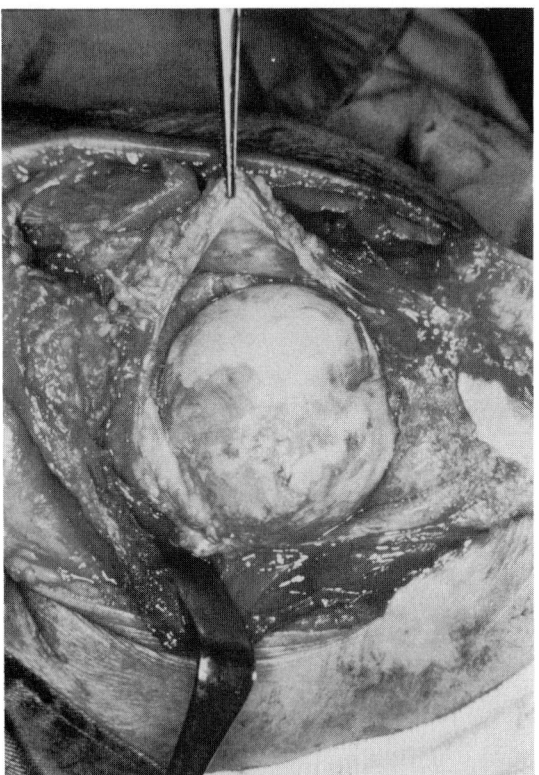

Figure 6b The humeral head is exposed and the torn rotator cuff edge had been retracted far under the scapular spine. The bicipital long tendon had also torn off the glenoid and retracted away. The tuberosities are bare.

Illustration continued on the opposite page

DISCUSSION

In case of moderate rotator cuff tear in which the edges cannot be sutured without tension, McLaughlin freshens the edge of the cuff and then attaches it to the humeral head at whatever point it reaches without tension.[7] We have been using this technique for the repair of almost all rotator cuff tears. However, on the repair of chronic massive rotator cuff tears, McLaughlin's technique cannot be applied, and many surgeons have developed their own method. Neviaser[8] used the intra-articular portion of the long head of the biceps, incising it to produce a sheet in order to close the defect. Bateman[2] used the coracoacromial ligament or fascia lata to close the residual defect, and Debeyre[3] devised a procedure of supraspinatus muscle advancement. However, these methods have not always been successful because the materials tend to wear and stretch. Furthermore, the supraspinatus muscle or biceps tendon may be too small to bridge the massive defect of rotator cuff. These problems could be avoided by the application of synthetic fabrics as described here. In our patients there is no sign of foreign body reaction and the follow-up study on 27 patients proved it to be a worthy procedure for the treatment of massive rotator cuff tears. In 25 out of 27 patients, pain relief and improvement of motion were uniformly obtained.

Moreover, we can conclude that the rotator cuff acts as the "tendinous glenoid" to substitute for the small and shallow osseous glenoid. According to the concept of the "tendinous glenoid," it is biomechanically substantiated that the use of synthetic fabrics to bridge the cuff defect leads to satisfactory functional results. On the basis of our biomechanical considerations, it can be conceived that the synthetic fabrics should become as thick as the normal rotator cuff in the shoulder. So we have used 3 mm to 5 mm thick Teflon felt as the substitute for the rotator cuff in our recent series.

Summary

Artificial materials have not been used as a substitute for the rotator cuff up to the present

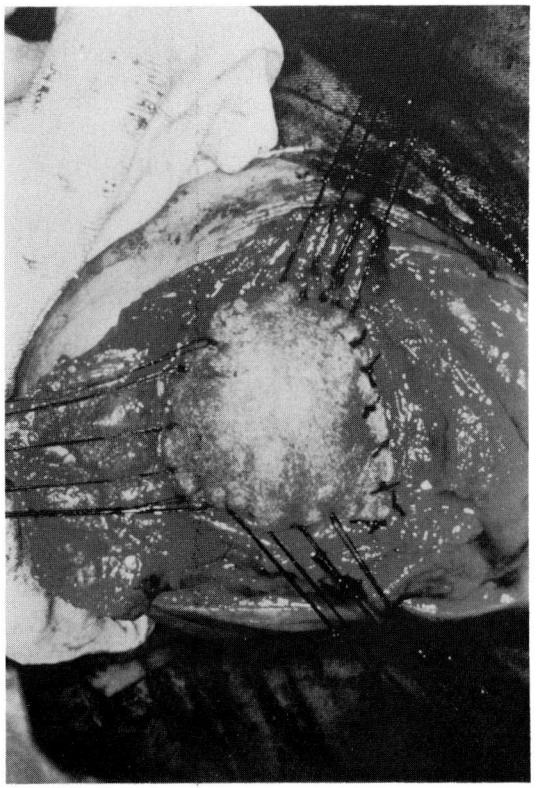

Figure 6c Teflon felt graft sutured in place.

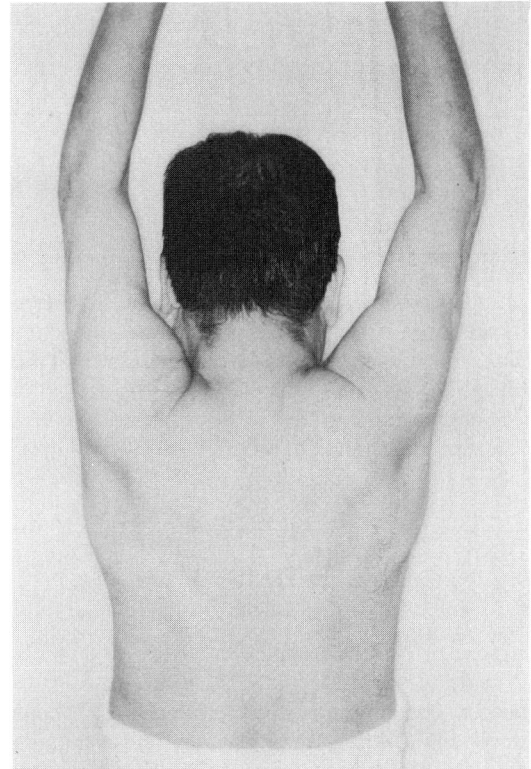

Figure 6d Three months after surgery, he was able to move his arm without experiencing pain. The result was very satisfactory.

time. In order to establish a reliable surgical procedure for chronic massive rotator cuff tears, fundamental and clinical studies were performed using synthetic fabrics.

Biomechanically, the rotator cuff acts as the "tendinous glenoid" substituting for the small and shallow osseous glenoid. In accordance with this concept, a new technique has been developed, applying synthetic fabrics, namely Teflon felt, to repair chronic massive rotator cuff tears. Clinically, in 27 patients with chronic massive rotator cuff tears, synthetic fabrics yielded satisfactory functional results in 25 patients. The clinical applications of synthetic fabrics prove to be of great significance in the treatment of chronic massive rotator cuff tears.

REFERENCES

1. Codman EA. The Shoulder. Boston: Thomas Todd, 1934.
2. Bateman JE. The Shoulder and Neck. Philadelphia: WB Saunders, 1972.
3. Debeyre J, Patte D, Elmelik E. Repair of rupture of the rotator cuff of the shoulder. With a note on advancement of the supraspinatus muscle. J Bone Joint Surg 1965; 47B:36.
4. DePalma AF. Surgery of the Shoulder. Philadelphia: JB Lippincott, 1973.
5. Kapandji IA. The physiology of the joints. Edinburgh: Churchill Livingstone, 1970.
6. Linge B, Mulder JD. Function of the supraspinatus and its relation to the supraspinatus syndrome. An experimental study in man. J Bone Joint Surg 1963; 45B:750.
7. McLaughlin HL. Rupture of the rotator cuff. J Bone Joint Surg 1962; 44A:979.
8. Neviaser JS, Neviaser RJ, Neviaser TJ. The repair of chronic massive ruptures of the rotator cuff of the shoulder by use of a freeze-dried rotator cuff. J Bone Joint Surg 1978; 60A:681.
9. Ozaki J. Shoulder mechanism. A study based on cineradiography and radiography with the arm elevated. J Jap Orthop Asso 1980; 54:1679.
10. Saha AK. Theory of shoulder mechanism. Springfield: Charles C Thomas, 1961.
11. Takagishi N. The new operation for the massive cuff rupture. J Jap Orthop Ass 1978; 52:775.
12. Usher FC, Allen JF, Crosthwaite RW, Cogan JE. Polypropylene monofilament. A new, biologically inert suture for closing contaminated wounds. JAMA 1962; 179:780.
13. Wesolowski SA. Evaluation of tissue and prosthetic vascular grafts. Springfield: Charles C Thomas, 1961.

REPAIR OF ROTATOR CUFF TEARS

ROBERT L. SAMILSON, M.D.

This chapter details the technique for repair of rotator cuff tear including the incision, deltoid detachment, subacromial decompression, cuff mobilization, cuff repair, flaps and grafts, deltoid repair and wound closure. We have discussed patient selection in a previous paper.[12]

TECHNIQUE

The Incision

An incision is made at the posterior acromial border, coursing along the acromial margin anteriorly and to the anterior clavicle above the coracoid process. It then swings inferiorly into the superior portion of the deltopectoral groove.

This incision is used for all primary cuff repairs. In those patients who have had unsuccessful repairs elsewhere, the incision may be modified to avoid skin necrosis at intersection with prior incisions, and to avoid long thin islands of skin between the prior incision and that used for secondary cuff repair.

A word concerning transacromial approach[3] for cuff repair. I believe that this approach is unnecessary, and potentially harmful. Postoperative subacromial impingement may occur from the occasional nonunion of the acromion, or from callus consequent to union of the iatrogenically induced acromial fracture. The relationship of an unfused acromial apophysis to impingement syndromes[2] has recently been reported. I have not found it necessary to advance the origin of the supraspinatus, and feel that such advancement necessitates delayed postoperative motion to allow time for healing of both the origin and the insertion of the cuff. The technique outlined in this paper has permitted perfectly adequate repair of the rotator cuff without these disadvantages.

Deltoid Detachment

Using an electrocautery knife, the origin of the deltoid is detached from the anterior clavicle and the anterior acromion. The soft tissue is detached from the superior portion of the anterior acromion and is preserved for subsequent deltoid repair. It is not necessary to remove a thin margin of bone with the deltoid origin for subsequent reattachment.

Identification of the anatomical septum between the anterior and middle deltoid will permit division of the deltoid in "T" fashion. The vertical split in the deltoid should not extend more than three finger-breadths below the acromial margin, in order to avoid any potential damage to the axillary nerve.

Small Richardson retractors are used to bring the anterior deltoid medially and the middle deltoid posterolaterally.

Lateral partial or total acromionectomy is to be condemned.[8] This results in weakened deltoid function consequent to a change in the length-tension diagram of the musculotendinous unit. Cosmetic deformity occurs because the rounded shoulder contour is no longer present.

Subacromial Decompression[7]

The coracoacromial ligament is identified at its origin and insertion. It must be remembered that the ligament is "Y" shaped, the acromial insertion having anterior and posterior arms. Both arms of the insertion must be identified and incised.

The anterior acromion anterior to the level of the clavicle is divested of soft tissue. A vertical cut is made in the anterior acromion with an osterotome[11] acromion projecting anterior to the clavicle is removed. The coracoacromial ligament is excised at the same time.

Rather than using an osteotome to perform an anterior acromioplasty, I prefer to use a pineapple-shaped burr on a power drill,[4] burring off the inferior half of the anterior acromion, and removing any subacromial spurs. The same device may be used to burr off the inferior aspect of the outer end of the clavicle if it seems to be an impingement factor. It is helpful to have a surgical assistant exert downward traction on the circumferentially draped forearm while the subacromial decompression is proceeding.

An acromial branch of the acromiothoracic artery[1] is often encountered directly beneath the coracoacromial ligament and must be controlled for hemostasis.

The subacromial bursa is excised within the confines of the exposure, being careful to remove its floor as well as its roof; this will expose the cuff tear. More than once, I have performed repairs on tears which had been operated upon elsewhere, only to find that the prior surgeon had sutured the bursa rather than repair the torn cuff. The differential thickness of the two structures should be sufficient to identify them.

Small exostoses may be present either at the greater tuberosity or on the margins of the biceps groove; these may be removed using the power burr described above.

Cuff Mobilization

Thorough visualization of the cuff tear is necessary for its proper repair. This is a principle which must be followed even for what appear to be small tears. Palpation of the cuff will sometimes reveal a horizontal cleavage tear far more extensive than that which is visualized on its superior surface. Vertical incision into such tears will permit visualization of the horizontal cleavage tear, and its repair.

Full thickness tears involve the entire vertical thickness of one or more components of the cuff. It is necessary to visualize the proximal apex of the tear in every case.

McLaughlin[5,6] has classified full-thickness tears into pure transverse ruptures, pure vertical rents or longitudinal splits paralleling the direction of the cuff fibers, tears with retraction, and massive avulsion. No two tears are identical, but adequate exposure is necessary in order to mobilize the cuff for proper repair without undue tension. Inadequate excision of the subdeltoid bursa within the confines of the wound and mistaking bursal tissue for the rotator cuff are common errors which may lead to failure to identify all components of the tear, and thus to inadequate repair.

Complete mobilization of the cuff by blunt dissection will also permit approximation of all components of the tear in most cases without undue tension. Pure transverse ruptures usually occur between the supraspinatus and infraspinatus tendons. The supraspinatus tends to slide anteriorly, and the infraspinatus and teres minor tend to slide posteriorly, but retraction may not be significant. This type of tear is uncommon in younger patients.

Vertical rents or longitudinal splits paralleling the direction of the cuff fibers occurs in the interval between the subscapularis and the supraspinatus and tend to occur in a somewhat younger age group than does the pure transverse tear.

Tears with retraction have an inverted "V" shape, with the apex of the "V" proximal and medial, and the base at the greater tuberosity laterally. The subscapularis tends to pull the anterior arm of the "V" anteroinferiorly, while the teres minor pulls the posterior arm of the "V" posteroinferiorly. Mobilization of this type of tear is particularly essential if repair without tension is to be achieved. Adhesions, which often fix the cuff in the retracted position, must be divided during the course of surgical mobilization. Thorough mobilization permits side-to-side approximation of the components of the tear. A tear with extensive retraction will appear as a crescentic defect until mobilization converts it into an inverted "V", prior to actual repair.

Massive cuff avulsions are sometimes accompanied by subluxation or dislocation of the intraarticular portion of the long head of the biceps. The entire greater tuberosity will appear bare, with fibrillated nubbins of tendinous insertions sometimes present. Most of these massive avulsions can be repaired, utilizing the principle of side-to-side approximation as much as possible, with augmentation by fascial or tendinous graft or flap development and rotation. Ultimately, reinsertion into bone as close as possible to the normal insertion is necessary. I have found that reinsertion into the humeral head cartilage proximal to the greater tuberosity does not produce a satisfactory result.

During the course of mobilization of the cuff, it is useful to put #1 Ethibond® stay sutures at the apex of the tear, so that traction on these sutures will assist in further mobilization.

Cuff Repair

Adequate repair is possible if the surgical steps previously mentioned are carried out. Nonabsorbable sutures must be used for repair, to permit early postoperative movement without compromising the repair. I prefer interrupted #1 Ethibond® sutures on a round, noncutting needle. Downward traction on the circumferentially draped forearm, will facilitate the repair by increasing the subacromial space and exposing the proximal apex of the tear.

Conversion of crescentic defects, retracted tears, or massive avulsions into inverted "Vs," to enable side-to-side approximation is essential. Mobilization of all components of the tear so that repair without undue tension is possible is equally essential.

Avascular margins of the tear should be cleanly excised back to healthy tendinous tissue. Starting at the apex of the tear, interrupted #1 Ethibond® sutures on a round, noncutting needle are placed, proceeding from the apex of the tear towards the insertion at the greater tuberosity. I prefer interrupted sutures to a continuous "shoelace" type suture because if one suture loosens or breaks, the integrity of the repair is not lost. It is always preferable to suture the cuff into bone except in the simple vertical rent tears, where side-to-side approximation will suffice.

The bony insertion at the greater tuberosity is prepared by using a small osteotome to remove fibrinous nubbins of avulsed cuff down to fresh bleeding bone. Care should be taken to remove any bony prominence over which the cuff must be drawn on its way to its insertion. Drill holes are made in the decorticated greater tuberosity and directed towards the lateral humeral cortex. The fully mobilized cuff, which has been approximated side-to-side from the apex towards the greater tuberosity, is sutured into the decorticated greater tuberosity. Nonabsorbable sutures are placed through the drill holes and tied firmly on the lateral humeral cortex, with the arm at the side. In most cases of cuff tears with retraction, this can be accomplished without undue tension, provided that mobilization of the cuff has been adequate. In a few instances, it will be impossible to bring the cuff down to its normal insertion with the arm at the side; in other instances, side-to-side approximation proceeding from the apex will leave a triangular gap near the greater tuberosity which must be bridged by some means. The technique for accomplishing this is discussed in the next section. This is a situation which occurs rarely, and only in the most massive tears. In isolated instances which are rarer yet, there will be found some massive avulsions which are irreparable. In these rare cases, subacromial decompression may provide symptomatic relief, but will not restore function.

Flaps and Grafts

Fascia lata, freeze-dried fascia, biceps tendon, and resected coracoacromial ligament have been utilized to bridge defects in cuff repairs, particularly in massive avulsions. Theoretical and practical considerations clearly indicate that the use of these materials represents a compromise, and that their use is indicated only where the standard side-to-side approximation leaves an unbridged triangular defect. The intra-articular portion of the long head of the biceps serves an important function as humeral head depressor with the arm externally rotated. This function is lost if the tendon is tenodesed in the biceps groove, and the intra–articular portion is excised and filleted to be used as a graft.

Fascia lata and coracoacromial ligament used as graft material tend to stretch out so that integrity and "water-tight" repair utilizing these materials is sometimes transient at best. Freeze-dried fascia or tendon has been utilized,[9] but its incorporation must be delayed because of its avascular nature.

Synthetic materials have been utilized on an experimental basis, but certainly at this stage, they cannot be recommended for general clinical use.

Microvascular muscolotendinous pedicles have been utilized, but I have had no experience with their use in cuff repairs, and know of no long-term studies that might enlighten us.

Superior shift of subscapularis and teres minor has been described[10] to bridge an irreparable cuff defect, and I have utilized this on occasion, but the results are less than optimal.

Deltoid Repair

Reconstitution of a functioning deltoid is as important as the cuff repair itself. The biomechanical force couple which permits glenohumeral elevation depends on the integrity of both the deltoid and the rotator cuff.

The deltoid is sutured to the preserved flap of soft tissue which had been dissected from the superior aspect of the anterior acromion prior to anterior acromioplasty. This will give a firm repair, utilizing nonabsorbable #1 Ethibond® sutures on a noncutting needle. I have not found it necessary to make drill holes in the remaining acromion to reattach the deltoid.

Wound Closure

Usually, it is not necessary to use suction tubes even on a temporary basis, provided that hemostasis is adequate during the procedure. Interrupted 3-0 plain catgut is used for subcutaneous tissue. Subcuticular continuous 3-0 Dexon® suture is utilized. Steristrips are applied to the wound prior to application of wound dressing.

REFERENCES

1. Bateman JE. The Shoulder and Neck. Philadelphia: WB Saunders, 1978.
2. Bigliani LV, Neer CS, Norris TR, Fischer J: The relationship between the unfused acromial apophysis and subacromial impingement lesions. Scientific Exhibit, Ann Meet Am Acad Orthop Surg, 1983.
3. Debeyre J, Patte D, Emelik E. Repair of ruptures of the rotator cuff with a note on advancement of the supraspinatus muscle. J Bone Joint Surg 1965; 47B:36–42.
4. Matsen F. Personal communication
5. McLaughlin HL. Repair of major cuff ruptures. Surg Clin North Am 1963; 43:1535–1540.
6. McLaughlin HL. Lesions of the musculotendinous cuff of the shoulder I. The exposure and treatment of tears with retraction. J Bone Joint Surg 1944; 26(L):31–51.
7. Neer CS. Anterior Acromioplasty for the Chronic Impingement Syndrome: A Preliminary Report: J Bone Joint Surg 1972; 54A:41–50.
8. Neer CS, Marberry TA. On the disadvantage of radical acromionectomy. J Bone Joint Surg 1981; 63A:416–419.
9. Neviaser JS, Neviaser RJ, Neviaser TJ. The repair of chronic massive ruptures of the rotator cuff of the shoulder by use of freeze-dried rotator cuff. J Bone Joint Surg 1978; 60A:161.
10. Neviaser RJ, Neviaser TJ. Transfer of subscapularis and teres minor for massive defects of the rotator cuff. In: Bayley I, Kessel L, eds. Shoulder Surgery. New York: Springer-Verlag, 1982.
11. Rockwood C. Personal communication
12. Samilson RL, Binder WF. Symptomatic full thickness tears of the rotator cuff, an analysis of 292 shoulders in 276 patients. Orth Clin North Am 1975; 6(2):449–466.

TRAPEZIUS TRANSFER FOR GLOBAL TEAR OF THE ROTATOR CUFF

MOTOHIKO MIKASA, M.D.

The aim here is to report a new procedure for global tear of the rotator cuff.

The treatment of massive rotator cuff tears is very difficult. It is especially so in those cases having no tendinous portion and in which the humeral head is completely exposed. Bateman[2] coined the term "global tear" for these massive cuff defects. For these conditions, I have performed a procedure since 1977 in which the upper fibers of the trapezius were transferred to the greater tuberosity.

Up to the present, I have performed this trapezius transfer in nine cases (Tab. 1), of which eight were men and one was a woman. The patients' ages ranged from 58 to 78. The right shoulder was involved in eight patients and the left shoulder in one patient. The follow-up period in seven cases was 1 year to 5 years and 5 months.

OPERATIVE TECHNIQUE

A skin incision is made from the anterior portion of the acromion to the scapular spine as shown in Figure 1. The acromion is temporarily osteotomized near the angulus acromialis, and the middle portion and a part of the anterior portion of the deltoid are detached from the acromion, and the upper fibers of the trapezius are detached from the scapular spine (Fig. 2). The distal stump of the acromion is pulled upward by a hook and the rotator cuff is observed. If the remnant of the tendinous portion of the supraspinatus is more than 1 cm long, either tendon advancement[5] or muscle advancement[4] can be carried out. If it is less than 1 cm long, the trapezius transfer is indicated. The elevated acromion is put back and the upper fibers of the trapezius are detached from the acromion and the clavicle. Next, they are freed and raised for rerouting and they are reflected proximally for 8 cm (Fig. 3).

The osteotomized acromion is again raised for the following procedure. The remnant of the cuff is incised longitudinally between the supraspinatus and the infraspinatus for the later reattachment of the infraspinatus to the transferred trapezius. After a trench is made by chisel in the greater tuberosity, the distal stump of the upper trapezius is anchored to it. The already freed infraspinatus tendon, if present, is pulled forward and sutured to the side of the transferred trapezius as far distally as possible. If possible, it is anchored to the greater tuberosity as shown in Figure 4. The posteriorly prominent portion of the clavicle needs beveling for easy rerouting of the trapezius (Fig. 5).

The osteotomized scapular spine is reapproximated and immobilized by a single K-wire (Fig. 6), and the deltoid is then reattached firmly to the acromion.

The shoulder is immobilized in a brace in about 100° abduction for four weeks. Passive and active exercises are started.

Results

The results were assessed as to pain, ROM, muscle strength (Tab. 2) and ADL (Tab. 3). The overall evaluation was done with the criteria advocated by Wolfgang (Tab. 4). All patients except one were pain-free at follow-up. The improvement in abduction was noted in all cases except one. The range of external rotation was not satisfactory. The muscle strength in active abduction was 5 in five cases, 4 in one and 3 in one case. The most difficult ADL postoperatively was to lift an object up from a shelf. It was possible for three patients. The next most difficult ADL was throwing, which was possible in four patients and impossible in three patients. Six cases were rated excellent by Wolfgang's criteria.

Some illustrative cases are presented:

Case 4. A 78-year old man fell and dislocated his right shoulder. The right shoulder was reduced but the range of motion was not recovered.

The active abduction was 30° and the active

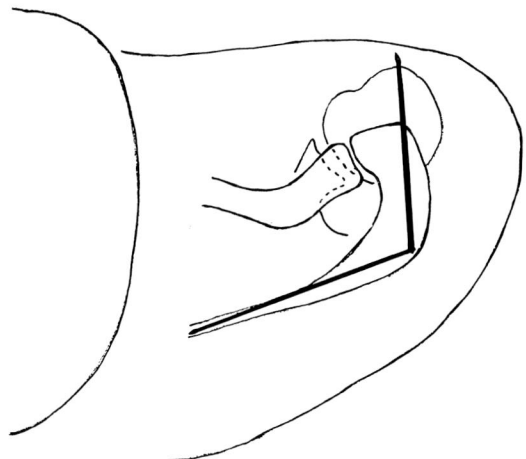

Figure 1 A skin incision is made from the anterior portion of the acromion to the scapular spine.

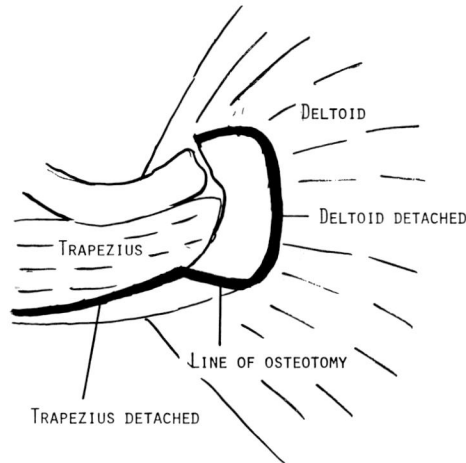

Figure 2 The acromion is temporarily osteotomized near the angulus acromialis, the middle portion and a part of the anterior portion of the deltoid are detached from the acromion, and the upper fibers of the trapezius are detached from the scapular spine.

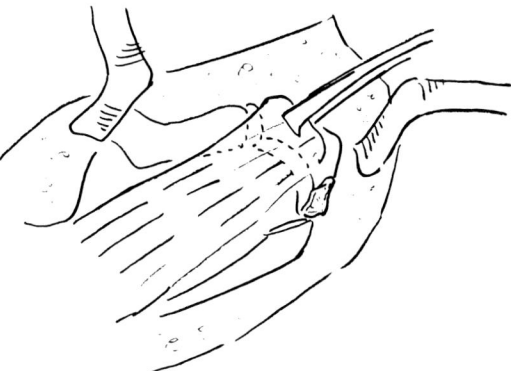

Figure 3 The elevated acromion is put back and the upper fibers of the trapezius are detached from the acromion and the clavicle, and they are reflected proximally 8 centimeters.

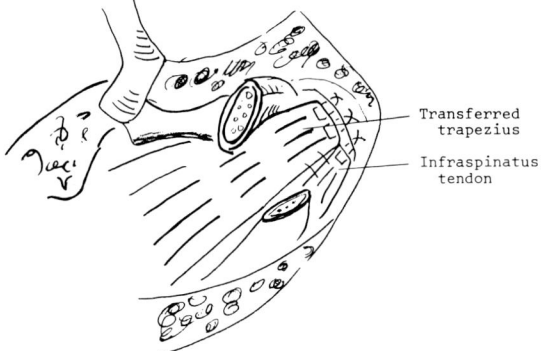

Figure 4 If the remnant of the infraspinatus can be pulled forward, it is sutured to the side of the trapezius and the greater tuberosity.

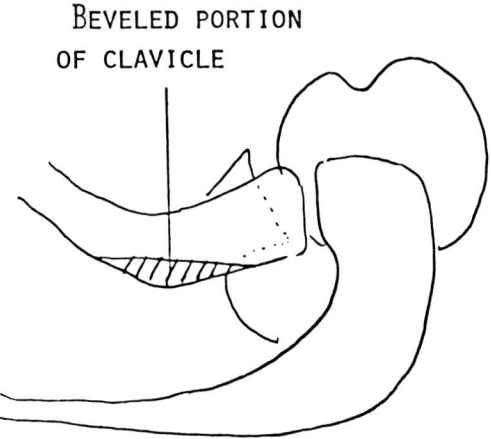

Figure 5 The posteriorly prominent portion of the clavicle needs beveling for easy rerouting of the trapezius.

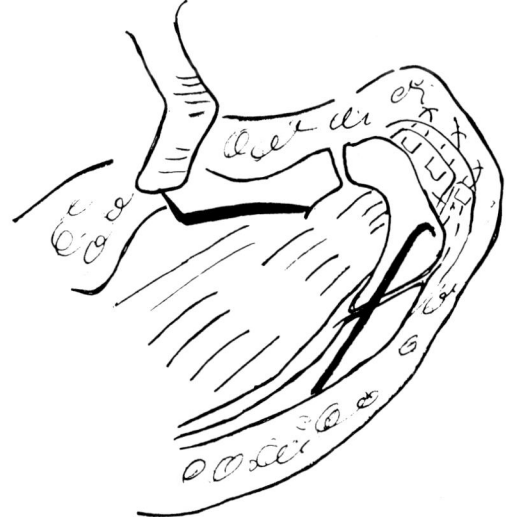

Figure 6 The osteotomized scapular spine is reapproximated and immobilized by a single K-wire.

TABLE 1 Materials

Case	Age	Sex	Side	Follow-up
1	67	female	rt	5 y 5 m
2	57	male	rt	5 y 2 m
3	53	male	lt	4 y 10 m
4	78	male	rt	3 y 9 m
5	67	male	rt	3 y 3 m
6	67	male	rt	3 y 1 m
7	72	male	rt	1 y
8	75	male	rt	
9	68	male	rt	

TABLE 2 Results 1

Case	Pain	Range of Motion		Muscle Strength ABD
		ABD	ER	
1	–	55° → 165°	–20° → –20°	3⁻ → 5
3	–	70° → 180°	0° → 20°	4 → 5
4	–	30° → 175°	0° → 10°	3⁻ → 4
6	–	170° → 170°	–20° → –20°	3⁻ → 5
				3⁻ → 3
				4 → 5
				3⁻ → 5

external rotation was 0°. The drop-arm sign and crepitus were positive. In the arthrogram (Fig. 7), the contour of the humeral head was continuous with that of the subacromial bursa, which was interpreted as evidence of a massive rotator cuff tear.[6] Surgery was performed three months after the dislocation. At operation, there was a global tear and the trapezius transfer was done (Fig. 8).

At follow-up, 3 years and 9 months postoperatively, the patient could abduct to 175° and externally rotate to 20° without pain. His muscle strength was 5 in both abduction and external rotation. He did not have any difficulty in ADL. This case was rated 17 points and excellent in Wolfgang's criteria.

Case 7. A 72-year old man tried to raise his arm while holding a parcel, when he suddenly felt severe pain in the right shoulder and became unable to move it. His preoperative ROM was 45° in both abduction and external rotation actively. The drop-arm sign was positive. The arthrogram was suggestive of a massive tear.

Surgery was undertaken three weeks after injury; there was no tendinous portion in the supraspinatus. The trapezius was transferred and the remnant of the infraspinatus tendon was sutured to it.

At follow-up, one year postoperatively, the patient could abduct to 165° and externally rotate to 45° without pain. His muscle strength was normal and he had no complaints in ADL. This case was rated 17 points and excellent in Wolfgang's criteria.

DISCUSSION

In my review of the literature, various procedures such as the patch graft,[1] supraspinatus advancement,[4] deltoid-rotator cuff suture,[7] shifts of the long head of biceps tendon[3] and others have been reported in an attempt to cover massive rotator cuff defects. However, the patch graft appears to have a disadvantage with two suture lines in the way of force transmission. In the supraspinatus advancement and deltoid-rotator cuff suture, the remaining portion of the tendon must be longer than at least 1 cm. Therefore, they are not indicated for the true global tear. As the long head of the biceps tendon may have been torn with the cuff, its shift procedure is not possible in all cases.

TABLE 3 Results 2

	Cases						
	1	2	3	4	5	6	7
Lifting an object up to the shelf	±	+	±	+	–	±	+
Throwing	+	+	–	+	–	–	+
Doing hair	+	+	+	+	±	–	+
Washing face	+	+	+	+	–	+	+
Perineal care	+	+	+	+	+	+	+

TABLE 4 Results 3

Evaluation by Wolfgang's Criteria		
Case 1	16 points	excellent
2	16 points	excellent
3	16 points	excellent
4	17 points	excellent
5	9 points	excellent
6	14 points	excellent
7	17 points	excellent

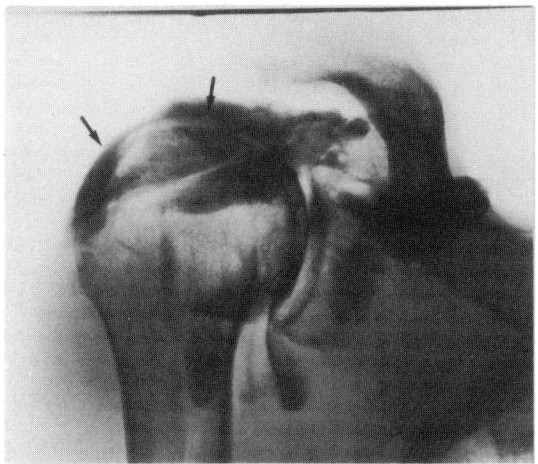

Figure 7 The arthrogram of the global tear in case 4. The contour of the humeral head (right arrow) is continuous with that of the subacromial bursa (left arrow).

The trapezius transfer has been devised to overcome those disadvantages.

The upper fibers of the trapezius are considered to have four advantages as the source of transfer for the supraspinatus. 1. They act as a synergist with the supraspinatus and the deltoid. 2. They are properly disposed for the substitute of the supraspinatus. 3. They are endowed with good power. 4. They are endowed with good compensatory property.

The preliminary results of this transfer are satisfactory and encouraging for both patients and surgeons.

REFERENCES

1. Bateman JE. Diagnosis and treatment of ruptures of rotator cuff. Surg Clin N Amer 1963; 43:1523–1530.
2. Bateman JE. The Shoulder and Neck. Philadelphia: WB Saunders, 1978.

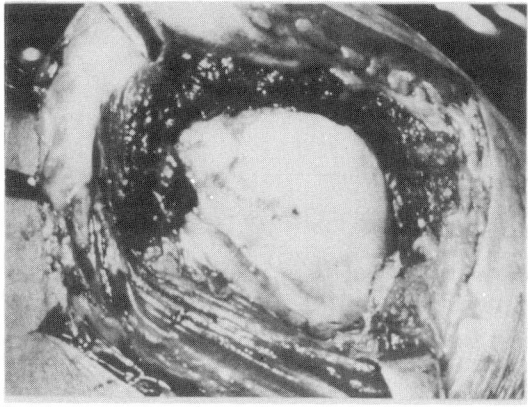

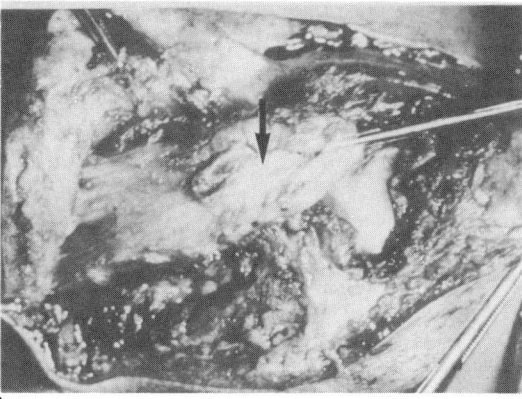

Figure 8 (a) The appearance of the global tear in case 4. (b) The upper fiber of the trapezius is freed for transplantation.

3. Bush LF. The torn shoulder capsule. J Bone Joint Surg 1975; 57A:256–259.
4. Debeyre J, Patte D, Elmelik E. Repair of ruptures of rotator cuff of shoulder, with note on advancement of supraspinatus muscle. J Bone Joint Surg 1965; 47B:36–42.
5. McLaughlin HL. Lesions of the musculotendinous cuff of the shoulder. J Bone Joint Surg 1944; 26:31–51.
6. Mikasa M. Subacromial bursography. J Jpn Orthop Ass 1979; 53:223–231.
7. Takagishi N, Okabe Y, Matsuzaki A, et al. Treatment of the rotator cuff tear. J Jpn Orthop Ass 1975; 49:698–699.

THE ACROPOLE PROSTHESIS

PAUL M. GRAMMONT, M.D.

Rotator cuff degeneration is a natural concomitant of aging; there is a very high incidence of cuff tears in the older population. Many of these are asymptomatic, but those that become symptomatic and are neglected can lead to a very disabling arthritis of the shoulder joint. It is for the purpose of salvage of this difficult situation that the Acropole prosthesis (Fig. 1) has been developed.

The prosthesis seeks to prevent the upward ascension of the humerus in situations where the deltoid is unopposed by the stabilizing influence of the other cuff tendons. This prosthesis controls pain and prevents the upward migration of the humeral head by restoring the normal fulcrum of movement beneath the subacromial arch. Indeed the Acropole prosthesis seeks to restore the normal mechanics of the subacromial articulation rather than making a primary assault upon the glenohumeral joint.

Three important principles are observed: (1) the function of the shoulder is greatly enhanced by restoration of the effective moment arm of the deltoid; (2) pain is eliminated by resurfacing the painful subacromial impinging surfaces; and (3) the prosthesis preserves the basic structure of the shoulder, making salvage to arthrodesis a very viable proposition. Should failure of the prosthesis occur, removal of the device does not disable the patient and further salvage reconstruction is possible.

The Basic Concept

The acromial vault is resurfaced by a vault hemiprosthesis replacing both the articulating acromion and coracoacromial ligament surfaces. Articulation is made with a prosthetic tuberosity replacing completely the area of the greater tuberosity from which the cuff tendons have become detached. Thus there is created a new subacromial articulation between a prosthesis spanning between the coracoid and the acromion, the undersurface which it lines, and the opposing tuberosity. As there is now no friction and the moment arm of the deltoid has been effectively restored, the deltoid very effectively acts as an abductor with the prosthetic surfaces gliding freely on one another.

Indications for the Acropole Prosthesis. These include all syndromes of pain and stiffness caused by subacromial impingement where active motion is impossible (especially in the elderly with major rotator cuff tears of an irreparable nature or those suffering from rotator cuff arthropathy) and rheumatoid arthritis which causes a similar disruption of cuff function, where restoration of a subacromial articulating surface is required.

SURGICAL TECHNIQUE

With the patient in the lateral position and the arm draped free, a saber incision is made over the front of the shoulder. The lateral edge of the acromion is osteotomized with a saw, the deltoid

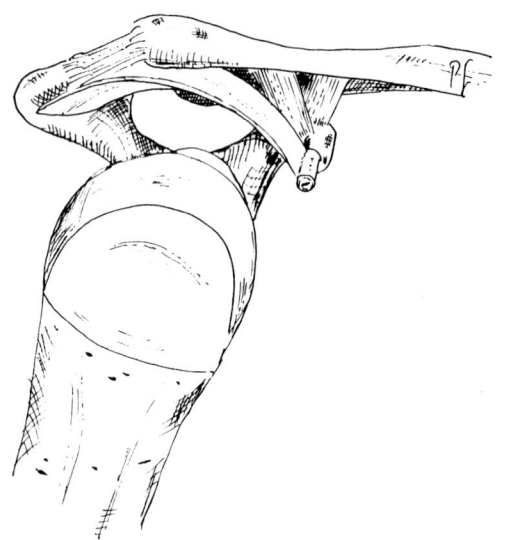

Figure 1 A new subacromial articulation is created between a prosthesis spanning between the coracoid and the acromion and the opposing tuberosity.

being carefully preserved, particularly anteriorly, to facilitate later reattachment. Care has to be taken in the drilling of the coracoid because of the unusual curvature of this structure and the rather fragile nature of the bone. Care must be taken; firm fixation utilizing the coracoid is an essential feature of the prosthetic stabilization. The undersurface of the acromion is carefully shaped and the prosthesis fixed in place with the tightening of two nuts and bolts. Cement may be used to facilitate the screw fixation if necessary. The preparation of the greater tuberosity is carried out with a vertical osteotomy and a transverse cut to remove tuberosity bone sufficient to fit the prosthesis in place with a securing hole in the tuberosity for cement fixation. Careful reconstruction of the deltoid completes the procedure, and routine closure includes the use of drains.

Following protection in a sling for two days, passive motion can be started, including simple activities of daily living such as feeding, or writing. Active motion and lifting are forbidden for four weeks, however, until the deltoid is secure.

Results

Twelve Acropole prostheses were implanted between December 1977 and January 1980. Of these, three men and nine women required surgery; three were in their 50s, the remainder were between 60 and 80 years of age. The results are summarized in Figure 2.

The results in terms of pain relief were very good; 10 achieved complete pain relief. The prosthesis was universally successful in alleviating disabling pain.

Active range of motion was poorly enhanced as indicated with only Grade 2 (on a 1–5 scale) improvement. Only one patient achieved good range of motion following the procedure.

Strength was rated 3 out of 5 in 11 cases, and while the results in terms of active range of motion and strength are not startling, the improvement in the patient's functional capability is nonetheless very gratifying because of the associated pain relief and enhanced ability to cope with daily activities.

With regard to stability, all proved stable and there was no incidence of dislocation.

Discussion

The Acropole prosthesis seeks to resurface the important subacromial articulation enhancing the effective moment arm of the deltoid in situations where the cuff has been irreparably destroyed. This is a circumstance poorly dealt with in conventional forms of shoulder arthroplasty and which is not generally benefitted even by recourse to procedures such as arthrodesis.

The results in terms of pain relief are excellent, instability is not a problem but the range of motion and the regaining of strength are generally poor. Nonetheless, functional improvement is very considerable and the benefits definitely exceed those which could be anticipated from arthrodesis, the only other possible surgical salvage procedure. In the majority of cases, the shoulder was painless but weak, the patient could not work overhead but was very satisfied with the freedom from disabling pain.

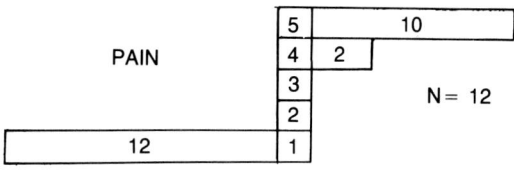
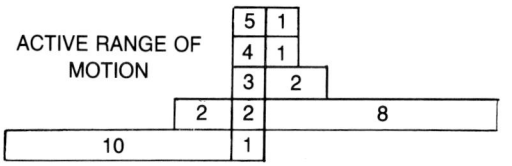
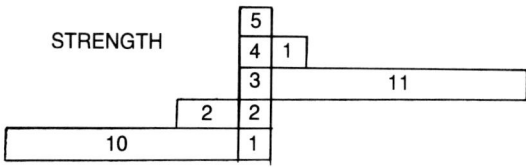
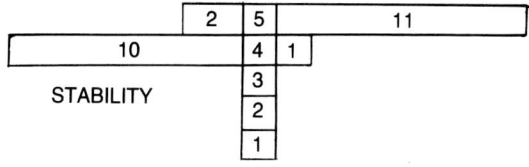

Figure 2 Summary of results.

A SURGICAL APPROACH TO ROTATOR CUFF TEARS

N. GSCHWEND, M.D.

In repairing 130 rotator cuff tears, we have employed nearly all the surgical approaches reported in the literature. There was none which gave us true satisfaction, particularly in cases where we had to deal with extensive tears. Incisions to release the clavicular portion of the deltoid muscle result in a weakening of flexion which is most important in everyday life. Release of the acromial part of the deltoid muscle with subsequent reinsertion carries the risk of tearing and weakening the abduction.[1] The transacromial approach,[2] particularly on the patient in prone position, complicates operative procedures in the ventral part. The "sabre cut" access with simple spreading of the clavicular and acromial portions of the deltoid muscle seems to be best esthetically, allowing easy removal of the impingement syndrome. However, when we have to mobilize a more retracted supraspinatus muscle or even to reinsert or transfer the infraspinatus, an additional incision[3] or the release of the deltoid are required. These difficulties coupled with unsatisfactory functional results have caused the surgical treatment of rotator cuff tears came to fall into disfavor. How else could we explain the fact that even nowadays some reputable authors doubt any possible success through surgery, while others suggest without hesitation the simple removal of the structures torn and degenerate—at least in elderly patients, the remaining pseudoparalysis being acceptable provided there is freedom from pain (Apoil, Dautry[4])? This attitude is one of resignation and in contradiction to the reconstructive aims which have always been foremost in orthopaedics.

MANAGEMENT OF THE ROTATOR CUFF TEAR

The indication for surgical treatment is not merely that a rotator cuff tear has been proved, but that there is persistent disturbing pain and/or a pseudoparalysis despite a good convervative treatment. It is only the very rare cuff tear in young people which we regard as an indication for early surgery.

The *aim* of managing the rotator cuff tear is to achieve:

1. Removal of pain which is mostly caused by an impingement under the coracoacromial ligament, the anterior part of the acromion, or by osteophytes arising from an osteoarthritic acromioclavicular joint. The anterior acromioplasty with resection of the coracoacromial ligament and possible also of the lateral end of the clavicle removes the disturbing défilé impingement of the damaged structures, allowing also a free inspection of the supraspinatus, the biceps tendon and the subscapularis.

2. The best possible restoration of the original anatomy by reinsertion of the torn muscles to their actual point of insertion, or, when possible, functional replacement by transferring neighboring muscles to the place of the irreparably impaired muscles. This occurs mostly by mobilization of the supraspinatus, possibly also of the infraspinatus in the mainly tendinous portion up to the crossing point of the suprascapular nerve. Under certain circumstances it may be necessary to shift the infraspinatus more cranially to the place of the supraspinatus. Transferring the subscapularis or the teres minor is rarely indicated.

Surgical Approach

The requirements of a good surgical approach include:

1. Easy anatomic orientation
2. Good comprehensive view
3. Minimal damage to the tissue; respect for the important muscles with regard to after-treatment and function
4. Minimum risk of damaging vital structures (nerves, vessels, etc.)

5. Possibility of extending access without additional incisions

6. Simple technique for those with less experience

7. Esthetically acceptable scar

Technique

The patient can be operated on in a semi-sitting position with the shoulder being completely free on the anterior and posterior aspect. We prefer the patient lying on his side in the anti-Trendelenburg position as indicated by Grammont (Fig. 1)[5] wherein one leg is extended on a foot-board and the other leg, with the knee in flexion, rests on a support. This positioning allows the operation to be performed ventrally and dorsally without impediment. As a rule, the surgeon stands on the patient's ventral side, the nurse to his right, an assistant on the patient's posterior side. A second assistant, placed ventrally or dorsally, holds the patient's forearm and hand and pulls or rotates the wanted part into the surgeon's field of vision. Before the cutaneous incision, we mark the clavicle, AC-joint, coracoid, acromion and the scapular spine.

Incision

Our approach is a modification of the Kessel approach. Generally, the length of the cutaneous incision is between 8 cm and 10 cm (Fig. 2). It is performed in the prolongation of the lateral part of the neck vertically to the acromion and bisects the triangle formed by the clavicle and scapular spine; 4–5 cm of the incision are effected proximally towards the center of the acromion, 3–4 cm distally from it parallel to the acromial muscle fiber of the deltoid. Without releasing the subcutaneous tissue any farther than necessary for the identification of the center of the acromion, the aponeurosis formed by the radiating fibers of the trapezius and deltoid muscles is incised here together with the periosteum in the direction of the skin incision. For hemostasis of the empirically well vascularized shoulder region, we prefer a hot Ringer solution. Further preparation is done with a sharp chisel, optimally with the Ombrédanne blade-chisel. With the inclusion of very thin slivers of bone, the soft tissue together with the periosteum is detached in one single layer ventrally in the direction of the anterior border of the acromion and the AC joint (Fig. 3). The joint capsule of the AC-joint can be lifted together with a bone sliver. Prior to com-

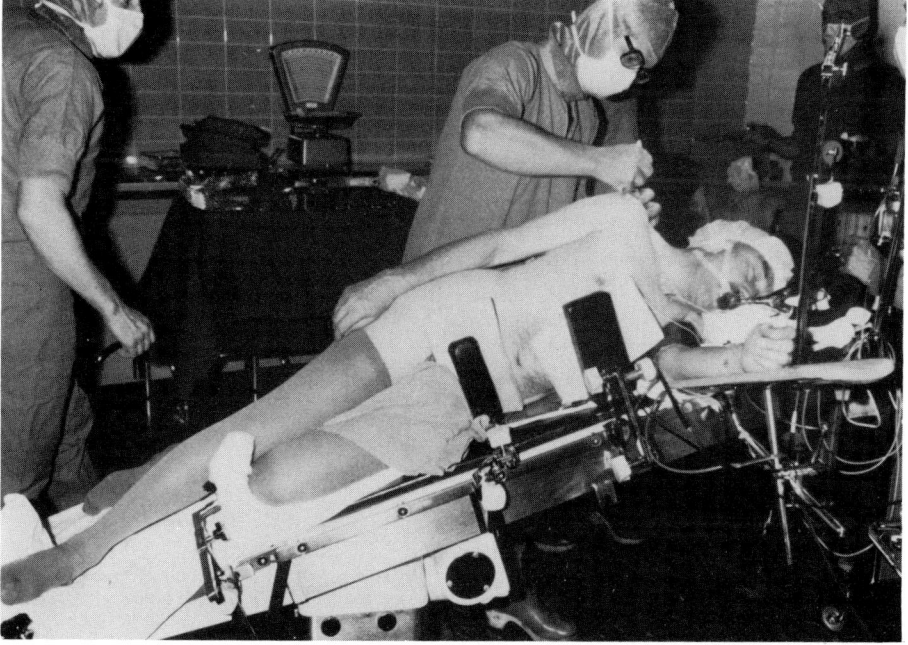

Figure 1 Patient's lateral positioning on the operating table according to Grammont.

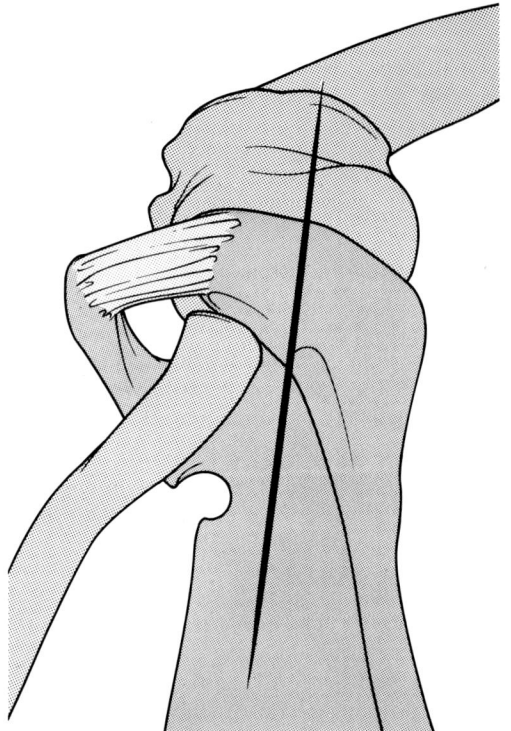

Figure 2 Skin incision.

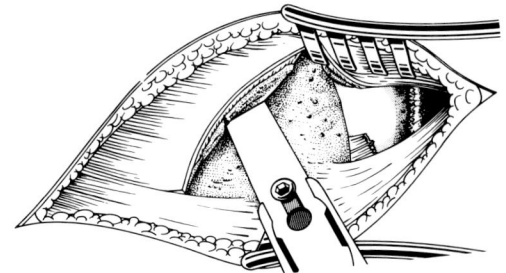

Figure 3 Detaching insertion of trapezius and deltoid muscle from the acromion with thin bone slivers. On the right, the deltoid muscle fibers are spread and the rotator cuff tear comes into view.

pleting this preparation, the fibers of the trapezius are bluntly separated proximally in the direction of the skin incision, and we thus reach the layer of adipose tissue covering the supraspinatus muscle. The same occurs distally with the fibers of the deltoid. Here one has to be strictly aware that the fibers are separated not more than 4 cm from the border of the acromion (to avoid a lesion of the muscle branches of the axillary nerve coming from behind) and that the insertion of the deltoid on the lateral acromial edge is always carried out with the chisel including thin bone slivers. This allows a rapid and good inspection of the frequently thickened subacromial and subdeltoid bursae as well as, after their splitting, the site of the tear and the greater tuberosity. A hypertrophic bursa is resected.

Once the surgeon has a good view of the region of the acromion and the AC joint, the acromioplasty can be undertaken as follows (Fig. 4): In a dorsalwards slanting plane an almost triangular piece of the acromion can be osteotomized from its anterolateral corner to the dorsal corner of the AC joint by the means of an oscillating saw and be removed together with the coracoacromial ligament. In case of osteoarthritic changes of the AC joint, or of caudally prominent osteophytes, previous subluxation or dislocation, we additionally resect 1 cm of the lateral end of the clavicle. The supraspinatus can now easily be exposed in the proximal part of the incision; an accurate definition of its limits is facilitated by pulling its torn end. If the defect refers exclusively to the supraspinatus, it can be mobilized up to the entrance of the suprascapular nerve. In case of greater retraction, this is managed by a ventral and dorsal release incision on the muscle border (Fig. 5). The transverse osteotomy of the acromion practised by Debeyre and Kessel[6] seems superfluous, since there is sufficient room and visibility to mobilize the supraspinatus without acromionotomy. The reinsertion is made in a transverse slot medially to

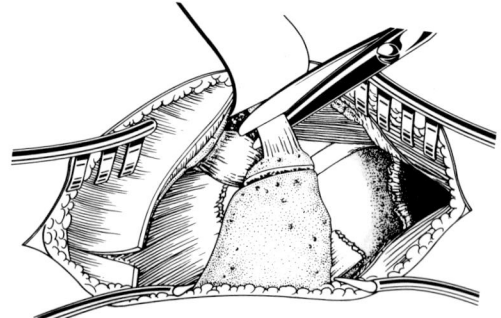

Figure 4 Anterior acromioplasty resecting a triangular piece of the acromion including the articular surface of the AC-joint together with the coraco-acromial ligament. Note that the capsule of the AC-joint should also be elevated with a thin bone sliver prior to the acromioplasty.

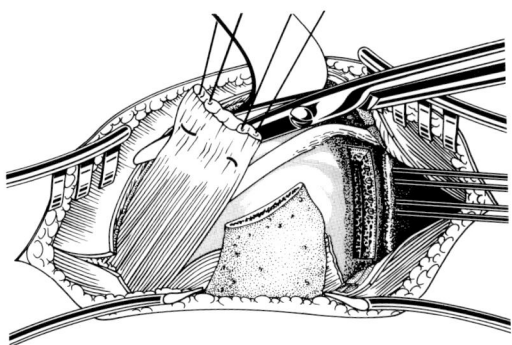

Figure 5 Mobilization of the retracted supraspinatus and preparation of the slot and transcortical holes for fixation of the freshened tendinous end.

the greater tuberosity and if possible in the region of the former tear. The strong threads issuing from the freshened edge of the tendon are pulled through the cortical bone distally from the greater tuberosity and tied there. If the infraspinatus is ruptured too, this muscle has to be mobilized in the same manner as the supraspinatus (Fig. 6). An osteotomy of the dorsally prominent acromion can be carried out and tilted dorsally, taking with it the deltoid. We thus gain a good view over the infraspinatus which is mobilized and reinserted in similar manner to that for supraspinatus. If the supraspinatus appears too much retracted or if it is irreparably damaged in its substance, the reconstruction of continuity is possible either by using autologous material such as skin or fascia lata or by foreign material (Lyodura, deep-frozen rotator cuff from the postmortem bank), or by artificial material (Dacron used in vascular surgery). Preferably, functional compensation for the failed supraspinatus should be achieved by a cranial transfer of the infraspinatus. If the biceps tendon is largely intact, it is left under the sutured rotator cuff. If it is severely damaged and frayed, it can be spread out to cover the ventral defect or be shifted over the rotator cuff sutures underneath. Whenever possible, the biceps tendon should not be removed because of its contribution to lowering and stabilizing the shoulder. In case of extreme impairment from a tear, we suture it in the intertubercular sulcus and shift it on to the coracoid.

Although it is possible to mobilize the teres minor and subscapularis muscles and to suture them over the humeral head instead of the irreparably injured supraspinatus and infraspinatus, this management should be considered only in those cases involving massive defects.

Closure

The closure is very simple—a further advantage of this incision. The dorsal acromionotomy is reinforced with a small-fragment cortical screw anteriorly inserted through the acromion, enhancing the mutually stabilizing trapezius and deltoid muscles to totally stabilize the osteotomy. The borders of the trapezius and deltoid muscles are approximated with strong resorbable sutures (Fig. 7). Due to the good vascular supply of the acromion,

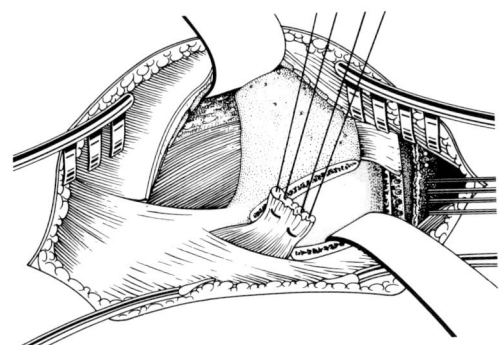

Figure 6 Posterior acromion-osteotomy reflecting the deltoid insertion. The infraspinatus can easily be mobilized similarly to the supraspinatus and fixed closed to same.

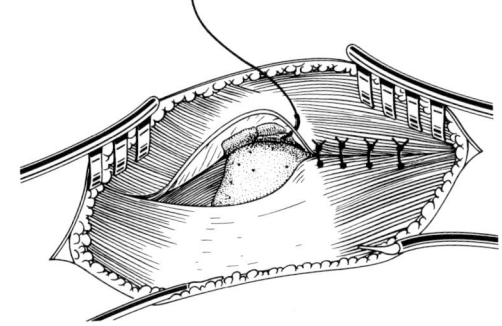

Figure 7 Simple suture by approximation of the trapezius and deltoid muscles. The bone slivers underneath are well vascularized as well as the acromion.

the thin bone slivers underneath the soft tissues will heal without difficulty.

The method and duration of immobilization (whether abduction splint or simple bandage) depend largely on the quality of the reinserted rotator cuff. To prevent adhesions, an early mobilization is always effected through careful passive rotation in the first postoperative days. As a rule, however, active exercise with flexion against gravity should not be carried out before the end of 4 to 6 weeks. In contrast to this, passive flexion-elevation in the supine position may start from the second week. During the first four weeks, exercise is increased avoiding the force of gravity and with increasingly more active participation. Only when the arm can be held in a 90° abduction without any help, and when external rotation is achieved also against gravity, is elevation practised from the zero-position of the shoulder. With proper wound healing and favorable geographic circumstances, outpatient treatment is possible from the second or third week. Treatment should only be discontinued when the patient can elevate his shoulder without difficulty.

REFERENCES

1. Henry AK. Extensile exposure applied to limb surgery. 2nd ed. Edinburgh: E & S Livingstone, 1957.
2. Debeyre J, Patte D, Elmelick E. Repair of ruptures of the rotator cuff of the shoulder with a note on advancement of the supraspinatus muscle. J Bone and Joint Surg 1976; 47B:36–42.
3. Patte D, Goutalier D, Debeyre J. Ruptures of the rotator cuff. Results and perspectives of the retrostruction. Orthopäde 1981; 10:206–215.
4. Apoil A, Dautry P, Moinet Ph, Koechlin Ph. A propos de 70 interventions pour syndrome dit de rupture de la coiffe des rotateurs de l'épaule. Rev Chir Orthop 1977; Suppl:11–63.
5. Grammont PM, Lelaurin G. Scapula-osteotomie und Acropole-prothese. Orthopäde 1981; IO: 219–229.
6. Kessel L. The transacromial approach for rotator cuff rupture. In: Bayley J, Kessel L eds. Shoulder surgery. Heidelberg, New York: Springer Berlin, 1982:39–44.

ARTHRODESIS/ ARTHROPLASTY

SHOULDER ARTHRODESIS—A.O. TECHNIQUE

JOHN P. KOSTUIK, M.D., F.R.C.S.(C), and JOSEPH SCHATZKER, M.D., F.R.C.S.(C)

Arthrodesis of the shoulder is a time-honored procedure used primarily in the treatment of paralytic problems to improve upper extremity function and to relieve pain in post–traumatic arthropathy.

The indications at the present time remain related primarily to those two major entities but also include postinfective problems, primary osteoarthritis and arthritis secondary to rheumatoid disease, and problems related to failed arthroplasty.

With reference to paralytic disorder about the shoulder, proximal brachial plexus injuries remain a paramount indication for operative intervention, particularly those secondary to traumatic lesions. Other paralytic indications are Erb's palsy, poliomyelitis, and paralysis about the shoulder and deltoid muscle paralysis, usually of traumatic origin.

The prerequisites for arthrodesis of the shoulder, and paralytic conditions about the shoulder, are that the patients generally have a good elbow, although Seddon[7,8] has shown that the addition of transfers to produce elbow flexion about the elbow can be done in conjunction with an arthrodesis of the shoulder.

Arthrodesis of the shoulder in the past has been fraught with a relatively high incidence of nonunion and has generally required the use of external immobilization, despite internal fixation.[1,2,3,9]

Charnley and Houston[4] used a technique of compression arthrodesis associated with external immobilization and, in 1964, reported a union rate of 22 out of 23 at eight weeks. Neer and Hawkins[5] more recently reported a 20 percent incidence of nonunion. They felt that arthrodesis of the shoulder was rarely indicated and that arthroplasty was preferable. Riggins,[6] in 1976, made the first North American report on the use of the A.O. compression arthrodesis technique; he reported the incidence of 100 percent union without external immobilization in a small series of cases.

OPERATIVE POSITIONING

In the literature, a considerable variation exists as to the operative positioning of the shoulder at the time of arthrodesis. The range reported is considerable, going from 50° to 90° of abduction to 20° to 90° of flexion and 25° to 90° internal rotation. It is recognized that every case must be individualized, particularly if there is paralysis of the serratus anterior, but generally the position used has been 60° of abduction using the vertebral border of the scapula as a base line. This will usually allow the patient up to 90° of scapulohumeral abduction and when this is associated with about 30° of flexion, the patient can easily raise his hand to his mouth or the top of his head with the contralateral shoulder especially when associated with approximately 30° of internal rotation of the shoulder. If the serratus anterior is paralyzed, it is generally recognized that abduction must be decreased to approximately 30°.

The desired functional goals in arthrodesis of the shoulder are to allow the patient to put his hand to his face, his arm to his side and his hand into the pants pocket on the ipsilateral side.

TECHNIQUE

We have employed the A.O. technique of arthrodesis of the shoulder for the past 14 years. In no case was external immobilization used and in no case were bone grafts other than local grafting applied to the site of arthrodesis.

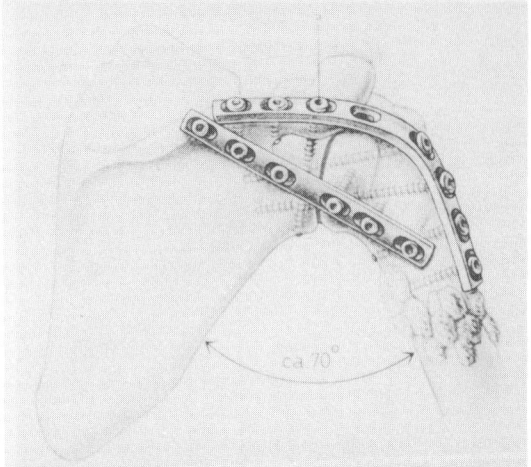

Figure 1 Schematic view of technique and abduction. The use of the vertebral border of the scapula at 60° abduction is easier.

The technique consists of the use of a narrow A.O. plate contoured from the spine of the scapula onto the lateral surface of the humerus. Heavy cancellous screws are used over washers to obtain the initial position of the head after decorticating the undersurface of the acromion and cutting the humeral head, where its remnant is of the appropriate shape, to fit a squared-off glenoid.

A posterior buttress plate to control rotation was added from the spine of the scapula along the posterior aspect of the glenoid and posterior aspect of the proximal humerus (Fig. 1).

MATERIAL

This report is a retrospective study of 18 patients who have undergone arthrodesis using this technique, 14 males and four females. The etiology has been divided equally between paralytic and arthritic cases. Age range was from 19 to 64 years with an average of 35 years. The etiology of the paralytic cases was brachial plexus palsy in 5, axillary nerve palsy in 2, Erb's palsy in 1 and a postpolio paralysis in 1 case.

The etiology of the arthritic cases included: two cases secondary to repeated recurrent dislocation of the shoulder of an anterior nature, four cases of post-traumatic fracture dislocations above the shoulder, one osteoarthritic postunipolar Neer arthroplasty, one radiation necrosis, and two chronic irreparable rotator cuff problems secondary to osteoarthritis.

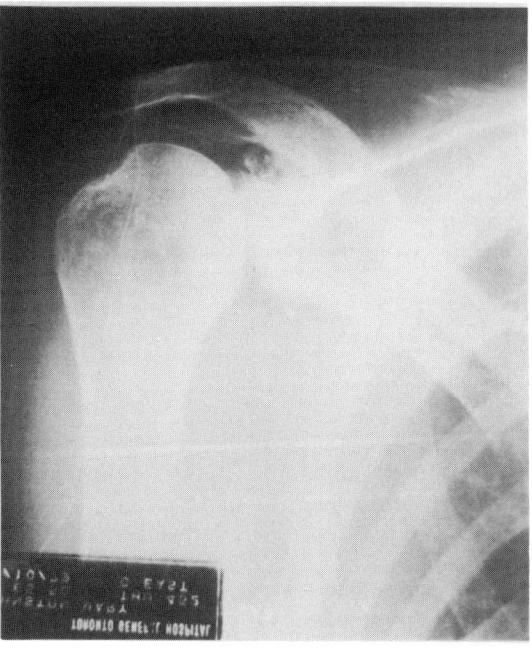

Figure 2 Patient with flail shoulder.

RESULTS

There was one minor wound infection which cleared with local dressings. One patient sustained a fracture below the internal fixation devices at a later time and was treated conservatively with no abnormal sequelae. Four patients required removal of their internal fixation devices some two years following their arthrodesis because of prominent screws along the spine of the scapula and the superior surface of the humerus. These were all paralytic cases where, because of absence of tissue, the internal fixation devices were prominent.

From the point of view of function, all patients were relieved of pain except for three all of whom were post-traumatic osteoarthritic cases on Workmen's Compensation. The patients' occupation postoperative continued at the preoperative level, one executive, six clerical workers, four housewives, one cabinet maker, one gardener, one labourer. One patient remained unemployed because of preoperative alcoholism. The three patients who were on Workmen's Compensation did not return to work despite a solid arthrodesis and their arm in a functional position, but continued to complain of pain unrelated to the internal fixation devices.

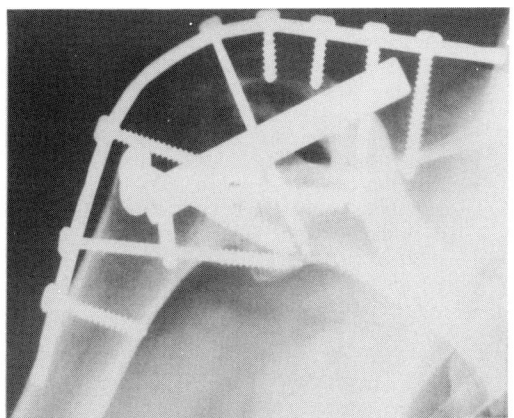

Figure 3 Sound union with internal fixation utilizing a double-plate technique.

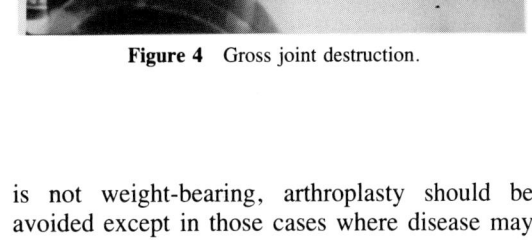

Figure 4 Gross joint destruction.

Union occurred in all patients. From an objective point of view, satisfactory function and relief of pain was obtained in 100 percent but subjectively in only 87 percent because of the continued problems with the Workmen's Compensation cases.

Six paralytic patients were somewhat unhappy because of atrophy about their shoulder.

DISCUSSION

The problems of shoulder arthrodesis are primarily those of loss of motion in that the procedure can only be done in patients with unilateral disease. The contralateral shoulder should be normal both clinically and radiologically. There may be difficulties if the extremity is required for reasons of personal hygiene; unless position is accurate, the patient may have difficulty in placing his hand in his pocket or reaching his mouth or the top of his head.

It is our feeling that nonunion and external immobilization are no longer major problems when the described technique is used. This is borne out by the statistics in this review which showed an incidence of union of 100 percent despite the absence of both extra graft material and external immobilization devices.

We would disagree with Neer and Hawkins[5] who stated that total shoulder arthroplasty is preferable, even in young people to arthrodesis of the shoulder. Given the high incidence of problems of arthroplasty in young people with lower extremity arthritis, we feel that, although the upper extremity is not weight-bearing, arthroplasty should be avoided except in those cases where disease may be bilateral or the patient suffers from associated problems such as the multiple joint problems of juvenile rheumatoid arthritis or hemophiliac arthritis.

The advantages of shoulder arthrodesis are that it is painless and offers a functional upper extremity that is strong and durable.

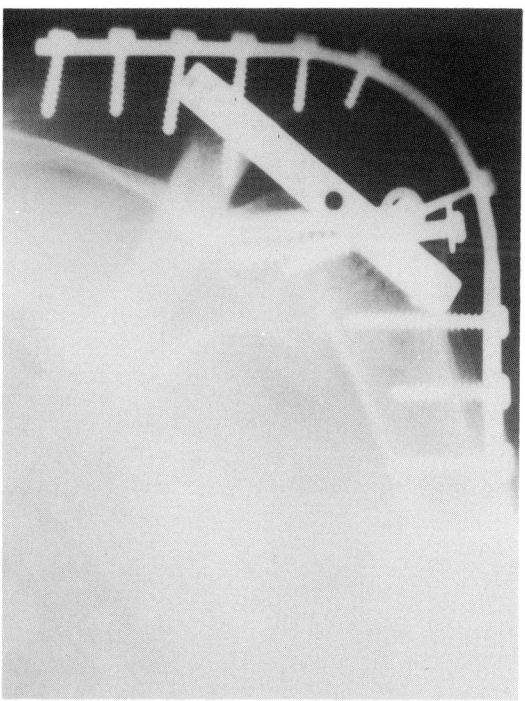

Figure 5 A.O. technique. Sound arthrodesis at 6 months.

REFERENCES

1. Barr JS, Freiberg JA, Colonna PC, Pemberton PA. A Survey of End Results on Stabilization of the Paralytic Shoulder. Report of the Research Committee of the American Orthopaedic Association, J Bone Joint Surg. 1942; 24:699–707.
2. Barton NJ. Arthrodesis of the Shoulder for Degenerative Conditions. J Bone Joint Surg. 1972; 54A:1759–1764.
3. Beltran JE, Trilla JC, Barjau R. A Simplified Compression Arthrodesis of the Shoulder. J Bone Joint Surg. 1975; 57A:538–541.
4. Charnley J, Jouston JK. Compression Arthrodesis of the Shoulder. J Bone Joint Surg. 1964; 46B:614–620.
5. Neer II CS, Hawkins RJ. A Functional Analysis of Shoulder Fusion. J Bone Joint Surg. 1977; 59B(4):508.
6. Riggins RS. Shoulder Fusion Without External Fixation. A Preliminary Report. J Bone Joint Surg. 1976; 58(7):1007–1008.
7. Seddon HJ. Reconstructive Surgery of the Upper Extremity In Poliomyelitis, Second International Poliomyelitis Congress, Philadelphia: JB Lippincott, 1952.
8. Seddon HJ. Transplantation of the Pectoralis Major for Paralysis of the Flexors of the Elbow. Proc Roy Soc Med. 1949; 12:837.
9. Watson-Jones R. Extra-articular Arthrodesis of the Shoulder. J Bone Joint Surg. 1933; 15:862.

BIPOLAR IMPLANT SHOULDER ARTHROPLASTY

ALFRED B. SWANSON, M.D.

The shoulder joint destroyed by arthritis has received relatively little attention from those interested in joint replacement. The painful shoulder presenting as an isolated symptom in an otherwise normal patient, receives a great deal of attention because of the patient's complaints and the severe loss of function that frequently accompanies bursitis, tendinitis and impingement syndromes in this area. Degenerative or osteoarthritic arthritis presents as a similar, though more chronic complaint, which does not respond to usual treatment methods, and is usually not treated satisfactorily. In the rheumatoid arthritic patient, whose sphere of functional activity has been largely restricted by multiple joint involvement, the disabilities of the shoulder joint are frequently ignored by both the patient and the physician. Severe disability of this joint is accompanied with marked destructive changes, but the patient will usually not complain unless he experiences severe crepitation or instability. Loss of shoulder movement results secondarily in limitation of normal functional activity of the hand. An armamentarium of surgical procedures has been developed to correct more obvious problems in the joints of the hand, wrist, elbow and lower extremity, but the surgical treatment of the arthritic shoulder has received little attention.[3,4] Evaluation and treatment of shoulder disabilities must be included in the rehabilitation and reconstructive surgery program for the arthritic upper extremity.

DESIGN CONSIDERATIONS

Anatomical Considerations

Knowledge of the physiology and anatomy of the shoulder joint is of great importance for anyone who would attempt reconstructive and rehabilitation programs. The shoulder girdle could be described as comprising five joints: the glenohumeral joint, the scapulothoracic joint, the sternoclavicular joint, the acromioclavicular joint, and the subdeltoid joint, which is not an anatomical joint, but consists of two musculotendinous surfaces moving on each other.

The scapulothoracic joint is not frequently involved in the arthritic process. Its function, however, is dependent upon its surrounding muscles and a stable glenohumeral joint if it is to add motion to the upper extremity. The acromioclavicular joint is frequently involved in the arthritic process, and its dysfunction may also limit potential shoulder motion through pain, incongruity and instability.

Resection of this joint should be considered frequently in reconstructive procedures. The glenohumeral joint is a true ball and socket articulation. The stability, movement and normal function of this joint depend not only upon adequate joint surfaces, but on exquisite interplay of motor tendon units along with ligamentous and capsular coordinated looseness and tightness and gliding planes that do not restrict motion. Superior dislocation of the humeral head, may be caused by excessively strong contraction of the long muscles across the disorganized joint; this tendency is prevented by the presence of a coracoacromial arch and contraction of the shoulder cuff muscles. The subdeltoid bursa forms a cleavage between the deltoid muscle and the underlying periarticular short cuff muscles. Adhesions in this area will prevent the important gliding required to achieve abduction, and will consequently restrict motion. During abduction, the greater tuberosity is pulled superiorly and medially by the action of the supraspinatus muscles, allowing the humeral head to slip under the coracoacromial arch. This point is extremely important in the pathomechanics of the arthritic shoulder.

Implant Design Considerations

The normal glenohumeral joint offers a great range of stable movement that is difficult to reproduce. The basic concepts for a joint replacement implant design require engineering, anatomical and physiological considerations, as well as evaluations of the implant material and of the patient's needs. An efficient implant arthroplasty procedure for the shoulder joint must be designed to simplify the joint's mechanism, because the complexity of the normal mechanisms cannot be completely reproduced.

The implants, or endoprostheses, used in the arthritic shoulder reconstruction can be categorized: (I) Hemiarthroplasty type, in which the head of the humerus is replaced with an intramedullary stemmed implant. Neer has reported his results with a metal hemiarthroplasty implant for replacement of the articulating surface of the humerus.[6,9,10] He feels that this implant works very well to restore the congruity of the humeral surface, and, thereby, decrease pain. It is especially useful in patients with the sequelae of a fracture dislocation of the upper end of the humerus; (II) So-called total joint type in which several basic implant types are presented. (A) nonconstrained type in which the humeral head and glenoid are resurfaced (Neer II, UCLA type),[9,10,11] (B) bipolar or bicentric implant type in which the humeral and glenoid components are joined, but the glenoid component is not fixed (Swanson type),[16] (C) semiconstrained type implant which has a conforming component for the glenoid (Macnab-English type),[8] and (D) constrained type implant in which the humeral and glenoid components are connected to each other and also fixed to the bone (Lettin-Stanmore, Post, Gristina types).[7,12]

The nonconstrained arthroplasty with two articulating components, one inserted in the humerus and one in the scapula, appears to have a reasonable potential for good results if the musculotendinous units are intact, or reconstructible. Stability of the glenoid component has been a problem because fixation is difficult in the presence of inadequate bone stock; this is especially true in the rheumatoid arthritic patient, and offers a potential for loosening at the cement-bone interface. The nonconstrained implant also does not protect against superior subluxation of the humeral head. The constrained implant in which the humeral and glenoidal components are connected, would simplify many of the movement problems of the deranged shoulder mechanism; however, our dependence on stabilizing the implant by current fixation techniques, makes the procedure applicable in only a small number of cases.

THE SHOULDER BIPOLAR IMPLANT

History, Development and Concept

Our concern for replacement of the humeral head in the arthritic began with our initiation of a research project to develop implants for arthroplasty of the joints of the upper extremity, in 1962.[14,15] It was our feeling that a humeral sphere of larger diameter than normal would decrease the force of the coupling action necessary to maintain the contact of the joint surfaces at the glenohumeral joint. We noted that, in most arthritic patients who have lost abduction and external rotation movement at the shoulder joint, there is a tendency towards vertical or superior displacement of the humeral head. This displacement frequently causes an impingement of the superior portion of the head of the humerus and the greater tuberosity against the acromion and the coracoacromial ligament. In the past, corrective procedures have included resection of the acromion and the coracoacromial ligament to decrease the symptoms of impingement. We believe that the coracoacromial arch should be preserved to maintain the head in position underneath it. The humeral head should contact not only the glenohumeral joint, but also the coarcoacromial arch. The leverage to move this large humeral head implant could then be achieved by the weaker cuff muscles, and with greater singular dependence on the strong deltoid muscle.

The large head humeral implant concept has the following theoretical advantages: (1) It provides a smooth concentric total contact for a potential entire shoulder joint cavity, which includes the coracoacromial arch as well as the glenoid. (2) It decreases the force concentration over any one contact area, thereby decreasing resistance to movement. (3) It lengthens the momentum arm between the fulcrum, or the joint contact point, and the muscle insertion, thereby increasing the efficiency of the muscle pull. (4) It prevents abutment of the greater tuberosity against the acromion. One-piece silicone and metal large-headed implants were designed and tested in 1965.[15] The results were good for pain relief, but inadequate from the point of view of motion and durability.

This concept of implant arthroplasty for the shoulder has been the subject of continuing study in our research department. In 1975, the possibility of using a bipolar implant at the shoulder was considered. Such an implant was designed, fabricated, tested and applied in clinical use. This report describes our experience with this implant procedure.

Definition

The bipolar, or bicentric, implant provides a self-contained ball and socket component, to allow joint motion between a distal extremity and a proximal part through two moving interfaces. In a ball and socket joint such as the shoulder or hip, this can be accomplished by the cup of a prosthetic device which moves within the "socket" (glenoid or acetabulum), and a ball attached to an intramedullary stem which articulates with a polyethylene bearing within that cup. This is a type of interposition arthroplasty, similar to the concept of the Smith–Peterson cup arthroplasty, where motion occurs between the reshaped head of the femur and the inner surface of the metal cup, and between the cup's outer surface and the acetabulum.[13] This bipolar motion concept was applied to hip endoprostheses by Giliberty, Bateman and Monk in 1974.[2,5]

The implant consists of a metal humeral component, and an articulating snap-fit glenoid resurfacing cup fabricated from plastic and metal. The

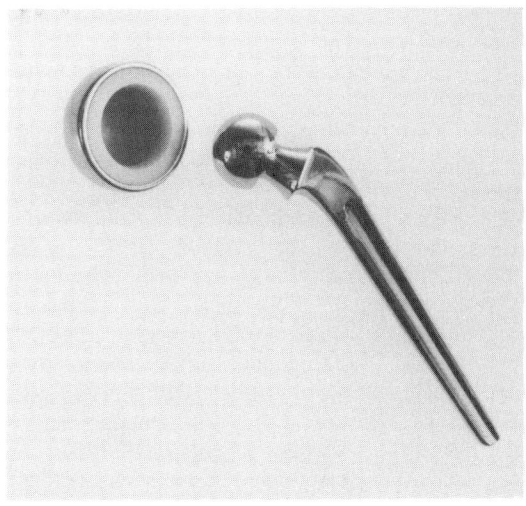

Figure 1A The bipolar shoulder implant allows motion between a distal extremity and a proximal part through two moving interfaces. The ball of the intramedullary stemmed humeral component articulates with a polyethylene bearing within the glenoid cup component. The glenoid component has the advantage of not being fixed to bone.

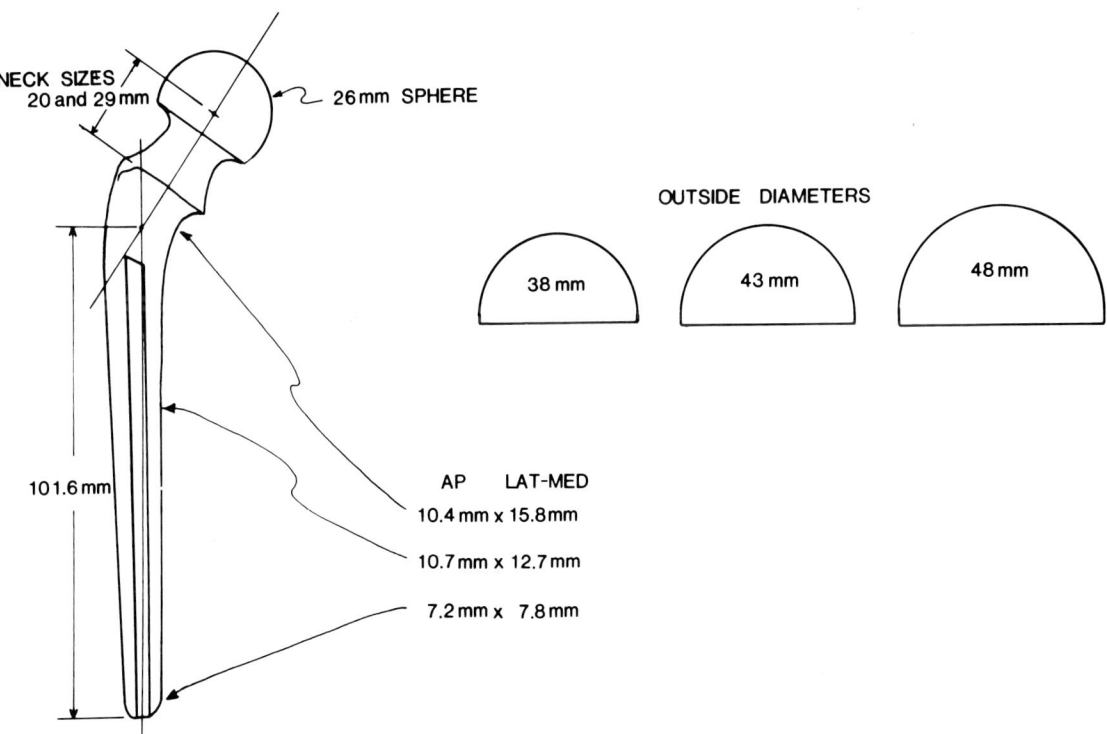

Figure 1B The glenoid cups are available in 3 diameters (38, 43 and 48 mm); the sphere of the humeral ball is 25.4 mm; two neck lengths, 20 and 29 mm, are available (manufactured by Zimmer Co.).

humeral component consists of a stem, collar, neck and ball. The cold-worked 316 LVM stainless steel humeral component is supplied in two different neck lengths: 20 mm and 29 mm. The diameter of the ball is 25.4 mm and the stem length is 10.16 cm. The stem is tapered distally and grooved, to enhance cement fixation (Fig. 1).

The cup component consists of a cold-worked LVN stainless steel shell and an ultra high molecular-weight polyethylene inner liner. The plastic cup is mechanically locked inside the shell through mating ridges located on the concave side of the metal shell, and the convex surface of the plastic cup. There are three diameters of the cup component: 38, 43, and 48 mm. The spherical head of the humeral component articulates with the concave, UHMW polyethylene bearing surface.

Advantages

The advantages of the bipolar shoulder implant are: (1) It provides new joint surfaces; (2) it provides concentric total contact for the shoulder cavity, which includes the coracoacromial arch, as well as the glenoid; (3) it acts as a spacer and prevents abutment of the greater tuberosity against the acromion, and moves the center of axis of rotation away from the coracoacromial arch; (4) it allows the cup to align itself in the glenoid, similar to a universal joint; (5) it requires no fixation of the glenoid component; (6) it decreases the wear between the device and glenoid because motion occurs both at the joint outer cup interface and also the ball-inner cup interface. The coefficient of friction is less between the metal ball and polyethylene liner of the metal cup, so that motion will selectively occur at the interface with the least friction (cinefluoroscopic studies of postoperative patients have demonstrated this); (7) it potentially increases the range of motion because of the two separate moving joint interfaces; (8) it dampens stress concentrations, thus minimizing wear changes on the implant and surrounding tissues; (9) it provides stability by the design of the glenoid component and its fit into the shoulder socket and the soft tissue operative reconstruction around it. This stability allows motion to occur within the glenohumeral implant and also the scapulothoracic joint; (10) it utilizes a standard anterior surgical approach and the procedure and soft tissues closure are straightforward and simple; (11) it has provided a stable, painfree, reasonably mobile arthroplasty, essentially free of complications as demonstrated in the long term review of clinical cases; and (12) this procedure can be used as a salvage method for the failed total joint procedure.

SURGICAL PROCEDURE

The bipolar shoulder implant arthroplasty is indicated for reconstruction of a severely painful, disabling arthritic shoulder, with evidence of joint destruction, incongruity and/or subluxation.

This method is contraindicated in the presence of: active or past sepsis in the shoulder, inadequate skin, bone or soft tissue structures or neuromuscular function; and in the uncooperative patient.

Familiarity with shoulder reconstruction and rehabilitation procedures should be a prerequisite for anyone who would undertake shoulder implant arthroplasty. Patients who are candidates for the bipolar implant may need anterior capsular reinforcement, and reconstruction of the rotator cuff; these should be considered in the surgical planning. All patients should have a medical review and clearance, and are interviewed and well counseled on the expectations of the procedure. They are informed on the immediate postoperative course and are instructed for the rehabilitation program. The usual meticulous program used for any total joint arthroplasty is used, with special emphasis to prevent infections; this includes the use of perioperative antibiotics and a laminar air flow apparatus in the room. General anesthesia with intubation is required.

The patient is placed in a semi-sitting attitude and positioned to the edge of the table, so that the extremity can hang freely. This gives a good presentation of the shoulder for the surgeon. The drapes are applied so that manipulation of the extremity can be accomplished as required.

A deltopectoral incision, 10 to 20 cm in length, is started at the level of the acromioclavicular joint and directed over the coracoid process and down the anterior medial aspect of the arm (Fig. 2A). The deltoid muscle is separated from the pectoralis and retracted laterally (Fig. 2B). The anterior deltoid muscle fibers are not incised from the clavicle unless absolutely necessary because these fibers are very important in the active flexion movement. The cephalic vein is identified between the deltoid and pectoralis major muscles and ligated. Development of the separation between the deltoid and pectoral muscles is continued down to the coracoid, which is identified. The tip of the coracoid is osteotomized and the combined tendons are dissected and retracted distally, taking care to protect the neurovascular structures (Fig. 2C and D). If the acromioclavicular joint is involved, the cutaneous incision is extended superiorly to expose and excise the lateral end of the clavicle. With the arm held in internal rotation, the deltoid muscle is carefully retracted and the subacromial bursa is identified and removed, if it is abnormal. As the arm is externally rotated, the insertion of the subscapularis tendon to the lesser tuberosity is identified. Bleeding points are controlled. The shoulder joint capsule and the subscapularis tendon are incised longitudinally 1 cm from the bicipital groove (Fig. 2E). The shoulder joint is identified, and with the extremity position controlled by an assistant, a synovectomy is performed as necessary. The long head of the biceps is released from its origin on the superior rim of the glenoid and dissected distally to gain length necessary for capsular reconstruction.

The head of the humerus is dislocated into the wound by careful passive external rotation and vertical lifting of the arm. The humeral surface is usually irregular and destroyed. The portion of the humerus covered with cartilage is excised with power saws or osteotomes, great care being taken to avoid injury to the remaining bone stock (Fig. 2F). It is best to leave the greater tuberosity intact; however, if more bone removal is necessary, the tuberosity with its muscle attachments may be osteotomized from the humerus (Fig. 2G). Following adequate humeral head resection, the synovectomy is completed and any osteophytes of the glenoid or humerus may be excised at this time. The intramedullary canal of the humerus is inspected and prepared to receive the stem of the appropriate size trial implant. The center of the head of the implant should be directed in 30° of retroversion and should be well seated against this aspect of the humeral neck (Fig. 2H). That part of the humerus can be marked with a small bite of a rongeur. The degree of retroversion can be determined by the implant relationship to the bicipital groove and the lesser tuberosity which face anteriorly, as well as by using the alignment of the transverse axis between the epicondyles of the humerus. With the proper implant size in place, passive range of motion is carried out to determine if more bone needs to be removed. Enough bone is removed to allow 90° of flexion, abduction and external rotation. The implant may require from 30° to 60° of retroversion to be stable when external rotation movement is applied. Trial implants of the three head sizes and regular and long neck sizes are used to obtain a proper concentric fit of the implant head in the shoulder joint cavity, and to ensure proper length of the neck so as to have no impingement of the proximal humerus in the joint. It is important at this time to be assured that there is no capsular loosening posteriorly, and that there is adequate capsule for repair anteriorly. A loose capsule can be sutured to the rim of the glenoid as needed.

If the greater tuberosity required removal, it is reattached utilizing Dacron tapes (Fig. 2G and I). Only a small wafer of bone of the tuberosity is left with the tendons for re-attachment. Two sets of drill holes approximately 2 cm from the end of the lateral humerus are made and Dacron tapes are passed through the tuberosity and humerus, and tied inside the canal. The tapes may be woven through the rotator cuff muscles before they are passed through the tuberosity and humeral shaft. Two Dacron tapes may also be placed through drill holes in the anterior surface of the proximal shaft to allow for re-attachment of the capsule and subscapularis tendon. The implant may also be tested for fit at this time.

The wound is thoroughly irrigated with saline and triple antibiotic solution before cementing the humeral component. An intramedullary plug for the humeral canal is fashioned, either from bone removed from the humeral head or with a silicone plug, to prevent distal flow of the cement and improve the cementing technique by applying the cement under pressure to obtain adequate bone filling. The intramedullary stem of the implant is fixed within the humeral canal in the appropriate degrees of retroversion with methylmethacrylate cement. After the cement has hardened, the implant is reduced into the joint, and the limb is taken through a range of motion to ensure stability of the implant in the glenoid cavity.

With the arm in neutral rotation, the medial capsule and subscapularis tendon are advanced to their previous attachments and held in position by the Dacron tapes (Fig. 2I and J). This capsulorrhaphy is also reinforced by weaving the biceps tendon into it (Fig. 2K). The shoulder is carried out through its range of motion to determine stability and appropriate tension of the soft tissue closure. The coracoid may be placed at the anterior rim of the glenoid, after the technique of Bristow, to act as a bony block to any tendencies for anterior dislocation in certain cases. The coracoid may also be attached either to the coracoacromial ligament or to its original anatomical position (Fig. 2L).

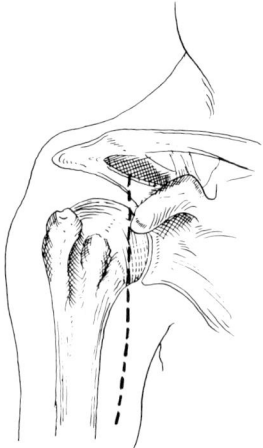

Figure 2A Anterior approach.

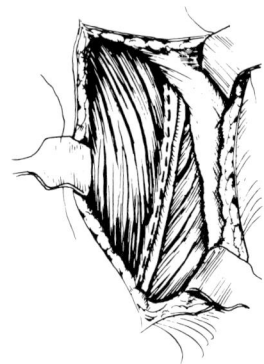

Figure 2B Muscle splitting incision between the deltoid and pectoralis muscles protecting the clavicular attachment of the deltoid anteriorly. The cephalic vein is occasionally tied off.

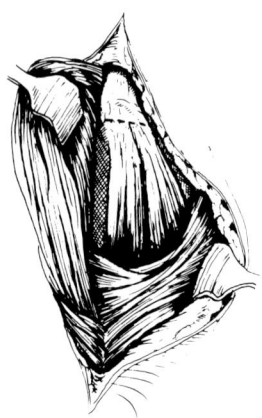

Figure 2C Exposure of the coracoid.

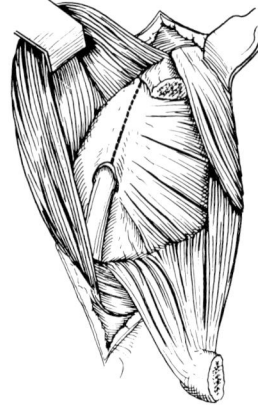

Figure 2D Osteotomy of coracoid and retraction of the attached musculature to allow exposure of the anterior shoulder and biceps tendon.

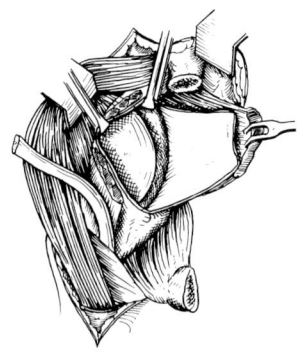

Figure 2E The shoulder joint is exposed through a longitudinal incision reflecting the anterior capsule and the overlying subscapularis muscle medially. The biceps tendon is shown separated from its glenoid attachment.

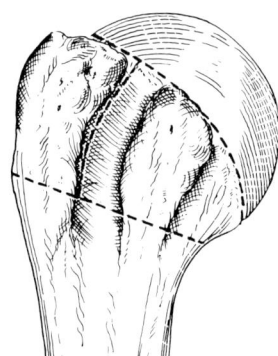

Figure 2F The amount of resection of the head and upper humerus depends on several factors; vertical displacement and adduction contracture require greater bone removal to provide a joint space for an adequate range of motion. If more than the head is removed, the greater tuberosity with its muscle and capsular attachments is detached and preserved. The implant tester may then be inserted and the range of motion tested passively; if not satisfactory, more bone is removed.

Arthrodesis/Arthroplasty / 217

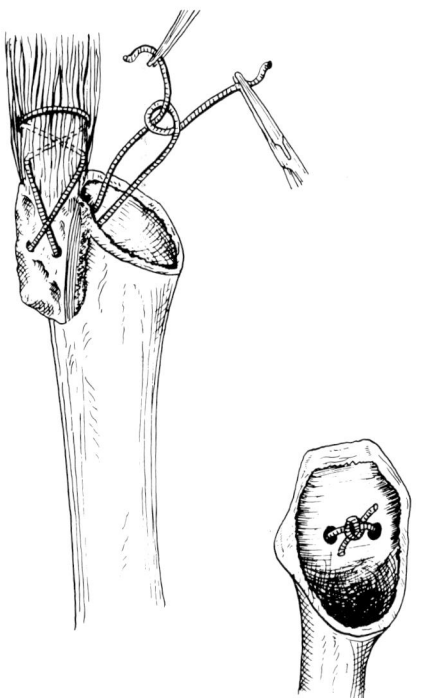

Figure 2G Reattachment of the tuberosity, shoulder cuff muscle and capsule is done utilizing a Dacron^R tape suture as shown. These attachments can be advanced distally and should also be placed slightly anteriorly to facilitate the final anterior capsule closure. Lesions of the shoulder cuff can be evaluated and treated as desired.

The deltoid and pectoral muscles are brought together with absorbable sutures, as are the subcutaneous tissues. The skin is closed over a Penrose drain or suction apparatus. A conforming dressing is placed over the wound, and the limb held in Velpeau type of dressing, or a sling and swathe.

Postoperative Care

The immediate postoperative care for the shoulder replacement procedure requires protection of the anterior capsular incision and the reattached shoulder cuff or deltoid muscles. Surgical variables may alter the postoperative plan and require further use of a Velpeau dressing, a shoulder spica cast or abduction brace. Most commonly, the extremity is positioned to avoid humeral abduction, to maintain some humeral flexion and to restrict motion with a sling-swathe dressing. When supine, the humerus should rest at the side on a foam wedge pillow placed under the arm to provide 20° of forward flexion of the shoulder; the forearm is placed across the chest. This position has been found satisfactory for patient comfort and for protecting the usual surgical repair. The patient is not usually expected to exercise the extremity until 3 to 5 days following surgery. Until that time, they are expected to accept the responsibility for

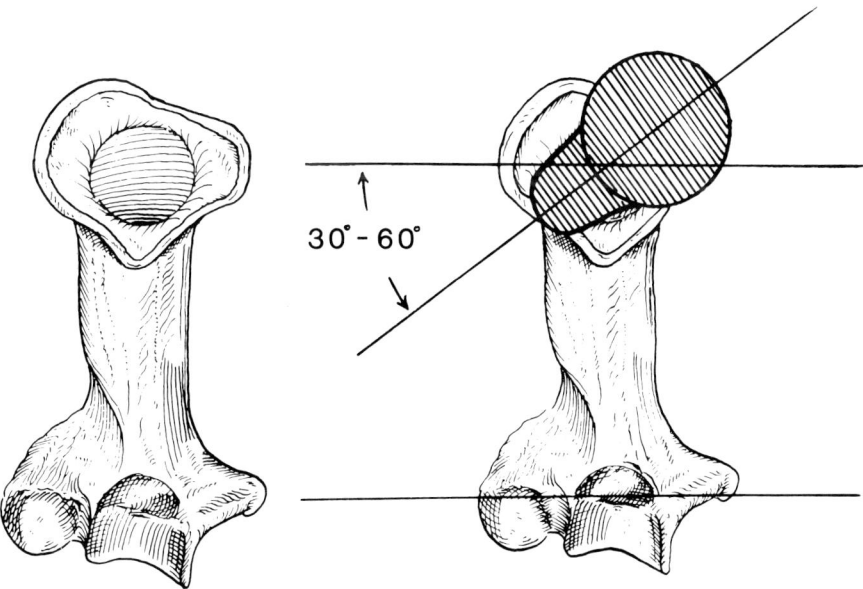

Figure 2H Axially oriented view of the humerus demonstrates the retroversion in which the implant is positioned relative to the transcondylar axis. With the implant tester inserted, the range of motion is tested, especially external rotation to evaluate the stability of the implant; 30° to 60° of external rotation are usually required.

Illustration and legend continued on the following page

218 / Surgery of the Shoulder

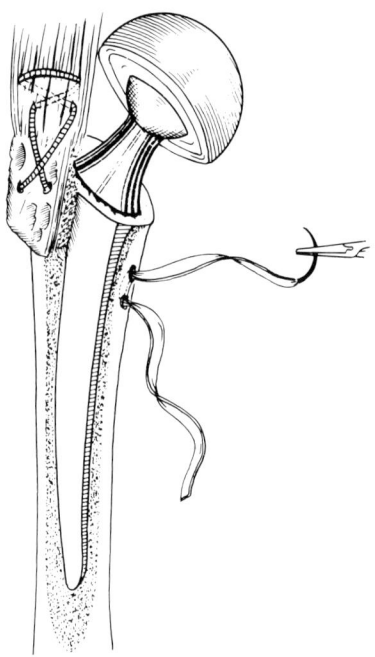

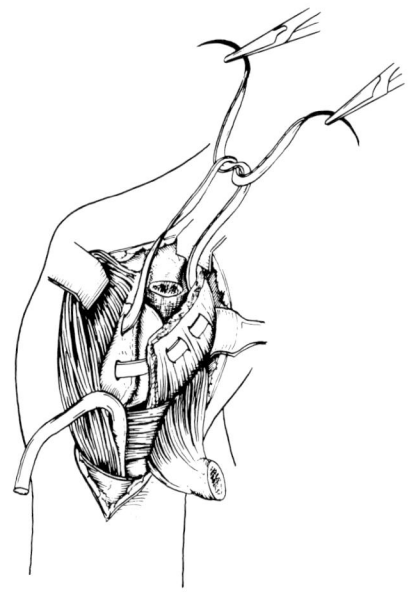

Figure 2J   The capsule is then closed with the Dacron^R tapes.

Figure 2I   One or two Dacron^R tapes are placed through drill holes for later closure of the capsule before cementing the implant in position. The intramedullary canal has been prepared in the usual manner to receive the cement. A bone graft or a silicone plug is used to block the intramedullary canal 2 cm from the tip of the implant to improve the cementing technique.

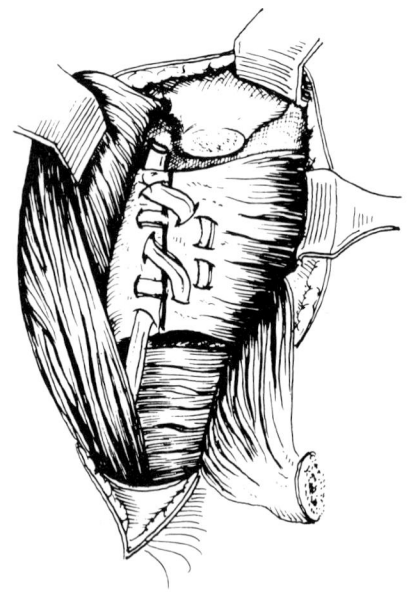

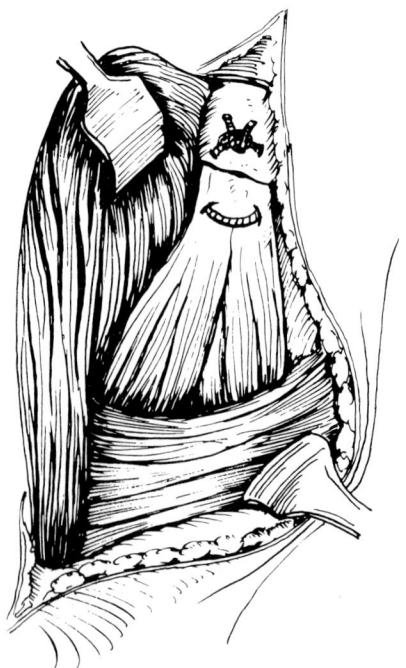

Figure 2K   The biceps tendon can be interwoven to provide fixation for the tendon and improve the capsular strength. Further closure can be done with heavy absorbable sutures. The closure is tested for stability of the implant by carrying the extremity through its range of motion.

Figure 2L   The coracoid process is reattached as shown and the muscle, subcutaneous tissues and skin are reapproximated; silicone drains are placed subcutaneously.

maintaining the position described and to learn to relax the muscles, avoiding tension in the neck, upper back and shoulder.

Three to five days postoperatively, an exercise program of passive forward flexion is started and carried out for 5-minute periods, 8 to 10 times daily; this is done in a supine position. During this period, the patient may ambulate with the arm placed in an appropriate sling to maintain the described position. Support of the arm is continued with the positioning pillow, and the elbow is now extended with the palm up.

During the first six weeks, it is imperative that the patient avoid active flexion or abduction or leaning on the operated extremity during activities of daily living. Excessive external rotation may disrupt the operative repair of the anterior shoulder.

At one week postoperatively two circumduction exercises are added. The sling may be removed at meal time permitting limited hand activity.

At two weeks, the sling may usually be discarded. The patient may allow the arm to hang naturally at his side. The circumduction exercises are continued, enlarging the circles. Flexion exercises are now done in a standing position and are guided through a passive range of motion with the nonoperated hand. Guarded passive external rotation to 20° is started.

At four weeks, active exercise of hyperextension and internal rotation are started from a standing position.

At five weeks, horizontal external rotation is added, to the patient's tolerance. Passive pulley exercises are introduced in addition to the passive exercises.

At six weeks, progressive resistive isometric exercises are initiated in forward flexion, internal and external rotation. If the greater tuberosity is intact, abduction exercises may also be started at this time. The opposite hand may be used to provide resistance.

Moist or dry heat may be beneficial prior to the exercise program, followed by pendulum and pulley exercises for relaxation, gradually progressing to the more difficult motions. If a greater range of motion is desired, the active exercises of forward flexion, external rotation and flexion with abduction can be done more vigorously.

At 12 weeks, active abduction of the shoulder is encouraged if there has been osteotomy and reattachment of the tuberosity. At this time, the patient is expected to achieve 70 percent of the normal range of motion in shoulder flexion and external rotation. Patients are encouraged to continue daily exercises up to one year postoperatively to maintain the range of motion and to develop additional strength.

It is imperative that the patient keep in close contact with his therapist. Twice daily visits by the therapist are routine while the patient is in the hospital, and, after discharge, the patient should be seen every week for two months. Visits may be spaced at greater and greater intervals, up to two years. The physiotherapy program and the willingness of the patient to follow through with the prescribed exercises to strengthen the muscles are very important to the success of the procedure. A patient guide has been developed so that patients will be well acquainted with the sequence of events that take place postoperatively.[16]

CLINICAL EVALUATION

Materials

The bipolar shoulder device was implanted by the investigator in 15 shoulders of 14 patients between November 1976 and July 1981 at Blodgett Memorial Medical Center in Grand Rapids, Michigan (Table 1). The follow-up period ranged from 14 to 75 months, with an average of 41 months. All patients, but 3, had a follow-up of more than

TABLE 1 Shoulder Implant Study—Swanson Design Bipolar

Case	Sex	Age at Surgery	Diagnosis	Follow-up Period (mos.)	Greater Tuberosity Transfer
1	F	56	RA*	75	+
2	F	64	RA	74	+
3	F	60	RA	69	−
4	F	54	RA	46	+
5	F	55	RA	33	+
6	F	65	RA	21	+
7	F	60	RA	27	+
8	M	69	RA	25	+
				14	+
9	F	74	RA	17	+
10	F	49	post-trauma + OA**	63	+
11	F	71	OA	44	+
12	M	74	OA	43	−
13	F	55	OA	34	−
14	M	66	OA	30	−

*RA = rheumatoid arthritis
**OA = osteoarthritis

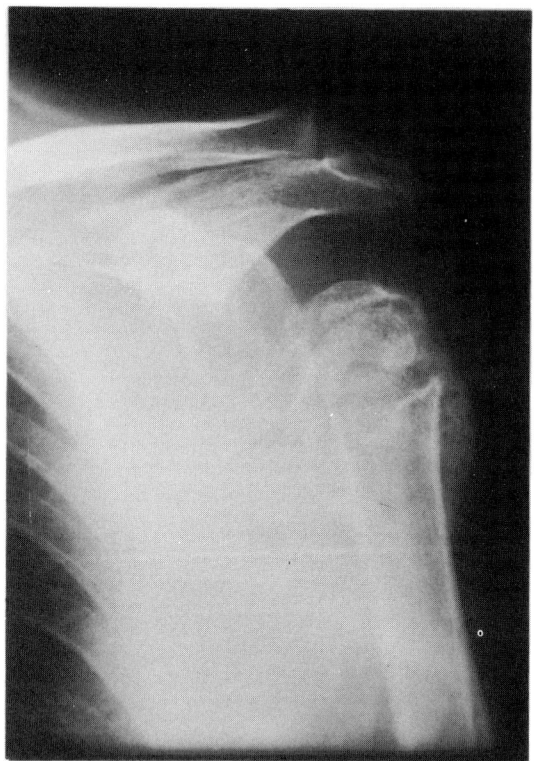

Figure 3A Preoperative radiogram of the shoulder of a 74-year-old male presenting with severe pain and disability of the shoulder secondary to osteoarthritis (Case #12).

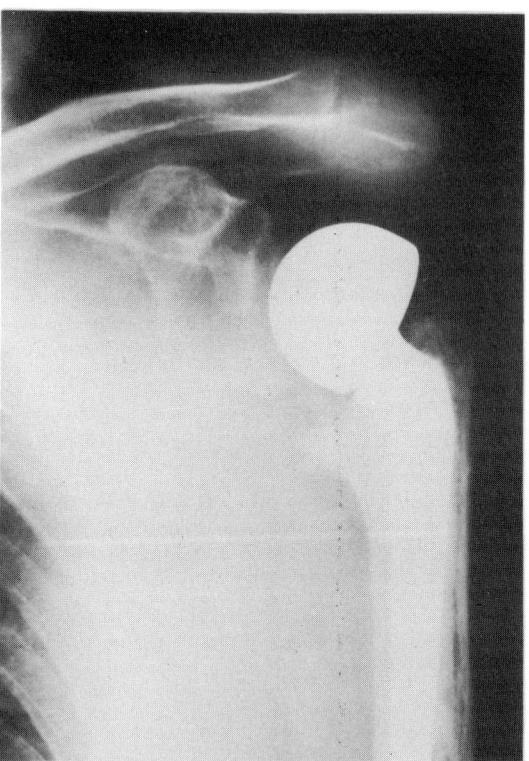

Figure 3B Three and a half years postoperative radiogram of shoulder in Figure 3A.

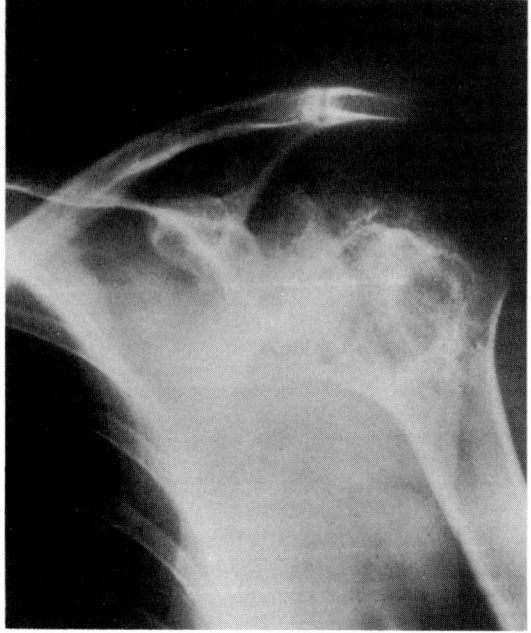

Figure 4A Preoperative radiogram showing the severe destruction of the humeral head and glenohumeral articulation of a 49-year-old woman who presented a post traumatic aseptic necrosis of the humeral head with acromioclavicular joint arthritis (Case #10).

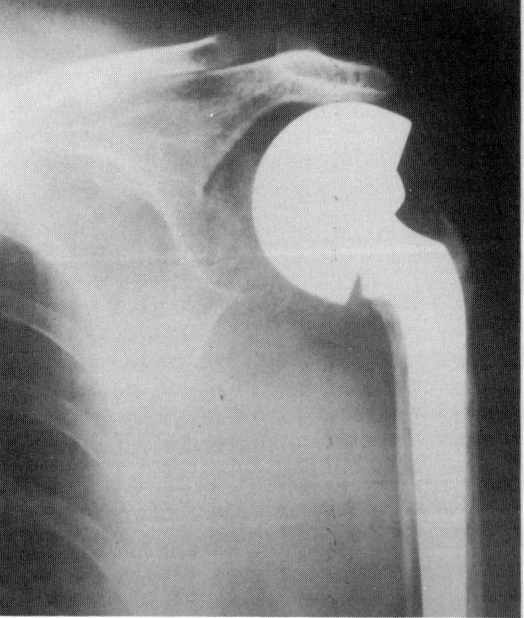

Figure 4B Five years postoperative radiogram showing the well tolerated bipolar shoulder implant used in Case 10. Note resection of the distal end of the clavicle. Three and a half years after surgery he remains painfree with an excellent functional result.

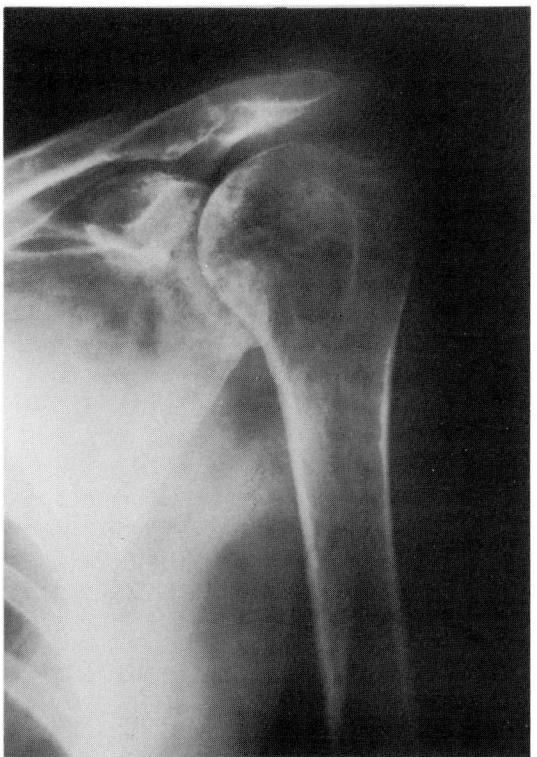

Figure 5A Preoperative radiogram showing erosive changes involving the glenohumeral joint with some tendency for vertical subluxation of the humeral head of a 60-year-old woman with rheumatoid arthritis presenting severe disability of the left shoulder including pain, loss of function and motion (Case #3).

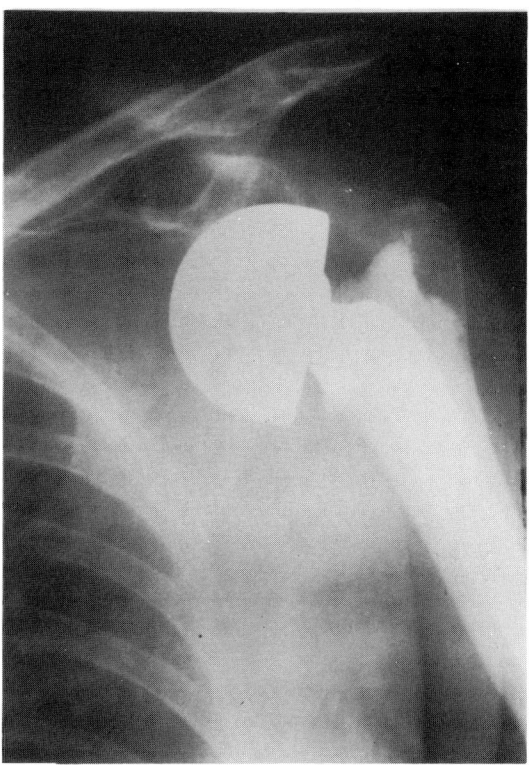

Figure 5B Two weeks following bipolar implant shoulder arthroplasty, the patient in Figure 5A presented a subcoracoid dislocation; attempts at reduction were unsuccessful. The radiogram shows the dislocation, which at four and a half years is not causing any pain and minimal loss of function. No neurovascular compromise occurred. Shoulder movement occurs between the metal ball and the polyethylene insert.

2 years. Of these three, two died of cancer and one in an automobile accident (Cases 6, 8, 9). Nine patients had chronic rheumatoid arthritis and five had osteoarthritis. One patient with rheumatoid disease had bilateral shoulder implants. Of the 14 patients, 11 were female and 3 male, their ages ranging from 49 to 74 years old with the average being 62. Severe pain at rest was the preoperative complaint in all patients. The majority of patients either had markedly limited or total inability to use the shoulder for activities of daily living through deformity and lack of range of motion (Table 2).

The bipolar implant arthroplasty method included osteotomy and distal reattachment of the greater tuberosity in eleven shoulders with a Bristow-type transfer of the conjoined short head of the biceps and coracobrachialis in two cases; the long head of the biceps was used to reinforce the anterior capsule in all cases.

Methods of Evaluation

Following surgery, careful follow-up evaluations were obtained; these included a clinical and a radiographic study.

A method of evaluation of the clinical results was devised to obtain more standard and accurate records. This included evaluation of pain, activities of daily living and shoulder range of motion. A certain number of points, up to a maximum of ten, was given in each category of evaluation according to the result obtained (Table 3).

The sum of points obtained in each category would correspond to the patient's "shoulder score." According to the score obtained, the results could then be classified as excellent (28–30), good (23–27.9), fair (18–22.9), and poor (<18).

The radiographic study included standard AP and lateral views taken preoperatively, immedi-

TABLE 2 Comparison of Pre- and Postoperative Range of Motion

Case	Pain Pre	Pain Post	A.D.L. Pre	A.D.L. Post	Abduction Pre	Abduction Post	Extension Pre	Extension Post	Flexion Pre	Flexion Post	Int. Rotation Pre	Int. Rotation Post	Ext. Rotation Pre	Ext. Rotation Post	Shoulder Score
1	2	8	2	8	30	90	10	30	30	90	30	90	10	25	25.6
2	2	8	2	4	25	30	15	30	10	60	60	30	10	30	17.8
3	2	8	2	6	40	65	15	45	40	60	60	90	10	30	20.5
4	2	10	4	8	50	80	25	30	85	110	0	80	25	30	27.0
5	2	10	4	8	15	60	20	60	70	70	90	90	15	45	26.2
6	2	10	4	8	30	90	20	45	60	90	30	90	20	30	27.8
7	2	10	6	8	60	90	20	45	70	100	85	80	20	50	28.0
8	2	8	4	8	50	65	20	45	60	80	30	70	10	30	24.2
	2	10	4	8	45	70	60	30	70	90	20	20	60	20	26.8
9	2	8	4	8	45	50	20	50	45	55	0	80	0	15	22.6
10	2	10	4	10	40	70	30	50	90	100	45	80	0	60	29.4
11	2	8	4	8	35	45	30	45	30	70	60	75	40	15	23.6
12	2	10	6	10	20	60	15	20	45	80	60	90	10	10	27.2
13	2	8	4	6	30	90	40	45	50	60	90	90	30	20	21.6
14	2	8	6	10	45	100	35	45	135	150	0	90	30	20	27.6
Average	2	8.9	4	7.9	37	70	25	41	59	78	44	79	19	27	25.0

TABLE 3 Shoulder Score System Devised by Swanson

ROM Score (10 pts.)			Pain Score (10 pts.)	
	Points	ROM	Points	Degree
Abduction (2 pts.)	0.4	<20°	10	Pain free
	0.8	21–40	8	Minimal pain after heavy work
	1.2	41–60	6	Pain with daily activity
	1.6	61–80	4	Pain with shoulder motion
			2	Pain at rest
Extension (1 pt.)	0.2	<0°		
	0.4	0–10	ADL* Score (10 pts.)	
	0.6	11–20	Points	Activity
	0.8	21–30	10	Independent, normal activities
Flexion (5 pts.)	1	<20°	8	Slight restrictions for heavy work overhead activity
	2	21–40		
	3	41–60	6	Most activities of daily living
	4	61–80	4	Light activities only, requiring assistance for some activities of daily living
Int. Rotat. (1 pt.)	0.2	<20°	2	Inability to use shoulder for function through deformity or lack of ROM
	0.4	21–40		
	0.6	41–60		
	0.8	61–80	Shoulder Score (30 pts.)	
Ext. Rotat. (1 pt.)	0.2	<0°	Excellent	28–30 points
	0.4	0–10	Good	23–27.9
	0.6	11–20	Fair	18–22.9
	0.8	21–30	Poor	<18

*ADL: activities of daily living

ately and early after surgery and long-term follow-up views. A cinefluoroscopy was done in a few cases to evaluate the dynamics of motion.

Results

Pain relief was good or excellent in all shoulders; complete pain relief was reported by seven patients and minimal pain after heavy work was reported by seven patients in eight shoulders. All patients had increased function of the shoulder and reported a greater ability to perform activities. Three patients were restored to independent normal activity; nine patients presented only slight restriction for heavy work and overhead activity; only two patients were restricted to light activities. The average improvement of motion obtained after surgery was most encouraging. Postoperatively, the average abduction was 70°, an increase of 33° over the preoperative value; forward flexion was 78°, an increase of 19°; internal rotation was 79°, an increase of 35°; extension was 41°, an improvement of 16°; and external rotation was 27°, an increase of 8°. One patient who had had a stroke did not show as good a range of motion as the average (Case 2). No significant differences were noted between the results obtained in the rheumatoid and osteoarthritic patients. The results were also surprisingly similar whether the greater tuberosity was transferred distally (11 cases) or not (4 cases).

According to the "shoulder score," pain improved from a score of 2 before to 8.9 after surgery; activities of daily living improved from 4 before to 7.9 after surgery; and the range of motion improved from 6 points to 8.2 points after surgery. The average shoulder score improved from 12/30 before surgery to 25/30 after bipolar shoulder implant reconstruction, following an average follow-up period of 41 months.

Roentgenographically, the response of the glenoid and the superior coracoacromial arch to the implant was satisfactory, with no erosive changes. No clinical or roentgenographic loosening of the cement fixed implant stem occurred in the proximal humerus (Figs. 3, 4, and 5). Two complications occurred. Subcoracoid dislocation occurred one week postoperatively in one patient (Case 3); closed manipulation was unsuccessful.

A decision was made to leave it in that position as it seemed to function adequately. At five years follow-up, the patient has pain-free motion, most of which occurs at the polyethylene humeral ball interface, and no neurovascular compromise. One patient with progression of acromioclavicular arthritis in the operated shoulder required resection of the tip of the distal clavicle four years postoperatively with complete relief of pain (Case 10). We now recommend routine resection of the distal end of the clavicle in cases with radiographic evidence of arthritis.

REFERENCES

1. Amstutz HC, Sew Hoy AL, Clarke IC. UCLA anatomical total shoulder arthroplasty. Clin Orthop. 1981; 155:7–20.
2. Bateman JE. Single-assembly total hip prosthesis—preliminary report. Orthop Dig. 1974; 15–22.
3. Clayton ML, Ferlic DC. Surgery of the shoulder in rheumatoid arthritis. A report of nineteen patients. Clin Orthop. 1975; 106:166–174.
4. Cofield RH. Status of total shoulder arthroplasty. Arch Surg. 1977; 112:1088–1091.
5. Giliberty RP. A new concept of a bipolar prosthesis. Ortho Rev. 1974; 3:40–45.
6. Hughes M, Neer CS II. Glenohumeral joint replacement and postoperative rehabilitation. Phys Ther. 1975; 55: 850–858.
7. Lettin AWF, Scales JT. Total replacement arthroplasty of the shoulder in rheumatoid arthritis. J Bone Joint Surg. 1973; 55B:217.
8. Macnab I. Total shoulder replacement. J Bone Joint Surg. 1977; 59B:257.
9. Neer CS II. Replacement of the humeral head. Indications and operative technique. Surg Clin North Am. 1963; 43:1581–1597.
10. Neer CS II. Replacement arthroplasty for glenohumeral osteoarthritis. J Bone Joint Surg 1974; 56A:1–13.
11. Neer CS II, Watson KC, Stanton, FJ. Recent experience in total shoulder replacement. J Bone Joint Surg. 1982; 64A:319–337.
12. Post M, Haskell SA, Finder JG. Total shoulder replacement. J Bone Joint Surg. 1975; 57A:1171.
13. Smith-Peterson MN. Arthroplasty of the hip: New method. J Bone Joint Surg. 1939; 21:269–288.
14. Swanson AB. Implant arthroplasty in hand and upper extremity and its future. Surg Clin North Am. 1981; 61:369–382.
15. Swanson AB. Flexible Implant Resection Arthroplasty in the Hand and Extremities. St. Louis: CV Mosby, 1973.
16. Swanson AB, Leonard J, Ziemba B, DeBoer M. Postoperative care and exercise program: Swanson bipolar shoulder replacement—Patient Guide. Unpublished.

EXPERIENCE WITH THE NEER TOTAL SHOULDER REPLACEMENT

ALAN H. WILDE, M.D., LESTER S. BORDEN, M.D., and JOHN J. BREMS, M.D.

Arthrodesis of the shoulder has been the accepted means of treatment of many shoulder disorders, including osteoarthritis, traumatic arthritis, paralytic disorders, bacterial infections and tuberculosis.[1,2] While it is still the treatment of choice for tuberculosis, residuals of septic arthritis, and paralytic disorders such as brachial plexus palsy and poliomyelitis, the choice of arthrodesis for the treatment of arthritis of the glenohumeral joint may be questioned.[2,5] Arthrodesis is not usually recommended in rheumatoid arthritis due to the likely involvement of other joints in the upper extremities and due to the prolonged immobilization required.[4] In osteoarthritis, a pseudoarthrosis rate has been reported as high as 40 percent.[1] The use of replacement of the shoulder joint has the prospect of a more rapid and hopefully complete rehabilitation.[5,6]

CLINICAL DATA

Between May 8, 1975 and May 26, 1983, 120 Neer total shoulder replacements were performed at the Cleveland Clinic Hospital. This chapter reports a consecutive series of 44 operations in 38 patients which were performed from May 8, 1975 until November 29, 1979. Six patients had bilateral operations.

The age at surgery ranged from 34 to 82 years with a mean age of 58 years. The diagnosis at the time of surgery was rheumatoid arthritis in 20 patients, osteoarthritis in 12, and traumatic arthritis in 7. Juvenile rheumatoid arthritis, avascular necrosis of the humeral head, nonunion of a fracture of the neck of the humerus, an acute 4-part fracture and a failed Stanmore shoulder replacement were indications for surgery in one patient in each instance.

Previous surgical procedures on the involved shoulder had been performed in 7 patients (18 percent). A total of 14 procedures had been performed on these patients and 4 patients had had more than one operative procedure on their shoulders prior to the Neer total shoulder replacement. The previous operative procedures were open reduction and internal fixation in 4 patients and shoulder manipulation in 2. Biopsy, excision of the humeral head, osteotomy of the humerus, Mumford procedure, debridement of the shoulder joint, Stanmore shoulder replacement, removal of a Rush rod and one undefined procedure had been performed on one instance in each case.

Follow-up was obtained in 38 operations. Two patients had died since shoulder replacement, of causes unrelated to their surgery. There was no follow-up on 4 cases. The follow-up period averaged 36 months; the range was from 8 to 69 months. Data concerning pain, range of motion and ability to perform certain activities of daily living were obtained pre- and postoperatively according to the shoulder evaluation form devised by Dr. Charles S. Neer II.

OPERATIVE APPROACH

The approach that was used in the early part of the series was the classical anteromedial approach described by Thompson and Henry. The anterior deltoid was released from the clavicle and acromion. The subscapularis was sectioned near its insertion into the lesser tuberosity and the supraspinatus tendon was incised to aid in the operative exposure. The coracoacromial ligament was excised and the clavipectoral fascia released This approach to the shoulder joint was utilized in 23 operations.

Later, the new approach described by Dr. Neer was employed. In this approach, a long oblique incision was made from the coracoid process to the insertion of the deltoid muscle. The deltopectoral groove was identified and the cephalic vein was doubly ligated and excised. The deltoid was dissected from origin to insertion but not released. The coracoacromial ligament was excised and the clavipectoral fascia incised. The subscapularis was lengthened in a "Z" fashion leaving approximately 2 cm of the subscapularis tendon attached to the lesser tuberosity when an internal rotation contracture existed. The capsule was dissected from the subscapularis. In most instances it was not necessary to incise the supraspinatus tendon. In a few cases, approximately 1 cm of the supraspinatus was released.

A Neer anterior acromioplasty was performed with either approach if there was anterior impingement, and a Mumford clavicular resection was usually performed if there was osteoarthritis of the acromioclavicular joint, particularly if an osteophyte impinged on the rotator cuff.

The preparation of the humerus and the glenoid was the same in both groups. In order to properly identify the angle of resection of the humeral head, it was important to remove all overhanging osteophytes. Only a thin wafer of bone containing the articular surface of the humeral head was removed. This line of resection was made so that the humeral head prosthesis was inserted in 35 to 40 degrees of retroversion. The medullary canal of the humerus was opened with a long curette. Grooves for the flanges on the stem of the humeral prosthesis were made on the humerus. The size of the stem of the humeral component was determined by measuring the width of the intramedullary canal of the humerus on the preoperative x-ray. The humeral prostheses that were employed in this series were the long (23 mm) and short (15 mm) heads with either a ½ inch, ⅜ inch, or ¼ inch diameter stem. Methyl methacrylate was inserted into the humeral canal only when there was a tendency for the prosthesis to rotate. The humeral component was cemented in place in nine cases and not cemented in 35.

A high density polyethylene glenoid component with an intramedullary stem was used in all cases. Only one size was available. All of the glenoid components were cemented in place with methyl methacrylate. The glenoid was prepared by removing any residual articular cartilage. The subchondral plate was preserved to give support to the glenoid component; removal of the subchondral plate would jeopardize the support and fixation of the glenoid component. A slot was cut into the glenoid. This was started with a high speed buff. Once the subchondral plate was penetrated, a curette was used to open the medullary canal of the scapula. It is helpful to depress the humeral head with a round Hohman retractor placed beneath the posterior portion of the glenoid in order to more easily prepare the medullary canal of the glenoid. It is quite easy to perforate the posterior cortex of the scapula if the proper angle for entering the medullary canal of the scapula is not used; a small curved curette is helpful in order to avoid this problem. Additional fixation can be obtained if the bone of the base of the coracoid is curetted. The glenoid and medullary canal of the scapula are lavaged with an irrigating system and dried with a sponge containing sterile 10 volumes percent hydrogen peroxide. The hydrogen peroxide is used to provide hemostasis before inserting the methyl methacrylate. After cementing the glenoid component and inserting the humeral prosthesis, the shoulder is reduced. The subscapularis is repaired; the capsule is not repaired. The deltopectoral groove is sutured, and a suction catheter is inserted to prevent a hemarthrosis.

POSTOPERATIVE REHABILITATION

Rehabilitation following total shoulder replacement is demanding. An organized program that is well instructed to a patient who is cooperative and diligent in its implementation is essential. The postoperative regime described by Hughes and Neer has been instituted at the Cleveland Clinic.[3] The impression of those professional people in contact with the patients who have undergone shoulder replacement is that the program is easier and more effective for the patient who does not have release of the deltoid muscle or a significant portion of the supraspinatus. During the early part of the series, when the anterior deltoid and the rotator cuff were released, external rotation, abduction or active forward elevation could not be started before the rotator cuff and deltoid attachment had healed or until 8 weeks postoperatively. With the new approach and the preservation of the deltoid and rotator cuff, abduction, external rotation and total elevation can be started within a few days after surgery. It is our impression that rehabilitation is more rapid with the new approach.

CLINICAL RESULTS

Pain Relief

Pain was subdivided into 6 categories. (1) Complete shoulder disability, interrupting sleep;

TABLE 1 Results of Shoulder Abduction

	No. of Operations	Range	Average	%
Gained	22	10°–160°	63°	79
Same	2			7
Lost	4	5°–25°	14°	14
Not Measured	10			
Total	38			

TABLE 2 Results of Total Elevation

	No. of Operations	Range	Average	%
Gained	31	5°–155°	68°	86
Same	1			3
Lost	4	15°–25°	20°	11
Not Measured	2			
Total	38			

(2) marked with serious limitation of shoulder activity, occasionally requiring medication and interfering with sleep; (3) moderate, interfering with some activities; (4) Only after unusual activity but disappears quickly; (5) Slight or occasional, no compromise in activity; (6) None. Using this scheme, it was found that postoperatively, 29 percent of patients had complete pain relief; 42 percent had almost complete relief of pain (category 5); 21 percent were improved (categories 3 & 4); and 8 percent had no relief.

Range of Motion

The results of shoulder abduction are shown in Table 1. In the early part of the series, abduction was not measured in 10 operations. Total elevation was measured in most cases as abduction is a combination of both elevation and rotation. Later, abduction was also included in the measurements as many surgeons are used to evaluating shoulder motion in that manner. It can therefore be seen that 79 percent of patients gained an average of 63° of abduction following shoulder replacement. An average of 14° of motion was lost in 14 percent of cases and 7 percent remained the same.

Total elevation was measured with the patient in the recumbent position in order to fix the spine. The results are shown in Table 2.

The results regarding external rotation are shown in Table 3.

The results concerning internal rotation are shown in Table 4.

The majority of patients achieved a greater range of motion postoperatively, especially in total elevation, external rotation and abduction. To a lesser extent there was also a gain in internal rotation.

Complications

There were five complications of the shoulder surgery in three patients. There was one probable infection manifested by heterotopic bone formation and chronic pain. There were three anterior dislocations of the humeral components in two patients. There was one patient with gross loosening of the glenoid component.

One patient dislocated the prosthesis on two occasions. She disrupted her rotator cuff repair and deltoid repair. She originally had a tear of the rotator cuff and a nonunion of a fracture of the humeral neck. This same patient also was the one with gross loosening of the glenoid component. The second patient who dislocated her prosthesis had had a Stanmore shoulder replacement. Her rotator cuff was found to be extensively scarred and her deltoid muscle was found to have been de-

TABLE 3 Results of External Rotation

	No. of Operations	Range	Average	%
Gained	32	5°–90°	40°	84
Same	3			8
Lost	3	10–30°	20°	8
Total	38			

TABLE 4 Results of Internal Rotation

	No. of Operations	%
Increased	25	70
Same	11	30
Decreased	0	0
Not Measured	2	

tached at the time of surgery. All three dislocations were related to problems with both the rotator cuff and the deltoid muscle.

Subsequent Surgery

Four additional surgical procedures were required in three patients. The combination of Neer acromioplasty and Mumford clavicular resection were required in two patients with osteoarthritis in which there was chronic pain due to impingement of the rotator cuff by the anterior acromion and osteophytes originating from the acromioclavicular joint. It was also necessary to recement a loose glenoid component and repair the rotator cuff in a patient who had disrupted the repair and dislocated the humeral prosthesis postoperatively. This same patient dislocated again and the glenoid component became grossly loose and was removed.

RADIOGRAPHIC EVALUATION

Humeral Component

Humeral components were cemented in place in nine patients and were not cemented in 29 patients. In 5 patients in which the humeral component was cemented in place, there were no follow-up x-rays obtained, leaving only 4 operations with radiographs for evaluation. This number was insufficient to provide any meaningful information.

In the 29 humeral components that were not cemented, sclerosis was noted at the tip of the humeral component in 44 percent. Forty-eight percent had no sclerosis at the tip of the prosthesis and 8 percent had sclerosis completely around the prosthesis. Subsidence was not observed during the period of follow-up. There were no fractures of the stem of the humeral component. Rotation of the humeral component was not observed.

Glenoid Component

An evaluation was made of the thickness of the radiolucent zone at the bone-cement interface around the glenoid component. This was measured immediately postoperatively and also at the time of follow-up. Table 5 shows the radiolucency found immediately postoperatively; this would be related to the cement technique itself. The bone-cement interface of the glenoid component, for purposes of evaluation, was divided into three zones (Fig. 1). Zone 1 comprised the interface

TABLE 5 Radiolucency of Glenoid Component Immediately Postoperative

	Zone 1	Zone 2	Zone 3
Percentage of cases	75	28	14
Average radiolucency	0.89 mm	0.35 mm	0.25 mm
Range	0–3 mm	0–4 mm	0–4 mm

between the subchondral bone of the glenoid and the collar of the prosthesis. The stem of the prosthesis was divided into 2 equal portions representing Zones 2 and 3.

Zone 1 includes the area between the shoulder of the glenoid component and the glenoid itself. It would not be surprising that a radiolucent zone would appear in this area as the hard subchondral surface does not permit interdigitation with the cement. There was a 28 percent incidence of radiolucency in Zone 2 and 14 percent in Zone 3. Most of the fixation could be expected to occur at Zones 2 and 3.

The radiolucency about the glenoid component was also evaluated at the time of follow-up examination. From Table 6, it can be seen that radiolucency increased in the number of cases to 89 percent in Zone 1, 75 percent in Zone 2, and 67 percent in Zone 3. The amount of average radiolucency in Zones 1, 2 and 3 also increased. This would indicate radiographic loosening.

The completeness or incompleteness of radiolucency about the glenoid component was also determined. The radiolucency was complete in 68 percent of cases, incomplete in 25 percent of cases, and there was no radiolucent zone in only 7 percent of cases.

As there was a significant percentage of cases that had radiolucency immediately postopera-

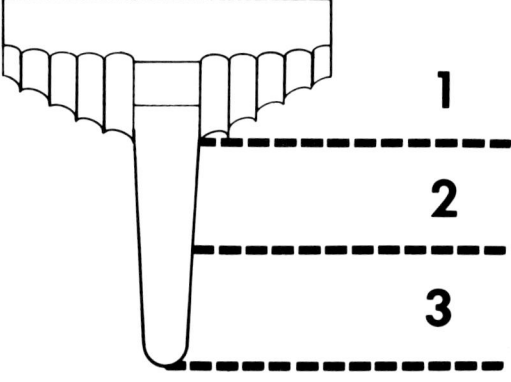

Figure 1 Bone-cement interface of glenoid component.

TABLE 6 Radiolucency of Glenoid Component at Follow-Up

	Zone 1	Zone 2	Zone 3
Percentage of cases	89	75	67
Average radiolucency	1.4 mm	1.1 mm	1.1 mm
Range	0–4 mm	0–5 mm	0–4 mm

tively, it would seem that improvements in cement technique might decrease the radiographic incidence of loosening in the future.

No mechanical failures of either the glenoid component or of the humeral component were noted in the postoperative follow-up.

DISCUSSION

The presence of active infection or a Charcot's arthropathy have been considered to be contraindications for this procedure.

The results thus far have been encouraging with regards to pain relief and improvement in range of motion. The high incidence of radiolucency at the bone–cement interface surrounding the glenoid component is disturbing. A significant portion of the cases with radiolucency are related to cement technique. Modification of the cement technique should decrease the incidence of this radiographic finding. The radiolucency at the bone-cement interface has not yet proven to be a significant problem. A longer follow-up is necessary in order to evaluate the significance of this finding.

It is our impression that results have been improved with the new approach described by Neer in which the deltoid muscle and the rotator cuff are not disturbed. The range of motion has been achieved more rapidly.

Soft tissue contractures should be released at the time of surgery. If there is an impingement by the anterior acromion, then an anterior acromioplasty should be performed at the time of replacement. Similarly, if there is any impingement of the rotator cuff by osteophytes originating from the acromioclavicular joint, a Mumford procedure should be performed. The operation is difficult and the results have improved as the surgeon's experience has increased.

REFERENCES

1. Barton NJ. Arthrodesis of the shoulder for degenerative conditions. J Bone Joint Surg. 1972; 54A:1759–1764.
2. Bateman JE. The Shoulder and Neck. Philadelphia: WB Saunders, 1972:269–292
3. Hughes M, Neer CS. Glenohumeral joint replacement and postoperative rehabilitation. Phys Ther 1975; 55:850–858.
4. Neer CS. The rheumatoid shoulder. In: Cruess RL, Mitchell N, eds. Surgery of Rheumatoid Arthritis. Philadelphia: JB Lippincott, 1971:117–125.
5. Neer CS. Replacement arthroplasty for glenohumeral osteoarthritis. J Bone Joint Surg. 1974; 56A:1–13.
6. Neer CS, Cruess RL, Sledge CB, Wilde AH. Total shoulder replacement, a preliminary report. Orthop Trans. 1977; 1:244–245.

TOTAL SHOULDER ARTHROPLASTY: ASSOCIATED DISEASE OF THE ROTATOR CUFF, RESULTS, AND COMPLICATIONS

ROBERT H. COFIELD, M.D.

Total shoulder arthroplasty can be used to treat various arthritic conditions. During the 7-year period 1975–1982, 205 Neer arthroplasties[1] were performed to treat rheumatoid arthritis, osteoarthritis, traumatic arthritis, cuff-tear arthritis, shoulders with previous operations that had failed, avascular necrosis, old sepsis, ankylosing spondylitis, and radiation necrosis. Of these shoulders, 165 (80%) were operated on for the treatment of rheumatoid arthritis, osteoarthritis, or traumatic arthritis due to old fractures or fracture-dislocations. This presentation reviews the pathologic findings in the rotator cuffs in the initial 176 total shoulder arthroplasties, analyzes the probability of prosthetic failure in these 176 shoulders, and reports in some depth the results and complications of 73 total shoulder arthroplasties performed between December 1975 and December 1979 for treatment of the three major diagnostic categories mentioned above.

DISEASE OF THE ROTATOR CUFF

When total shoulder arthroplasty was in its infancy slightly more than a decade ago, disease of the rotator cuff was expected to be parallel and proportional to the degree of disease of the intraarticular cartilage. Experience has shown, however, that this expectation is not necessarily true. The pathologic findings identified at operation in the initial 176 Neer II total shoulder arthroplasties are presented in Table 1. Tears of the rotator cuff are unusual in osteoarthritis but, when present, are usually typical of subacromial impingement and are confined to the supraspinatus tendon. Patients with rheumatoid arthritis often have thinning of their rotator cuff tendons with some scar formation. Only 18 of the 66 patients with rheumatoid arthritis had actual tearing of their rotator cuffs. Pathologic findings in rotator cuffs vary considerably in trauma, but tearing is usually associated with displaced or non-united tuberosities of the humerus. Cuff-tear arthritis is thought to be arthritis of the glenohumeral joint secondary to longstanding and severe disease of the rotator cuff; by definition all shoulders with cuff-tear arthritis will have massive tearing of the rotator cuff. Of the 176 shoulders, 48 (27%) had tears of the rotator cuff present. Not all of the tears were large; but they did vary in size, as do tears of the rotator cuff in the absence of glenohumeral arthritis. In 10 shoulders, the tears were small (less than 1 cm in greatest length), in 10 they were medium (1–3 cm), in 7 they were large (3–5 cm), and in 21 they were massive (more than 5 cm). Repair of the tears required tendon-to-tendon or tendon-to-bone suturing in 14, subscapularis transposition in 17, a local muscle transfer in 2, fascia lata grafting in 9, and a cup-shaped glenoid component in 6. Thus, of the 176 shoulders, only 17 (9.7%) necessitated some unusual or complex surgical technique to treat the tears of the rotator cuff. This figure speaks quite strongly for the use of an unconstrained or resurfacing prosthesis for most persons who require total shoulder arthroplasty.

SURVIVAL OF THE PROSTHESES

The survival of arthroplastic prostheses can be analyzed in much the same way as oncology patients are analyzed for survival. Although this method is not the usual one for analyzing total joint replacement, it does offer some advantages in that all patients can be included in the analysis up to their most recent time of follow-up and trends can be more easily appreciated.

TABLE 1 Pathologic Findings in Rotator Cuffs (176 Shoulders)

Diagnosis	Pathologic Findings			Osteotomy of Tuberosity
	None	Thin	Torn	
Osteoarthritis	46	1	6	
Rheumatoid arthritis	11	37	18	
Old trauma	6	2	3	10
Cuff-tear arthritis			14	
Miscellaneous	13	2	7	
	76	42	48	10

Of the initial 176 Neer II total shoulder replacements, 56 have been followed up for less than 1 year, 34 for 1 to 2 years, 27 for 2 to 3 years, 27 for 3 to 4 years, 23 for 4 to 5 years, 8 for 5 to 6 years, and 1 for 6 to 7 years. Of these shoulders, eight (4.5%) have necessitated a major reoperation: three for the treatment of early dislocation associated with retearing of the rotator cuff, three for glenoid loosening (at which time a glenoid component was recemented), one for paralysis of the axillary nerve, and one for infection. The probability of prosthetic failure (that is, the need for a major reoperation) from the time of surgery to the most recent follow-up evaluation or reoperation was determined with the use of nonparametric estimation (Fig. 1). Although the current need for a major reoperation in these 176 shoulders is only 4.5 percent, analysis of this graph reveals that should the current experience continue, the need for a major reoperation when all shoulders have been followed up for 5 years will be 9.6 percent.

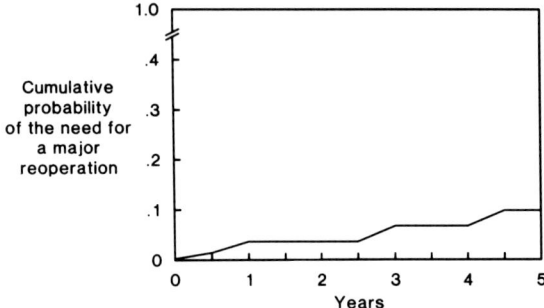

Figure 1 Failure of total shoulder arthroplasty (nonparametric estimation). Of 176 Neer total shoulder arthroplasties, 8 (4.5%) have necessitated a major reoperation. This graph relates chance for prosthetic failure after operation (that is, the need for a major reoperation) from the time of operation to the most recent follow-up evaluation or reoperation. The cumulative probability of failure by 5 years postoperatively, given the information currently available, is 9.6%.

RESULTS AND COMPLICATIONS

Between December 1975 and December 1979, 77 shoulders were treated with a Neer II total shoulder arthroplasty because of osteoarthritis, rheumatoid arthritis, or traumatic arthritis due to old fractures or fracture-dislocations. At least a physical examination at 1 year and a roentgenographic examination at 2 years after operation were performed on 73 (95%) of the shoulders. The average duration of follow-up at the most recent physical examination was 39 months (range, 12–73 months); and the average duration of follow-up at the most recent roentgenographic evaluation was 46 months (range, 24–77 months).

The study group included 29 patients with 31 shoulders treated for osteoarthritis, 24 patients with 29 shoulders treated for rheumatoid arthritis, and 12 patients with 13 shoulders treated for traumatic arthritis. The average age of the patients at the time of operation was 56 years (range, 22–75 years). There were 39 women and 26 men. Previous operations had been performed on 14 shoulders, 8 of which had had fracture-fragment repositioning for old fractures or fracture-dislocations. Preoperatively, pain was moderate in 22 shoulders and severe in 51. The average preoperative active abduction was 76° and the average preoperative external rotation was 22°.

An anterior surgical approach was used. Early in the series, anteromedial exposure with release of the deltoid origins on the clavicle and anterior acromion was used; later in the series, an extended deltopectoral exposure was used; and presently, the anteromedial exposure is used only when osteotomy of a greater tuberosity and repositioning or extensive repair of a rotator cuff are necessary. The humeral component is seated in 30° of retroversion, and as much glenoid bone as possible is preserved. Subchondral bone is roughened but not removed; and in cutting the glenoid slot, a minimal amount of bone is removed from the subchondral region. Soft cancellous bone is curetted before the cement and component are introduced.

Postoperatively, most shoulders are placed in an immobilizer, as were 53 shoulders in this series. An abduction splint was used to position 19 shoulders, and a spica cast was used to support one shoulder. In this series, patient cooperation with postoperative physical therapy was good in 44 shoulders, fair in 24, and poor in five.

Associated procedures performed at the time of prosthetic replacement, when the pathologic findings dictated their necessity, were anterior acromioplasty in 38 shoulders, distal excision of the clavicle in 23, and repair of the rotator cuff in 12. These procedures included a fascia graft in three, osteotomy and repositioning of a tuberosity in eight, and biceps tenodesis in three.

Analysis of the rotator cuffs revealed that 32 shoulders did not have significant disease, the rotator cuff was thinned in 21 shoulders, the tuberosities were malunited in 8, and the cuff had major tears in 8 and minor tears in 4. Thus, 20 of the shoulders necessitated either repositioning of a tuberosity or repair of a tear of the rotator cuff. This amount of disease of the rotator cuff parallels that seen in the larger group of 176 shoulders.

Postoperatively, 59 of the shoulders had no pain or slight pain, and 67 of the shoulders had no pain, slight pain, or pain only after unusually vigorous activity. Postoperatively, the average active abduction was 120° for the entire group. In those patients with osteoarthritis, the average active abduction was 141°; in those with rheumatoid arthritis, it was 102°; and in those with traumatic arthritis, it was 109°. Of the 73 shoulders, 28 had between 150° and 180° of active abduction, 9 had between 120° and 149°, 16 had between 90° and 119°, 16 had between 60° and 89°, and 4 had less than 60°. The amount of active abduction was associated with the severity of disease of the rotator cuff. The average active abduction of the shoulders according to severity of disease was as follows: no significant disease, 141°; minor tearing of the rotator cuff, 158°; thin rotator cuffs, 102°; osteotomies of a tuberosity, 93°; and major tearing of the rotator cuff, 63°. Twenty shoulders had active abduction of less than 90°. This degree of active abduction was usually associated with severe progressive rheumatoid arthritis, the presence of complications, or with major disease of the rotator cuff.

Rotational movements were also improved: the average postoperative external rotation was 48°, and internal rotation improved from the preoperative median ability to touch the sacrum to the postoperative median ability to touch L-2.

Limb function was assessed by asking the patients if they could accomplish certain activities easily or only with slight difficulty. Table 2 analyzes these preoperative and postoperative capabilities. The preoperative to postoperative change in limb function was statistically significant for all activities except for the ability to do usual work.

When asked for their response about the operation, patients stated that their shoulders were much better (51), better (16), the same (4), or worse (2)—thus, 67 shoulders benefited from operation.

TABLE 2 Preoperative and Postoperative Limb Function (71 Shoulders)

Function	% Able to Accomplish Task	
	Preoperatively	Postoperatively
Eat with utensil	80	99
Dress	69	97
Perform activities of personal hygiene	68	96
Sleep on side	56	90
Carry 10–15 lb	68	85
Do usual work	76	83
Comb hair	38	79
Use limb at shoulder level	25	75

There were 14 complications in 13 shoulders. Five shoulders had retearing of the rotator cuff. Only one of these retears was associated with significant pain; the other shoulders had less ample function than those of the remainder of the patient group but the patients did not want to consider reoperation because of the satisfying degree of pain relief. Three shoulders had glenoid loosening; in two shoulders, a reflex dystrophy developed postoperatively; one shoulder had an intraoperative injury to the axillary nerve; one shoulder had a hematoma postoperatively; one middle-aged man had a nonfatal pulmonary embolus; and one shoulder with traumatic arthritis in which the tuberosities were repositioned had nonunion of a tuberosity.

Five reoperations were necessary: three to replace loose glenoid components at 48, 70, and 73 months postoperatively, one to perform a trapezius transfer in the patient with the injury to the axillary nerve, and one to evacuate the postoperative hematoma. Figure 2 illustrates the usual changes that are seen when the glenoid component loosens. Histologic study at the time of operation showed an intense histiocytic response in the fibrous tissue that surrounded the loosened component and fragmented methyl methacrylate.

In addition to the three shoulders with glenoid loosening which required revision, roentgenograms of five other shoulders showed indications of glenoid loosening. This loosening was revealed by a shift in the position of the glenoid component in four of the shoulders and by a 2 mm radiolucent line at the entire bone-cement interface in the other shoulder, which also had moderate pain. The di-

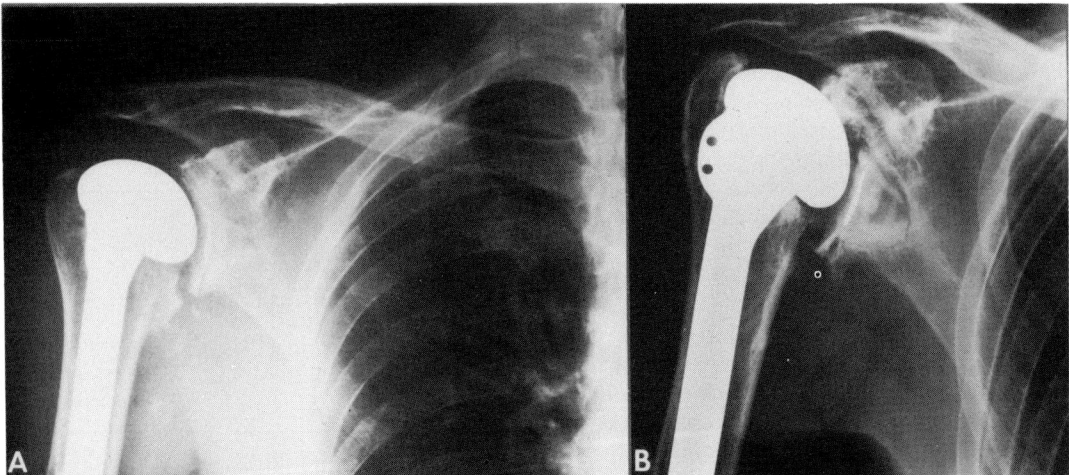

Figure 2 A. Roentgenogram of shoulder (40° posterior oblique view) of 67-year old man with osteoarthritis who had Neer II total shoulder arthroplasty (roentgenogram was obtained 1 month postoperatively). B. Roentgenogram of same shoulder 5 years postoperatively, showing medial migration of glenoid component and upward tilting of articular surface. Patient had moderate pain and underwent revision 6 years after initial operation.

agnoses for the eight shoulders with glenoid loosening were osteoarthritis in seven and rheumatoid arthritis in one.

Of the 65 shoulders without distinct roentgenographic evidence of loosening at the glenoid bone-cement junction, 52 showed some degree of radiolucent lines. In no instance, though, was this line more than 1.5 mm in width. Of the 52 shoulders with glenoid radiolucent lines, the lines were observed to begin between 0 and 2 weeks postoperatively in 14 shoulders, between 2 weeks and 2 months postoperatively in 17 shoulders, and more than 2 months postoperatively in 21 shoulders. The radiolucent lines at the glenoid bone-cement junction involved the entire interface in 24 of the 52 shoulders. Analysis of sequential roentgenograms in the 52 shoulders with radiolucent lines revealed stability of the lines in 35 shoulders, and the lines continue to progress in extent or thickness in 17 shoulders.

Of the 73 shoulders operated on between 1975 and 1979, the humeral component was cemented in only seven. Fifty humeri had no prosthetic-humeral or cement-humeral radiolucent lines. Of the humeri that did have radiolucent lines present, none was complete or more than 2 mm in width. Symptoms related to loosening of the humeral component have not been recognized.

One would conclude from this review that relief of pain and patient satisfaction are obtained with Neer II total shoulder replacement unless complications occur. Active abduction is dependent on disease of the rotator cuff and capsule, rehabilitation, and the avoidance of complications. The ability to do daily functions is significantly improved. Loosening of the glenoid component is a problem, but it occurs late.

We recommend the continued use of the resurfacing type of arthroplasty and also strongly recommend improvement in the design of the glenoid component. The role of replacement of the proximal humerus alone in the treatment of the arthritides needs to be carefully explored and defined.

SUMMARY

Between December 1975 and December 1982, 205 total shoulder arthroplasties were performed. Before the initiation of this series, disease of the rotator cuff was thought to be parallel and proportional to the degree of disease of the intra-articular cartilage. However, this belief was not true. In the initial 176 shoulders, tearing of the rotator cuff occurred in 48 (27%). Nonparametric estimation of survival of the prostheses was used for these 176 shoulders, which have been monitored for up to 7 years; only eight shoulders (4.5%) have required a major reoperation. However, if the current experience continues, failure of the prostheses will approximate 10 percent at 5 years.

Seventy-three total shoulder arthroplasties performed in 65 patients for the treatment of osteoarthritis, rheumatoid arthritis, or traumatic arthritis had an average follow-up of 46 months at the latest roentgenographic evaluation (range, 24–77 months). Postoperatively, pain was absent, slight, or moderate only after vigorous activities in 67 shoulders. The average active abduction increased from 76° to 120° (range, 30°–180°). The amount of abduction was related to the diagnosis and to the severity of disease of the rotator cuff. The average external rotation increased to 48° postoperatively (range, 0°–90°). Patients believed that the results of their operations were better or much better in 67 shoulders. Complications developed in 13 shoulders, and five reoperations were necessary: three to revise loose glenoid components, one to perform a muscle transfer, and one to evacuate a wound hematoma. Five additional glenoid components showed roentgenographic evidence of loosening. Of the 65 shoulders without evidence of glenoid loosening, 52 had some degree of radiolucent lines at the glenoid bone-cement junction.

REFERENCE

1. Neer CS II, Watson KC, Stanton FJ. Recent experience in total shoulder replacement. J Bone Joint Surg 1982; 64:319–337.

TEN YEARS OF EXPERIENCE WITH UNCONSTRAINED SHOULDER REPLACEMENT

E. ENGELBRECHT, M.D.

This account concerns a 10-year period during which shoulder arthroplasties of an unconstrained type have been performed. The results have led to changes in design and operative approach with a consequent lack of homogeneity but it has seemed appropriate at this stage to review the cases and conclude certain instructive points as a result. The earliest operations began with the Neer prosthesis in 1966 and the relatively small number of operations performed over a long period of time indicates that arthroplasty of the shoulder is uncommonly indicated and considerable time is needed to obtain a meaningful series for evaluation.[6] The lack of homogeneity and consequent difficulty in assessment of clinical results lies not only in the differing models used but in the many different preoperative conditions.

In nearly all shoulders selected for arthroplasty, destruction of the tendinous rotator cuffs and restriction in deltoid function must be expected especially when there have been previous operations. In unconstrained systems the pathological changes of the joint and lack of strong bone for firm fixation of the glenoid component prejudice fixation and stability. We have used various designs with different degrees of builtin restraints (Fig. 1, Table 1). Improvement in surgical technique has concentrated on the repair of the damaged rotator cuff with preservation of what remains as well as the anterior portions of the deltoid important for the restoration of function.[3,4,8]

OPERATIVE TECHNIQUE

It became apparent that a standard anterior approach, used routinely until 1978, may well jeopardize function of the anterior part of the deltoid and rotator cuff, particularly in revision cases. Poor active anteversion and abduction are likely. Accordingly, after 1978 we have used, exclusively, a modified dorsal Kocher approach which includes an osteotomy of the acromion.[5] The posterior part of the rotator cuff is detached from the tuberculum with a small bone lamella. This approach provides an excellent view of the joint while the anterior portions of the deltoid, the rotator cuffs and the tendon of the long head of the biceps are preserved intact. The anterior structures are also accessible and in some instances we attempt a capsular repair using lyophylised dura. Finally, rehabilitation is more rapid. Early follow-up indicates that function is improved and there is a reduced risk of dislocation (Fig. 2).

The anterior approach is used only in cases of fractures of the humeral head treated previously by internal fixation from in front, upper humeral head pseudoarthrosis and tumors in which special prostheses are required. After either approach the operated arm is immobilized in an abduction splint for 4-6 weeks before physiotherapy is instituted.

CLINICAL MATERIAL

110 primary shoulder replacements were performed from 1966 to 1983. Of these, 22 have required revision while four revisions have been performed on referred patients (Table 2). The relatively high number of revisions indicates clearly that shoulder replacement is still in the experimental phase.

Indications included traumatic arthritis with intractable pain, acute fracture dislocation in older patients, rheumatoid arthritis with severe destruction, osteoarthritis and tumors. Because of a particular interest in the treatment of infected hip and knee-endoprostheses with antibiotic-loaded acrylic cement, we included two cases of old osteomyelitis[2] (Table 2).

Contraindications to the use of an unconstrained prosthetic shoulder replacement were neurological lesions, axillary palsy, and gross destructions of the deltoid muscle because of feared loss of stability. In young patients only rheumatoid arthritis and bone tumors were regarded as justifiable indications for shoulder arthroplasty.

Arthrodesis/Arthroplasty / 235

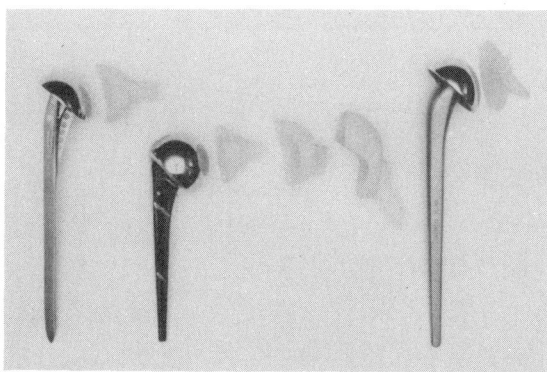

Figure 1 Different types of unconstrained designs used from 1966 to 1983.

TABLE 1 Different Types of Unconstrained Shoulder Replacements Used

1966–1974	Neer prosthesis	14
1971–1974	Neer prosthesis + "Stellbrink" cup	8
1974–1975	St.Georg prosthesis Mark I	17
1976–1979	St.Georg prosthesis Mark II	24
1979–1981	Endo-model with HDP cup	13
1979–1983	Endo-model hemiarthroplasty	37
1974–1983	Tumor endoprosthesis	8
1976–1982	Total humerus replacement	3

RESULTS

Due to the unhomogeneity of the clinical cases, detailed statistical evaluation of the results according to diagnosis is impossible. At the present time, the overall results offer some indication of what can be achieved with the unconstrained shoulder prosthesis with respect to pain and function and most importantly, where emphasis should be placed in further developments.

Fifty-one shoulder arthroplasties were evaluated in 45 patients at the time of review. The average follow-up was longer than four years, ranging from 1 to 8 years. Evaluation has been made with respect to pain and function (Table 3).

Pain

More than one-third of the patients in this series were pain-free and one-half reported minimal or tolerable discomfort, regarding their final result as a significant improvement over their preoperative state. Residual pain was located predominantly in the anterior capsule. In 14 percent of patients having residual pain this related to glenoid component loosening. Two patients had an axillary

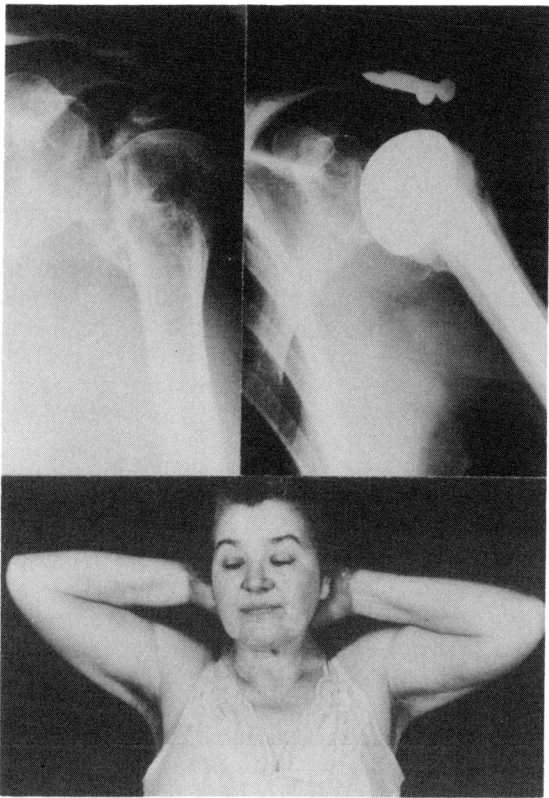

Figure 2 Conservative treatment of fractured dislocation. Severely restricted function (above left); hemiarthroplasty through a dorsoproximal approach (above right); pain-free function one year postop (below).

TABLE 2 Clinical Material—136 Operations

Indications	
Traumatic arthritis	30
Severe fracture dislocation	26
Rheumatoid arthritis	24
Osteoarthritis	15
Tumors	13
Osteomyelitis	2
Revisions	
Exchange of both components – our own patients	9
referred patients	4
Glenoid exchange to a special model	2
Removal of the glenoid cup + osteotomy of the glenoid + autogenous bone grafting	9
Removal of both components	2

TABLE 3
Clinical Results (51 arthroplasties in 46 patients) Follow-up: 1-8 years (mean 4 years)
Pain:
Painfree 36 % ⎫
Tolerable discomfort 50 % ⎬ 86 % remarkably improved
Severe pain 14 % ⎭
Gain in range of motion: (mean total value 80 %)
Retroversion 15°
Anteversion 15° hand-to-back 72 %
Abduction 25° hand-to-neck 42 %
Rotation 25°
Patient satisfied with surgery - 90 %

TABLE 4		
Complications 1966-1978 (N=99)		
Infection	2	
Glenoid loosening	31	(50 %)
Early antero-inferior dislocation	10	
Late antero-superior dislocation	6	
Late superior subluxation	7	
Topic bone formation	4	
1979-1983 (37 hemiarthroplasties)		
Late superior subluxation	2	

nerve palsy which had been present before operation.

Following experience with hemiarthroplasty over the past four years we have revised our assertion made in the early 1970's that pain relief could only be achieved when the articular surfaces of both sides were replaced. To date, no marked difference has been observed with respect to pain when the glenoid was not replaced. Further review is necessary for evaluation of later methods of management of the acetabulum (molding, osteotomy, autogenous bone grafting) comparable to the double osteotomy described by Benjamin.[1,7]

Function

We decided to measure total shoulder function because evaluation of function of the glenohumeral joint in isolation is not easy. The generally poor preoperative condition was improved by an average of only 15°-25° of range of motion; particularly discouraging was the small gain in the range of anteversion and abduction. The results of range of motion tests correspond generally to the typical tests of function: while hand-to-back and hand-to-shoulder was possible in 72 percent, hand-to-neck and care of hair was only possible in 42 percent. In nearly all patients with a small range of anteversion and abduction the anterior deltoid and the rotator cuff were grossly damaged contributing to instability and possible upward subluxation or even dislocation.

Complications

In a study of complications and failures are found the lesions which indicate pathways for improvement (Table 4). In two patients deep infection was controlled by removal of the entire prosthesis. Mechanical loosening only affected the glenoid component and the incidence relates strongly to the degree of congruency of the articulating surfaces. Thus, the glenoid component of the St. Georg Mark II prosthesis, a model with the greatest builtin restraint, had the highest rate of loosening. After a short to medium term follow-up period of 1 to 6 years 50 percent of all glenoid components were loose. In some of our earlier patients with glenoid loosening a special cup with additional support against the acromion was inserted.

During the last four years, we have removed only the loose glenoid component. The glenoid surface showed a large central defect and in most cases this was widened by longitudinal osteotomy in either the transverse or sagittal direction. The site of osteotomy and all defects within the glenoid floor, particularly within the superior region, were filled with autogenous bone graft in order to form a new trough-shaped bed with superior support to accommodate the humeral prosthetic component (Figs. 3, 4). (Special sockets designed were inserted previously but presented a problem regarding shape and fixation because of different anatomical conditions; they are no longer used).

Seven out of nine patients were significantly improved in function and pain compared with their preoperative state when they had a firmly fixed glenoid component. Encouraged by these positive results, we have used this bone grafting procedure principle in different ways in primary interventions in addition to replacing only the humeral head. In this way two shoulders with gross rheumatoid arthritic destruction of the anterior part of the glenoid surface have been treated successfully (Fig. 5).

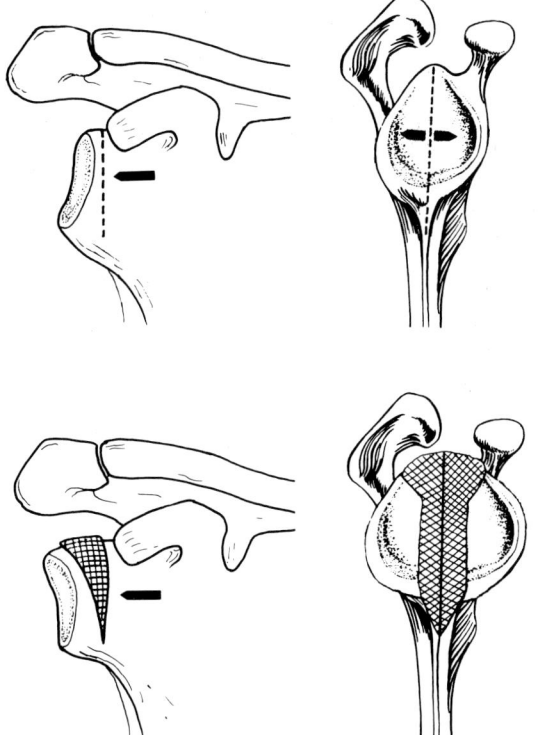

Figure 3 Different types of osteotomy and bone grafting at the glenoid.

We believe that further improvement in this technique is possible.

Specific complications of an unconstrained system are *early* and *late dislocation*. It has become apparent that early postoperative dislocation is not the main problem, as was first assumed, but rather late dislocation. With increased experience in repairing grossly destructed rotator cuffs, early postoperative, in most cases anteroinferior, dislocation has become rare; it has not occurred in the last 37 operations performed over a four-year period. Late superior subluxations and anterosuperior dislocations are a result of gross destruction within the anterior portions of the tendinous rotator cuff and perhaps of the anterior portions of the deltoid.

In prostheses with minimal constraint the risk of glenoid loosening is relatively low because of the small shear loads exerted across a very shallow socket. Severe capsular destruction will cause inadequate stabilisation of the center of rotation leading to unsatisfactory function of the deltoid and enhancing the risk of a then typical upward subluxation.

Efforts to obviate dislocation by increasing the degree of constraint at the articulating surfaces have failed. A glenoid component with a roof, as in the St. Georg Mark II model prosthesis, will

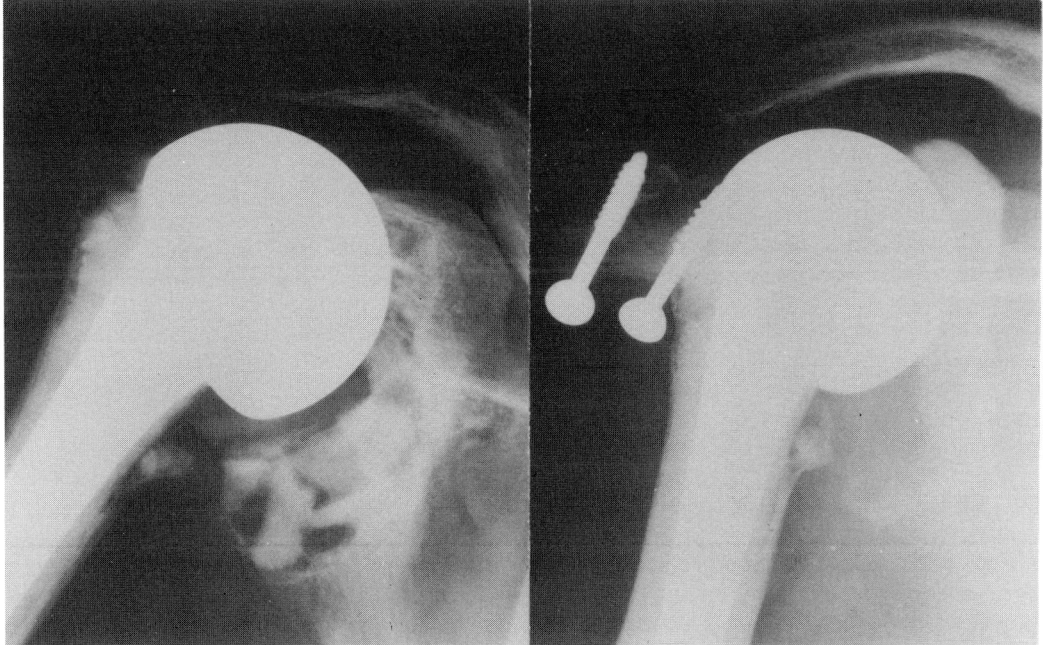

Figure 4 Radiograph of a 46-year-old female rheumatoid patient. Loosening of the glenoid cup 5 years postop (left); removal of cup, osteotomy and bone grafting at the glenoid with new bone bed formation 1 year postop (right).

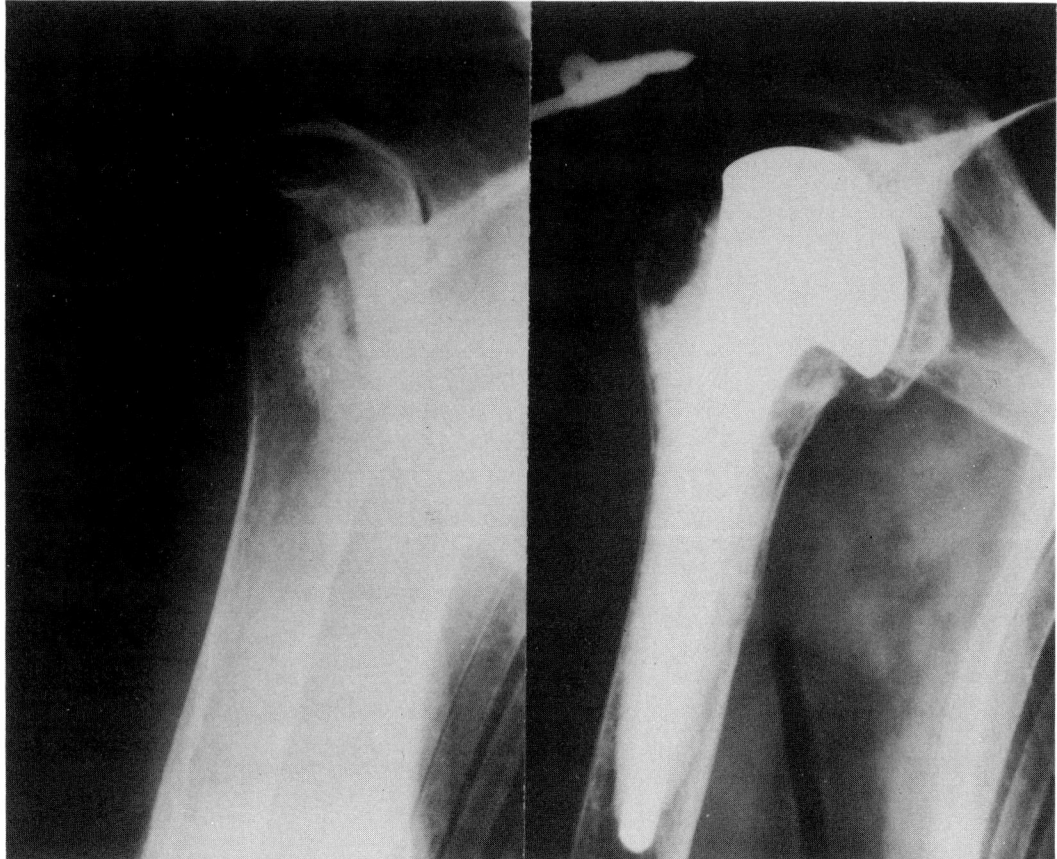

Figure 5 Radiograph of a 66-year-old female rheumatoid patient. Neurosis of the humeral head and anterior parts of the glenoid (left); hemiarthroplasty and reconstructed glenoid (osteotomy, bone grafting) with new bone bed formation 3 years postop (right).

provide temporary stability but at the same time the increased load on the glenoid fixation enhances the risk of loosening. Loose sockets tend to displace superomedially in the main direction of load, and in advanced cases late secondary total displacement is likely to occur.

The number of late dislocations in 37 hemiarthroplasties performed within the past four years has amounted to only two upward subluxations and this is attributed to increased experience in the reconstruction of tendinous rotator cuffs, the additional nonalloarthroplastic measures performed at the glenoid and the posterior operative approach to the joint that we now favor in order to preserve the anterior structures.

Heterotopic bone formation has been an occasional cause of loss of range of motion in 3 percent of cases.

No damage to the axillary vessels or brachial plexus was observed associated with either the anterior or the posterior approach to the joint. One patient developed a Sudeck atrophy following compression of the brachial plexus because of delay in the treatment of early postoperative dislocation. Special indications for shoulder arthroplasty have included neoplasms necessitating excision of the upper humerus. Stability now depends entirely upon the integrity of the remaining muscles, especially the deltoid.

CONCLUSIONS

Mechanical loosening of the humeral component of a shoulder arthroplasty is unlikely. The high rate of mechanical glenoid component loosening no longer justifies its use. Indications for hemiarthroplasty may be more generous in the light of encouraging late results. Additional measures are useful for the repair of glenoid damage:

molding, transverse or sagittal osteotomy, and autogenous bone grafting in order to fashion a new supporting bony roof to the glenoid. Particularly in primary operations, the dorsal approach modified by Kocher with osteotomy of the acromion is of great advantage leading to better joint function; the anterior approach should be confined to special cases. Hemiarthroplasty is a valuable procedure if the indications are chosen carefully. Improved clinical results can be expected from these measures and we are encouraged by the initial findings.

REFERENCES

1. Benjamin A. Double osteotomy of the shoulder. Scand J Rheumatol 1974; 3:65.
2. Buchholz HW, Engelbrecht E, Lodenkämper H, Röttger J, Siegel A, Elson RA. Management of deep infection of total hip replacement. J Bone Joint Surg 1981; 63B:342.
3. Engelbrecht E, Siegel A, Heinert K. Erfahrungen mit der Anwendung von Schultergelenksendoprothesen. Chirurg 1980; 51:794.
4. Engelbrecht E, Stellbrink G. Totale Schulterendoprothese Modell "St. George". Chirurg 1975; 47:565.
5. Kocher T. Excisionen und Resectionen, Obere Extremität. Chirurgische Operationslehre. Vol. 4, Fischer, Jena (1902)
6. Neer CS, Watson KC, Stanton FJ. Recent experience in total shoulder replacement. J Bone Joint Surg 1982; 64A:319.
7. Bayley I, Kessel L, eds. Shoulder Surgery. Springer, Berlin Heidelberg New York: Springer, 1982.
8. Siegel A, Buchholz HW, Engelbrecht E, Röttger J. The non-blocked shoulder-endoprosthesis. In: Joint Replacement in the Upper Limb. Conference sponsored by the Med Eng Sect of the Inst Mech Eng and the Brit Orthop Assoc, London, 18–20 April, 1977. London, New York, Mech. Eng. Publ. 1977.

UNCONSTRAINED SHOULDER ARTHROPLASTY

CHARLES S. NEER, II, M.D.

Shoulder replacement is in a stage of development that is ahead of replacement of other joints, considering not only movement and function, but also durability.[3] This chapter discusses the design of the implant and indications for shoulder replacement as well as some principles of technique.

DESIGN

It has long been the opinion of the author that a replacement operation should retain normal anatomy as much as possible. In 1951, a humeral head prosthesis was designed with a 44 mm radius of curve. This was the average size of the humeral head in 50 cadaver specimens. A long stem to diffuse force through a large segment of bone was thought imperative. This was used with the concept of reconstructing the tuberosities and cuff around the prosthesis to reproduce normal anatomy. The head of the implant was flattened slightly on top to avoid encroachment on the rotator cuff; fenestrations were placed in the proximal end of the prosthesis for the ingrowth of bone; and the stem was made in five diameters so that a firm press-fit could be obtained (Fig. 2A). There was never a problem of loosening of this prosthesis. When there was a good rotator cuff, good deltoid, good glenoid, and a good rehabilitation regime, an excellent result was obtained. This implant had great durability, and, unlike an acetabulum, wear on a normal glenoid was never a problem. However, the results were not as good when there were weak muscles or the articular surface of the glenoid was involved, and it was hoped a total shoulder replacement might solve this problem.

In the early 1970s several types of fixed-fulcrum total shoulders were designed. The third and last type of fixed-fulcrum prosthesis which I designed with Mr. Robert Averill, and which is shown in Figure 1, was made with complete axial rotation within the shaft of the humerus, to avoid rotary constraint. Even so, mechanical failure continued to be a problem. In addition to the problem of mechanical failure, it was realized that a fixed-fulcrum would not solve the problem of an inadequate rotator cuff. External rotation is necessary for use of the arm above the horizontal, and since the infraspinatus supplies 90 percent of the power of external rotation, the preservation of this muscle is essential for good function. I have not used a fixed-fulcrum replacement in recent years.

In 1973 the original humeral head design, Figure 2A, was revised as shown in Figure 2B. In this Mark II humeral component, the flattening on the top of the head was removed, the edges of the head were rounded, two lengths of head were provided, and the stem was redesigned for use with acrylic cement. A polyethylene glenoid component also with a 44 mm radius of curve was made with the dimensions similar to an average glenoid. During the past ten years of design development, nine different glenoid components have been used, including one 200 percent larger than the average human glenoid and one 600 percent larger in an effort to give more constraint in special situations where the cuff was extensively destroyed. At the present time, I continue to use the 200 percent glenoid component very occasionally (in cuff-tear arthropathy and in the very worst rheumatoids), but have not used a 600 percent glenoid in the past four years. The 200 percent glenoid component, when used with the short head humeral component, allows repair of the supraspinatus tendon in most cases; however, the 600 percent component precludes this. Most patients who have extreme loss of the rotator cuff also have a scapula so deficient that these larger glenoid components cannot be used. It is difficult to install even the standard polyethylene glenoid component in many of these patients. We have come to rely more on soft-tissue reconstruction and "limited goal" rehabilitation (discussed later) in advanced cases. Fortunately, these do not represent more than 10 percent of the indications. The other 90 percent can be given the full rehabilitation program. Recently, I have been using a metal-backed standard-sized glenoid component in patients who have a sloping glenoid and in those who are younger and more active. I be-

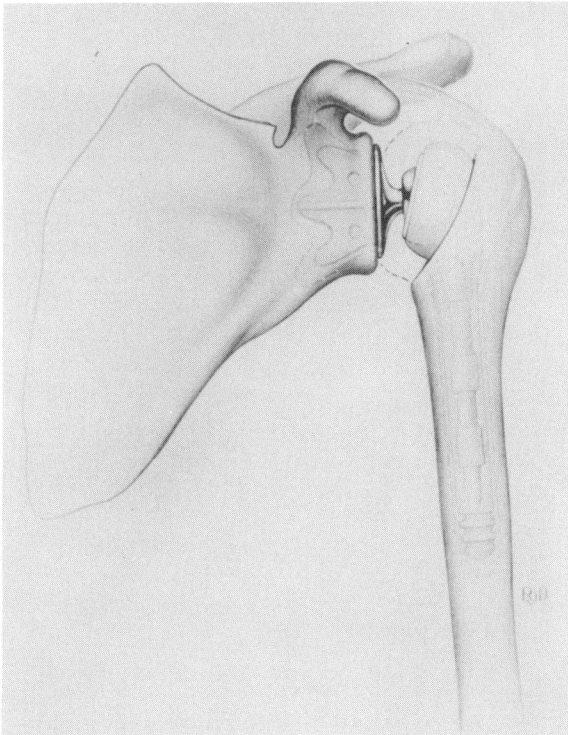

Figure 1 A constrained fixed-fulcrum prosthesis, Mark III, designed by CS Neer with Mr. Robert Averill, which allowed complete rotation of the stem within the shaft to avoid constraint. We concluded in 1974 that fixed-fulcrum invited mechanical failure and did not eliminate the need for repairing the rotator cuff.

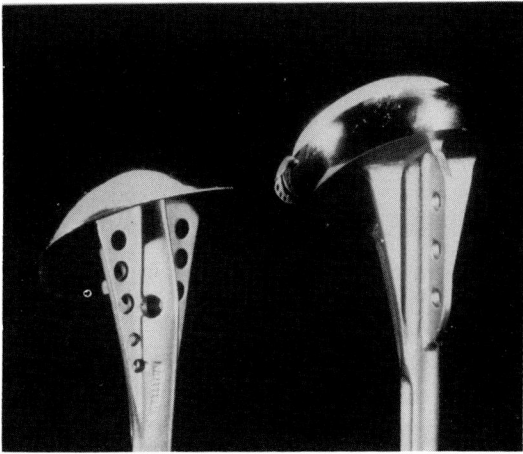

Figure 2 The Neer I and Neer II proximal humeral prostheses.

lieve this type of glenoid component has been sufficiently perfected so that it will soon be released for general use. We continue to use the standard polyethylene glenoid component, however, in those with a smaller scapula. In keeping with the current interest in "cementless replacements," we have designed three types of glenoid components for bony ingrowth; however, since we have never revised one of our own cemented glenoid components because of loosening, we have to date been unwilling to begin a clinical trial of cementless glenoid components. Motion and rehabilitation of the soft tissues around an implant is of crucial importance in shoulder replacement; an ingrowth component requiring any sort of special protection or immobilization would be most detrimental.

TECHNIQUE

Since 1977 we have used a long deltopectoral approach as illustrated in Figure 4. It is extremely important to avoid detachment of any portion of deltoid origin, especially the anterior deltoid. Some of the insertion of the deltoid is detached to free the muscle so retraction does not damage the muscle. An arm board for support of the arm in the abducted position is used for much of the procedure to reduce the amount of traction required on the deltoid. When the anterior structures (including the subscapularis) are contracted, they are released to obtain the length needed for external rotation. Otherwise the rotator cuff is left intact. Details of surgical technique vary with each indication.[3]

It is now appreciated that stability depends not only on the version of the implant but also on the length of the implant to place tension on the myofascial sleeve. If the proper length of head is selected, stability of the unconstrained implant is obtained. Active motion depends on the power of the muscles.

When the rotator cuff is intact, a closely supervised exercise program is advanced as rapidly as possible beginning first with passive exercises to recover movement and, within two weeks, adding strengthening exercises. When the rotator cuff has been torn, the rehabilitation program is the same as that for tears of the rotator cuff. Passive exercises are begun early but active exercises are deferred depending on the extent of the rotator cuff repair. The rehabilitation goal in 90 percent of our patients is near-normal movement, strength, and function. In only 10 percent is a "limited goals" rehabilitation program given.

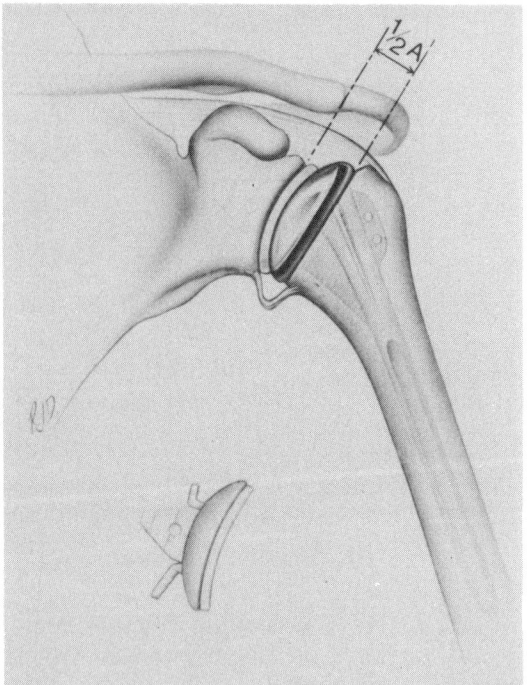

Figure 3 Illustrating some of the unconstrained total shoulder replacements used in this series. The humeral component is made with two lengths of head and 14 varieties of stem. Five different glenoid components have been used; one with a metal backing and 200% larger articular surface is shown (Inset). A half-sized implant of this design, made for Dr. Robert Cofield for juvenile rheumatoids, is available.

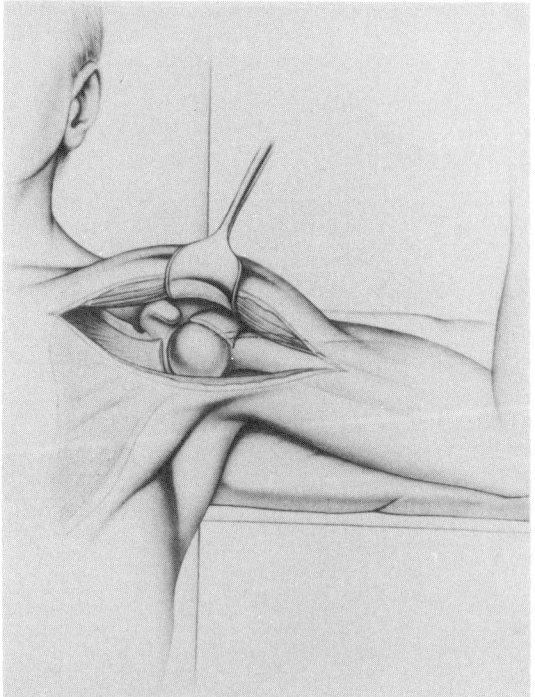

Figure 4 The long deltopectoral approach used for all replacement arthroplasties. The origin of the deltoid is left intact, but some of the insertion may be released if necessary. The arm is abducted on an armboard to relax the deltoid as necessary. Only the subscapularis tendon is divided and it usually requires lengthening. The long head of the biceps is left intact. The arm is extended off the side of the table when inserting the humeral component.

INDICATIONS

The indications and type of implant in the last 500 consecutive shoulder replacements are shown in Table 1. We continue to use a humeral component without a glenoid component in the 25 percent of replacements where there is a good rotator cuff and good glenoid, as in avascular necrosis, acute trauma and a few other conditions. Very rarely, a large-head humeral component is used alone when the glenoid is so destroyed a glenoid component cannot be installed. In approximately 75 percent (377 patients of this series), an unconstrained total shoulder replacement was performed. The addition of the glenoid component, in addition to eliminating incongruity, seems of value in situations where there has been destruction of the glenoid and where muscles have been weakened by injury or disease. The improved fulcrum offered by the glenoid component is thought to aid in the rehabilitation of weak muscles. No fixed-fulcrum prosthesis was used after the first year of this series.

Humeral Head Replacement Arthroplasty

The surgical approach, treatment of the soft tissues, postoperative rehabilitation program, and the rehabilitation goals are the same when the humeral component is used alone as when a glenoid component is added.

Avascular Necrosis

Avascular necrosis due to steroids or other causes treated prior to arthritic changes on the glenoid are ideal for humeral head replacement without a glenoid component. Many of these patients are younger and, since they have thick cortices of the humerus and intact tuberosities, can usually be treated with a press-fit of the humeral component.

TABLE 1 Indications and Type of Implant for Total Shoulder Replacement*

Indications	Humeral Head	TSR	Fixed Fulcrum
Trauma			
Acute	52		
Old	33	91	3
Avascular necrosis	19		
Osteoarthritis (1° & 2°)	6	89	
Arthritis of disloc.	2	30	
Rheumatoid	1	85	
"Elsewhere" prosthesis	3	43	
Cuff-tear arthropathy		25	
Miscellaneous (fusion, neoplasm, dysplasia, etc.)	4	14	—
	120	377	3

*500 consecutive shoulder replacements

This is a very conservative operation since it is done without the introduction of any foreign matter other than a metal humeral component which has a known long-term follow-up of over 30 years.

Severe Proximal Humeral Fractures

Severe proximal humeral fractures with crushing or detachment of the head segment are also treated without a glenoid component require repair of the cuff and tuberosities.[3] When the tuberosities and cuff have been repaired, the rehabilitation program is longer and more difficult; however, the goals should be the same: near-normal motion and function. Our standards have risen a great deal through the years. We now prefer nonmetallic, nonabsorbable sutures to repair the tuberosities. Some patients with old injuries, particularly those who are younger and with good articular surface of the glenoid, are also treated without a glenoid component. However, when the glenoid is abnormal and surrounding rotator cuff muscles are contracted and weak, a glenoid component is added.

Total Shoulder Arthroplasty (Head with Glenoid Component)

The surgical technique and the method of aftercare varies according to the indication. Let us briefly consider the special features of each category.

Osteoarthritis, Primary and Secondary

The functional result following replacement arthroplasty is determined by the strength of the muscles, and since the muscles are normal in osteoarthritis, it is predictable that a near-normal shoulder can be obtained with a properly performed arthroplasty and rehabilitation program. In the exposure we use for replacements, all muscles are left intact, with the exception of the subscapularis. It is lengthened. The long head of the biceps is left intact. A typical patient regains at least 90 percent of normal range of motion and strength and resumes full activities.

Arthritis of Dislocations

This is a newly-recognized entity[3] which presents three special problems: a scarred deltoid (from previous surgery), shortened or contracted subscapularis tendon (from prior surgery), and severe wear with bone loss on the posterior glenoid. Special steps in the operation entail deltoidplasty, lengthening of the subscapularis, and leveling off of the glenoid which may require a bone graft. Since the average age of these patients is slightly below 40 years, we now tend to use a standard-sized, metal-backed glenoid component in this group.

Rheumatoid Arthritis

The special features of rheumatoid arthritis include muscle disease, acromioclavicular joint destruction, subacromial bursal involvement, and, in about 30 percent, a tear of the rotator cuff. The intensity of the disease varies, however, and the prognosis for at least 80 percent of these patients is for a near-normal shoulder provided they work hard in their rehabilitation program to strengthen the diseased muscles. The rotator cuff tears are usually small and easily repaired and present a special problem in only about 10 percent. The glenoid involvement is less predictable than in degenerative arthritis because granulation tissue may destroy bone in an unpredictable way. Bilateral shoulder replacements were necessary in 20 percent of our series, and elbow replacement in 10 percent. Only 10 percent of rheumatoids have the type of pathology that requires limited goals rehabilitation; more patience is required in the rehabilitation program of rheumatoids.

Old Displaced Fractures

These lesions have usually had previous surgery; this introduces a special risk of infection. They are also difficult because of extensive scar tissue, retracted tuberosities, loss of bone and shortening that weakens the deltoid, and surgical incisions that have weakened the deltoid. Nerve injuries may also add to the difficulty. Detachment of the deltoid from previous surgery, especially radical acromionectomy, may make reconstruction for a good functional result impossible. Special cases have to be given limited goals rehabilitation; however, the full exercise program can be given the majority, but must be closely supervised and individualized for optimum results.

Failed Prosthesis

Of the 46 failed prosthetic procedures listed in Table 1, only 6 had been performed in our hospital and the rest referred from elsewhere. This was the most difficult category of all because of deficiency or actual excision of the rotator cuff, deficiency of scapula, loss of humerus, scarred and detached deltoid, and the special risk of infection. These problems illustrate the difficulty of revision and emphasize the need for a good replacement the first time.

Cuff-Tear Arthropathy

This is a newly-described condition[3] and is a term applied only when the articular surface of the head has collapsed and become distorted due to disuse and poor nutrition in association with a massive tear of the rotator cuff. All of the patients in this category required limited goals rehabilitation. A fusion might be an acceptable alternative in an atypical patient; however, since bilateral shoulder disease is usually present and the patients are older, a fusion usually cannot be done. The glenoid is too eroded and soft to consider a fixed-fulcrum.

Miscellaneous

Two patients with fusions had successful revisions to total shoulder arthroplasty although their active motion was limited by rotator cuff deficits. Nine patients with neoplasms were treated with long humeral components and bone grafts. The key to tumor replacement is to retain length of the arm for tension on the myofascial sleeve for stability and reattach the muscles for function. Until there is a satisfactory method for porous ingrowth for reattachment of tendons to the prosthesis, bone grafts serve the purpose.

DURABILITY AND FUNCTION

When the muscles are normal, as in osteoarthritis, the predictable results should be an essentially normal shoulder. This is also true of 90 percent of the patients with the arthritis of dislocations and 75 percent of those with rheumatoid arthritis. Only 45 percent of those with old fractures obtained an excellent rating; and only 33 percent of those with failed prostheses obtained excellent results. Those with cuff-tear arthropathy, and extensive tumor surgery usually required limited goals rehabilitation.

The Full Exercise Group

Ninety percent of the 500 patients in this series were in this group and obtained excellent or satisfactory ratings. Their results were graded prospectively and were as previously described.[3] Activities included golf, tennis, and other noncontact sports.

Limited Goals Group

Ten percent of this series were treated with a rehabilitation program directed at a more limited range of movement but more stability. The indication for this special form of rehabilitation was massive defects of the rotator cuff and deltoid or loss of bone. The results of these patients were graded separately. In this group the postoperative regime was limited to passive exercises which were restricted to not over 110 degrees of elevation and 20 degrees of external rotation. Ninety-five percent of this group achieved satisfactory freedom from pain and function for the activities of daily living with the arm at the side. This special program was used in only 10 percent of rheumatoids, 8 percent of old fractures, 30 percent of prosthetic revisions, and was necessary for all of those with cuff-tear arthropathy and extensive resections for tumors.

Roentgen Follow-up

In the 1982 report,[3] lucent lines around the glenoid component were seen in 31 percent. However, all but six of these patients exhibited the same lucent lines in their initial postoperative films and there was no tendency for enlargement. In the more recent cases, apparently because the cement technique has improved, we very rarely see roentgen evidence of lucent lines. I consider the high instance of lucent lines at the glenoid component reported by some other surgeons to represent differences in surgical technique. Factors may include presence of blood, loose bone or motion at the time of cementing, or failure to preserve the subchondral bone. In any case, we have never done a revision for loosening of the glenoid component in our own series.

REFERENCES

1. Neer CS II, Brown TH Jr, McLaughlin HL. Fractures of the neck of the humerus with dislocation of the head fragment. Am J Surg. 1953; 85:252–258.
2. Neer CS II. Articular replacement for the humeral head. J Bone Joint Surg. 1955; 37A:215–228.
3. Neer CS II, Watson KC, Stanton FJ. Recent experience in total shoulder replacement. J Bone Joint Surg. 1982; 64A:319–337.
4. Cofield RH. Personal communication.
5. Neer CS II, Rockwood CA Jr. Fractures and dislocations of the shoulder. In: Rockwood CA Jr, Green DP, eds. *Fractures*. Philadelphia: JB Lippincott, 1975; 1:585–623.

NEUROMUSCULAR DISORDERS

THORACOSCAPULAR FUSION FOR FACIOSCAPULOHUMERAL DYSTROPHY

S. A. COPELAND, M.B., F.R.C.S.

Seventeen thoracoscapular fusion operations have been done on nine patients. The indication is symptomatic winging of the scapula caused by thoracoscapular muscle paresis with intact function in the deltoid. This situation almost exclusively occurs in facioscapulohumeral dystrophy. The operation used is successful in achieving stability of the scapula and in greatly improving function and cosmesis. Although the course of this type of muscular dystrophy is variable, the benefits of operation have not deteriorated with progression of the disease over a maximum follow-up period of 23 years.

This paper describes the technique of thoracoscapular fusion using tibial cortical grafts with screw fixation.

Duchenne[3] in 1868 described the clinical course of a progressive muscular atrophy in 13 patients, and his name has been associated with the early onset sex-linked recessive form of muscular dystrophy. In 1884 Landouzy and Dejerine[4] reported on a small group of cases in which muscular involvement was initially limited to the face and shoulder girdle. This form of the disease has since been known as facioscapulohumeral dystrophy; it is transmitted as an autosomal dominant with a wide range of expressivity. The age of onset is usually 15 to 30 years, commonly involving the serratus anterior, trapezius, rhomboids, and latissimus dorsi muscles and the muscles about the eyes and mouth. This form of the disease runs a very variable course but is generally benign and a normal life span is probable.[7]

Fortunately, the deltoid muscle is nearly always spared or only partially involved. Without a stable origin the deltoid loses its mechanical advantage, and in attempted abduction, the scapula rotates and active sustained abduction and flexion is severely limited. If the scapula can be stabilized, the deltoid can exert a powerful action on the humerus. Several methods of achieving stability of the scapula have been described but unfortunately they have come from small series with short periods of follow-up. Putti[5] (1906) described an interscapular fixation which apparently caused compression of the vessels under the clavicle. Rinaldi[6] (1964) fixed the scapula to the thorax using a fascial band taken from the fascia lata and passed around the spinous processes of the second and third and fifth and sixth thoracic vertebrae and then through a hole in the spine of the scapula. This was a modification of the techniques used by Whitman[8] (1932) and Dewar and Harris[2] (1950). They considered it necessary to retain some thoracoscapular movement. Although the initial results are satisfactory, the fascial slings stretch and function deteriorates. More recently one case was described by Bunch[1] (1973) in which true bony fusion had been achieved between the scapula and thorax using wire and bone grafts. It was noted that after a bilateral procedure vital capacity was reduced.

The technique here described was first carried out using tibial cortical grafts alone, but subsequently, cancellous iliac crest grafts alone were used. Bony union has been achieved in all patients. The technique and early results of the first three cases were reported to the British Orthopaedic Association in 1960.[10] A long term follow-up of these and further patients is presented. Later results were reported by Copeland and Howard in 1978.[9]

248 / Surgery of the Shoulder

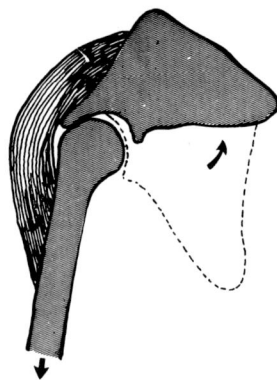

Figure 1 Winging of the scapula. The scapula rides upward and locks the stabilizing muscle control.

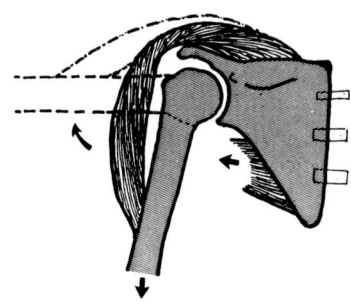

Figure 2 With scapula stabilized, a firm fulcrum is established for shoulder abduction.

MATERIAL AND METHODS

There were nine patients, eight of whom had had bilateral operations giving a total of 17 thoracoscapular fusions. The average age at the time of operation was 24 years (range 15 to 59 years). There were seven women and two men. All had a diagnosis of facioscapulohumeral dystrophy and were complaining of symptoms related to winging of the scapulae.

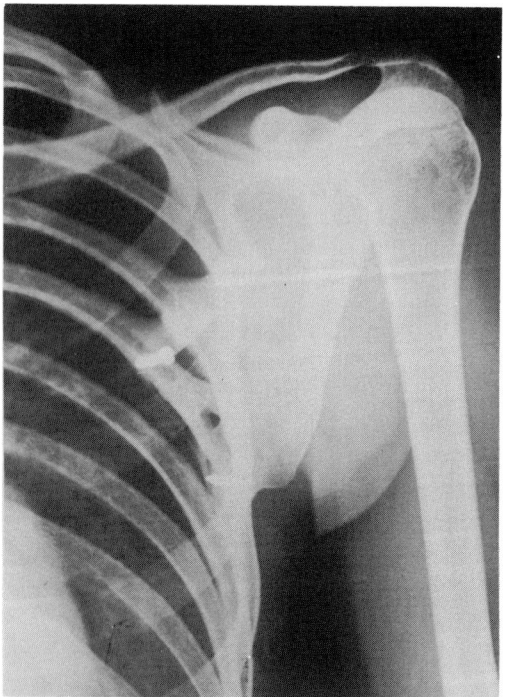

Figure 3 Roentgenogram showing failure of abduction with winging of the scapula.

Operative Technique

The patient lies supine and a cortical tibial bone graft 9 cm × 1 cm is taken. Cancellous bone from the proximal tibia is scooped out at the same time. This wound is closed, and the patient is then turned to lie prone with the arm hanging over the side of the table. This almost always brings the scapula into the ideal position for fixation to the ribs with the vertebral border lying parallel and 5 to 7 centimeters lateral to the spinous processes. The incision is made along the medial edge of the scapula. The underlying muscles, which are sometimes atrophied, are divided and the deep surface of the vertebral border of the scapula is denuded of tissue for 2 cm laterally, detaching part of the origin of the subscapularis. The superficial medial margin of the scapula is also cleared of muscle attachment for about 2 cm laterally. Three ribs lying under the most convenient part of the scapula are chosen: these are usually the fourth, fifth and sixth ribs. The periosteum is incised in the line of the rib, and the periosteum and parietal pleura are separated so that a retractor can be put under the ribs to prevent damage to the pleura.

The tibial graft is divided into two or three struts, and a hole is drilled at each end. Each graft is then fixed to the scapula and the underlying rib by means of screws passing through the whole thickness of the ribs but obviously not allowed to stand proud of their deep surface. Any gaps left between the scapula and the ribs are then packed with cancellous bone chips. If more cancellous graft is needed, this can be taken from the posterior superior iliac crest. In the last four operations cancellous bony graft only was used. Sound fixation of the scapula to the ribs is achieved at the end of

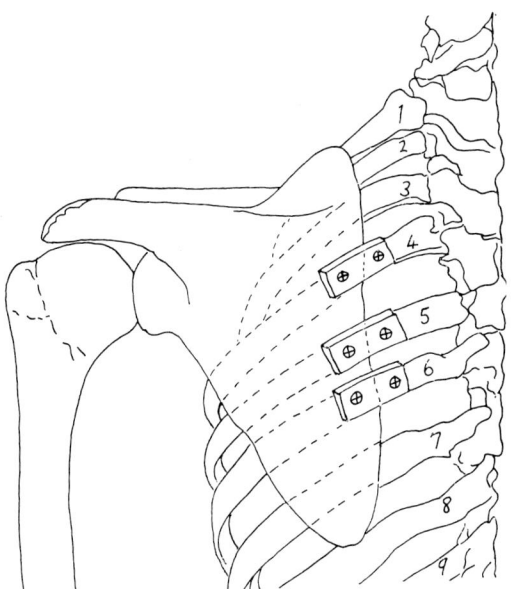

Figure 4 Stabilization of the scapula with rib grafts.

the operation. The wound is closed, with drainage, and the patient is carefully turned over, with an assistant holding the arm. A shoulder spica is applied with the arm at 80° abduction and 30° forward flexion, the hand being in front of the mouth. The patient is nursed after the operation in a sitting position. The average length of stay in hospital was 17 days.

Three months after operation the arm section of the spica is bivalved so that the upper section may be removed and the patient can start active abduction. Once control of abduction has been regained, the plaster of Paris is removed. A triangular pillow may be placed under the arm to allow gradual adduction of the arm over a period of one week. Physiotherapy is then needed to help regain full glenohumeral movements and to strengthen the deltoid muscle.

On two occasions, at surgery, the scapular muscles were found to be hypertrophic and the scapula could not be made to lie against the ribs. Some of the muscle belly of the subscapularis was excised, and the tibial grafts were used as spacers and placed between the ribs and scapula; screws were used in the same way. The number of ribs involved and the number of struts used varied, depending upon the shape of the chest wall and scapula and the fixation achieved.

Results

Eight of the nine patients were seen personally; the other was contacted by letter. The longest follow-up was 25 years and the shortest six months (average 11.2 years). The time between the onset of symptoms and operation was an average 7.6 years (range 2 to 19 years).

The main complaints before operation were of weakness of the arm and inability to sustain the arm in the abducted or flexed position, as it would just flop down after a short time (for example, patients complained that they could not reach things out of high cupboards nor get books from high shelves); of cosmetic deformity—the scapula would ride up in the neck and wing posteriorly, looking very ugly and causing great difficulty with clothing; and of a dragging sensation in the shoulder and aching and pain after use.

Power and Function

The power of the deltoid muscle did not diminish over the years and in fact became stronger. All patients experienced aching in the deltoid for several months after the operation but this gradually disappeared. Three of our patients had had a slow relentless progress to their disease and were severely affected at the time of follow-up, both eventually having involvement of the lower limb. They both, however, managed to do sedentary part-time jobs involving reaching upwards and forwards. All patients were independent before operation and could do most things but great effort was required in any movements involving the shoulder girdle. The operation allowed them to do sustained maneuvers involving the shoulder, and simple tasks such as getting dressed and cooking were achieved without pauses for rest, which was not possible before operation. Three patients who could not wash their hair or backs before operation could do so afterwards.

Cosmesis

The majority of our patients were women and cosmesis was a big factor in their decision to accept operative treatment. Before operation the scapulae not only winged but were elevated on attempted flexion or abduction, giving an ugly appearance of widening of the base of the neck. Although fixation of the scapula leaves a considerable scar the patients were happy to accept this because of the general improvement in appear-

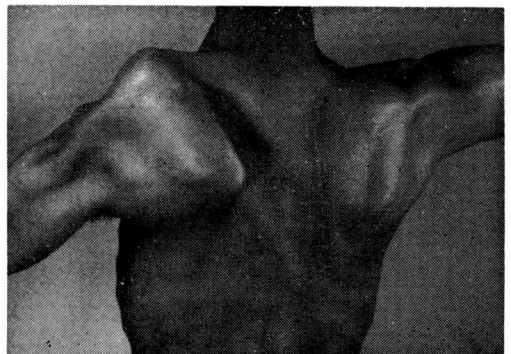

Figure 5 The appearance after unilateral operation. The left scapula is seen winging, the right side is fixed.

ance. The scapulae were fixed in the position previously described, which gives maximum range of active movements. This position is further lateral than the natural position of the scapula, and tends to produce a slightly square-shouldered appearance. This was noted by us but was never remarked upon by the patients.

Pain

Pain was never a major factor in that the most described was a persistent aching discomfort before operation. This was relieved in all patients.

Range of Movements

It is interesting to note the range of movements that these patients can achieve, all of which obviously takes place at the glenohumeral joint alone and is remarkably consistent. The average range of movement was: abduction 100°, flexion 90°, extension 35°, external rotation 20°, and internal rotation 90°. The ability to sustain abduction or flexion was, to the patient, the greatest improvement.

Complications

Early: Two patients complained of pleuritic pain but in both it settled within a week. This was presumably due to protruding screws on the deep surface of the ribs but could not be demonstrated radiographically due to the difficulties of radiography in the plaster spica. Two patients developed localized pain in the chest wall while in plaster, and subsequently this was thought to be due to stress fractures of the ribs that were later seen on radiography to have healed.

Late: One patient complained of pain at the site of fusion and the graft was shown to be nonunited. She had a successful secondary graft with iliac cancellous bone. Two patients had to have screws removed as they were causing superficial irritation. No particular anesthetic difficulties were experienced with these patients.

Discussion

Eight out of the nine patients returned to have a thoracoscapular fusion done on the remaining shoulder. This fact alone speaks for the success of the operation to the patient. The ninth patient had other disabilities of greater priority.

Often it appears that the disease is not symmetrical in its onset and only one shoulder may require treatment; several years may elapse before the other shoulder needs the operation. When the disease is asymmetrical the patient complains of feeling "unbalanced"; this balance is restored by operation. This complaint may recur later when the other shoulder is affected and again is corrected by thoracoscapular fusion. Lung function studies done on some of the earlier patients in the series showed only minimal loss of vital capacity. None of the patients at review had any functional problem related to this; they were limited by peripheral muscle weakness rather than by any diminution in respiratory reserve.

REFERENCES

1. Bunch WH. Scapulo-thoracic fusion for shoulder stabilization in muscular dystrophy. Minnesota Medicine 1973; 56:391–394.
2. Dewar FP, and Harris RI. Restoration of function of the shoulder following paralysis of the trapezius by fascial sling fixation and transplantation of the levator scapulae. Annals of Surgery 1950; 132:1111–1115.
3. Duchenne GB. Recherches sur la paralysie musculaire pseudo-hypertrophique ou paralysie myo-sclerosique. Archives generales de Medecine, 6s. 1868; 11, 5–25, 179–209, 305–321, 421–431 and 552–588.
4. Landouzy L, and Dejerine J. De la myopathie atrophique progressive (myopathie hereditaire, debutant, dans l'enfance, par la face, sans alteration du systeme nerveux). Comptes Rendus hebdomadaires des Seances de l'Academie des Sciences 1884; 98:53–55.
5. Putti V. L'osteodesi interscapolare in un caso di miopatia atrofica progressiva. Archivio di ortopedia 1906; 23:319–331.
6. Rinaldi F. Terapia chirurgica nella forma "facio-scapulo-

omerale'' della distrofia muscolare primitiva. Clinica Ortopedica 1964; 16:233–243.
7. Walton JN. Muscular dystrophy and its relation to the other myopathies. Research Publication of the Association for Research into Nervous and Mental Disease 1961; 38:378–421.
8. Whitman A. Congenital elevation of the scapula and paralysis of serratus magnus muscle. Journal of the American Medical Association 1932; 99:1332–1334.
9. Copeland SA, and Howard RC. Thoracoscapular Fusion for Fascio Scapulohumeral Dysrophy. J Bone Joint Surg 1978; 60B:547–551.
10. Howard RC. Thoraco-scapular arthrodesis. J Bone Joint Surg 1961; 43B:175.

PECTORALIS MINOR TRANSPOSITION IN SERRATUS ANTERIOR PARALYSIS

M. VASTAMÄKI, M.D.

Isolated, complete paralysis of the serratus anterior muscle appearing as a winging scapula is rather rare. It can cause severe disability in the function of the shoulder.

ANATOMY

The innervation of the serratus anterior muscle is supplied by the long thoracic nerve. The nerve courses across the scalenus medius and posterior muscles beneath the clavicle. It passes obliquely downward and laterally along the chest wall, and becomes angulated as it courses over the prominent second rib medial to the coracoid process.[8] Because of its vertical course to the axilla the long thoracic nerve is prone to being stretched if the shoulder is depressed or if the neck is flexed to the opposite side. The nerve is also susceptible to compression if lateral pressure is exerted against the scapula.

The serratus anterior is a large, broad and flat muscle which covers much of the lateral aspect of the thorax. It arises from the upper eight or nine ribs and attaches to the deep surface of the scapula along its vertebral border. The primary function of the serratus anterior muscle is to draw the scapula forward.

The pectoralis minor muscle originates from the second, third, fourth and fifth ribs and is inserted into the coracoid process medial to the origin of the coracobrachial and biceps muscles. The pectoralis minor is innervated by the medial anterior thoracic branch of the brachial plexus, which enters the middle third of its muscular portion.

CLINICAL PICTURE OF SERRATUS ANTERIOR PALSY

Paralysis of the serratus anterior has been noted following a severe blow, fall, or sudden malforming twist and strain which forces the shoulder downward and backward, or after prolonged heavy weight bearing, strenuous games of tennis, or chronic strain of the neck and shoulder.[2,3,5,6] The marked preponderance of cases occurring on the right side in the literature could provide some clue to the etiology.

In a number of cases the condition has developed after operative or obstetrical procedures or after certain infections or viral diseases or after the injection of sera, vaccines or antibiotics.[4,9] Wood and Frykman[12] reported six injuries to the long thoracic nerve during first rib resection.

In general, there is first noted an aching or burning pain of varying degrees of severity in the neck and shoulder. The pain may radiate down the arm and toward the scapular area and the chest wall. This is followed by inability to raise the arm above the horizontal plane and by winging of the scapula.

Careful muscle examination is important, especially in differentiating isolated paralysis of the serratus anterior from other paralyzing conditions involving the shoulder region. The simplest method of testing the serratus anterior is to have the patient standing and pushing hard against the wall with outstretched arms. In a paralyzed case the winging of the scapula will be instantly apparent.

TREATMENT

Many conservative and surgical methods of treatment have been recommended. In most cases the long thoracic nerve will recover spontaneously over a period of about one year. Therefore, therapy should be directed toward protecting the serratus anterior from overstretching. According to Horwitz and Tocantins,[3] derotation of the scapula is the most important means of restoring the tonicity of the paralyzed muscle. They devised the elevation and derotation brace method which was improved by Wolf[11] and Johnson and Kendall.[4] During this therapy patients are instructed to avoid any strenuous activity which would cause further damage to the weakened structures. Physical therapy with stretching of contracted antagonist muscles, such as the rhomboids and the pectoralis minor, is combined with brace protection.

If conservative treatment has been ineffective after about two years and the condition causes marked inconvenience to the patient surgical treatment should be considered. Various operations to correct paralysis of the serratus anterior muscle are described.

The ideal procedure in treatment of serratus anterior paralysis is one which restores scapular movement. This goal is achieved by muscle transposition procedures. Chaves,[1] emphasized the role of the muscles attached to the coracoid process in accentuating the winging of the scapula by muscle contraction. He concluded that transfer of the pectoralis minor from its coracoid insertion to the vertebral border of the scapula is beneficial in two ways: it will control scapular displacement directly by affording an adequate parallel substitute for the serratus anterior, and it will reduce the opposing action of the muscles attached to the coracoid process. Chaves reported one case of the pectoralis minor transfer. Later, Rapp[7] reported one case and Truchly[10] eight cases.

Pectoralis Minor Transposition

The patient is positioned on the operating table on his unaffected side. Two incisions are necessary, one at the coracoid process and one in the axilla. The tendon of the pectoralis minor is isolated and detached from the coracoid process with a piece of bone. The upper part of the belly of the pectoralis minor is freed, preserving the nerve supply to the muscle. One or two holes are made through the margin of the scapula into the lower third of it. The pectoralis minor muscle is tunneled under the pectoralis major muscle to the axilla and tethered to the scapula by means of a six– to eight–fold plantaris longus tendon graft. The muscle should not be overstretched, and passive movements of the arm should be unlimited after fastening the muscle to the scapula. Normally, gap of a few centimeters remains and a free tendon graft is necessary. After closure and dressing, the limb is immobilized in a Velpeau bandage. Mobilization is started by weight-free pendular motions of the shoulder four weeks after surgery. One to two weeks later flexion and abduction exercises are started.

I have performed a pectoralis minor transposition in six cases of serratus anterior paralysis. All patients were female, aged 22–45 years (mean age 37 years) at the time of the operation. In all cases the paralysis was on the right side. The etiology of the paralysis in two cases was a fall onto the shoulder, in one case a tractor accident, and in one case traumatic depression of the shoulder. In one case presumably strong exertion and in one case infection caused the paralysis.

Symptoms and signs were typical. No supporting splints or bandages had been used in any cases. The operative delay was 2–12 years (mean 6.5 years). At the time of surgery all of the patients were disabled in terms of their jobs due to pain upon exertion and poor range of motion. The pectoralis minor transposition was performed as described herein.

Following the operation the scapula did not wing anymore in any of the patients. After three months the motions of the shoulder were normal or almost normal in five patients. Four of the patients no longer had significant pain. Two patients still had pain primarily in the shoulder from an injury to the rotator cuff which had been previously diagnosed. In one 22-year-old patient the scapula began to wing after a two week mobilization period. A paralysis of the pectoralis muscle was demonstrated upon electroneuromyography. The transplanted muscle in this well built woman was branched and looked quite fragile and apparently was unable to meet the demands of the transposition, which subsequently caused too much tension on its innervation. The patient's scapula is currently supported by a light splint with the intention of giving both the nerve and the muscle a chance to recover. A transient complication of surgery in one patient was a peripheral weakness of the hand occurring over a three month period, apparently as a result of tension on the plexus during surgery. In two patients there were transient symptoms attributed to the short head of the biceps, the pain radiating to the biceps as a result of the manipulation of the coracoid process. Five of the patients operated on returned to their work after about four months of sick leave.

Case Report

A 22-year-old office worker had a prolonged wound infection following Cesarean section. Six

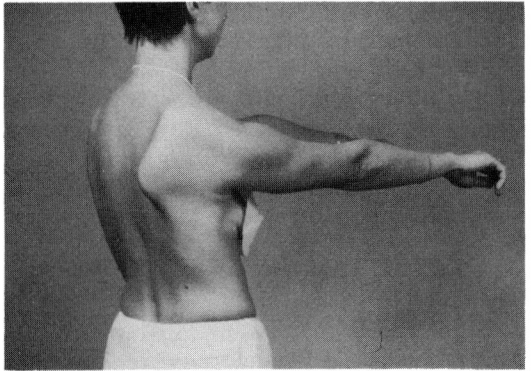

Figure 1 Patient demonstrating severe scapular winging.

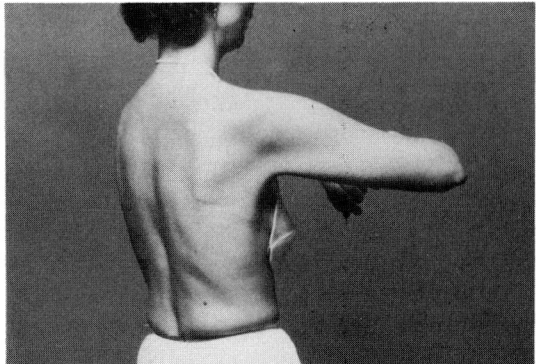

Figure 2 Complete control of scapular position.

weeks later she had severe pain in the shoulder region and shoulder motions deteriorated. The patient was able to perform her moderately light work, but after ten years the pain in the shoulder region had increased and the shoulder motions deteriorated such that the patient sought treatment once again. A winging scapula was demonstrated (Fig. 1). A transposition of the pectoralis minor was performed close to the lower corner of the scapula using six-fold plantaris longus tendon grafts for fixation. The upper extremity was immobilized using a Velpeau bandage for four weeks. After four months the motions of the upper extremity were normal, there was good strength, the scapula no longer winged and the patient was free of pain (Fig. 2).

Discussion

Paresis of the serratus muscle may cause symptoms which lead to work disability. By means of transposition of the pectoralis minor muscle it is possible to substantially alleviate the condition. In light of the cases described herein we can see, however, that the operation does not always lead to recovery, apparently due to weakness of the transposed muscle. The use of the splint to support the scapula in the early recovery stages should be emphasized. Generally paresis spontaneously disappears to a satisfactory degree over a period of two years and thus the operation should not be recommended at an earlier stage.

REFERENCES

1. Chaves JP. Pectoralis minor transplant for paralysis of the serratus anterior. J Bone Joint Surg 1951; 33B:228–230.
2. Fitchet SM. Injury of the serratus magnus (anterior) muscle. N Engl J Med 1930; 203:818–823.
3. Horwitz MT, Tocantins LM. Isolated paralysis of the serratus anterior (magnus) muscle. J Bone Joint Surg 1938; 20:720–725.
4. Johnson JTH, Kendall HO. Isolated paralysis of the serratus anterior muscle. J Bone Joint Surg 1955; 37A:567–574.
5. Kaplan PE. Electrodiagnostic confirmation of long thoracic nerve palsy. J Neurol Neurosurg Psych 1980; 43:50–52.
6. Lindström N, Danielsson L. Muscle transposition in serratus anterior paralysis. Acta Orthop Scand 1962; 32:369–373.
7. Rapp IH. Serratus anterior paralysis treated by transplantation of the pectoralis minor. J Bone Joint Surg 1954; 36A:852–854.
8. Struthers JW. The anatomy of the long thoracic nerve with special reference to paralysis of the serratus magnus muscle. Rev Neur Psychiatr 1907; 1:731–736.
9. Thorek M. Compression paralysis of the long thoracic nerve following an abdominal operation. With report of a case. Am J Surg 1926; 40:26.
10. Truchly G. (1981) Reconstruction of the "winging scapula" deformity: An improvement of an old procedure. Sicot-81 Rio. XV World Congress. Abstracts, 175–176.
11. Wolf J. The conservative treatment of serratus palsy. J Bone Joint. Surg 1941; 23:959–961.
12. Wood VE, Frykman GK. Winging of the scapula as a complication of first rib resection. A report of six cases. Clin Orthop 1980; 149:160–163.

THORACIC SCAPULOPEXY FOR RESTORATION OF ARM ELEVATION IN FACIOSCAPULOHUMERAL TYPE MUSCULAR DYSTROPHY

MINORU SAKURAI, M.D.

Facioscapulohumeral type muscular dystrophy is characterized by the gradual onset early in the second decade of muscular atrophy involving the shoulder girdle and orbicularis orcis muscles. Careful observation reveals a winging of the scapula as an attempt is made to elevate the arm and a tendency to scapula alata on initiation of arm elevation (Fig. 1). Deltoid function is well retained, however, and it has been found that the instability of the scapula can be controlled by means of fastening it to the thorax so that the pulling power of the deltoid muscle can be utilized to exert a powerful action on the humerus. Thoracoscapular fusion was first described by Howard in 1954, the results achieved being reported by Copeland and Howard in 1978.[1] A similar operation was introduced by Ketenjian[2] in the same year and it is this procedure which we have used for the basis for our own experience.

Clinical Material

Two girls and one boy ranging in age from seven to 15 years of age were operated on because of inability to elevate the arm without a winging of the scapula[3] (Fig. 2).

A modification of Ketenjian's technique was employed. The medial margin of the scapula was stripped of its muscle attachment and the surface of the fourth to sixth ribs exposed and roughened with an osteotome. The scapula was then secured with Tetron^R (polyester-polymer) lace passed through drilled holes in the scapula and adjacent ribs.

Depending on the shape of the scapula and the curvature of the adjacent thorax, two methods of fastening were employed (Fig. 3). The first method employed four holes in the medial margin of the scapula. A second method employed two holes in the spine of the scapula, through which Tetron lace was passed in order to secure the scapula to the fourth rib, and two holes at the medial margin facing the fifth and sixth ribs.

In order to ensure a wide range of abduction, the scapula was fixed in a position of 30 degrees abduction. The detached muscles were then sutured in layers and the skin closed routinely.

Following surgery, it was necessary to immobilize the arm in 60 degrees of abduction and 60 degrees of flexion for six weeks. Thereafter, an active program of rehabilitation therapy could be instituted.

Results

All of the patients achieved significant improvement in their ability to elevate the arm. As shown in Table 1, the preoperative abduction ranged from 45 to 90 degrees whereas postoperatively, it reached 135 to 145 degrees. The range of flexion before surgery was 40 to 80 degrees, but postoperatively was greatly improved to 130 to 150 degrees (Fig. 4).

Winging of the scapula was completely controlled following surgery, and, with freedom from pain, activities of daily living were greatly improved with enhanced ability to participate in sports such as swimming and basketball.

While the follow-up period is relatively short, the muscle strength of the deltoid already appears to have been markedly increased. Radiographically, hyperostotic reactive bone formation is seen around the ribs to which the scapula has been fastened and this phenomenon was recognized as early as 6 to 8 months following surgery.

The one effect of vital concern following sca-

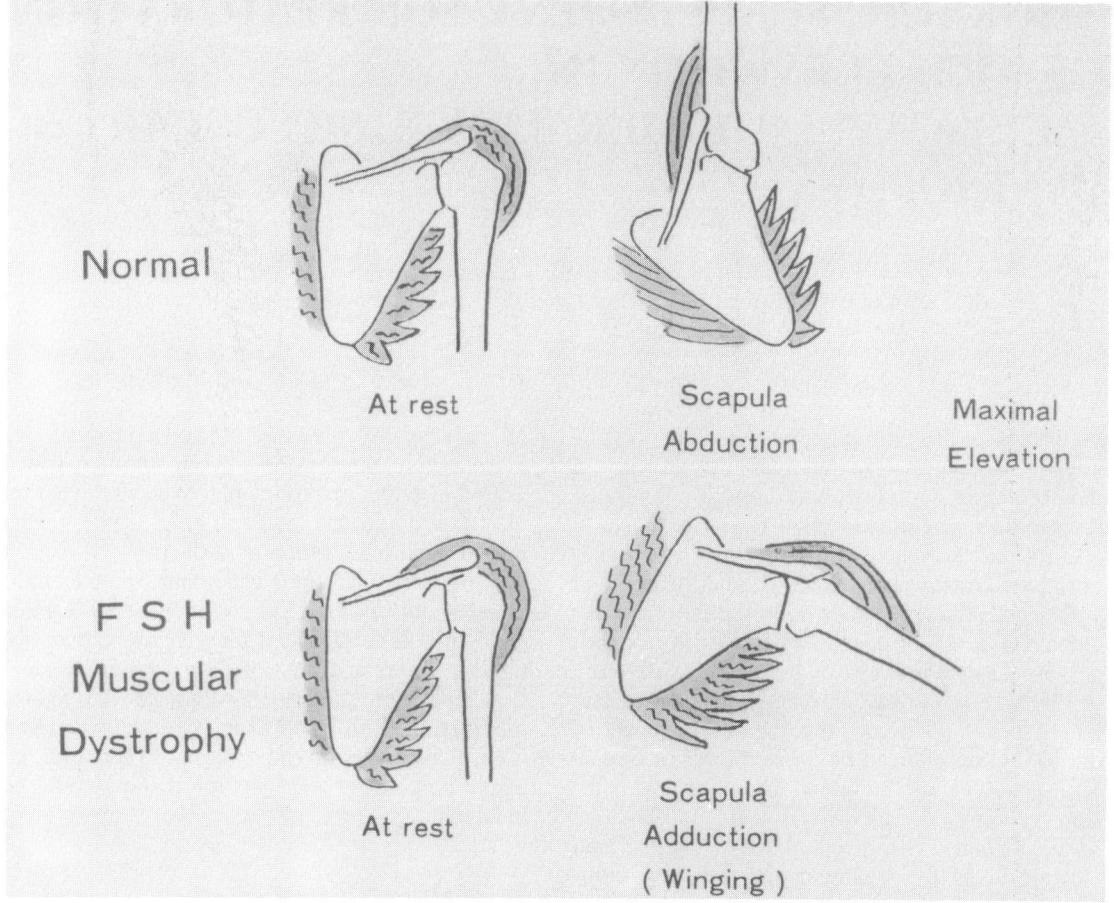

Figure 1 Winging of the scapula in FSH muscular dystrophy.

pulodesis with the thorax is a diminution in pulmonary function. Vital capacity was noted to be decreased to 78, 89 and 73 percent respectively following the primary procedure and fell further to 65, 85 and 50 percent after the second surgery. Although apparently diminished, there has been no functional limitation in day–to–day activity.

DISCUSSION

The great improvement in the day–to–day activity of individuals suffering from this nonprogressive muscular dystrophy is very gratifying. Greatly enhanced function of the whole shoulder joint is enjoyed, particularly the restoration of the strength of the deltoid muscle. Other observers have confirmed that there is not a deterioration of deltoid function with time as this muscle group is not involved in the primary process which involves only the orbicularis oris, sternocleidomastoid, pectoralis major, serratus anterior and rhomboid muscle groups.[4]

TABLE 1 Improvement of Active Range of Motion

Case (Sex)	Age at Operation (yrs)	Side	Pre-operative		Post-operative	
			ABD	FLX	ABD	FLX
C.M. (F)	12	L	70°	80°	130°	130°
	14	R	85	75	130	130
S.T. (M)	14	R	60	70	140	150
	15	L	90	80	145	145
N.W. (F)	7	R	65	40	130	130
	7	L	45	60	130	130

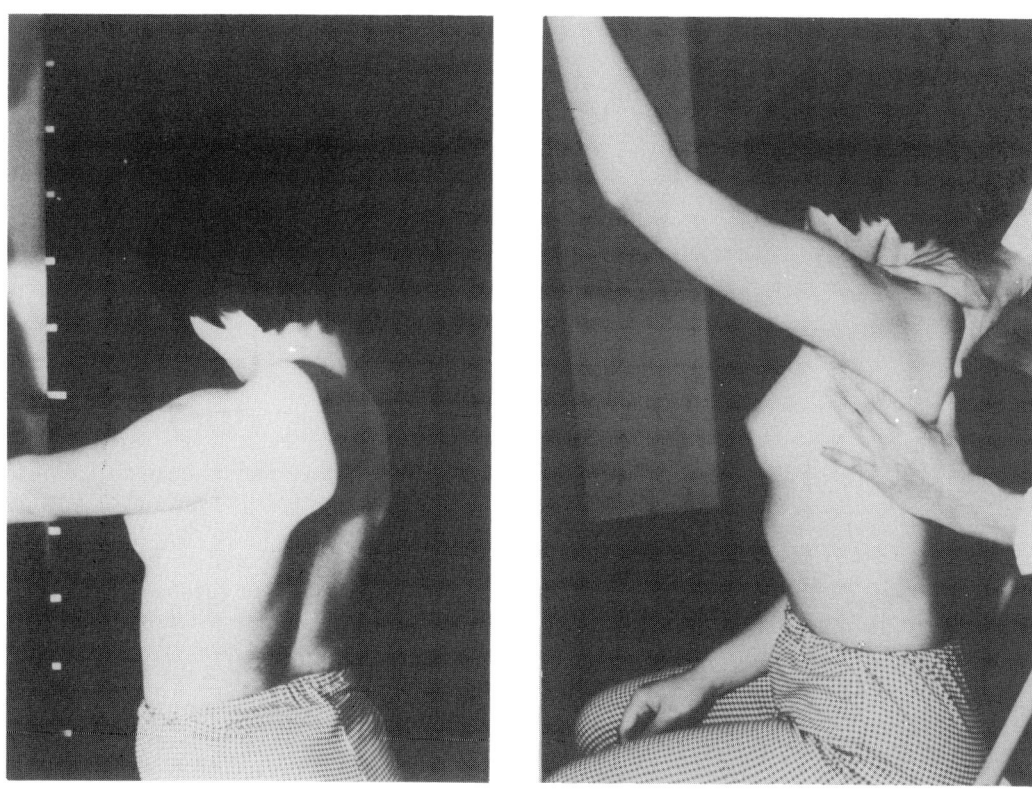

Figure 2 (a) Scapula alata and scapular winging, (b) Control of the winging allows arm elevation.

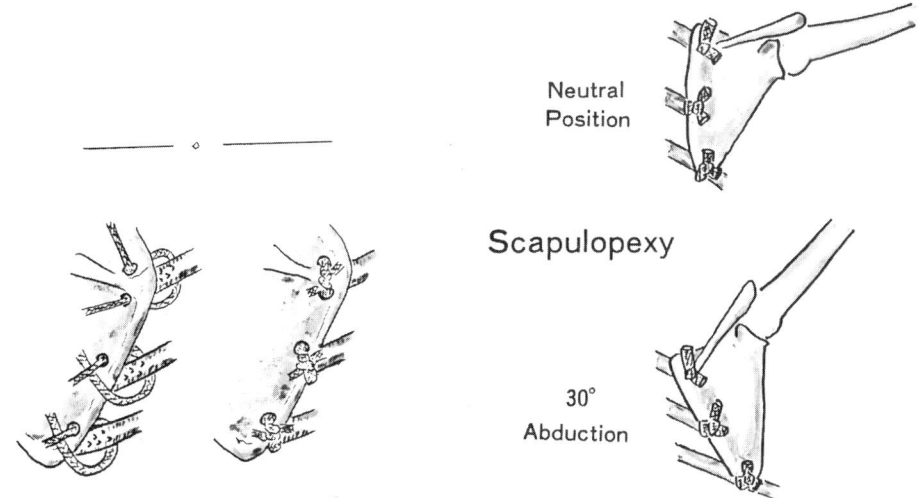

Figure 3 (a) Fixation of the scapula with Tetron^R lace, (b) 30° abduction of the scapula facilitates arm elevation.

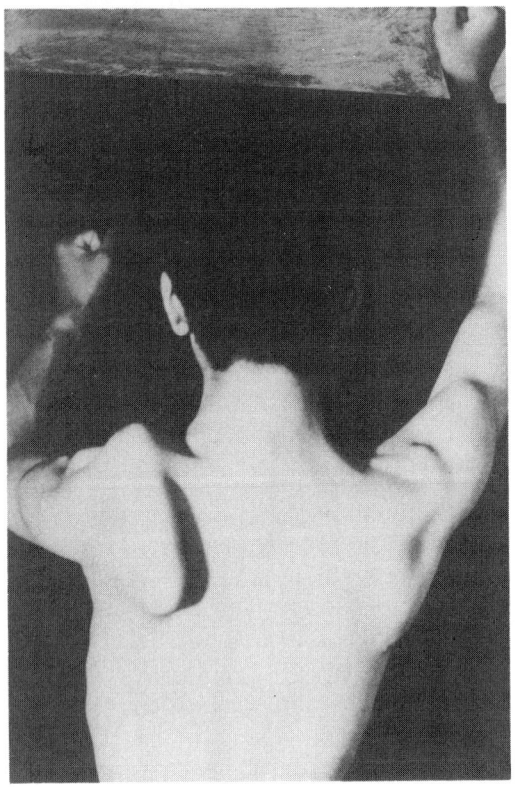

Figure 4 Scapulopexy on the right; presurgical state on the left.

Stabilization of the scapula on the thorax reliably controls the winging of the scapula. This is more than just a cosmetic improvement for it greatly enhances the function of the upper extremity.

The surgical technique described overcomes some of the problems previously encountered by other surgeons where utilization of bone grafts secured with screws had given rise on occasion to pleural irritation. The use of Tetron^R lace facilitates early fixation; the roughening of the opposing surfaces of ribs and scapula ensures an active hyperostotic reaction sufficient to reliably produce a solid fusion between the scapula and ribs.

There has been some discussion by previous authors with regard to the position of the scapula at the time of fixation. Copeland and Howard fixed the scapula in a neutral position, while Ketenjian secured it in 20 degrees abduction. In the present series, scapulopexy was carried out in 30 degrees abduction with excellent results.

It is contended that the scapulopexy procedure should be undertaken in early adolescence in order to avoid some of the problems encountered by Ketenjian where in patients operated on over the age of 20, restriction of glenohumeral movement became apparent with advancing years. In only one case was there a slight modification of 5 to 10 degrees in abduction and flexion, the others maintaining their normal range. It is therefore indicated to undertake this procedure at an early age before joint contracture has become established, joint contracture being otherwise a natural effect of the untreated disease. Psychologically, the benefit to these patients is immense for they are now able to participate freely in normal activities at school and in sports. The one negative feature to note has been the diminution of pulmonary function which is inevitably suppressed by the restriction of rib motion. Happily, while the vital capacity has been decreased, this has not appeared to be of functional consequence. It should nonetheless be noted as an important sequela of the procedure.

REFERENCES

1. Copeland SA, Howard RC. Thoracoscapular fusion for facioscapulohumeral dystrophy. J Bone Joint Surg 1978; 60B:547–551.
2. Ketenjian Y. Scapulocostal stabilization for scapular winging in facioscapulohumeral muscular dystrophy. J Bone and Joint Surg 1978; 60A:476–480.
3. Sakurai M et al. A case of facioscapulohumeral type muscular dystrophy who retained elevation of the arm by scapulodesis (in Japanese). Tokohu Arch Orthop Surg Traumat 1980; 23:206–209.
4. Walton JN. Muscular dystrophy: Some recent advances in knowledge. Brit Med J 1964; 1:1271–1274.

RESULTS OF SURGICAL TREATMENT FOR DELTOID MUSCLE CONTRACTURE

TOMOMITSU KUTSUMA, M.D. and KAZUO TERAYAMA, M.D.

Seventy-nine cases of deltoid muscle contracture (involving 116 shoulder joints) were seen during the last 10 years beginning in 1972. Among these, 83 joints were treated surgically. This paper will report the results of operation on 70 joints with one year or more follow up.

All the patients had some history of intramuscular injections into the deltoid muscle during infancy or childhood. The ailments which originally occasioned the injections were mostly common cold, influenza, tonsillitis, bronchitis, etc. The medicaments injected in many cases were antibiotics or antipyretics.

In all cases, tense fibrous bands were palpable in the lateral fibers of the deltoid muscle, and winging of scapula and abduction contracture were observed.

The chief complaints before surgery were, in many cases, winging of scapula, abduction contructure, restriction of shoulder movement (restriction of adduction), and dull pain in the shoulder region (Fig. 1).

Twenty-six cases were male, 22 cases were female, 17 cases involved the left shoulder, six cases involved the right shoulder and 23 cases were bilateral. Age at operation ranged from 6 to 16 years, (the average was 11 years and 2 months) (Fig. 2), and the follow—up term after surgery ranged from 1 to 9 years (the average was 4 years and 6 months).

The operative methods employed were of four types, that is, simple transverse section of the main fibrous band at its acromial origin in 1 case (involving 1 joint), detachment of the lateral fibers in 4 cases (involving 6 joints), detachment of the lateral and posterior fibers in 41 cases (involving 60 joints), and detachment of lateral and posterior fibers plus transfer of the posterior fibers in 2 cases (involving 3 joints) (Tab. 1).

The results of surgery were generally satisfactory, and among 48 cases (involving 70 joints), there was recurrence in only one case (involving 1 joint), in which only simple transverse section of the fibrous band had been performed. In this case, reoperation was carried out one year after the first operation (the reoperation consisted of excision of the fibrous band and detachment of the lateral fibers), and the results seven years after reoperation were satisfactory, with no recurrence.

Except for this one case of recurrence, the angle of abduction contracture was improved, from the average of 25 degrees before surgery to zero degrees after surgery, the angle of adduction was improved from zero to 28 degrees, and the angle of horizontal flexion was improved from 93 to 120 degrees.

Residual winging of the scapula was observed in 1 out of 6 joints (16%) in the cases in which the lateral fibers were detached, and in 20 out of 60 joints (33%) in the cases in which lateral and posterior fibers were detached. However, in all those cases, the residual impediments were of very mild degree, only projections of the inferior angle of the scapula being observed, and these posed no clinical problems (Tab. 2).

The abduction contracture disappeared in all cases except for the one case of recurrence mentioned above.

As shown in (Fig. 3), the restriction of horizontal flexion was satisfactorily improved, even though some relapse was observed after two to five years following surgery.

Dent deformity of the deltoid was observed in 3 out of 6 joints (50%) in the cases where detachment of the lateral fibers was performed, and in 30 out of 60 joints (50%) in the cases where both lateral and posterior detachment were carried out. In the cases treated by transfer of the posterior fibers, dent deformity was relatively rare and was not conspicuous (Tab. 3).

Keloids were observed in 2 out of 6 joints (33%) of the lateral detachment cases and 7 out of

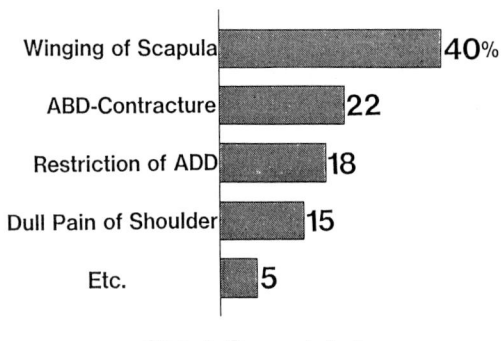

Figure 1 Chief complaints of patients with deltoid contracture.

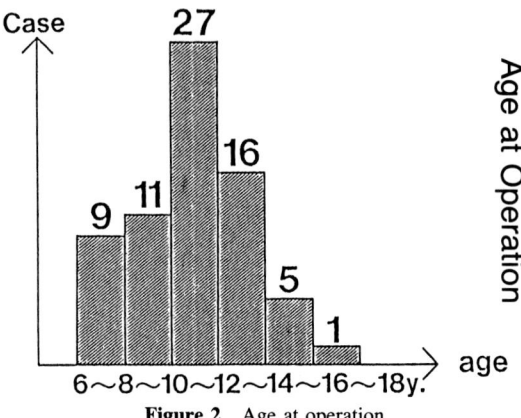

Figure 2 Age at operation.

60 joints (11%) in cases of both lateral and posterior detachment (Table 3).

Now, let us examine some representative cases.

Case 1

The first case is a nine-year old female. The abduction contracture angles were 25 degrees on both sides before surgery (Fig. 4a): the fibrous band in the left shoulder, and the lateral fibers in the right shoulder were detached. However, as a recurrence was observed in the left shoulder, reoperation was performed one year after the first operation (Fig. 4b). Observations during the reoperation showed that the fibrous band which had been detached in the previous operation had become completely continuous, like a tendon (Fig 5a), and about 2 cm extending from the origin were excised in the second operation. Furthermore, finely stretched tendonlike objects were intermingled in the muscular tissue which at first sight had seemed normal in a cursory inspection of the lateral and posterior fibers. Therefore, these objects were thoroughly detached while forcing adduction and horizontal flexion (Fig. 5b). Seven years have passed since the reoperation on the left shoulder, and eight years since the operation on the right shoulder, and the results are quite satisfactory.

Case 2

The second case is a 13-year old female. The abduction contracture angles before surgery were 35 degrees on the right and 40 degrees on the left, and even when the elbow was lifted from the flank of the body, the fingers could not reach the opposite shoulder. The left shoulder was dislocated anteriorly in some positions. (Fig. 7a, b, c). Observation at surgery showed that the entire lateral fibers were indurated like a plate (Fig. 8a); this was partially excised, starting from its origin, and the posterior fibers were detached (Fig. 8b).

Three years after surgery, results are satisfactory, the dislocation has disappeared and the patient can grasp the opposite shoulder (Fig. 9a, b, c).

TABLE 1 Operative Method

(1) simple transverse section of fibrous band	1 patient	1 joint
(2) cutting & detachment of lateral fibers	4 patients	6 joints
(3) cutting & detachment of lat & post. fibers	41 patients	60 joints
(4) (3) + post. fibers transfer	2 patients	3 joints

TABLE 2 Winging of Scapula

	Post Op.
(1) simple transverse section of fibrous band	1 joint, 100%
(2) cutting & detachment of lateral fibers	1 joint, 16%
(3) cutting & detachment of lat. & post. fibers	20 joints, 33%
(4) (3) + post. fibers transfer	0 joints, 0%

TABLE 3 Dent Deformity and Keloid

Operative Method	Dent Deformity	Keloid
(1) simple transverse section of fibrous band	0%	0%
(2) cutting & detachment of lateral fibers	50%	33%
(3) cutting & detachment of lat. & post fibers	50%	11%
(4) (3) + post. fibers transfer	0%	0%

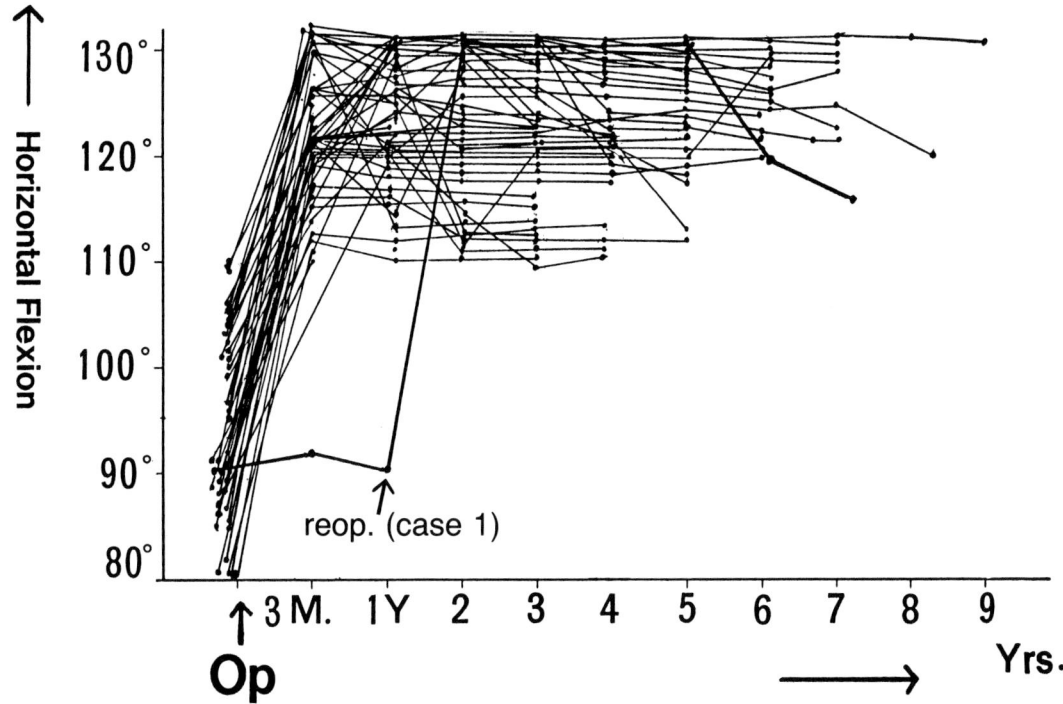

Figure 3 Improvement in horizontal flexion after operation.

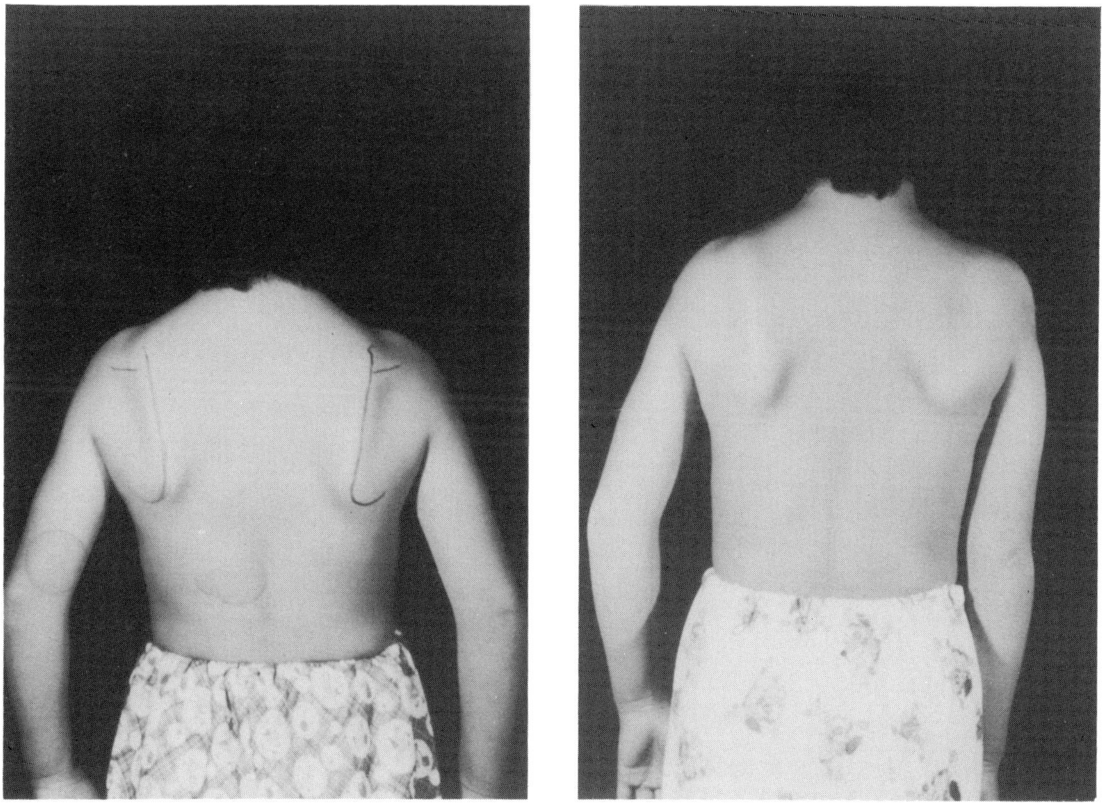

Figure 4 Pre- and postoperative appearance of 9-year-old child after bilateral correction.

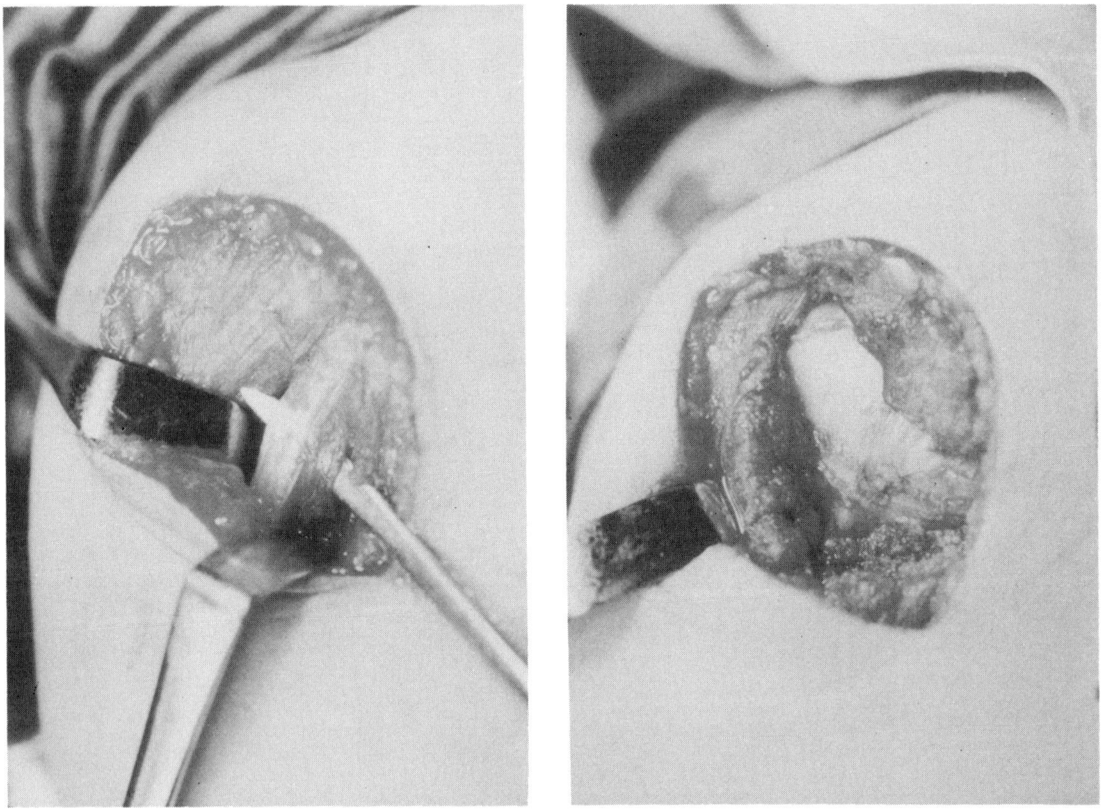

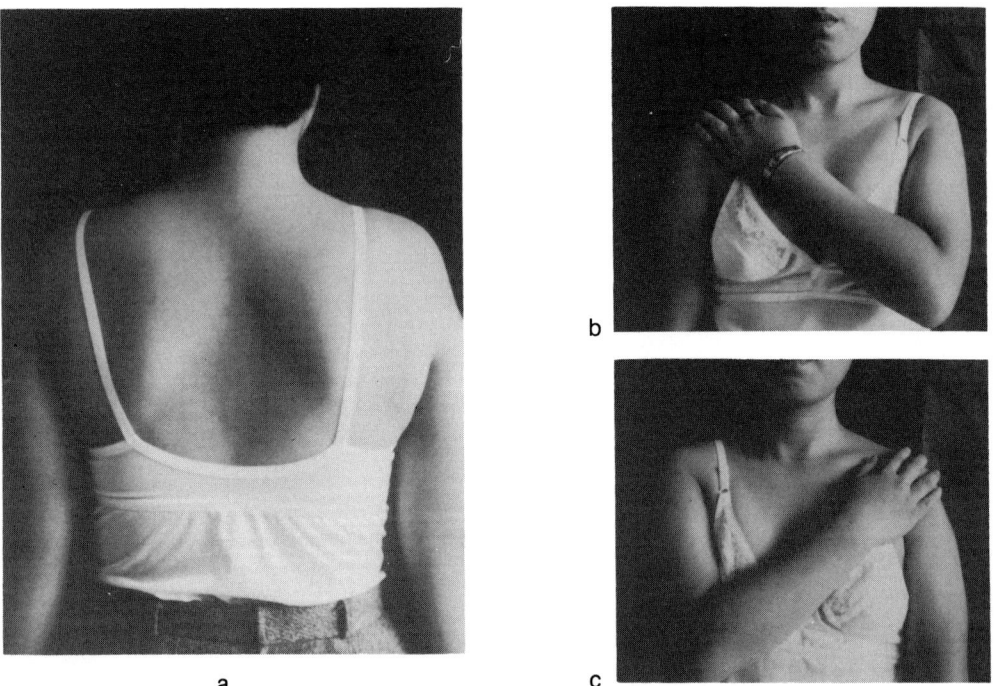

a b

Figure 5 The fibrous bands are almost tendon-like in appearance, requiring surgery.

a c

Figure 6 A 13-year-old girl demonstrating preoperative restriction of motion.

a b c

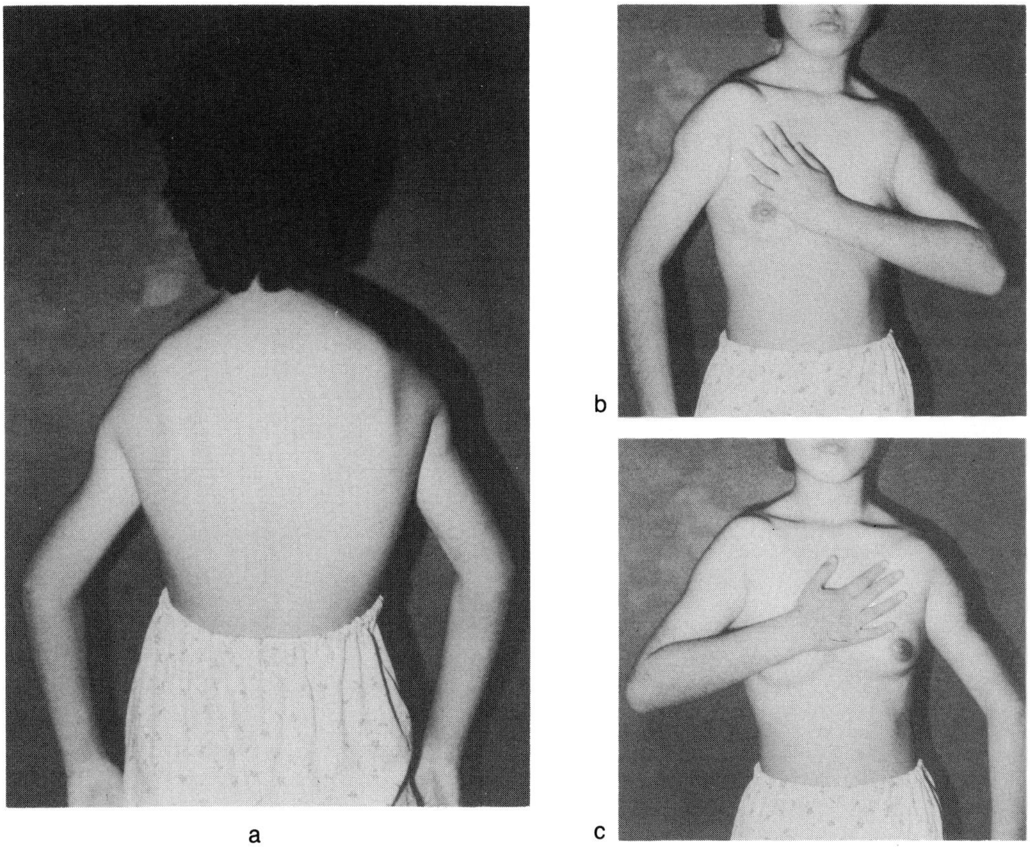

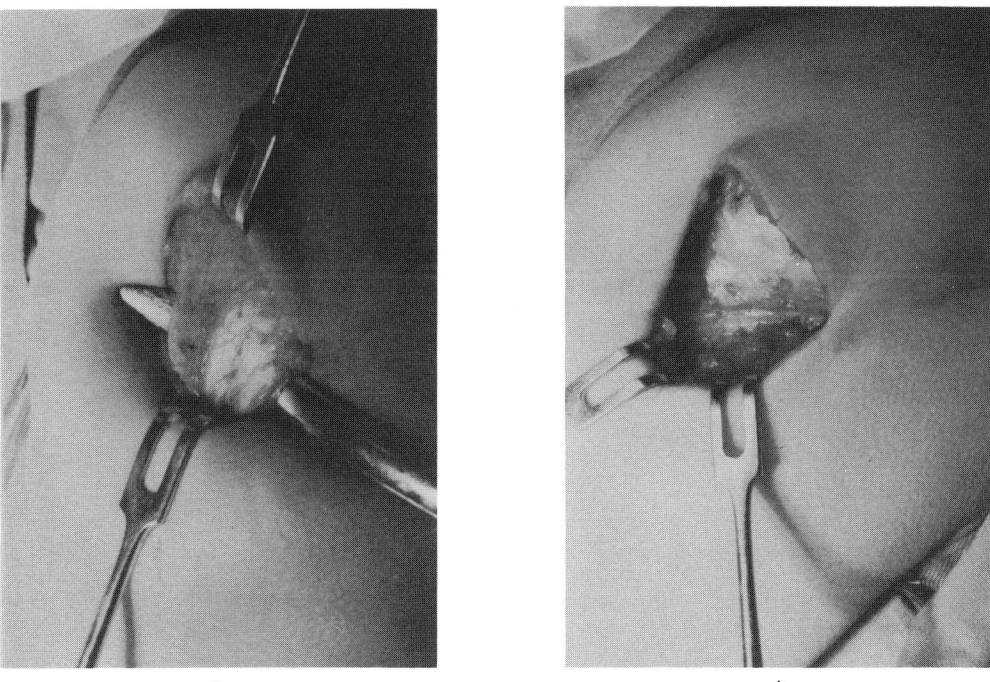

Figure 7 The left shoulder is seen to dislocate anteriorly.

a b

Figure 8 Lateral fibers of deltoid are indurated and plate-like.

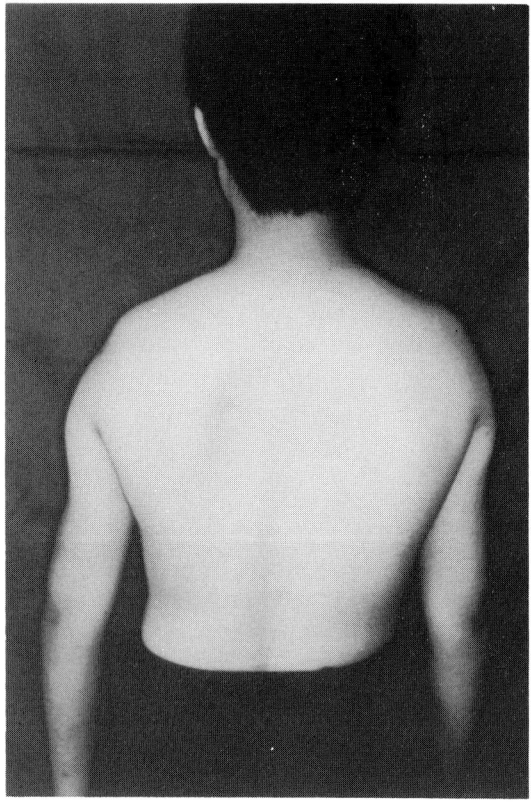

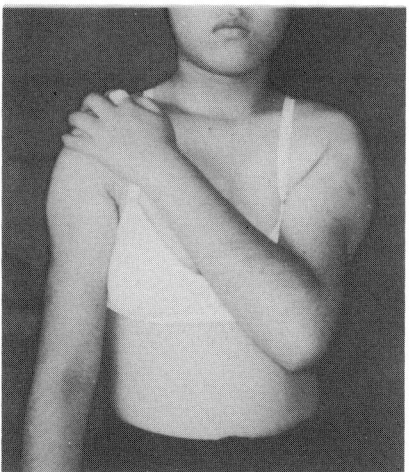

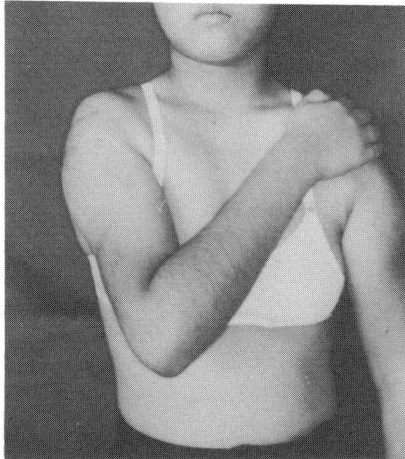

Figure 9 Function is greatly improved 3 years later.

Case 3

The third case is a 15-year old male. The abduction contracture angles before surgery were 35 degrees on both sides (Fig. 10a). In this case, the lateral and posterior fibers were detached and the posterior fibers were transferred to the lateral side.

Two years after surgery, the results are satisfactory and the dent deformity of the deltoid muscular region is slight and inconspicuous (Fig. 10b, c, d).

Case 4

The fourth case is a 16-year old female with abduction contracture of 35 degrees on both sides (Fig. 11a). The lateral and posterior fibers in the left shoulder were detached and after detachment of the lateral and posterior fibers in the right shoulder, the posterior fibers were transferred to the lateral side. One year after surgery, there is only a slight dent deformity in the deltoid on the right shoulder, in which transfer of the posterior fibers was performed (Fig. 11b).

DISCUSSION

We regard the overall results of surgical treatment of deltoid muscle contracture as generally satisfactory. However, simple transverse section of the fibrous band is insufficient and tends to result in recurrence.

In principle, we perform detachment of the lateral and posterior fibers in cases below 15 years of age. No recurrence was observed in 60 joints in which this surgical method was applied, and the

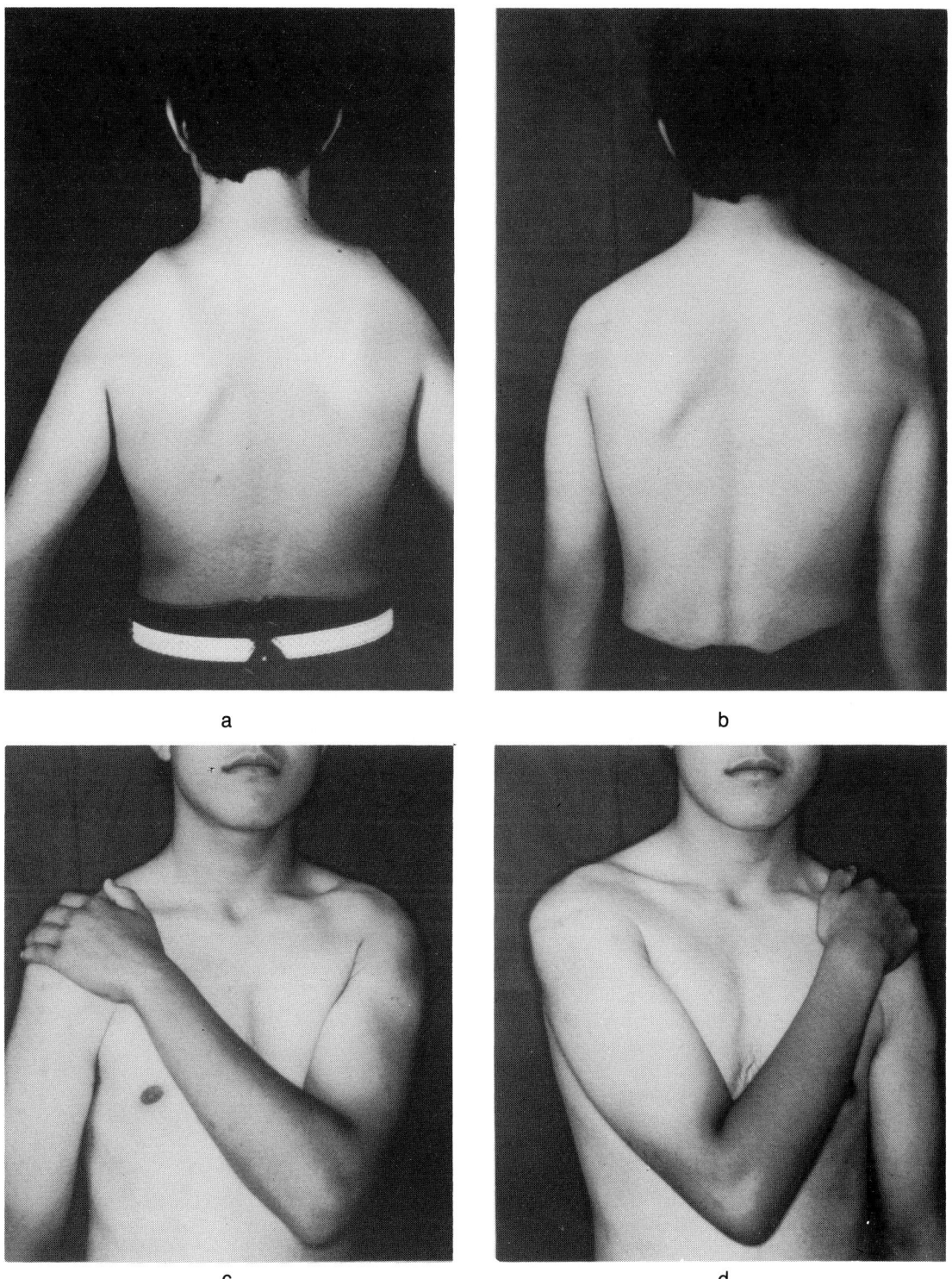

Figure 10 A 15-year-old male. Preoperative (a) and postoperative (b, c, and d) photographs.

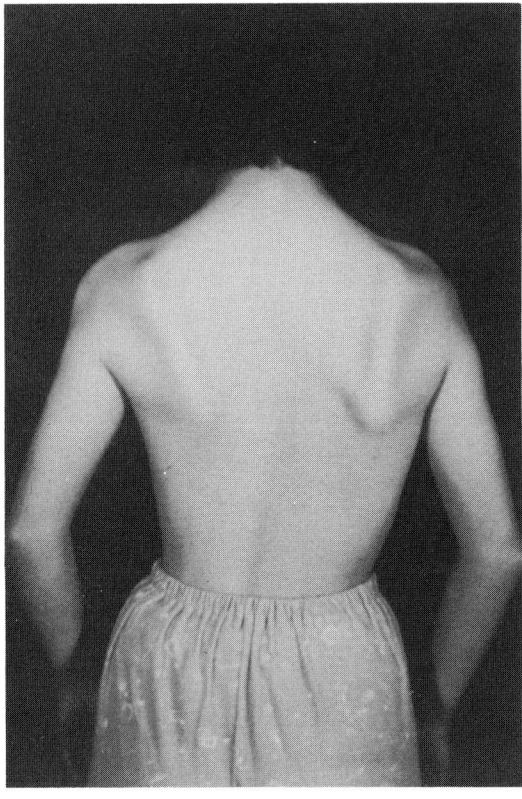
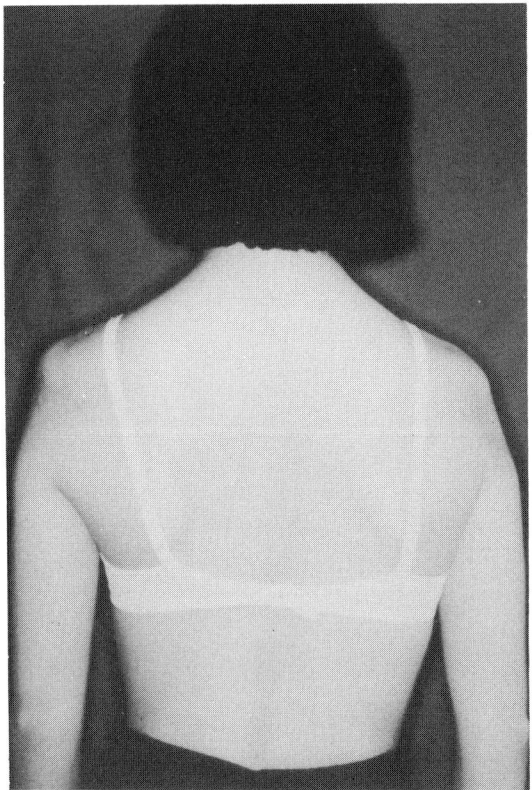

a   b

Figure 11 Pre- and postoperative photographs of 35° abduction contracture.

results were generally satisfactory. However, in 50 percent of this group, dent deformity of the deltoid muscular region was observed (Fig. 12a).

In cases over 15 years of age, we detach the lateral and posterior fibers and transfer the posterior fibers to the lateral side. In the three joints in which this method of surgery was employed, dent deformity of the deltoid muscular region after surgery was relatively slight and inconspicuous. We consider it preferable to transfer the posterior fibers in cases 15 years of age or older, in which the possibility of recurrence is slight (Fig. 12b).

Keloids constitute a problem for female patients in particular. To prevent keloids, we excise the adhesions between the subcutaneous tissue and fascia over an extensive region before detaching the contracted portion, in order to reduce the tension in the sutural area of the skin after surgery, and also use continuous intradermal sutures, as in plastic surgery, to close the incision.

Figure 13a shows the formation of keloid eight years after the use of ordinary single interrupted sutures, and Figure 13b shows the condition four years after the use of continuous intradermal sutures. In the latter case, the wound is clear and free from keloid formation.

According to the results of histological examinations, all the fibrous bands were indeed highly fibrotic and displayed a tendonlike struc-

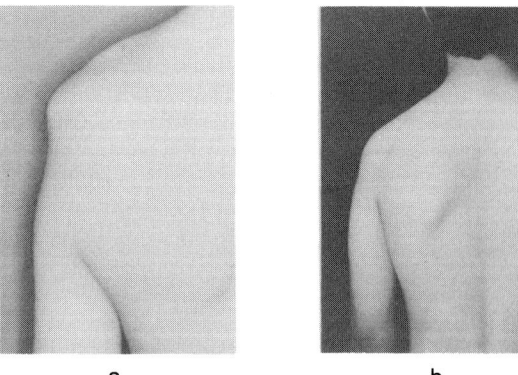

a   b

Figure 12 Severe dent deformity before and after surgery.

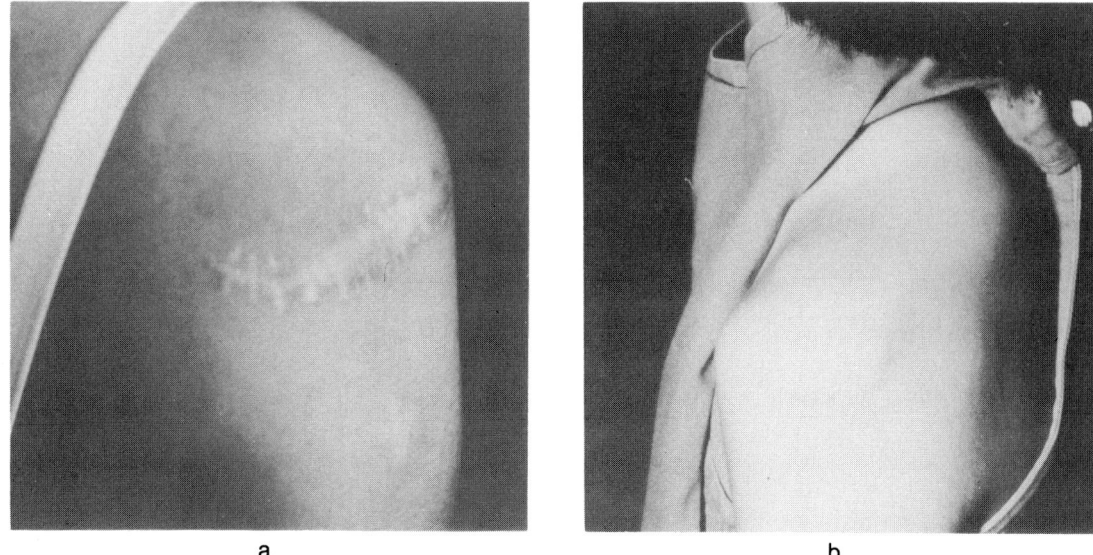

Figure 13 (a) Keloid complicating surgical treatment. (b) After revision with intradermal technique.

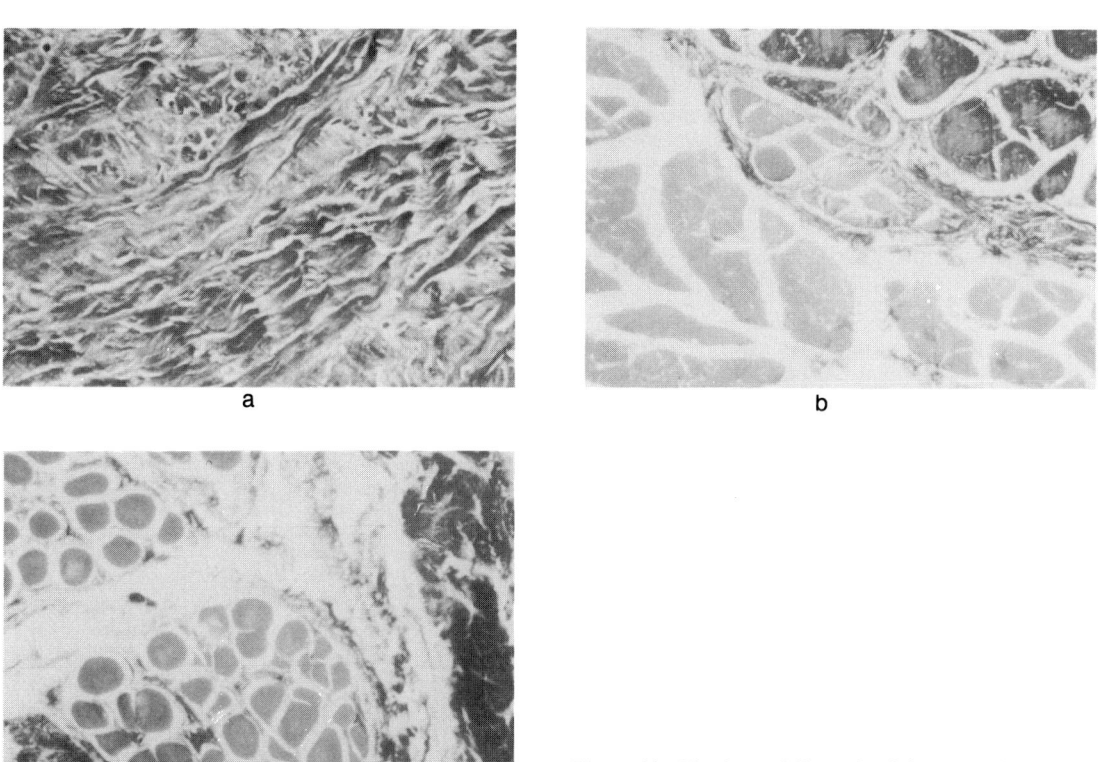

Figure 14 Histology of fibrous band tissue. (a) Mallory azar stain. (b) Fibrosis in perimysium and endomysium. (c) Fibrosis in posterior fibers is less pronounced.

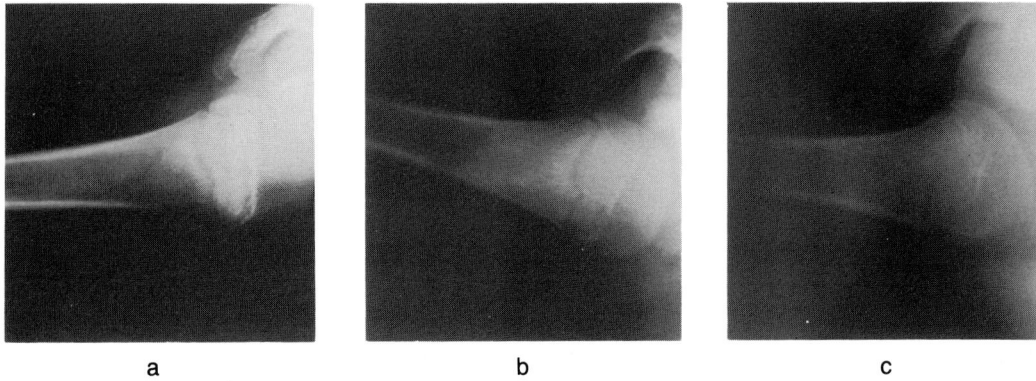

Figure 15 Appearance of the humeral head. (a) Normal. (b) Oval. (c) Flattened.

ture. Figure 14a shows a transverse section of a fibrous band treated with Mallory azan stain.

In all cases, fibrosis was observed in the perimysium and endomysium of the lateral fibers of the deltoid muscles, which, at first sight, had appeared macroscopically normal (Fig. 14b).

A similar appearance was observed in the lateral areas of the posterior fibers of the deltoid muscles (Fig. 14c). However, the degree of fibrosis was less pronounced than that in the lateral fibers.

The roentgenographic findings of pathological changes before surgery were observed from lateral view of the humeral head. Figure 15 shows images of normal, oval shaped and flattened humeral head. The flattened deformity in the posterior part of the humeral head is quite pronounced, and anterior subluxation is evident. We observed a high incidence of these changes, that is, oval shaped deformation in 45 percent, flattened changes in 36 percent, and anterior subluxation in 80 percent of the cases (Tab. 4).

As regards the relation between the deformation of the humeral head and the angle of abduction contracture, oval shaped and flattened deformations appeared when the angle exceeded 20 degrees, the oval shaped deformations increased to 61 percent in the range from 20 to 29 degrees, and for angles of 30 degrees or more, the flattened deformations were observed with a high frequency of 88 percent (Tab. 5).

We believe that surgery should be carried out at an early stage in cases with pronounced deformation of the humeral head.

TABLE 4 Roentgenographic Findings

(1) humeral head deformity	
type 1 (oval-shaped)	45%
type 2 (flattening)	36%
(2) anterior subluxation	80%

TABLE 5 The Relation Beween Head Deformity and ABD Contracture

	ABD Contracture		
Head Deformity	*15° ~ 19°*	*20° ~ 29°*	*30° ~*
type 1 (oval-shaped)	40	61	12%
type 2 (flattening)	0	28	88%

ARTHRITIC DISORDERS

SURGERY OF THE RHEUMATOID SHOULDER

N. GSCHWEND, M.D. and A. KENTSCH, M.D.

Frequency of Involvement

The shoulder joint ranges in place 7 or 8 regarding its frequency. Laine and Vainio found shoulder symptoms in 57 percent of their patients.[1] In a follow-up study of 300 patients with rheumatoid arthritis and a disease duration of 10 years, we identified clinical symptoms of shoulder involvement in 58 percent.

Radiological Changes of the Shoulder Joint

We have recently examined 144 shoulder joints in a noninterrupted series of 73 polyarthritic patients (two had undergone a previous arthrodesis).[2] This has been a selection of patients, insofar as a great majority came to the clinic for the performance of some kind of surgery, not referring to the shoulder yet. As criteria of evaluation, we used the 6 stages of Larsen-Dahle-Eek (Fig. 1) being used in most European rheumatoid centers, where 0 indicates normal conditions and 5 the most severe degree of destruction.[3] Table 1 shows the various degrees of severity in the 144 shoulder joints approximating a Gaussian curve. Table 2 assesses the generally known symmetric onset of changes in polyarthritis. Table 3 contains a graph of symmetry and severity of the alterations. We thus notice how symmetry correlates with degree of severity, with a few exceptions.

Pain

Clinically the pain, particularly on movement, can be named as a most striking symptom. As expected, pain and limited movement correlate with the degree of severity of radiological changes (Table 4a,b). The internal rotation appears to be somewhat less frequently reduced to a severe extent than the external rotation (Table 5a, 6c). This is probably due to the fact that the internal rotation is the appropriate position of work for self-care, being thus more important than the external rotation.

Functional Impairment

The consequences of shoulder disability involvement in everyday functions are impressive. In a former study of 35 patients with rheumatoid arthritis who were most severely handicapped in self-care, the question was investigated as to which joints of the upper extremities were mainly responsible. In 17 cases, i.e. in almost 50 percent it was the shoulder, whereas the elbow was found to be mainly responsible in only 5 cases. For further investigation of this question, 73 patients were subdivided into 3 groups, separating those showing destruction on both sides to severity degree 5. They were compared with a second group in which both shoulders were intact, and a third group in which only one shoulder was involved.

In group 1 with 8 patients (Table 6a), there were 3 in functional class ARA IV, 2 in functional class ARA III, 1 in functional class ARA II. This means that nearly all were highly impaired.

In group 2 with 6 patients (Table 6b), there were 4 in functional class 2, and 2 in class 1; in other words, they were only slightly handicapped. Group 3 with 7 patients, among whom there was only one shoulder involved, is in a medium position with regard to disability.

This leads to the conclusion that *severe destruction of both shoulder joints occurs nearly exclusively in the very severe forms of rheumatoid arthritis, where the other joints are not spared either* (Fig. 2) Conversely, those with healthy shoulders may reveal but a few changes in the other joints (Fig. 3), e.g. such as in group 2 with

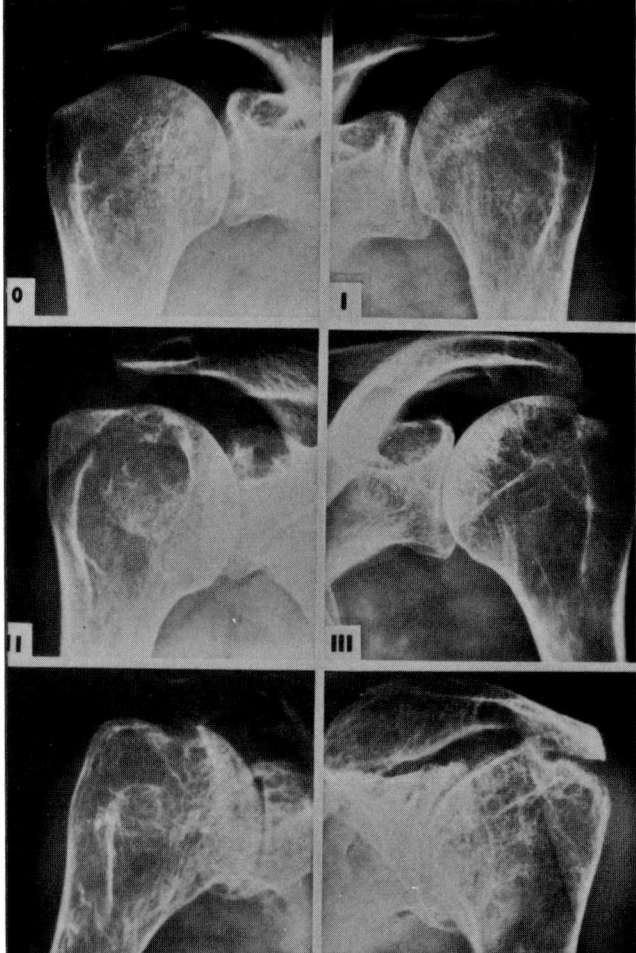

Figure 1 The 6 radiological stages of shoulder involvement according to Larsen-Dahle-Eek (LDE).

pauciarticular cases only, half of which referred to juvenile rheumatoid arthritis. On the other hand, the shoulder joints may still look normal, whereas most other joints show severe destruction. An opposite example in which the shoulder joints were destroyed while the other joints were mostly intact, could not be found in this series. In nearly all patients with shoulder involvement, we found that destruction appeared much later than in the other joints. These findings explain most surgeons' hesitation in regard to operative treatment of the shoulder.

SURGERY

Indications for Surgery

The patient whose hands are grossly and painfully changed, or who has an obvious limp will only agree to an operation of the shoulder, when there is no other choice and when he experiences a loss of independence. Taking into account the central functional significance of the shoulder, this reluctance is most unfortunate. In rheumatoid arthritis, the art of surgical treatment does not so

(Text continued on page 276)

TABLE 1 Pattern of Disease Severity

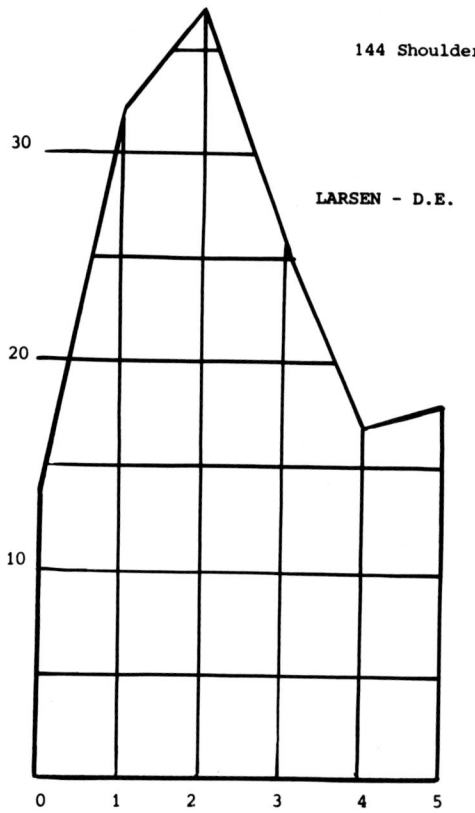

TABLE 2 Symmetrical Involvement in Polyarthritis

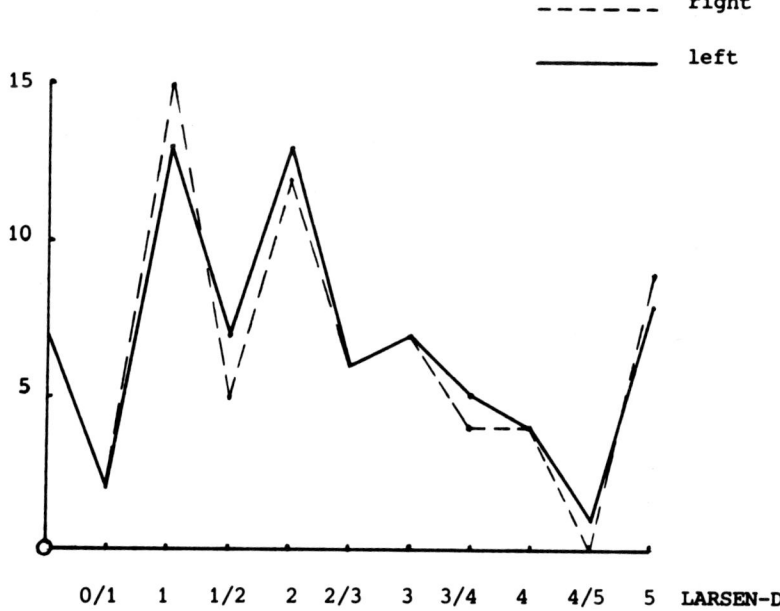

272 / Surgery of the Shoulder

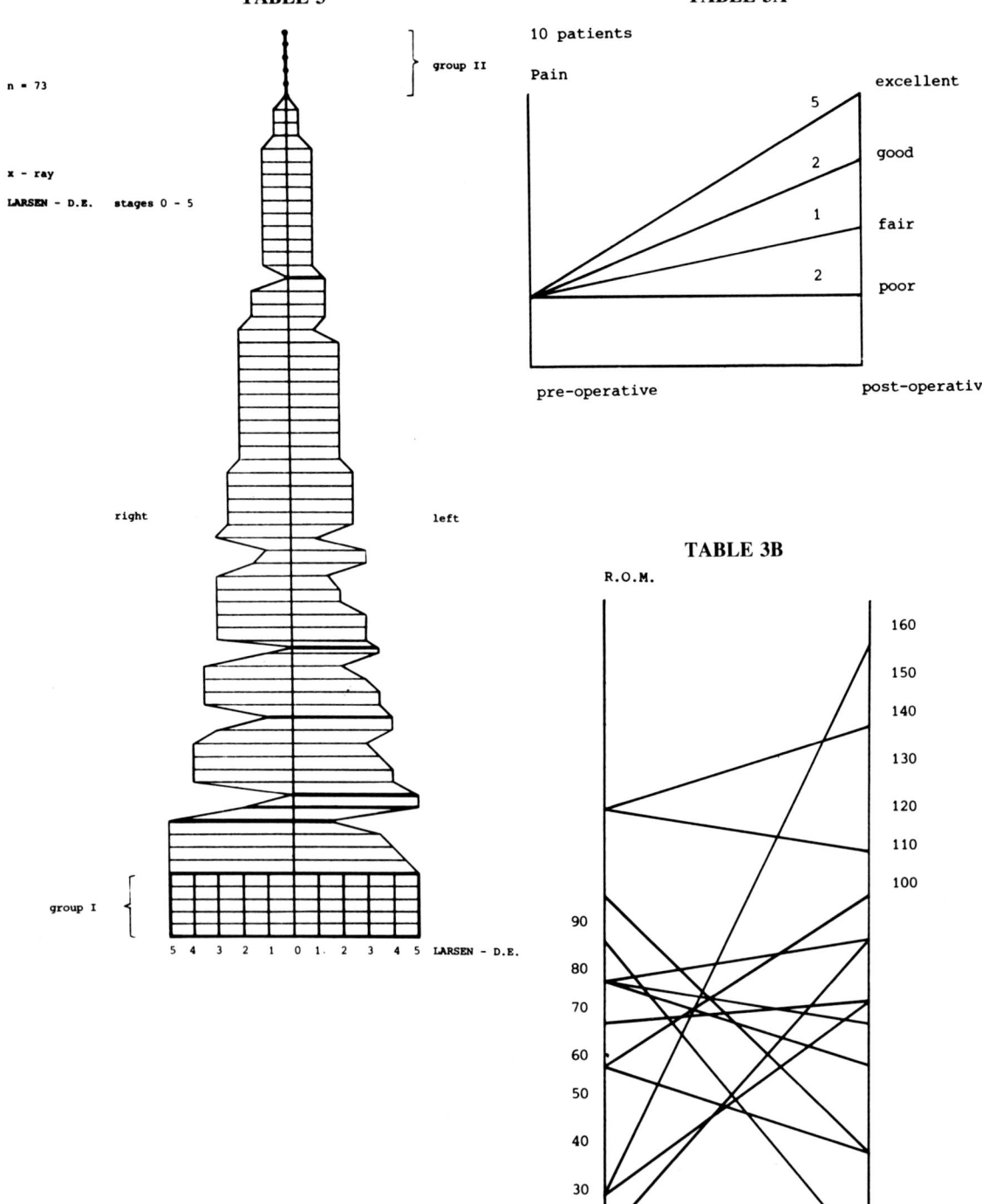

TABLE 4A Group I* Pain Severity in Larsen-Dahle-Eek Stage 5 Impairment

Severe	Moderate	Slight	None
80%	10%	10%	0

*6 patients, 12 shoulders

TABLE 4B Group II* Pain Severity in Larsen-Dahle-Eek Stage 0 Impairment

Severe	Moderate	Slight	None
0	0	0	100%

*6 patients, 12 shoulders

TABLE 5A Group I* Range of Motion in Larsen-Dahle-Eek Stage 5 Functional Impairment

flexion	min. 30° / max. 150°	average 95°
external rotation	min. 20° / max. 70°	average 40°
internal rotation	min. 30° / max. 80°	average 50°

*6 patients, 12 shoulders

TABLE 5B Group II* Range of Motion in Larsen-Dahle-Eek Stage 0 Functional Impairment

flexion	min. 180° / max. 180°	average 180°
external rotation	min. 80° / max. 100°	average 85°
internal rotation	min. 80° / max. 100°	average 90°

*6 patients, 12 shoulders

TABLE 5C Group III* Patients with Unilateral Involvement

Right				Left			
Rotation Ext/Int	Flexion	Pain	Larsen Stage	Larsen Stage	Pain	Flexion	Rotation Ext/Int
20-0-70°	100°	severe	5	1-2	slight	150°	60-0-90°
90-0-80°	160°	slight	2	5	moderate	140°	60-0-60°
70-0-80°	90°	moderate	1	5	severe	60°	50-0-60°
80-0-80°	180°	slight	1	4	severe	180°	60-0-60°
60-0-80°	180°	none	1	3-4	slight	160°	10-0-90°
80-0-80°	180°	painless	0	3-4	slight	180°	80-0-80°

*6 patients, 12 shoulders

TABLE 6A RA Shoulder Joint

Group 1	n = 8	ARA	
(LDE 4-5 bilateral)		I	0
		II	1
		III	2
		IV	5
			8

TABLE 6B RA Shoulder Joint

Group 2	n = 6	ARA	
(LDE 0 bilateral)		I	2
		II	4
		III	0
		IV	0

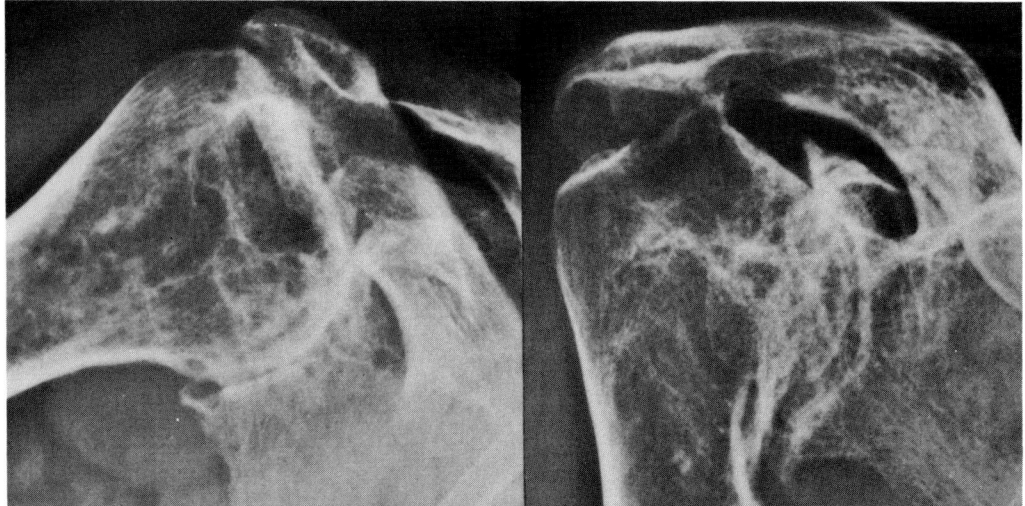

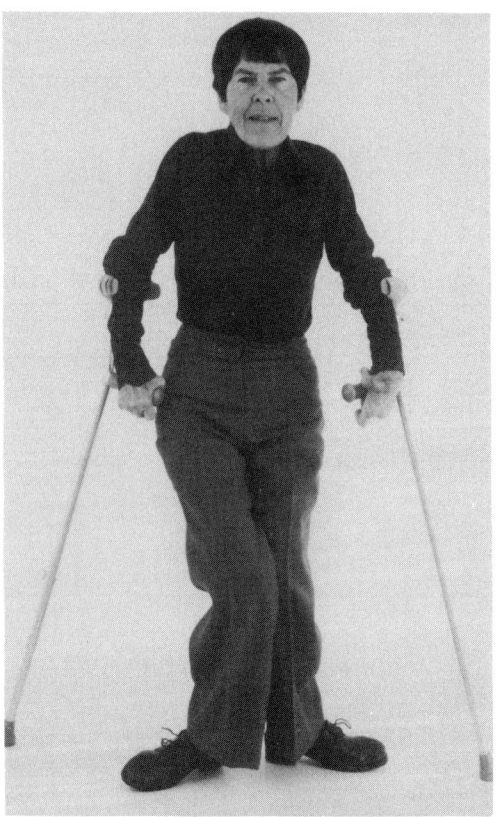

Figure 2a, 2b Patient with bilateral shoulder-involvement LDE 5. Functional class IV.

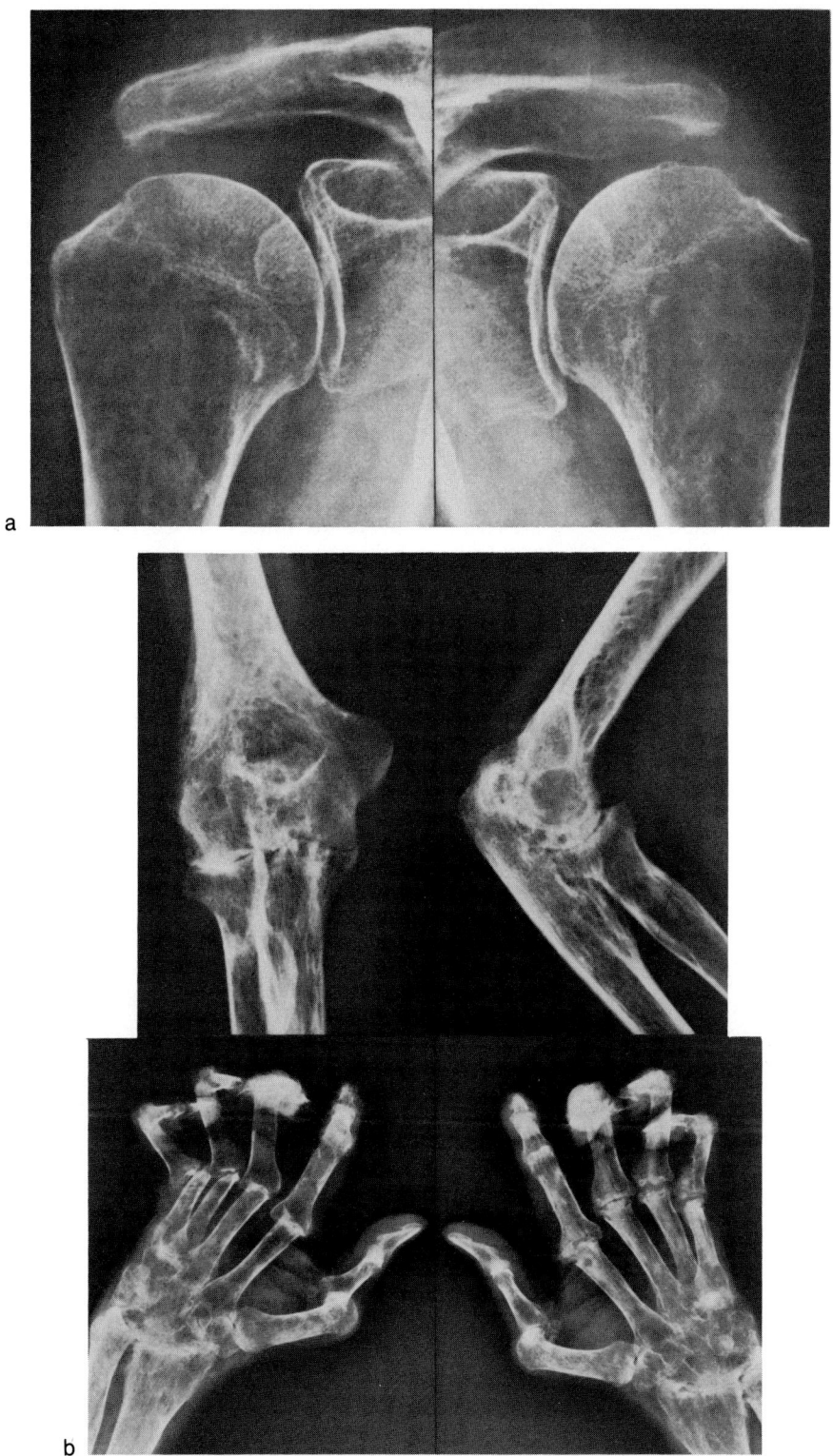

Figure 3a, 3b Severe destruction at various joints especially wrist-, finger- and elbow joints, whereas the shoulder joint looks really normal.

much consist of mastering surgical techniques—which is an obvious stipulation—but rather in setting up a list of priorities. The shoulder merits high priority. This is evident from our tests of occupational therapy that have been systematically performed for years. All polyarthritic patients coming to our clinic for surgery are tested, enabling us to define the degree of handicap as well as the main cause of disability.[5] We were amazed to see how patients got along reasonably well with severely destroyed shoulder joints, provided the scapular mechanism was compensating without too much pain and that enough rotation was retained as in cases shown in Figure 4a and b.

In 5100 operations for rheumatoid arthritis performed at our clinic, there were only 45 carried out at the shoulder. On the basis of our experience, we shall attempt to illustrate our attitude towards synovectomy, double osteotomy, arthrodesis and arthroplasty.

Synovectomy

Reports on shoulder synovectomies are few. Early synovectomies are the great exceptions. The highest figures come from the Scandinavian area (Pahle, 35 cases in 1981) and from Germany (Mohing et al, 39 cases in 1980). Most of these are bursectomies with concomitant synovectomy. The explanation is self-evident. Clinically, it is difficult to diagnose a synovitis. The swelling only becomes visible, alarming the patient and his doctor, when the joint involved starts communicating with the surrounding bursae via a rotator cuff tear. Out of almost 2000 synovectomies done at our clinic, only 12 were at the shoulder. There was only one case, when we could not trace a rupture of the rotator cuff. As a further consequence of the rotator cuff tear, the biceps tendon invaded by tenosynovitis is under additional mechanical strain, leading to typical anterior shoulder pain on movement, until spontaneous rupture of the tendon occurs. The relationship with the Baker cyst, respectively the rupture of the posterior knee capsule, becomes also obvious by the remarkable frequency of fibrinous content in the bursae which can be amorphous or in the form of melon seeds (Fig. 5).

Results. Our results of synovectomies in 12 cases correspond largely to those of Pahle and Mohing. Pain and swelling are essentially reduced. This is the reason why about 80 percent of the patients are personally satisfied with the outcome. Mobility depends largely on the absence of a rotator cuff tear and how it will be repaired. Mostly

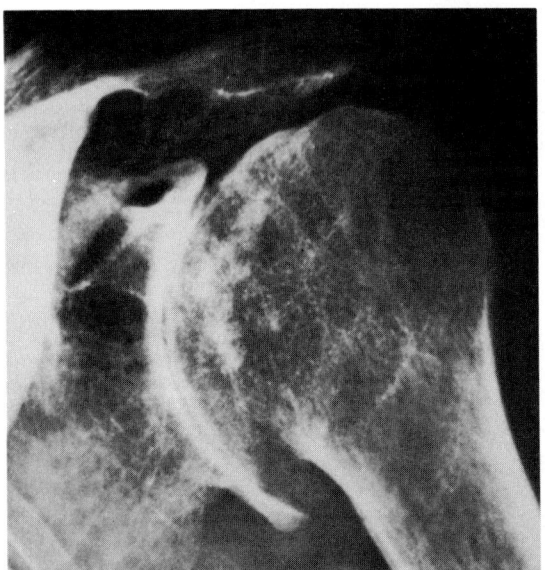 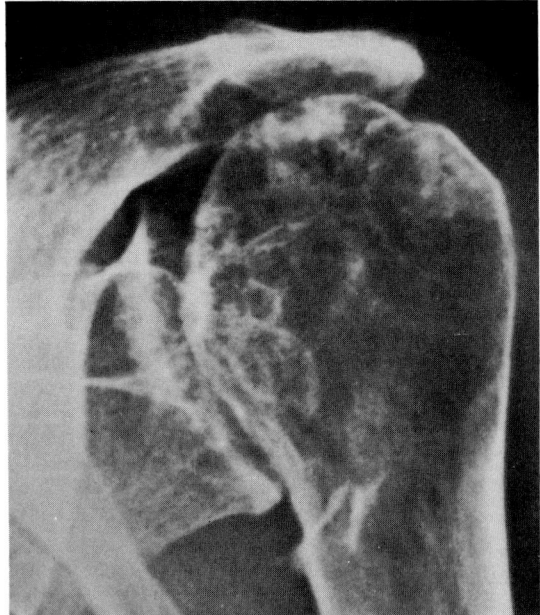

Figure 4a, 4b Severe radiological shoulder joint involvement with pseudo-arthroplastic-like adaptation of the joint surfaces. In Figure 4b the action of the rotator cuff has been taken over by a groove in the acromion. Function relatively good.

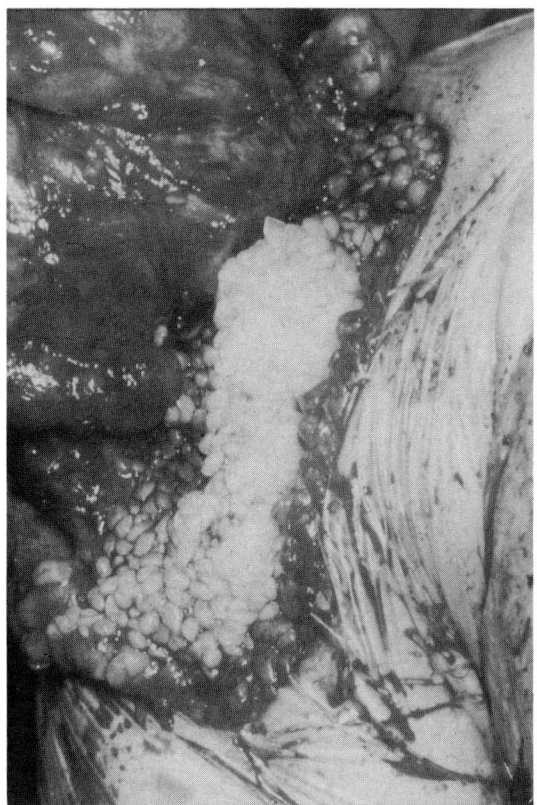

Figure 5 Synovitis and bursitis of the shoulder joint with massive melon seeds.

we found an improved range of movement which, however, diminished over several years as the radiographs also changed for the worse.

The *results* are of particular interest. At the ERASS (European RA Surgical Society) Congress 1983 in Moscow, one topic dealt with late (that is more than 10 years) results of early (Larsen-Dahle-Eek 0-3) synovectomy. Pahle reported on 10 late cases. In the meantime, two of them had died and two patients had had the shoulder joint replaced by a total prosthesis. For the remaining six, it was remarkable that all declared themselves satisfied, complaining of little pain, if any, and showing merely a slight reduction of range of motion and muscular strength. The radiograph had become worse by one Larsen's degree on the average. This result was completely in line with the late results after synovectomy of all the other joints which we assessed for the same Congress. The radiological picture of the shoulder operated on looks much the same after ten or more years as that of the non-operated shoulder. The type of rheumatoid arthritis is decisive for the final stage. However, a majority of patients complain of much less pain and functional impairment in the operated shoulder; this proves that precious time can be gained by synovectomy. Therefore, it is our opinion that synovectomy should be performed more frequently and earlier. Since other operations are often given priority, radioisotope synovectomy (synoviorthesis) should be carried out prior to the surgical synovectomy. This can be done concurrently with other surgical measures on the upper and lower extremity.

Menkes (1979) achieved in 70% of early cases (stages 1 and 2) an improvement regarding pain and swelling. Today there are even more effective β-ray emitters available.

The requirement of early synovectomy (respectively) synoviorthesis requires early diagnosis of synovitis. Pain in the shoulder, where other causes may also be implicated, is not an absolutely reliable criterion. To wait for the onset of visible swelling with bursitis means to lose precious time. We, therefore, have increasingly attempted to diagnose synovitis by means of technetium pertechnetate scanning or by gallium scintigraphy (Fig. 6). We were able to prove the reliability of this method by arthroscopy, and we shall use the former together with the synoviorthesis more often in the future. In case of failure of the synoviorthesis, we advocate surgical synovectomy if possible in Larsen's stage 0.1 or 2.

Double Osteotomy

Double osteotomy according to Benjamin[11] has been suggested widely as an alternative to arthroplasty in less advanced cases. We performed it 13 times, eight times in rheumatoid arthritis, five times in osteoarthritis, two cases of which revealed a humeral head necrosis. The operative technique followed Benjamin's description. The response was remarkably positive in all osteoarthritic joints, except in one case of dyschondroplasia. This method failed in four of eight patients with rheumatoid arthritis. In the failed cases, either a highly active disease with a high sedimentation rate was noted, or there was less involvement of the joint itself but more of the surrounding soft tissues. In the future we shall reserve double osteotomy for patients with juvenile polyarthritis suffering from secondary osteoarthritic pain with less activity of the disease, or osteoarthritis where in view of the age of the patient, we feel more hesitant about

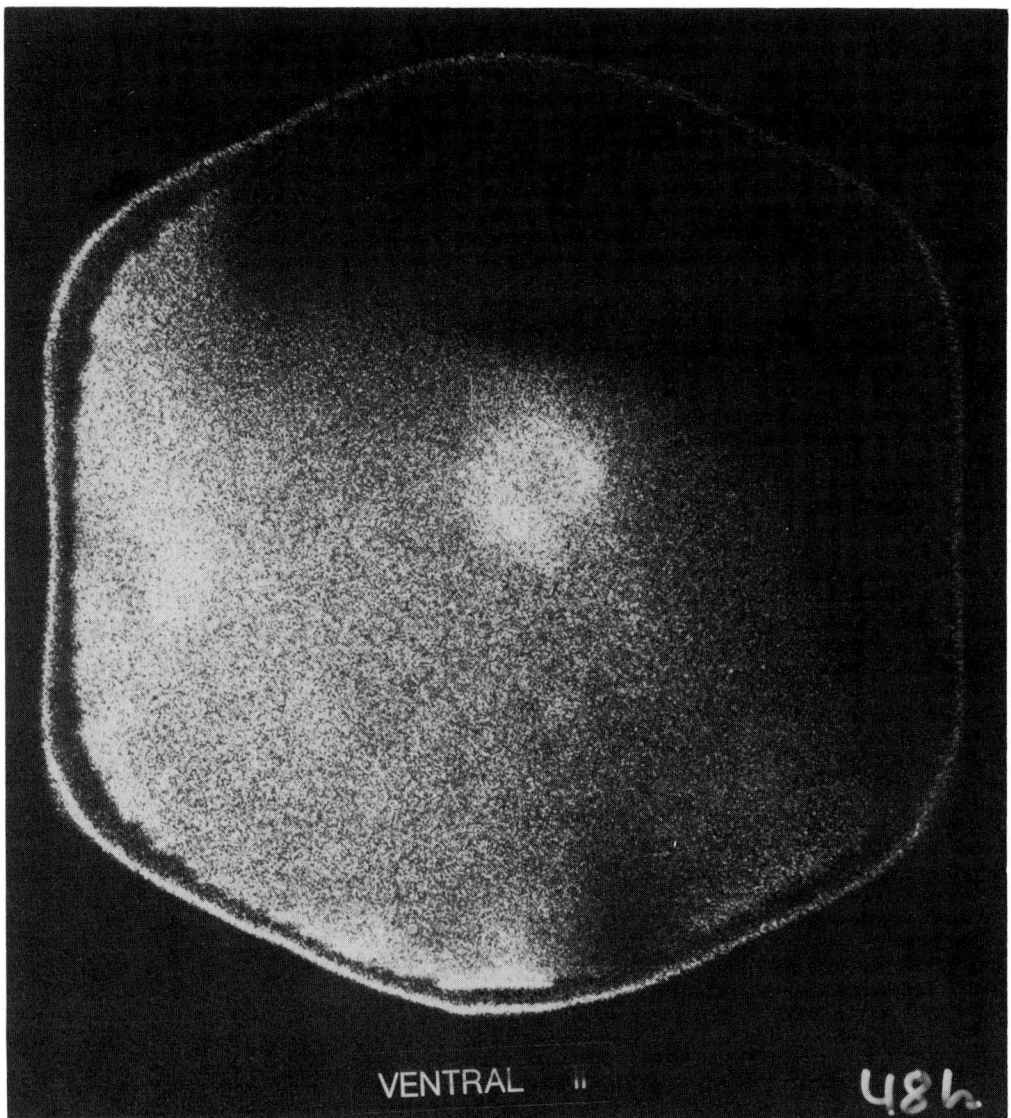

Figure 6 Gallium scintigraph showing shoulder joint synovitis.

replacement by an artificial joint. We expect pain relief and a functionally useful increase of motion (Table 6).

Arthrodesis

Arthrodesis of the shoulder joint which we performed on three patients may yield favorable long-term results, provided its performance does not subsequently require prolonged fixation, and if a medium position is chosen between external and internal rotation.[16] Satisfaction was expressed by our 3 patients. On the other hand, arthrodesis can hardly be regarded as a serious alternative to the rapidly improving arthroplasties.

Arthroplasty

This is the method of choice for the shoulder joint destroyed by rheumatoid arthritis in Larsen's stage 4 and 5, if the patient suffers from pain and functional impairment. The latter assessment is of particular importance, since the indication for surgical management in rheumatoid arthritis often is not based on the patient's real needs, but rather on the surgeon's personal interest and capacity. Especially, arthroplasty of the shoulder joint requires a thorough preoperative investigation to find the crucial point of disability. This is vital, since severe changes of the shoulder joint are often associated with no less severe destruction of the hand and elbow. If elbow flexion does not reach 90°, an improved external rotation by arthroplasty is of little use to the patient. Similarly, a painfully limited *prosupination* cannot be improved by arthroplasty, rather, a much less difficult resection of the ulnar head is the procedure of choice. "Start with a winner," is the slogan of W. Souter of Edinburgh in view of surgical management of rheumatoid arthritis. This means that we should start with a surgical procedure of first order, that is with a high chance of success. Based on recent international literature and also on our own experience, we would like to classify arthroplasty of the shoulder in the second of the three groups of successful surgical approaches. Arthroplasty can be remarkably successful, but the possibility of failure should not be underestimated, apart from the fact that there are not yet any long-term studies referring to socket loosening. Opportunities of withdrawal are by no means as easy as in other joints.

To our and our patients' satisfaction the Neer prosthesis is used in our clinic. I would like to mention the kinds of prostheses we do not use any longer on the basis of our negative experience.

In 4 cases we inserted the Zippel prosthesis, a fully constrained one. All of the four prostheses led to fracture in the region of the humeral neck associated with a painful functional loss of the shoulder. The Kölbel prosthesis has advantages compared with the other constrained prostheses, mainly regarding the fixation on the scapula, the fulcrum and the theoretical extension of motion. However, this prosthesis, implanted 3 times in our clinic, also shows a high degree of strain producing loosening and migrating of the scapular component, because of the mostly poor quality of bone. The problem of loosening also with non-constrained prostheses has not been solved yet, particularly where we have to compensate a non-restorable rotator cuff tear by a cranial lip. The acropole prosthesis developed by Grammont[20] was not really intended to be used for patients with rheumatoid arthritis. Nevertheless, the patient in Figure 7 illustrates the sound idea of functional replacement of the rotator cuff by a subacromial support and an artificial gliding surface on the greater tuberosity. Her scapulo–humeral joint had been largely destroyed and no replacement was made. However, thanks to the Acropole prosthesis, a remarkable improvement of function and relief of pain were achieved.

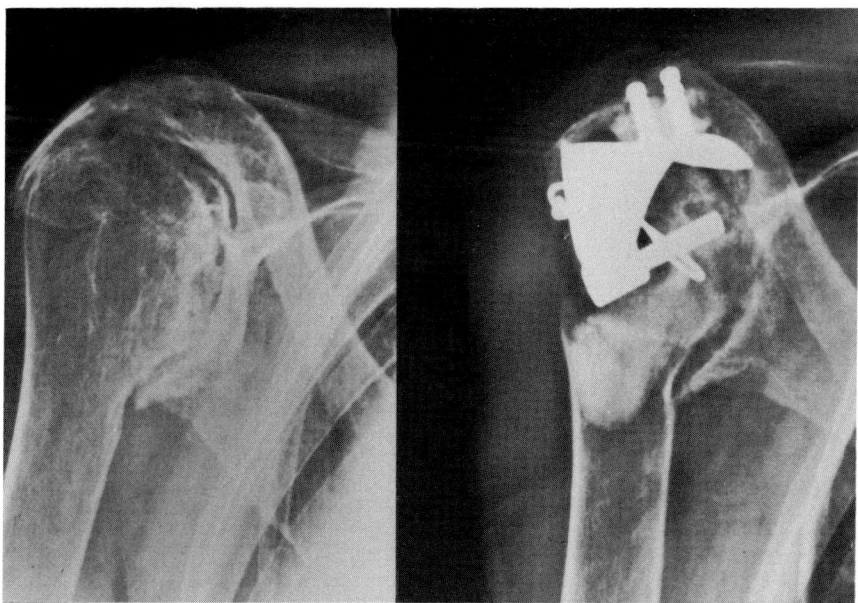

Figure 7a Grammont's Acropole prosthesis for compensation of a non-reparable rotator cuff.

(Illustration continued on the following page)

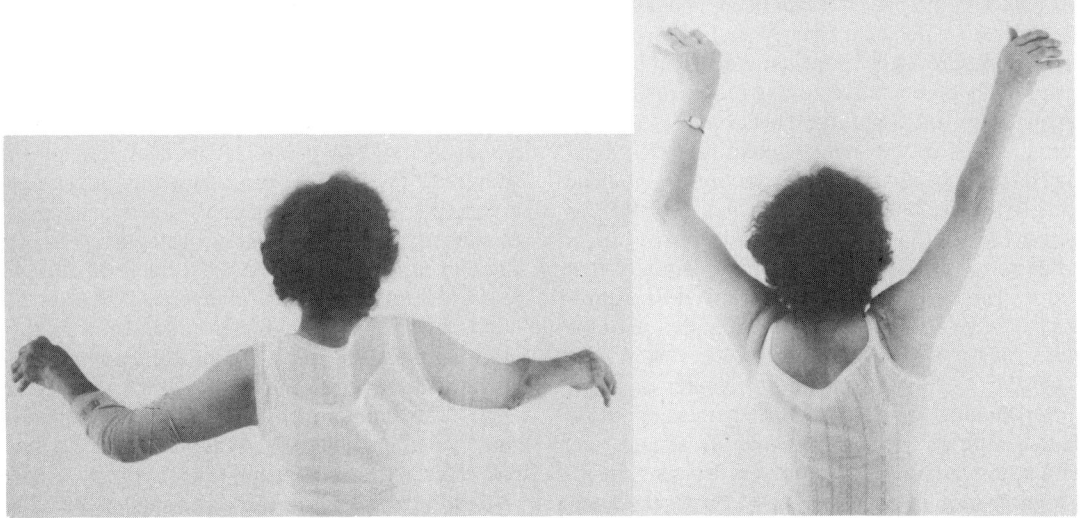

Figure 7b Clinical result: before and after operation.

Summary

Together with Grammont, we are working out a new technique that will enable us to replace functionally the joint surfaces as well as the rotator cuff, without the current high risk of socket loosening.

With any kind of reconstruction, even in an optimal case, we have to take into account long term stability and restricted opportunities for withdrawal. We, therefore, believe that we must concentrate increasingly on the early diagnosis of shoulder synovitis and its local treatment.

REFERENCES

1. Laine V, Vainio K. Shoulder in rheumatoid arthritis. Symposium on early synovectomy in rheumatoid arthritis. ISRA Amsterdam, 1967.
2. Gschwend N, Raaflaub B, Dybowski R. Häufigkeit und Art der Deformitäten bei Polyarthritikern. Schweiz. Rheumatologenkongress Fribourg 1975.
3. Larsen A, Dahle K, Eek M. Radiographic evaluation of rheumatoid arthritis and related conditions by standard reference films. Acta Radiologica Diagnosis 18, 1977.
4. Gschwend N. Surgical Treatment of Rheumatoid Arthritis. 1980 WB Saunders, Philadelphia.
5. Gschwend N, Ehrensperger E, Moser D. Occupational therapy in Rheumatoid Arthrits. Occupational therapy today-tomorrow, in: Proc. 5th Int. Congress WFOT, Zurich, 1970. Karger, Basel 1971.
6. Gschwend N. General surgical principles in rheumatoid arthritis: Priorities. The Canadian Journal of Surgery, Vol. 26, 1983.
7. Pahle JA. The shoulder joint in rheumatoid arthritis: Synovectomy. Reconstr. Surg. Traumat., vol. 18, Karger, Basel, 1981.
8. Köhler G, Schmidt F. Zur Synovialektomie des Schultergelenks bei chronischer Polyarthritis. Act. Rheumatol. 5, 1980.
9. Pahle JA. Late results in synovectomy of the shoulder. ERASS Congress, Moscow 1983, to be published.
10. Menkes CJ. Is there a place for chemical and radiation synovectomy in rheumatic diseases? Rheumatology and Rehabilitation Vol. XVIII 1979.
11. Benjamin A. Doppelosteotomie am Schultergelenk. Orthopäde 10, 1981.
12. Atefie K, Ammer K. Dynamische Gelenkszintigraphie in der Rheumadiagnostik. Akt. Rheumatol. 8, 1983.
13. Albrecht HJ, Westerburg KW, von Wilmovsky H. Beurteilung des intraartikulären Entzündungssubstrats mit Hilfe der Computer-tomographie. Akt. Rheumatol. 7, 1982.
14. Pfannenstiel P, Semmler U. Die diagnostische Bedeutung der Szintigraphie bei entzündlichen Erkrankungen der Gelenke. Der Nuklearmediziner 1, 1978.
15. Ostendorp U, Wiedmer U. Gelenknahe Knochenpunktion als Behandlungs-möglichkeit bei Schultersteife. Akt. Rheumatol. 1, 1980.
16. Rybka V, Raunio P, Vainio K. Arthrodesis of the shoulder in rheumatoid arthritis. J. Bone Jt Surg. 61-B, 2, 1979.
17. Souter WA: Planning treatment of the rheumatoid hand. Hand 1979; 11:3–16.
18. Zippel J. Die luxationssichere Schulterendoprothese Modell BMW, in Burri C., Rütter A. (ets): Aktuelle Probleme in Chirurgie und Orthopädie: Prothesen und Alternativen am Arm I: Schultergelenk. Huber, Bern 1977.
19. Kölbel R, Friedebold G. Schultergelenkersatz. Z. Orthop. 113, 1975.
20. Grammont PM, Lelaurin G. Die Scapula-Osteotomie und Acropole-Prothese. Der Orthopäde 10 (3) 1981.

STABILIZATION OF SHOULDERS WITH BONE AND MUSCLE DEFECTS USING JOINT REPLACEMENT IMPLANTS

REINHARD KOELBEL, M.D.

Instability at the shoulder severely limits the use of the arm and hand. It causes pain and an unsightly appearance. In the context of tumors, these sequelae of resection surgery have had to be accepted for lack of tissue stock for restoration of stability.[5] Tumors of the upper end of the humerus are an exception provided the rotator cuff can be reconstructed. After resection, implants for hemialloplasty can be used to restore bone length.[1,6] We have used this method, adding a free vascularized graft of the fibular shaft (Fig. 1). Expectations as to the active range of motion are limited.

Combined defects of bone length (humerus or scapula) and of the stabilizing or moving muscles are not amenable to this type of reconstruction. With regard to such cases I propose that semiconstrained implants for total joint replacement can alleviate problems related to instability. With further advance of tumor chemotherapy and limb-preserving surgery, more cases may be seen in which partial retention of the scapula is feasible. In these, reconstruction and stabilization of the shoulder with an implant may be of greater functional benefit than resection surgery alone.

This report results from experience with a series of 23 patients in whom a semiconstrained implant (Fig. 2) was used for a variety of indications. There is a detailed account of five cases in which the implant was used with modifications (Fig. 3) to reconstruct shoulders with tissue defects. In the other 18 patients, the implant in its original form was used to replace the joint surfaces. In these 18, the indications were: osteoarthrosis in 5, cuff tear arthropathy in 3, rheumatoid arthritis in 4, fresh and old trauma in 5 and revision of a total shoulder in 1. There occurred errors in surgical technique related to implant position in 1, unrelated to the implant in 2, and early death unrelated to surgery in 1.

The remaining 14 patients were followed closely for an average 4 years and 8 months (maximum 8 yrs. 4 mths., minimum 2 yrs.) The average age was 57 years (28 yrs. to 76 yrs.) There was one early failure of the fixation to the scapula in a vigorous 68-year-old woman with cuff tear arthopathy and a tiny scapula. The pin for cement fixation in the glenoid had to be shortened. The cement around this pin broke, initiating failure which resulted in removal of the implant after 3 years.

In the 14 patients, pain was reduced in 10, unchanged in 2, and 2 were acute trauma cases. Function was improved in 11, unchanged in 1 and 2 were acute trauma cases. Details of the ranges of motion, problems and intraoperative complications and of the late sequelae are given in Tables 1 to 4.

There were radiolucent lines or seams along all cement borders and around all steel and cobalt-chrome implants. It is remarkable, however, that except for the one early failure of scapular fixation there was no other case of loosening of either component.

While the implant in its original form has not been used for joint surface replacement since 1979, this experience has shown functional results second only to the ones achieved with the Neer II implant and technique (Fig. 4). It has confirmed clinically our impression from extensive experimental investigations of the quality of its mode of fixation (Koelbel et al 1972, 1977, 1982). It has encouraged us to make use of the implant design and its particular fixation to the scapula for those patients in whom inherent stability is required.

The experience in 5 cases with bone and muscle defects at the shoulder in which the semiconstrained implant was used follows.

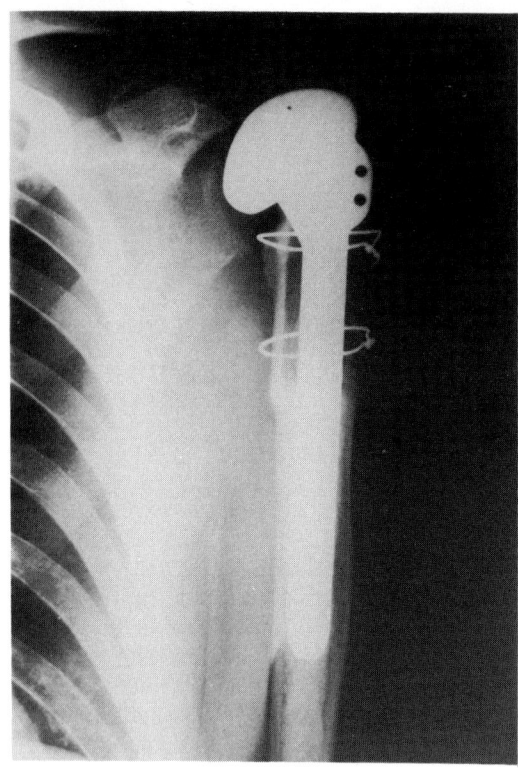
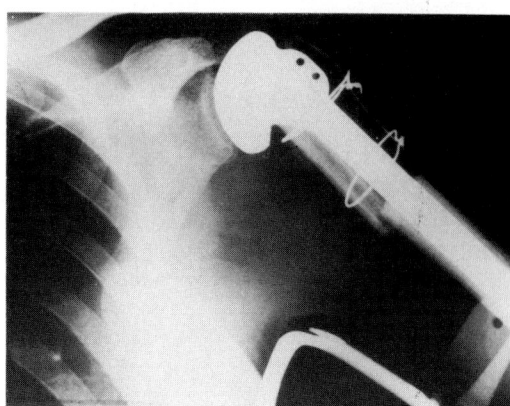
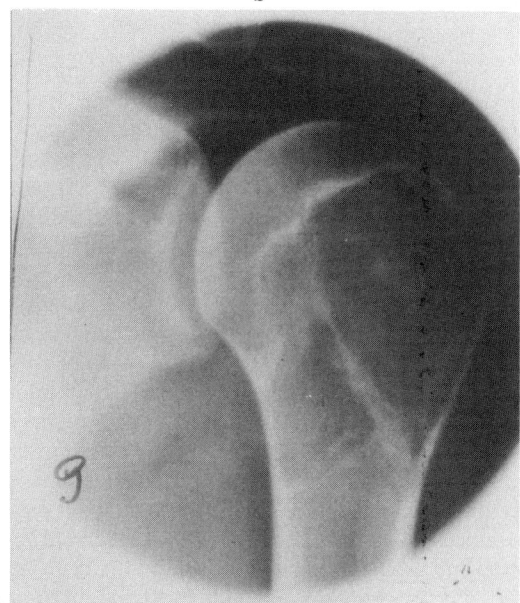

Figure 1 a) Chondrosarcoma in a 36-year-old male; b) 2 months after resection, replacement with cemented Neer II AF 03, free vascularized fibular graft and iliac grafts, reconstruction of rotator cuff; c) 1 year 1 month after surgery, incorporation of fibular graft and iliac grafts (overexposed film).

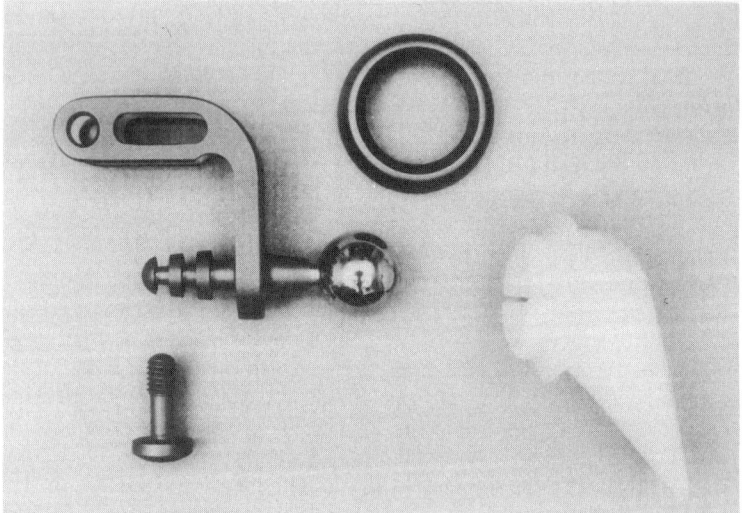

Figure 2 MK II total shoulder implant: scapular component, retaining ring and bolt of titanium-vanadium alloy, humeral component of HDP.

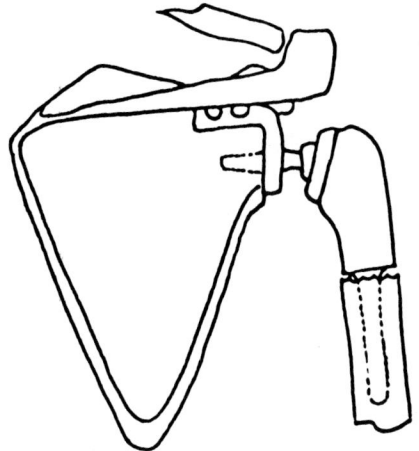 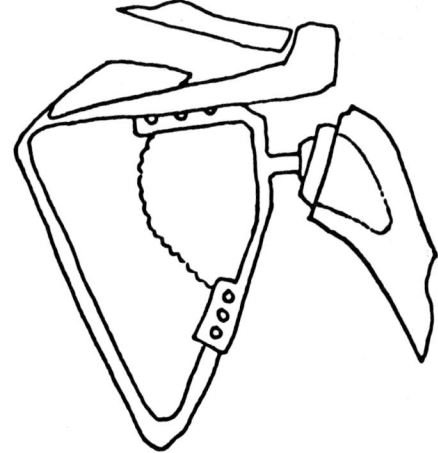

Figure 3 Modifications of humeral and scapular components for defect reconstruction.

Defects of the Proximal End of the Humerus with Rotator and Deltoid Muscle Defects

In a 74-year-old woman with painful instability after resection of the humeral head through the surgical neck, the semiconstrained, reverse-anatomy implant was first used. Only parts of the acromial and spinal parts of the deltoid were preserved. The patient was satisfied for 5 years. In the sixth year, she dislocated the joint with a heavy load. Radiographs from the fourth year showed some metal fragments. Clinical photographs show that she uses her trapezius to rotate her shoulder into abduction of the arm. She used the implant as an arthrodesis in this plane. This explains the mode of failure. At revision surgery, the inferior rim of the socket and the ring were heavily worn. The scapular component, however, was found solidly fixed to the bone. So was the humeral component.

In a 76-year-old woman, a similar situation existed after head resection for nonunion, head replacement and a Putti-Platt procedure. Pain was the reason to attempt stabilization with the reverse-anatomy implant plus a medullary nail-cum-receptacle for the plastic socket. The fracture of the osteoporotic shaft upon removal of the Neer-prosthesis was managed in the anticipated fashion. This patient was free of pain and is now three years post surgery.

(Text continued on page 292)

TABLE 1

14 Total Shoulder—Active ROM

FLEX: 8 improved, 3 unchanged, AV. 55.4° → 86.8°
ABD: 9 improved, 2 worse, AV. 51.3° → 80°
(N = 11; 2 AC TR., 1 S Preoperative Data)
Neck: 3− → +, 1+ = +, 9− = −
Back: 5− → +, 5+ = +, 3− = −
(N = 13; 1 S Preoperative Data)

TABLE 2

14 Total Shoulder—Passive ROM

Rotation: 11 improved, AV. 19.5° → 79°
Flex/ABD: 7 pass > ACT ROM
∴ Muscular Weakness

TABLE 3

14 Total Shoulder—Intraop. Problems:

1 tendon LHB cut
1 screw not engaged
1 error in position, impinges in adduction
1 ring not properly applied

TABLE 4

14 Total Shoulders—Late Sequelae:

1 dislocation—revised, reduced
1 failure of fixation—removed
1 impingement GR. tuberosity—revised
2 deltoid fixation detached
Radiolucent lines: all steel & CO/CR

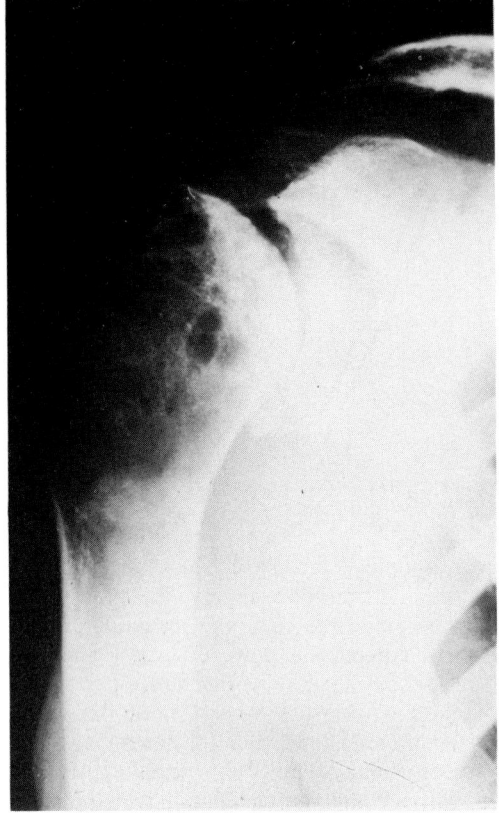
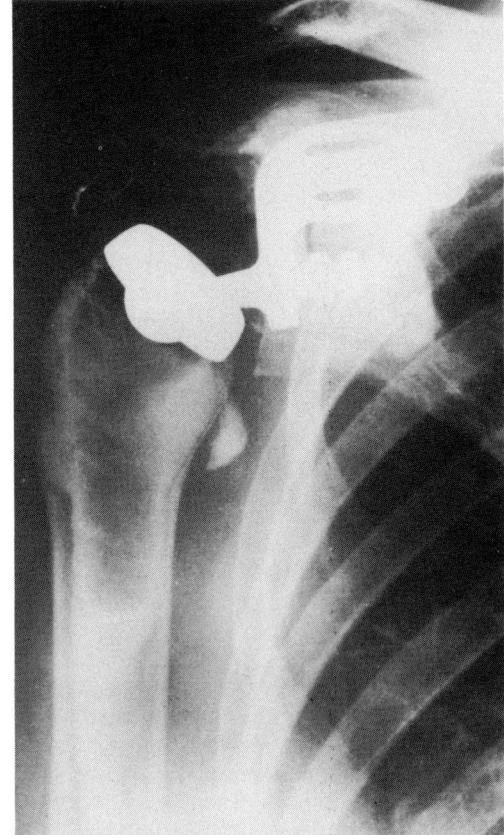
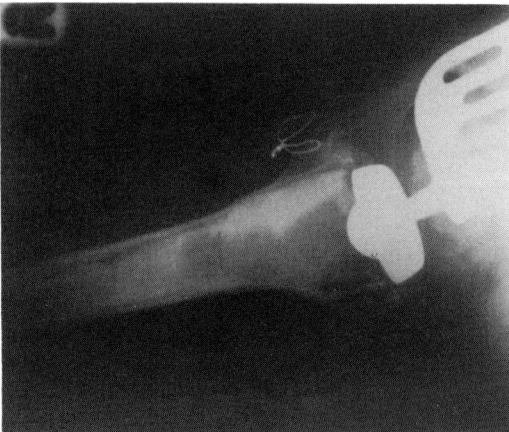

c

Figure 4 A 58-year-old female with rheumatoid arthritis: (b–c) 3 years after joint replacement right shoulder.

Illustration continued on the opposite page

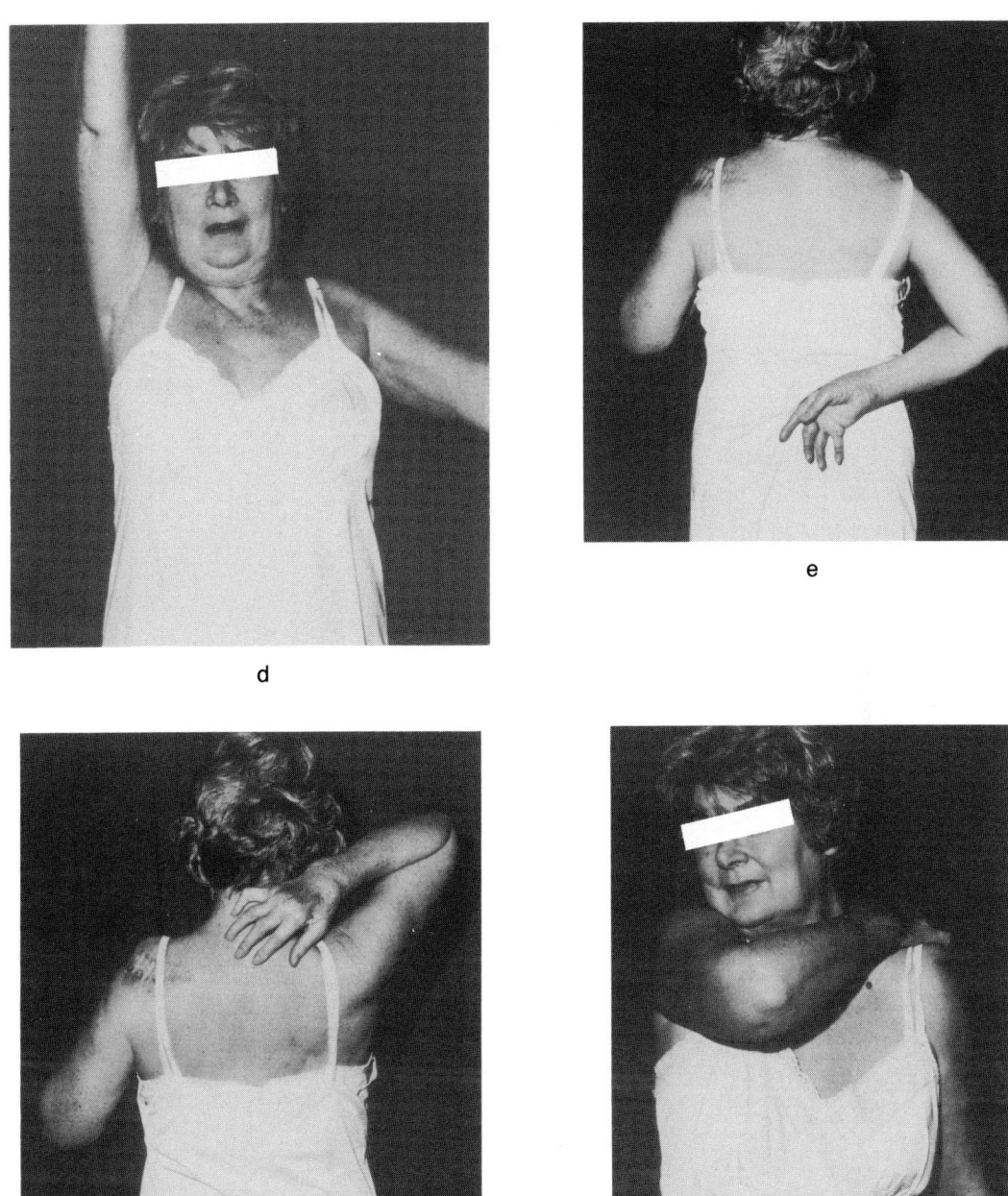

Figure 4 *(Continued)* (d–g) Active range of motion 6 years after surgery.

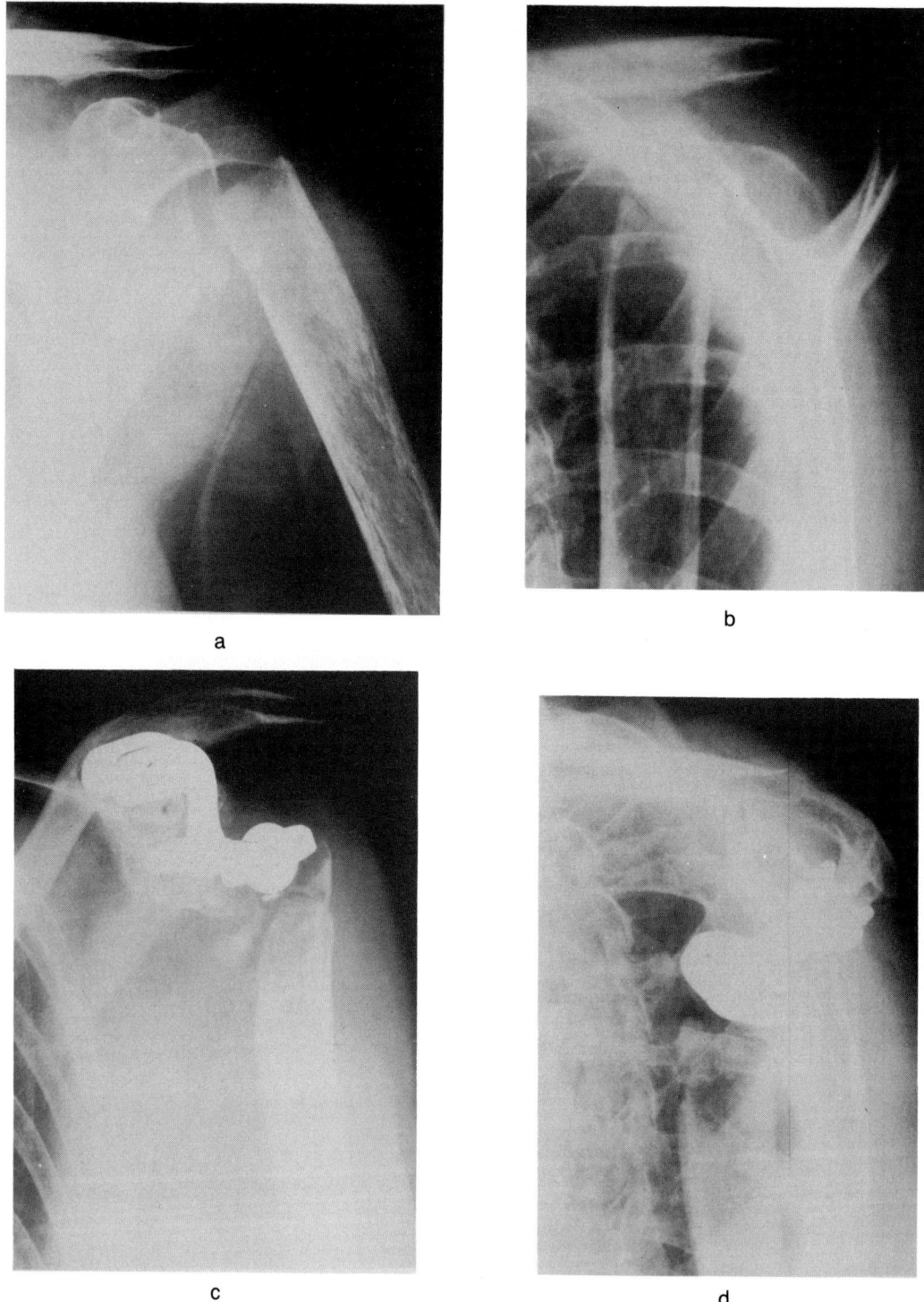

Figure 5 A 74-year-old female after humeral head resection. (a) AP radiograph, attempted active abduction; (b) tangential view to show base of spina scapulae; (c) up to the 5th postoperative year, the passive ROM of the implant increased, metal fragments of the ring appeared due to impingement in adduction; (d) tangential view to show purchase of the forked outrigger on the base of the spina.

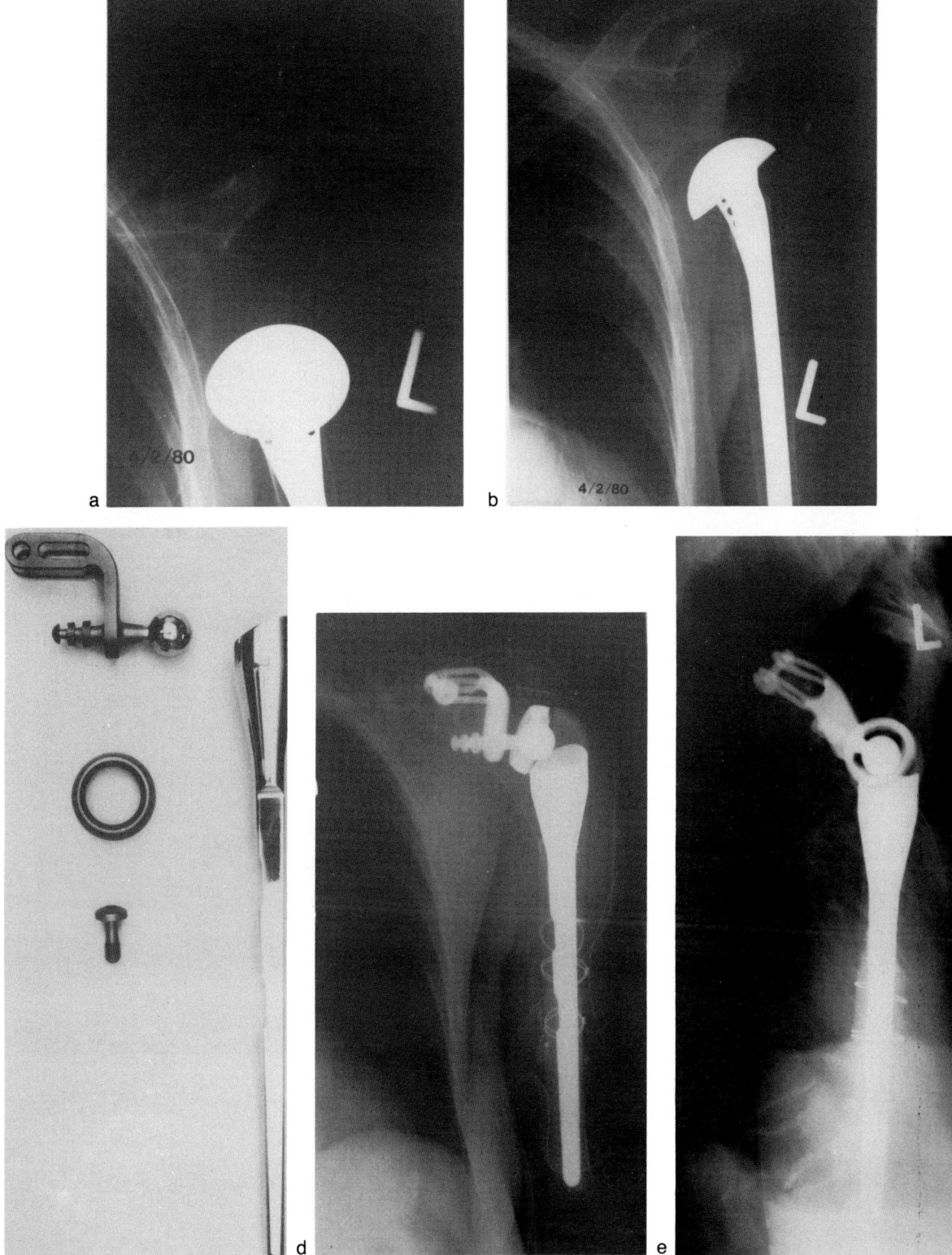

Figure 6 A 76-year-old female with bone defect of proximal end of humerus, rotator cuff and deltoid muscle. (a–b) Metal parts of implant shown; (c) humeral plastic component was inserted in medullary pin with radiopaque bone cement; (d–e) postoperative films.

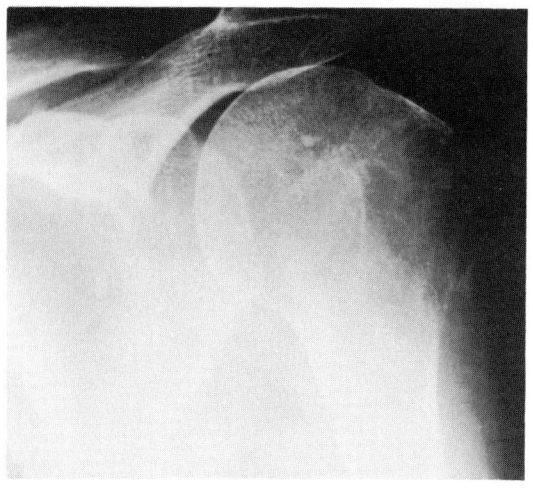

a

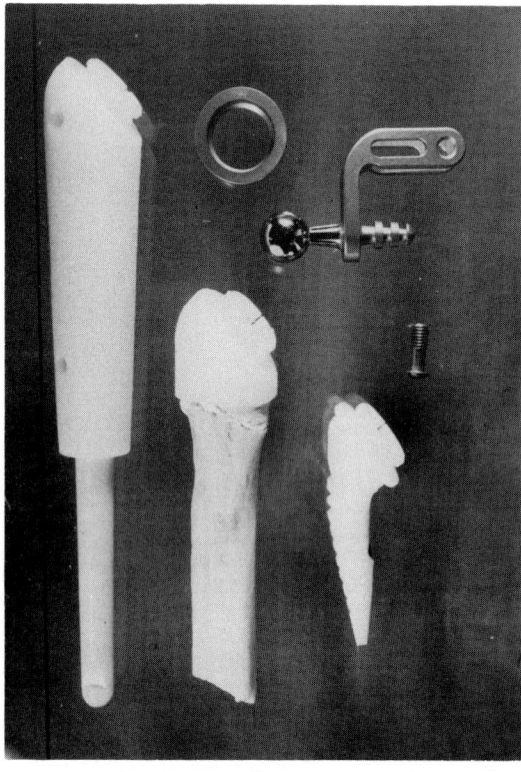

b

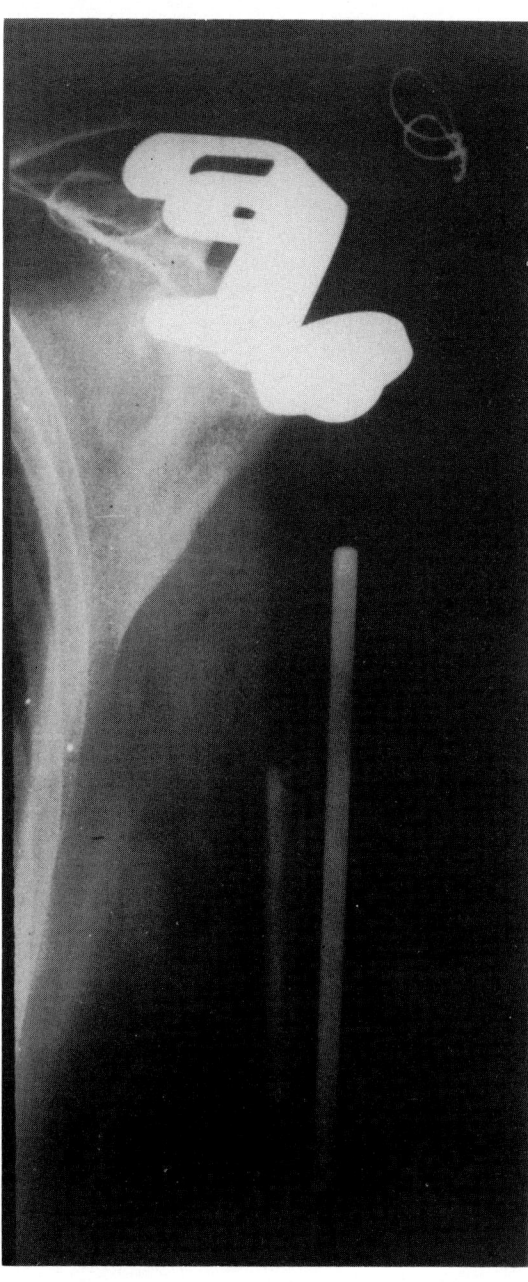

c

Figure 7 (a) Metastatic tumor in a 74-year-old female; (b) modifications of humeral component for joint surface, surgical head and proximal one third replacement; (c) postop film showing metal reinforcement of intramedullary stem.

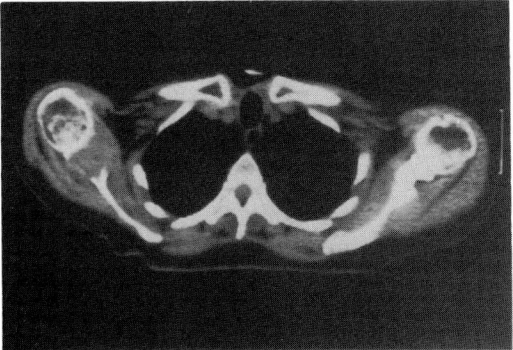

a

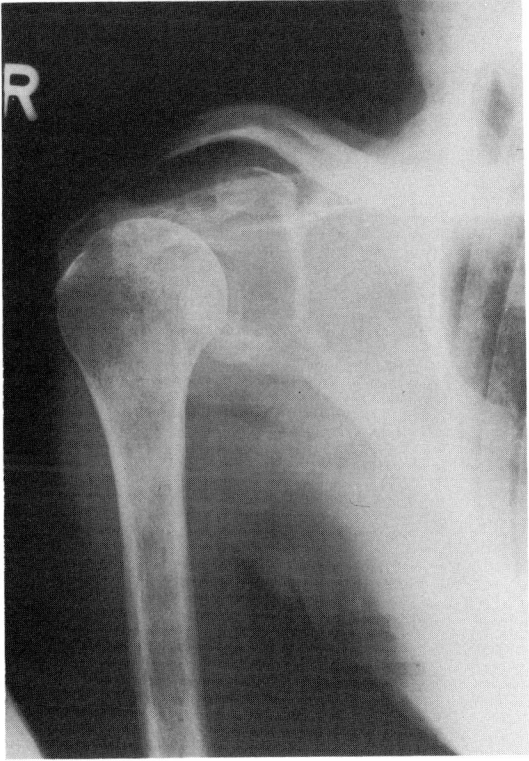

b

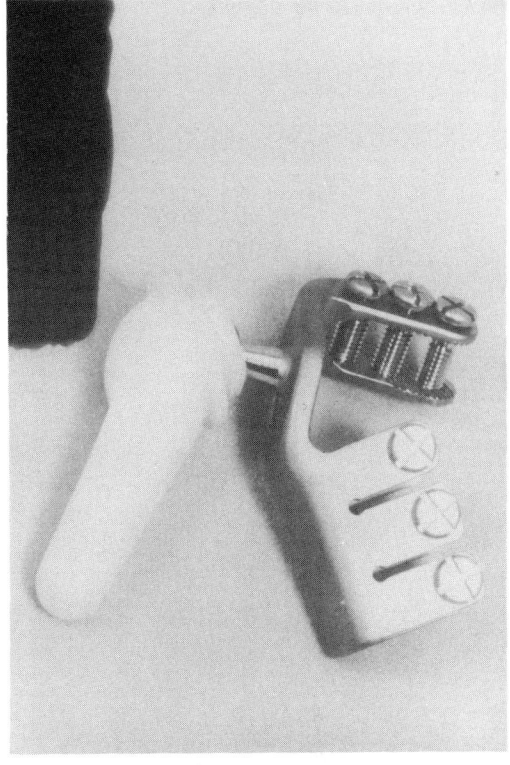

c

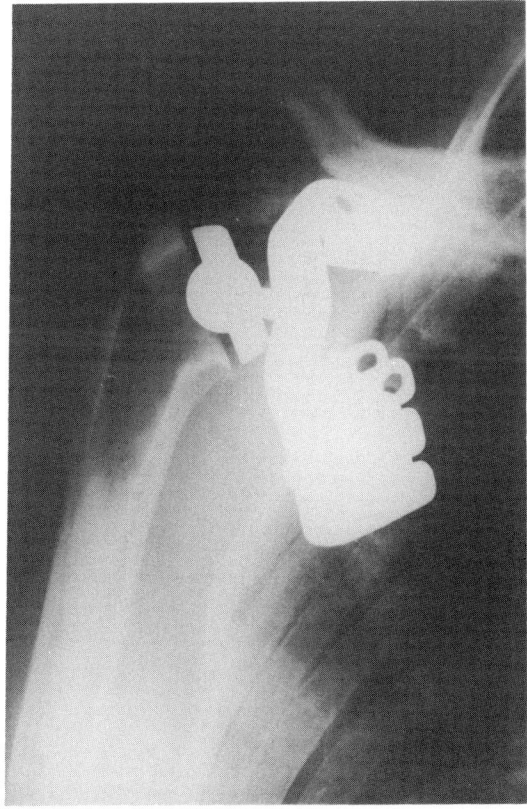

d

Figure 8 Solitary metastasis of thyroid carcinoma in a 56-year-old female. (a) CAT scan shows involvement/destruction of glenoid, neck and body of scapula; (b) plain AP film; (c) modification of scapular component; (d) radiographs 10 months after partial scapular resection and reconstruction.

(Illustration continued on the following page)

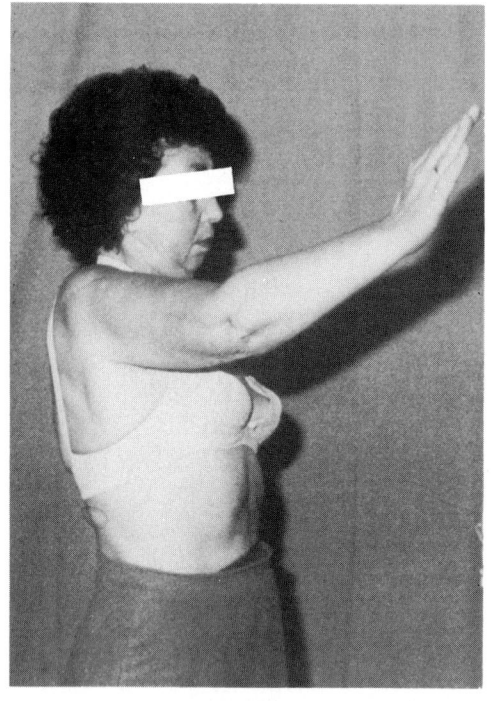
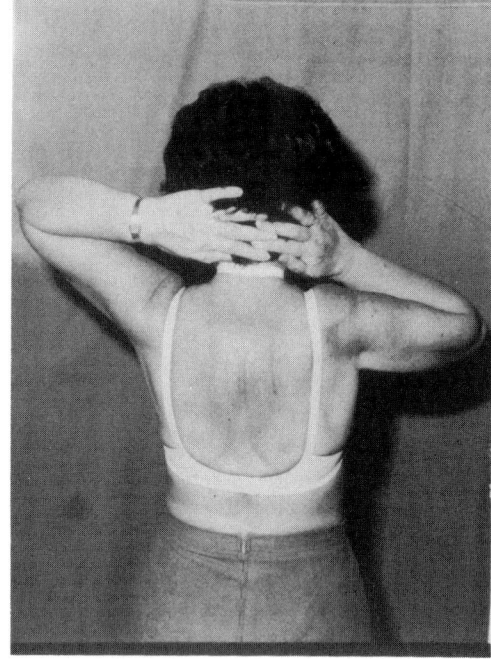

Figure 8 *(Continued)* (e–g) active range of motion 2 years after surgery.

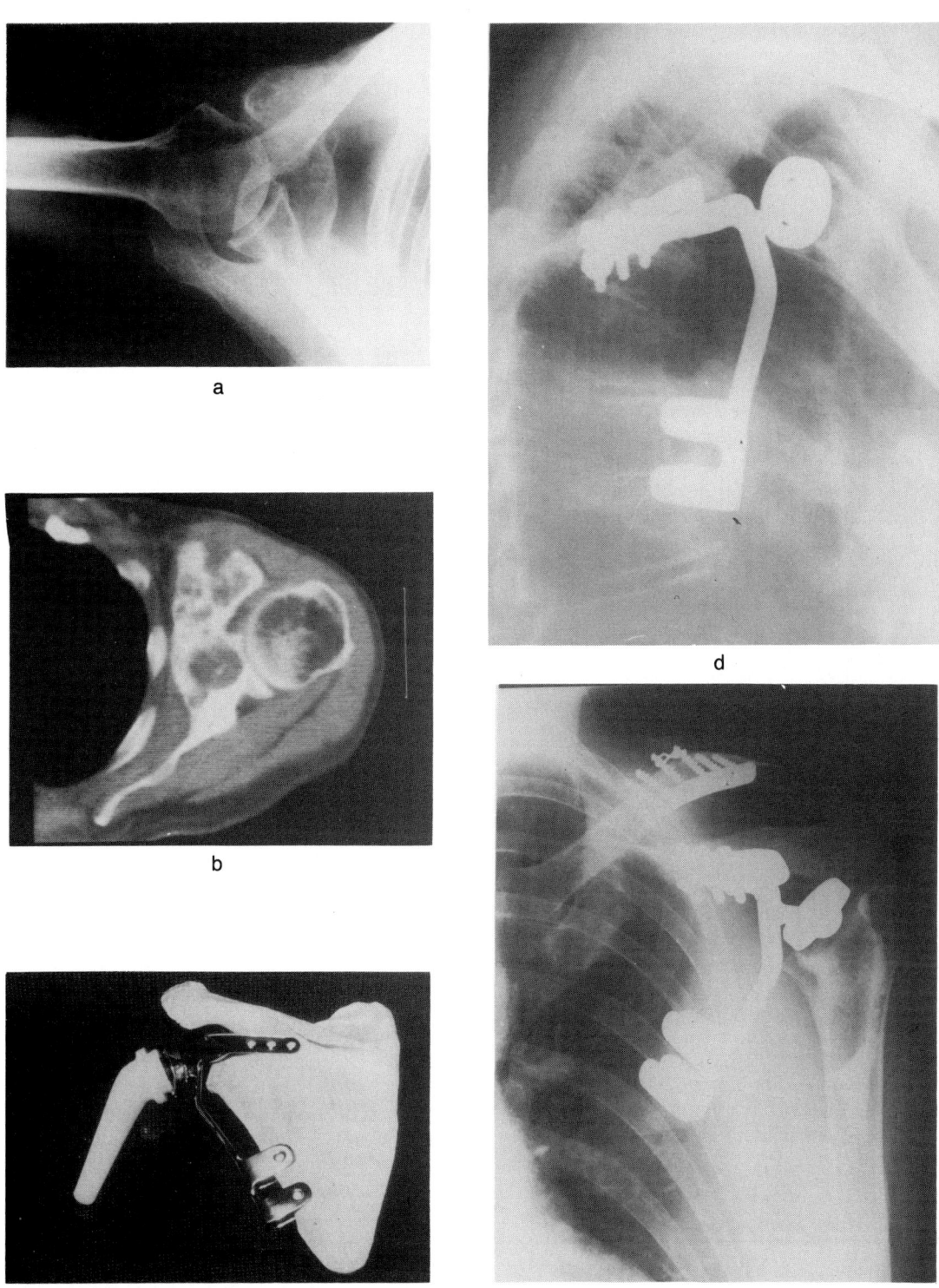

Figure 9 (a) Chondrosarcoma of the coracoid process and glenoid in a 54-year-old male patient; (b) CAT scan after biopsy from coracoid process; (c) modified scapular component; (d) transthoracic view of implant; (e) AP view of implant fixed to base of spina scapulae and lateral margin, internal fixation of clavicular osteotomy.

(Illustration continued on the following page)

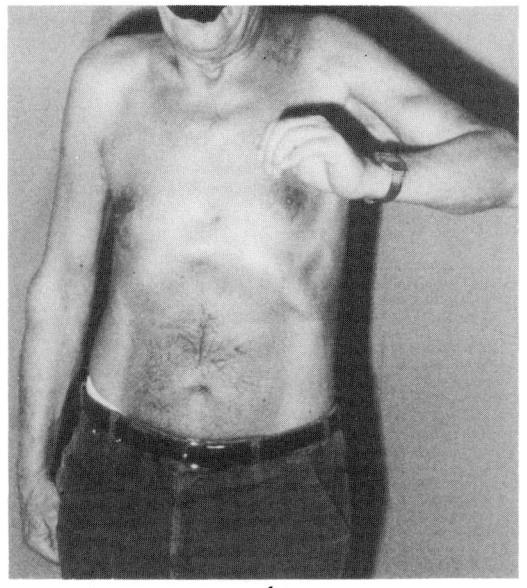

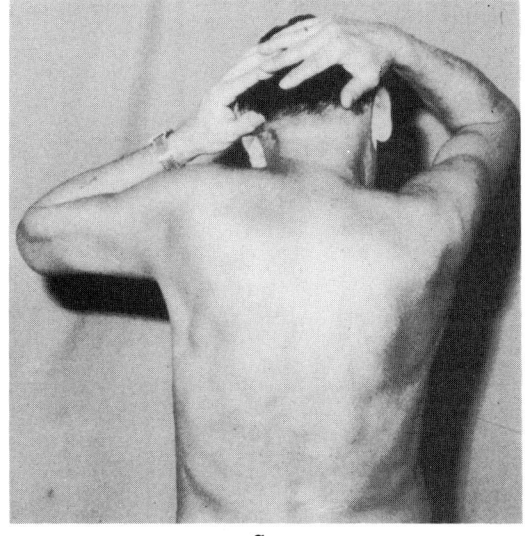

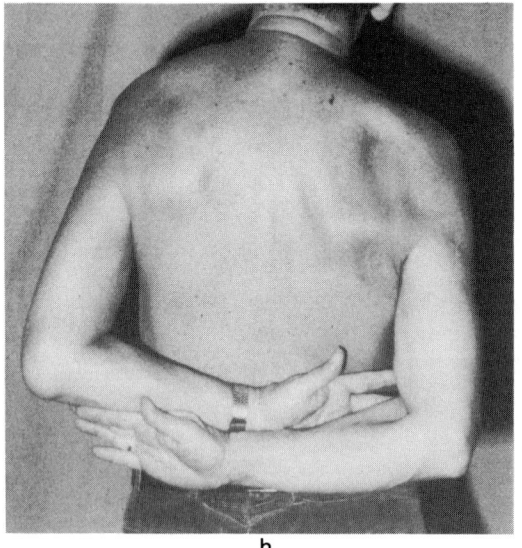

Figure 9 *(Continued)* (f–h) active range of motion after three months.

In a 64-year-old woman with an extremely painful metastasis, we elected to replace the upper end of the humerus. The axillary nerve was cut. The patient was free of pain and survived for six months.

Defects of the Scapula and the Rotator Muscles

A 56-year-old woman had received maximum radioiodine and radiation for local recurrences and regional metastases of a thyroid carcinoma. Radiotherapists suggested resection for this solitary painful metastasis. CT scans showed destruction of the glenoid body and coracoid process of the scapula. The base of the spina scapulae and the lateral margin were preserved. An implant was supplemented with an outrigger for fixation to the lateral margin. After resection of the tumor with the suprascapularis branch to the infraspinatus, the scapular component was fixed with a screw and a cerclage to the lateral margin and two screws through the base of the spina. Local radiation was instituted because the tumor was fractured during removal. The patient is 2 years post surgery and her shoulder functions well.

A 54-year-old man had a low grade chondrosarcoma involving the glenoid, coracoid process and body of the scapula. The tumor was resected en bloc with the suprascapular nerve. The remainder of the base of the spina was just wide enough to anchor three screws. The remainder of the body of the scapula cracked and was unstable. By fixation of the scapular component, the frame of the scapula was reconstituted and quite stable. This patient is 9 months post surgery and the shoulder functions satisfactorily.

There were no infections or other complications.

Conclusions

Tumor resection has first priority; reconstruction must take second place. If this is respected, there appear to be few disadvantages to using joint-replacement implants in similar cases. A stable shoulder with limited function and all other limits of alloarthroplasty is a reasonable alternative to a flail and painful shoulder.

REFERENCES

1. Neer CS, Watson KC, Stanton FJ. Recent experience in total shoulder replacement. J Bone Joint Surg. 1982; 64A:319–337.
2. Kölbel R. Total shoulder joint replacement. thesis. University of Surrey, 1972.
3. Kölbel R, Rohlmann A, Bergmann G. Biomechanical considerations in the design of a semiconstrained total shoulder replacement. In: Bailey I, Kessel L, eds. *Shoulder Surgery.* Berlin, Heidelberg, New York: Springer, 1982:144–152.
4. Kölbel R et al Shoulder joint replacement. In: Burri C, Coldewey J, Rüter A, eds. *Endoprostheses and Alternatives for the Arm.* Bern, Stuttgart, Vienna: Hans Huber, 1977:47–60.
5. Marcove RC. Neoplasms of the shoulder girdle. Orthop Clin N Am. 1975; 12:541–552.
6. Sim F. Limb salvage procedures for primary malignant tumors of the shoulder. 2nd Int Conf Surg Shoulder, 1983.

LONG TERM RESULTS OF NEER TOTAL SHOULDER REPLACEMENT

HARRY A. BADE III, M.D., RUSSELL F. WARREN, M.D.,
CHITRANJAN S. RANAWAT, M.D., and ALLAN E. INGLIS, M.D.

Over the past decade, total shoulder replacement has evolved as a solution for the severely painful shoulder caused by destruction of the surface of the glenohumeral joint. Because most shoulder pathology involves the surrounding musculotendinous tissues, initial prosthetic designs were constrained with a fixed fulcrum to replace both the joint surface and the rotator cuff. Unfortunately, this resulted in a high degree of mechanical failure due to the high stresses on the materials and the transfer of forces to the bone-cement interface.

In 1973, Neer redesigned his humeral head hemiarthroplasty to articulate with a polyethylene glenoid component.[6] This nonconstrained or resurfacing prosthesis has the advantage of simulating normal shoulder anatomy. Maximum return of shoulder motion is achieved with an intact rotator cuff and a functioning deltoid muscle. Stresses at the bone-cement interface are reduced because motion is now restricted by the surrounding soft tissues rather than the prosthesis. Potential mechanical problems such as metal failure, dislocation, fracture, and loosening, particularly of the glenoid component, are thus minimized.

This chapter reviews and discusses our initial consecutive series of Neer nonconstrained total shoulder replacements. It is a reexamination of a previous study to evaluate long-term results.[9]

INDICATIONS

The prime indication for surgery is pain due to destruction of the shoulder joint and unrelieved by the usual conservative programs of physical therapy and antiinflammatory medications.[9] Many disease entities are involved, but rheumatoid arthritis is the most frequent. Careful evaluation of the entire upper extremity is necessary, since a functional hand, wrist, and elbow are prerequisites to total shoulder replacement. In rheumatoid arthritis, the rotator cuff may be torn or involved by the disease process; this often compromises the end results. Approximately one-third of the patients with osteonecrosis of the humeral head have severe shoulder pain requiring either hemiarthroplasty or, if there is glenoid destruction, total shoulder replacement. Osteoarthritis has been an increasingly frequent indication for total shoulder replacement, both primarily and secondary to instability. If the rotator cuff is generally intact and of good quality, an excellent end result can be anticipated to follow total shoulder replacement. Traumatic arthritis may result from displaced fractures or fracture dislocations with resulting damage to the articular cartilage. These pose a potentially difficult problem to the reconstructive surgeon because of the contractures and scarring in the musculotendinous tissues. Rotator cuff arthropathy from long-standing massive tears also presents a difficult reconstructive problem. In addition, total shoulder replacement may be indicated in failed hemiarthroplasty and en bloc excisions in tumor surgery.

MATERIALS AND METHODS

Between 1974 and 1980, 38 Neer nonconstrained total shoulder replacements were implanted in 34 patients. A minimum 2 year postoperative period was our criterion for follow-up examination. Twenty-seven shoulders were examined; 11 shoulders were not (10 deaths and one patient lost to follow-up). The average follow-up was 4.5 years (range 2.0 to 7.3 years). The average age was 50 years.

Thirteen patients (48%) have rheumatoid arthritis. Three patients (11%) have osteoarthritis, three patients (11%) have post-traumatic arthritis while five patients (30%) including three bilateral total shoulder replacements have nontraumatic avascular necrosis.

The humeral component consisted of either the Neer I (8) or the Neer II (19) design. (Fig. 1) All glenoids were replaced with the standard polyethylene component which was developed in 1974.[6] A 100-point scoring system was devised to numerically evaluate each shoulder. The categories of pain, function, range of motion, and muscle strength contribute to the final score (Fig. 2).

SURGICAL TECHNIQUE

We currently use the long deltopectoral approach as described by Neer. Several technical considerations should be discussed for better surgical exposure and easier positioning of the components.

The patient is adjusted in a beach-chair position, sitting upright at 45 degrees angulation. Thus, the weight of the arm helps open the subacromial space. The arm is draped free for mobility and the shoulder moved just off the edge of the table to allow hyperextension for insertion of the humeral component. A folded towel is placed beneath the ipsilateral scapula to angle the glenoid cavity anterior for better visualization.

After the incision is made, better exposure is obtained by releasing the conjoined tendon, the superior 1 cm of the pectoralis major insertion, and the anterior one-third of the deltoid insertion on the humerus. The level of the humeral head osteotomy is aligned using a trial prosthesis (23 mm head) positioned just above the greater tuberosity with the humerus externally rotated 35 to 50 degrees. This allows simple anterior to posterior osteotomy, producing the desired retroversion for the humeral head prosthesis while preventing possible postoperative impingement problems. Great care must be taken to avoid either extending the osteotomy to the greater tuberosity or injuring the posterior rotator cuff.

The glenoid fossa must be well visualized by inserting specific retractors in positions inferior, posterior, and anterior to the glenoid. All soft tissue is removed from the surface of the glenoid. Release of the capsule may be necessary if there is marked loss of motion. A power burr is used to cut a slot through the subchondral bone of the glenoid cavity. Remaining cortical bone must be preserved. The slot is almost vertical, aiming for the base of the coracoid process. Curettes are used to deepen and undercut the slot, to avoid perforating the cortex of the scapula. The trial glenoid component must sit firmly against the subchondral bone without any toggling. Occasionally, with the severe protrusio type glenoid seen in rheumatoid arthritis, the fin needs to be shortened or bone grafting of a deficient glenoid may be necessary.

Postoperative Program

Postoperative rehabilitation is essential and depends on the condition of the rotator cuff and deltoid muscle. Immediate immobilization is achieved with either a sling and swathe or an abduction splint if a more relaxed position is needed after a large rotator cuff repair. Physical therapy is divided into two stages. The first is passive and assisted range of motion which is generally begun about the fourth postoperative day. If an abduction splint is necessary, the therapy is started passively from the splint in a range that is judged to be safe at the time of surgery. The second stage is active

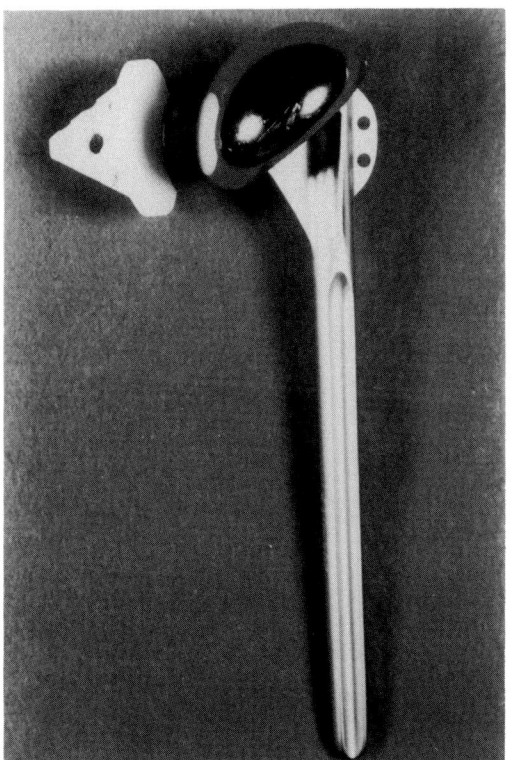

Figure 1 Neer II nonconstrained total shoulder replacement. The humeral components are made with two head sizes, 15.0 and 23.0 mm, and three stem diameters, 6.3, 9.5, and 12.7 mm. The radius of curvature of both heads is 44 mm which matches the standard glenoid component. Larger semiconstrained glenoid components are available.

THE HOSPITAL FOR SPECIAL SURGERY
Score Sheet for Total Shoulder Replacement

DOMINANT ARM _____
INVOLVED ARM _____

	SCORE	LEFT							RIGHT						
		PRE	6M	1Y	2Y	3Y	4Y	5Y	PRE	6M	1Y	2Y	3Y	4Y	5Y
PAIN ON MOTION (15 points - Circle one)															
None:	15														
Mild: Occasional, no compromise in activity	10														
Moderate: Tolerable makes concession, uses ASA	5														
Severe: Serious limitations, disabling, uses Codeine, etc.	0														
PAIN AT REST (15 points - Circle one)															
None: Ignores	15														
Mild: Occasional, no medication, no affect on sleep	10														
Moderate: Uses ASA, night pain	5														
Severe: Marked medication stronger than ASA	0														
FUNCTION (20 points - Circle all appropriate)															
Comb hair	5														
Lie on shoulder	5														
Hook brassiere (back)	5														
Toilet	5														
Lift weight in pounds 1 - 10 1 point per pound - Maximum 10 pounds															
None															
MUSCLE STRENGTH (15 points - Rate each) (Normal = 3, Good = 2, Fair = 1, Poor = 0)															
Forward Flexion															
Abduction															
Adduction															
Internal Rotation															
External Rotation															
RANGE OF MOTION (25 points - 1 point per 20° of motion)															
Forward Flexion (Maximum 8)															
Abduction (Maximum 7)															
Adduction (Maximum 2)															
Internal Rotation (Maximum 5)															
External Rotation (Maximum 3)															
RECORD RANGE OF MOTION (NO POINTS)															
Backward Extension															
Glenohumeral Abduction (scapula fixed)															
TOTAL															

PATIENTS NAME: _____ HISTORY NUMBER: _____

Figure 2 Shoulder score sheet for preoperative and postoperative evaluation.

range of motion and muscle strengthening. Therapy begins during the second week since the long deltopectoral approach is now used and we need not worry about deltoid muscle healing. Patients with large cuff tears remove their abductor splints at 4 to 6 weeks to begin the second stage of therapy. With satisfactory motion, patients are discharged from the hospital to be carefully followed on an outpatient basis to achieve maximum strength and active range of motion. This may require at least six months of therapy.

RESULTS

Using our 100-point rating system, the average score improved 51 points from a preoperative 27 points to a postoperative 78 points. There was no deterioration of our results with time.

When analyzed with respect to the preoperative diagnosis (Fig. 3), the best results occurred with the younger, avascular necrosis patients whose average score was 92 points. With relief of their pain they achieved excellent motion. All were noted to have a healthy rotator cuff at surgery.

The osteoarthritic group scored second highest with 77 points, followed closely by the rheumatoid group at 73 points. Since a previous study which included the same three patients, the osteoarthritic score has decreased considerably due to the development of anterior impingement pain in a female patient. The other two patients both have excellent results, each scoring 90 points. Rheumatoid patients benefited most in that significant pain relief modestly improved their active forward flexion to 93 degrees.

Patients with traumatic arthritis scored lowest due to postoperative scarring and stiffness. Two had revision surgery for failed Neer hemiarthroplasties and one had a stiff shoulder preoperatively.

Clinical results were graded excellent (85–100), good (70–84), fair (50–69), and failure (less than 50 points). Twenty-one patients (78%) were rated good to excellent. There were two failures.

Pain Relief

Patients subjectively evaluated their degree of pain both at rest and with motion. Overall, 16 patients (59%) had no pain, nine patients had mild pain with motion requiring an occasional aspirin, and two patients had moderate pain with motion. All patients improved. Pain relief was one of the prime indicators for surgery and accounted for 43 percent of the improvement in the total score. Avascular necrosis and rheumatoid patients had the best results, the former showing the greatest improvement.

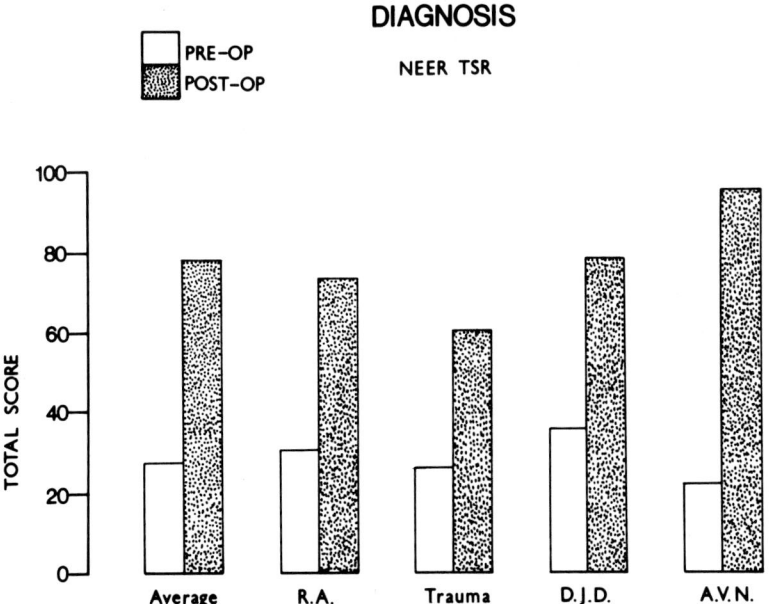

Figure 3 Preoperative and postoperative scores with respect to diagnosis.

Range of Motion

Range of motion was evaluated with respect to active foward flexion. The average improvement was from 68 degrees preoperatively to 118 degrees postoperatively (Fig. 4). Avascular necrosis patients had near normal motion. No patients lost motion. In our evaluation, several factors were noted. First, there was equal postoperative motion using either the Neer I or Neer II design. Second, the deltopectoral approach resulted in twice the postoperative motion when compared to the superior and posterior approaches. Third, when the deltoid muscle was not detached, postoperative forward flexion averaged 132 degrees while, with partial detachment, it averaged only 90 degrees. Four patients in the latter group had rotator cuff tears. Lastly, patients starting physical therapy during their first postoperative week averaged 128 degrees forward flexion while those starting after one week averaged only 100 degrees. The delay in therapy had been to allow rotator cuff repairs and partial deltoid muscle detachment to heal.

Function

Shoulder function was evaluated using a standardizing rating sheet for shoulder prostheses described by Cofield.[2] Each function (Fig. 5) was numerically graded from zero to a normal score of three. The preoperative score averaged ten points and increased to 25 points postoperatively (Fig. 6). Although avascular necrosis and osteoarthritic patients scored highest, significant improvement was noted with trauma patients.

Failure

Two patients were rated as failures of surgery, scoring less than 50 points postoperatively. Both were noted to have major rotator cuff tears at surgery. One patient has severe rheumatoid arthritis and, although now pain free, has very little function due to muscle weakness. Her active forward flexion remains only 30 degrees. The other patient had a revision of a Neer I hemiarthroplasty implanted for a 4–part shoulder fracture. She complains of moderate shoulder pain with motion. At surgery, part of her middle deltoid muscle was excised; she continues to have weak deltoid muscle power.

Roentgenographic Results

Follow-up roentgenograms were carefully evaluated for the presence of progression of radiolucent lines about the glenoid and humeral components. Those components with a progressive radiolucency greater than 2 mm were considered radiographically loose.

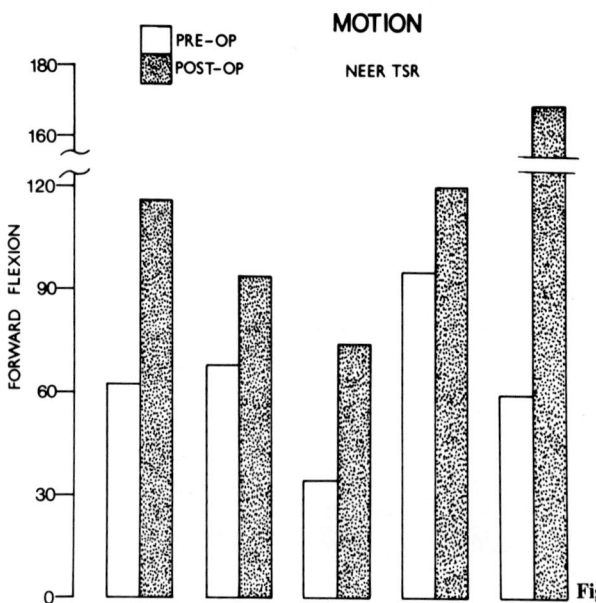

Figure 4 Active flexion of Neer prosthesis measured preoperatively and postoperatively for each diagnostic group.

*Function
(0–30)*

Use back pocket
Perineal care
Wash axilla
Eat
Comb hair
Arms at shoulder
  level
Carry 10–15 lbs
Dress
Sleep on side
Do usual work

Figure 5 Ten specific functions involving the shoulder were evaluated and graded; unable-0, with aid-1, difficult-2, normal-3.

All but one of the humeral prostheses were cemented using methylmethacrylate. Radiolucent lines at the humeral bone-cement interface are present in seven shoulders (26%). The majority are incomplete, remaining less than 1 mm in width. Two components are radiographically loose. The first has developed a progressive radiolucency at the prosthetic tip beginning 2¼ years postop with concommitant midlateral arm pain (Fig. 7). The second humeral loosening occurred after revision surgery for a humeral hemiarthroplasty in which the prosthesis was cemented proud to reestablish proper humeral length. The component has painlessly settled 1 cm into the humeral shaft.

The glenoid components have a 67 percent incidence of radiolucent lines at the bone-cement interface. In most, it was found to be complete on the immediate postoperative roentgenogram and has remained nonprogressive. One component is loose. It has occurred in a juvenile rheumatoid patient who is an avid hand ball player. At two years, he has developed a progressive radiolucency to 2 mm about the entire glenoid component (Fig. 8A, B).

COMPLICATIONS

At follow-up examination, a total of 17 complications were recorded (Fig 9). There are no infections or dislocations. One patient developed a neuropraxia of the lateral cord of the brachial plexus; the neuropraxia resolved spontaneously over six weeks. Three components are radiographically loose. Two have clinical pain, and one of these will require revision of the humeral component.

Five patients have developed rotator cuff tears. In each, the postoperative acromion-to-prosthetic head distance has decreased to less than 3 mm with two humeral heads abutting directly against the acromion (Fig. 10A, B). Each pa-

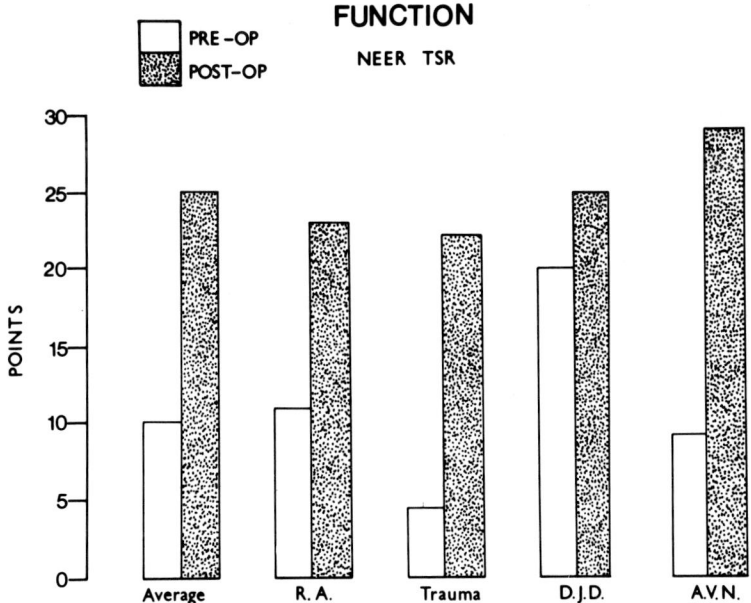

Figure 6 Preoperative and postoperative numerical comparison of function.

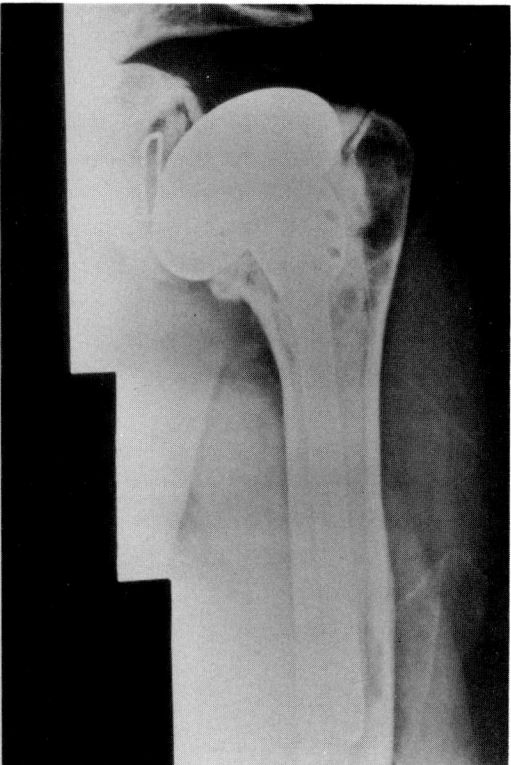

Figure 7 A progressive radiolucency is noted lateral to the prosthetic tip.

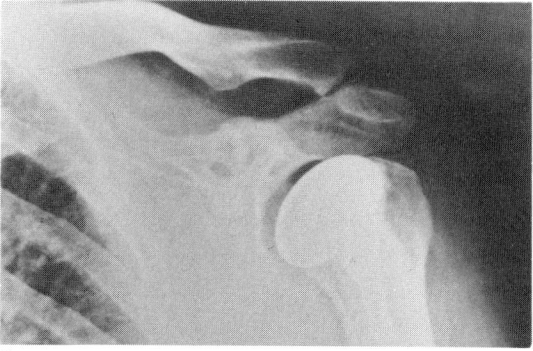
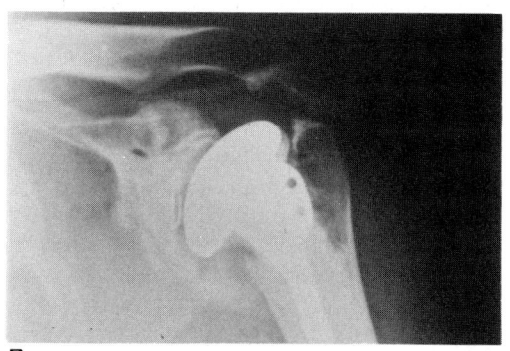

Figure 8 Anterior-posterior roentgenogram of the glenohumeral joint demonstrating a progressive lucency of 2 mm about the entire glenoid component 2 years 4 months after surgery.

tient demonstrated a decrease in external rotation strength and arc of motion. Four patients have severe rheumatoid arthritis while one had a failed Neer I hemiarthroplasty for a 4-part humeral head fracture. Four of these tears are recurrent and demonstrate a 100 percent failure rate for our four rotator cuff repairs performed at the time of shoulder replacement. All of the cuff tears were noted to be major, with the repairs described as difficult. This group has an average score of 55 points, an average 72 degrees of forward flexion, and includes both our failures. Despite their poor function, three patients regard themselves improved since they are now pain-free.

Impingement is present in two patients. One has a painful anterior impingement syndrome which has been relieved by physical therapy and a subacromial bursa injection. The other has a mechanical impingement caused by excessive humeral head resection which seated the prosthetic humeral head 7 mm below the greater tuberosity. Another had postoperative acromioclavicular joint pain which was treated by distal clavicle excision.

DISCUSSION

Overall, it appears that the Neer prosthesis functions adequately in the majority of patients. However, since our initial study, several problems have developed. Three components are now loose,

Complications	
	No.
Component Loosening	3
Rotator Cuff Tears	5
Greater Tuberosity Impingement	1
Anterior Impingement Syndrome	1
Acromioclavicular Pain	1
Biceps Tendon Rupture	1
Neuropraxia	1
Excessive Blood Loss	1
Hematomas	2
Gastric Ulcer	1

Figure 9 Immediate and long term complications following total shoulder replacement surgery.

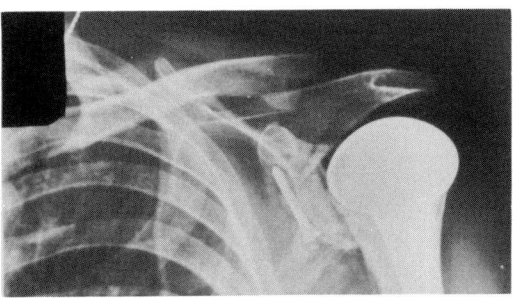

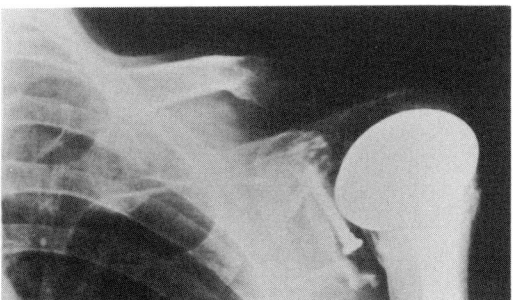

Figure 10 Superior migration of the humeral head with acromial erosion indicates a rotator cuff tear seen here in a rheumatoid patient 5 years 6 months after total shoulder replacement surgery.

two humeral and one glenoid. One humeral component has loosened without identifiable cause; the other has occurred as a result of poor cement fill coupled with positioning the humeral prosthesis proud without circumferential support. To avoid this problem, we have now begun to use cement plugs in the medullary canal to improve our cementing technique. We also recommend custom–made humeral prostheses to substitute for deficient humeral bone stock. This will inhibit subsidence of the humeral component and reestablish the proper length of the humeral shaft. In patients whose proper humeral length is not restored, the deltoid will be unable to support the humerus, resulting in inferior subluxation that can be very difficult to treat.

Sixty-seven percent of the glenoid components have postoperative radiolucent lines. Again, cement technique must be improved by controlling bleeding, debriding the glenoid bone with a Water-Pik, and pressurizing the cement with the glenoid component. One patient with a loose glenoid continued to play handball following surgery; this probably played a role in the development of his loosening due to overactivity. A second problem involves massive rotator cuff tears. These are most prevalent in patients with rheumatoid and post-traumatic arthritis where there is considerable damage to the soft tissues and rotator cuff either from disease or trauma. Careful preoperative evaluation should be carried out to predict the possibility of large rotator cuff tears or significant loss of bone stock. A thorough physical examination with proper roentgenographic evaluation is essential. A double contrast arthrotomogram will often give excellent visualization of the size of a rotator cuff defect, thus guiding the surgeon in his choice of a prosthesis.

Although the thinner 15 mm Neer II head size aids in closing difficult cuff repairs, adequate repairs may be impossible in these patients, due to poor tissue quality. Thus, it appears that, in some patients, a more constrained prosthesis is needed to substitute for rotator cuff function to improve postoperative motion if there is adequate bone stock. At present, this takes various forms: increased superior coverage by an oversized glenoid component,[1,7] a separate, smaller subacromial component, or a fixed fulcrum prosthesis.

Unfortunately, the use of fixed-fulcrum prostheses has led to a high rate of complications. Currently, we favor increasing superior coverage with an enlarged polyethylene glenoid component. However, the increased lever arm may potentiate stresses at the bone-cement interface resulting in an increased incidence of loosening with time. Maintaining proper humeral length is essential to optimizing deltoid muscle power and avoiding greater tuberosity impingement. As seen in our study, excessive humeral head resection must be avoided. Reestablishment of normal humeral length in a humerus shortened by revision surgery, tumor resection, or trauma is necessary. Bone graft or a custom-made neck will be needed.

Evaluation of the acromioclavicular joint is essential in the preoperative examination. It is frequently arthritic, especially in the rheumatoid patient and, if symptomatic, excision of the lateral 2 cm of the clavicle should be performed at the time of surgery. Occasionally, a large inferior osteophyte will cause pain. If possible, it should be removed with a power burr since this will avoid detaching part of the anterior deltoid muscle.

Finally, the role of physical therapy in the postoperative period cannot be overemphasized. A detailed program both in hospital and at home will assure the surgeon and patient of attaining and maintaining maximum function.

REFERENCES

1. Clarke JC, Sew Hoy AL, Gruen TA, Amstuts HHC. Clinical and radiographic assessment of a non-constrained total shoulder. Internat Orthop (SICOT) 1981; 5:1–8.
2. Cofield RH. Total joint arthroplasty, the shoulder. Mayo Clin Proc; 54:500–506.
3. Neer CS II, Watson KC, Stanton FJ. Recent experience in total shoulder replacements. J Bone Joint Surg 1982; 64A:319–337.
4. Post M, Haskell SS, Jablan M. Total shoulder replacement with a constrained prosthesis. J Bone Joint Surg 1980; 62PA:327–335.
5. Warren RF, Ranawat CS, Inglis AE. Total shoulder replacement indication and results of the Neer non-constrained prosthesis. AAOS Symposium on total joint replacement of the upper extremity. New York: CV Mosby, 1982:56–67.

SPECIAL CONSIDERATIONS

COMPARATIVE STUDY OF BONE LESIONS IN TRAUMATIC RECURRENT DISLOCATION OF THE SHOULDER—THEIR IMPORTANCE AND TREATMENT

CARLOS E. deANQUIN, M.D. and CARLOS A. deANQUIN, M.D.

The anatomic lesions associated with recurrent dislocation of the shoulder were well described in the late 19th century. In particular was the defect in the humeral head well documented, but it was not until the paper of Hill and Sachs that surgeons of this century became reawakened to the significance of this lesion which they described more as a radiologic phenomenon than for its clinical importance. Unfortunately there has tended to be an overemphasis on the soft tissue lesions associated with this condition and in particular a preoccupation with the so-called Bankart lesion. This has tended to make surgeons overlook the significance of the humeral defect and other bone lesions commonly seen with recurrent dislocation of the shoulder. The anatomic lesions noted include:

A. Soft tissue lesions:
  1. Capsular defects with detachment of the glenoid labrum
  2. Capsular distension
  3. A preglenoidal recess
B. Bone lesions:
  1. Humeral head defects (anterior and posterior).
  2. Glenoidal distortion:
      a) rim fracture
      b) erosion
      c) narrowing
      d) obliquity

Only by a complete understanding of the true pathology can an appropriate surgical procedure be selected for each case. Indeed, in surgery there are few conditions which have more procedures described than that for recurrent dislocation of the shoulder. Unfortunately, not all take into account the requirements of individual situations, and not all necessarily address directly the pathology associated with a particular case. While there is generally reported a failure rate of 3 to 12 percent with regard to surgical treatment of this condition, this takes into account only those failures due to dislocation. Many more would be rated unsatisfactory if consideration of those with restricted motion or persistent rim syndrome were also included.

Techniques for stabilization of the shoulder include: soft tissue procedures, bony procedures, and combined procedures. Each may be with or without joint exploration. In reality, the correct procedure can only be chosen if a complete understanding of the active pathology has been first defined. To this end, it is important to choose the most suitable procedure and this requires thorough clinical and radiographic evaluation.

Radiologic Studies

Since 1951 60k bone lesions and soft-tissue lesions have been studied radiographically. The bone lesions by a special posterior tangential x-ray, the soft–tissue lesions by arthrography.

The posterior tangential view is taken with the cassette placed on the shoulder and the beam directed along the posterior aspect of the arm. This is the only view that shows both the posterior humeral head and the glenoid cavity. From data collected from 1000 subjects in both dislocated and normal shoulders, our conclusions are that the normal shoulder shows a small notch corresponding to the anatomic neck while in cases of recurrent dislocation there is invariably a larger humeral defect. This technique allows a comparative evaluation of the size of the bone lesion. Three sizes of defects have been demonstrated: Grade 1: small, 1 cm in size; Grade 2: moderate, 2 cm; Grade 3: severe, more than 2 cm. The Grade 3 lesions include the flat defect, a very severe lesion in which there is absence of almost one-third of the posterior surface of the head of the humerus. This lesion in fact has been described by some as due to anteversion of the humeral head thereby predisposing to recurrent dislocation. In reality, it is a planar lesion produced by traumatic episodes of dislocation which cause a flattening out of the humeral head.

Significance of the Notch Defect

A notch defect predisposes to a catching of the head on the anterior rim of the glenoid. This may occur with or without labral detachment. This humeral defect occurs with the first dislocation and increases with successive recurrences as a result of compounding compression fractures. The significance of this notch defect is well demonstrated in an axillary x-ray taken in the military salute position. This will show how only a very small increase in the degree of external rotation will produce a catching of the humeral head on the glenoid rim.

In cases of posterior recurrent dislocation of the shoulder the lesions are reversed. There is an anterior notch and a posterior labral detachment on arthrography.

The significance of the humeral defect is that it effectively reduces the area of useful sliding surface for glenohumeral contact, facilitating a locking at the limit of the greatly reduced arc of contact. This accounts for failure in many cases in which a soft tissue reconstruction alone has been carried out. In this regard it should be noted that a flat defect can be quite deceptive; it is not so much the depth of a lesion which is significant as the overall size of the lesion involved, reducing as it does the effective glenohumeral gliding contact surface.

Surgical Data Regarding the Humeral Defect

In 232 patients with traumatic recurrent dislocation of the shoulder, the results of the radiographic studies were compared with the surgical findings. Accurate correlation was found between the radiologic grade of defect and that found at surgery. Even in those instances where there had been a negative tangential view, posterior fibrillation of the humeral head was generally identified.

It is significant that in 28 percent of the surgical explorations the labrum had not been detached. The sizes of the defects identified included:

Grade 1 (small): 106 shoulders (52%)
Grade 2 (moderate): 75 shoulders (28%)
Grade 3 (severe): 21 shoulders (10%)

Bone Lesions Affecting the Glenoid

Increasing emphasis has been placed in recent years on the significance of changes affecting the glenoid cavity. Carter Rowe estimated that changes in the glenoid affect 73 percent of patients coming to surgery. The lesions identified in our series included: (1) Fractures of the glenoid rim (much more frequently observed than often clinically suspected); (2) Erosion of the glenoid as a consequence of repeated impaction (always present in cases with labral detachment); and (3) Glenoid narrowing and glenoid obliquity—these were more frequently noted in nontraumatic instances. There may here be a congenital abnormality in the development of the glenoid predisposing to episodes of recurrence.

In traumatic cases associated with glenoid obliquity, erosion and a humeral head defect, we define what we call a malignant triad in which surgical repair has to be extremely well planned indeed.

Soft-Tissue Lesions—Evaluation by Arthrographic Study

Careful arthrographic study will determine, if films are correctly taken in the tangential posterior view, the absence of a labral image wherever there is a labral detachment. In the series studied, approximately 30 percent showed a normal image indicating the labrum to be still attached. At surgery, however, partial lesions could often be found although the main rim remained intact.

DISCUSSION

By utilizing the tangential posterior view and an arthrographic picture taken in the same position, the predominant lesion or the association of lesions can be appropriately determined. The grade of the humeral defect, the state of the glenoid and the presence or absence of a labral lesion can be fully evaluated so that the appropriate surgical procedure can be adopted.

In just over 50 percent of our patients, the radiographic review showed labral detachment, a small humeral defect and no alteration of the glenoid cavity. This group of patients can be very adequately dealt with by a technique such as Bankart's procedure, particularly if associated with the modifications introduced by Rowe. However, one cannot expect such procedures as the Putti-Platt technique to deal as effectively with this group, since it restricts considerably the external rotation.

Rowe in his series of cases treated with the modified Bankart technique had a failure rate of 3.5 percent in 145 shoulders. In the Rowe et al. series they were able to compare the recurrence rate after surgery with the size of the defect noted radiographically and at surgery. The results are found to directly correlate with the size of the humeral head lesion. Thus, with small defects there was no recurrence while with moderate defects 4.7 percent recurred. Severe defects were responsible for a 6 percent recurrence rate.

It is our conclusion, therefore, that with a Grade 3 type defect and many of those associated with a Grade 2 lesion, a Bankart repair alone may not be successful and attention may have to be given to dealing with the glenoid as well. This becomes especially important with a large humeral defect associated with a narrow glenoid, reducing as it does the useful sliding index ie. the effective area of surface contact between glenoid and humerus. In this case, a preglenoid graft combined with a capsular reattachment may have to be considered. Alternatively, a procedure to rebuild the humeral defect might be required particularly if the lesion is fairly large. To this end, we have endeavoured to obliterate the humeral defect by transfer of the infraspinatus tendon with a piece of bone from the greater tuberosity. For 12 years this has proved a reliable procedure for this difficult lesion.

The Grade 2 or moderate-sized defects produce 4.7 percent of failures but we believe that this could be eliminated with some form of grafting to the anterior rim associated with capsular repair. Such a graft may be taken from the posterior angle of the acromion, as we have used since 1951 with great success. The coracoid process could also be transferred as in the Bristow technique; or a modification of the old Eden-Hybinette operation can be employed using an iliac crest bone graft. This last procedure should be reserved for those with marked alteration in the glenoid, for it has been found that a simple grafting of the glenoid rim is enough to impede dislocation in those cases associated with minor alterations of the cavity with a moderate-sized defect of the humeral head.

Where there is a marked alteration of glenoid obliquity, techniques such as those described by Saha should be considered. This osteotomy of the scapular neck redirects the glenoid and corrects its marked obliquity. This is appropriate, however, more to situations of nontraumatic origin where there is a small humeral defect and no associated labral lesion.

Conclusions

It is our contention that many of the procedures now employed for recurrent dislocation of the shoulder should be abandoned. These include the techniques which do not explore the joint, because they risk leaving a detached labrum which will give rise to a postoperative rim syndrome. Similarly, techniques based on restriction of external motion bypass the pathology, completely missing both the bony lesion and the soft-tissue pathology.

Instead we would recommend the use of the Bankart repair for traumatic cases with small defects, and enhancement with preglenoidal grafting in patients with Grade 2 defects. A similar procedure may be used for those with glenoidal narrowing or marked obliquity, but a Grade 3 lesion will require refilling of the humeral defect if complete success is to be achieved.

THE PLACE OF COMPUTED ARTHROTOMOGRAPHY IN UNSTABLE SHOULDER

PATRICK KINNARD, F.R.C.S.(C), DOUGLAS GORDON, M.D.,
RÉJEAN-YVES LÉVESQUE, F.R.C.P.(C), and DENIS BERGERON, F.R.C.P.(C)

The diagnosis of recurring dislocating or subluxing shoulder is relatively straightforward if there is a clinical history of well documented recurrent shoulder dislocations or if the patient is clearly aware of his subluxation; but this is often not the case. Instead, there may be complaints of episodes of paralysing pain called the "dead arm syndrome" by Rowe[3] which must be differentiated from nerve root pain, thoracic outlet syndrome, rotator cuff tear, etc. . . . or the patient may already have had surgery for his recurring dislocations and more information is therefore needed to clarify the diagnosis.

Materials and Methods

At the University of Sherbrooke, in an ongoing prospective study begun in 1980, 17 patients complaining of unstable shoulder were evaluated. There were 13 males and four females with a mean age of 27 years. Previous history of documented dislocations or subluxations was present in 14 cases and absent in three cases. Two patients had already had surgery for their problem. The apprehension test was positive in all 17 cases. Routine radiography with varying degrees of internal rotation and axillary views demonstrated Hill-Sachs defect of glenoid rim fractures in 10 cases and was negative in seven cases.

Computed arthrotomography was done in all cases using 4 cc of 60% iodine solution and 10 cc of room air. Fifteen to 30 minutes later, each underwent CT scanning of the shoulder using a GE CT/T 8800 high resolution scanner. Six to eight, 5 mm contiguous cuts through the articulation were obtained. Generally, the CT study was completed in less than 15 minutes.

Results

Computed arthrotomography detected soft tissue and/or bony anomalies in all patients (Table 1) but one, where artifacts from a metallic staple rendered the evaluation inconclusive. The films were interpreted by a radiologist who was not familiar with any patient's history. The anterior capsular recess was increased in volume in 16 patients (Fig. 1). Septae or post-traumatic adhesions were visible in 10 patients (Fig. 2). Amputation of the glenoid labrum had occurred in seven patients (Fig. 3). Fractures of the glenoid rim were seen in four patients (Fig. 4). Three of these fractures were not detected with the plain and special incidence x-rays but were easily visualized with the CT scan.

All these findings were substantiated at surgery in 14 patients while three other patients are currently awaiting their surgical treatment.

Two patients had previous surgery on the shoulder and while one patient's study was inconclusive due to the presence of a metallic staple, the second patient's shoulder demonstrated an increased anterior recess, an objective clue detected with conventional techniques (Fig. 2).

Discussion

Though this is a small series we conclude that arthrotomography is the most sophisticated and

TABLE 1 CT Scan Findings

Increased anterior capsular recess	16/17
Septae	10/17
Labral amputation	7/17
Fracture of the glenoid rim	4/17

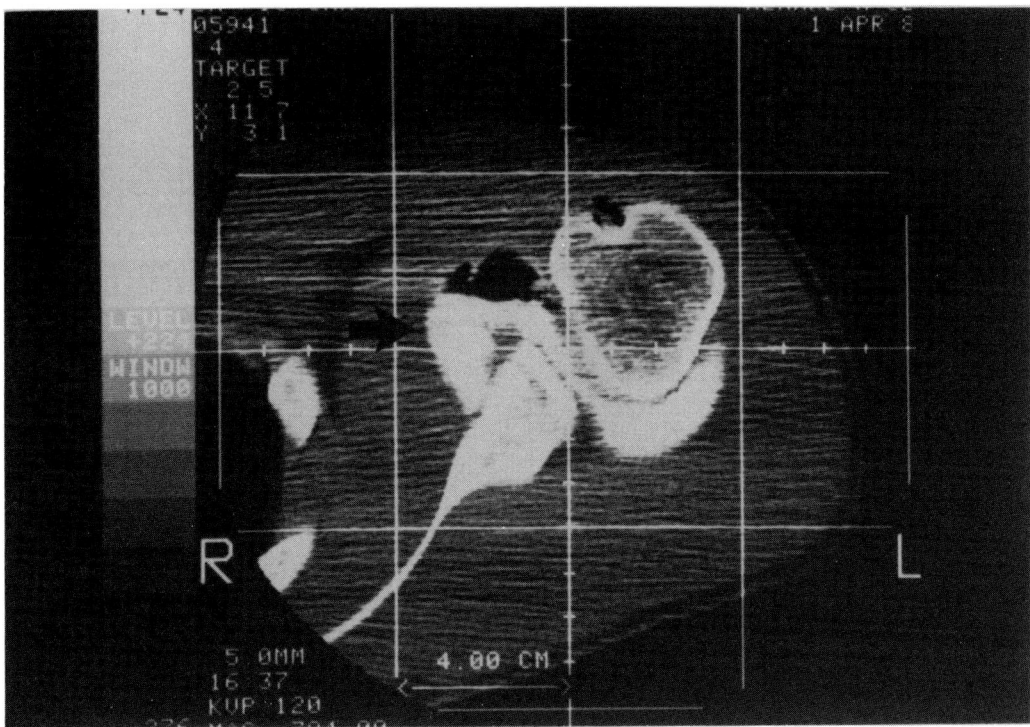

Figure 1 Increased anterior capsular recess.

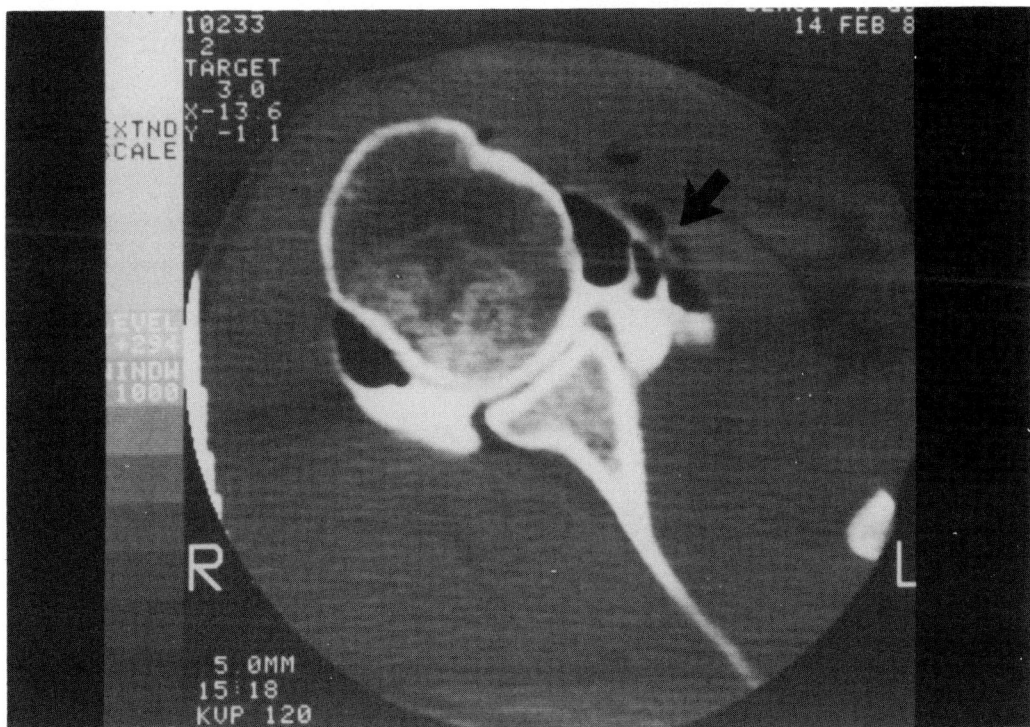

Figure 2 Increased anterior capsular recess and septae despite previous surgical treatment.

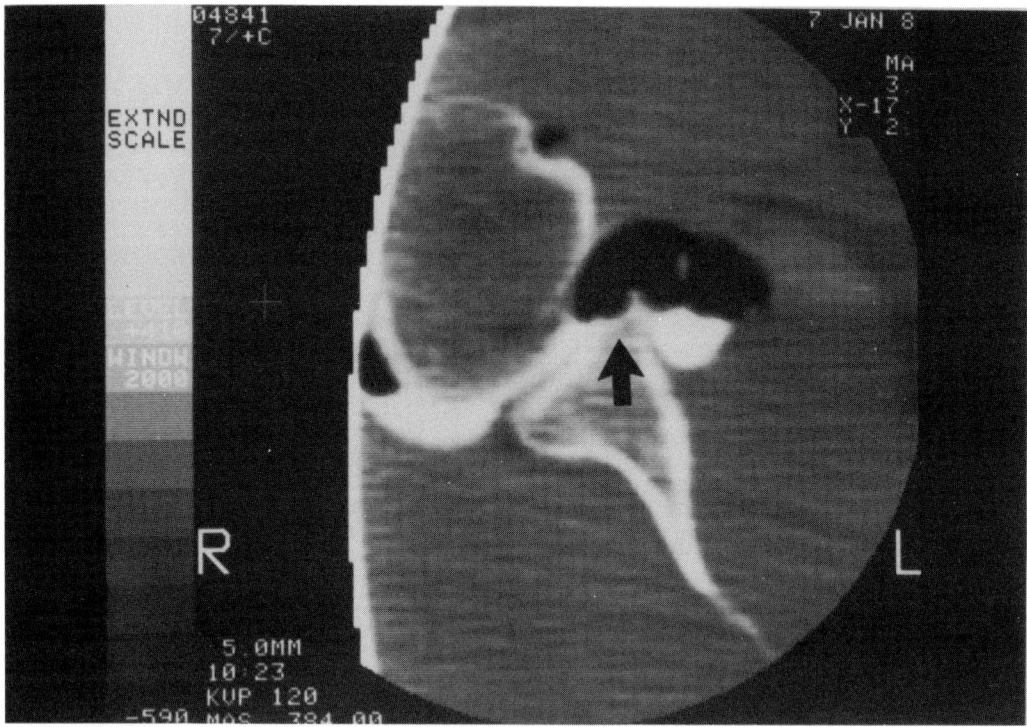

Figure 3 Labrum amputation.

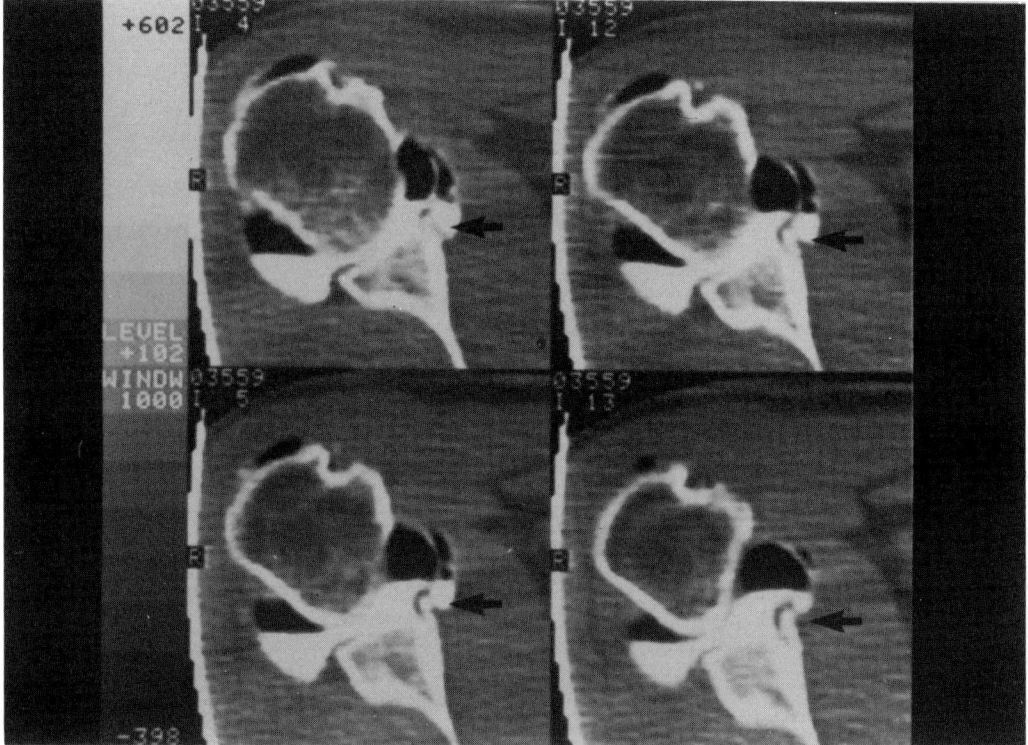

Figure 4 Glenoid rim fracture not detected by standard x-rays.

precise method of investigation currently available in the evaluation of the unstable shoulder. This procedure is capable of discovering objective clues to instability that would go undetected with conventional techniques.[1] Still one must not lose sight of the fact that shoulder instability remains primarily a clinical diagnosis; the history and physical examination will be conclusive in a large number of instances.[4]

Some cases, however, remain uncertain after plain x-rays and even arthrography or arthrotomography may be negative. This is especially true in the so called "dead arm syndrome,"[3] where a careful differential diagnosis is essential, and in patients having recurring symptoms despite surgical treatment of their condition.

The importance of objective assessment is evident when evaluating patients for surgical intervention. Detailed knowledge of the anatomical defects involved may be of tremendous help in determining the best treatment for a given patient.

Due to the actual cost of this technique, computed arthrotomography must be indicated in patients with an uncertain diagnosis or with recurring symptoms following previous shoulder surgery.

REFERENCES

1. Kinnard P, Tricoire JL, Levesque RY, Bergeron D. Assessment of the unstable shoulder by computed arthrography. Am J Sports Med. 1983; 11:158–159.
2. McGlynn F, El Khoury G, Albright J. Arthrotomography of the glenoid labrum in shoulder instability. J Bone Joint Surg. 1982; 64A:506–517.
3. Rowe C, Zarins R. Recurrent transient subluxation of the shoulder. J Bone Joint Surg. 1981; 63A:863–871.
4. Rockwood CA. Dislocation about the shoulder in fractures. Rockwood CA, Green DP, eds. Philadelphia: JB Lippincott, 1975:645.

LIMB SALVAGE PROCEDURES FOR PRIMARY BONE TUMORS OF THE SHOULDER REGION

MICHAEL G. ROCK, M.D., FRANKLIN H. SIM, M.D., and EDMUND Y. S. CHAO, Ph.D.

Advances in preoperative investigative measures, reconstructive surgery, implant design and a greater appreciation of the natural history of bone sarcomas have created renewed interest in limb salvage attempts. This interest is of great import in the shoulder area where amputation causes functional deficits which are inadequately compensated by any prosthetic devices available today. To provide a viable alternative to amputation, limb salvage procedures must afford comparable tumor control while allowing for maintenance of a functional status that represents an improvement over that achieved with ablative surgery.

Of 160 patients with primary bone tumors who underwent limb salvage attempts at the Mayo Clinic, 24 had tumors in the shoulder region. Each tumor was staged according to the recommended classification of Enneking and Spanier. This encompasses the pathological grade as well as the anatomical site of the tumor with reference to the compartment of origin. In our series, there were 16 chondrosarcomas, 7 osteosarcomas and 1 fibrosarcoma. The majority of chondrosarcomas were low grade while the osteosarcomas were high grade. Generally speaking, intraosseous or intracompartmental low grade and high grade lesions are suitable for limb salvage, as are low grade extracompartmental lesions. We have used these guidelines in our selection of candidates for limb salvage procedures.

There were 15 tumors in the proximal humerus, eight in the scapula and one in the distal clavicle, which had been subjected to various attempts at en bloc resection that adhered to well established principles of orthopedic oncologic surgery which mandates eradication of the tumor and biopsy tract with sufficient margins. This necessitates wide or radical margins around the tumor, including, according to Enneking, 2 cm of normal tissue between the margin of resection and the tumor pseudocapsule. There is no place for intralesional or marginal resection in malignant bone sarcomas.

The patients comprising this series were followed for an average of 33 months. At the time of follow-up, 19 patients were alive without disease, 1 patient had inoperable pulmonary metastases and 4 patients had died. Three of the four deaths were unrelated to the tumor; one patient who had had a low grade extraosseous chondrosarcoma had died of his disease. This patient was the only one in the series who experienced a local recurrence.

The principal advantage of limb salvage procedures is maintenance of extremity function. Judged by this criterion, the procedures performed in this series have been successful. All patients continued to enjoy near-normal elbow, forearm, wrist and hand function. Sufficient mobility existed in the shoulder area to maximize function of the distal extremity. This represents a marked improvement over available prosthetic devices. Serial assessments of these patients afforded the opportunity to evaluate shoulder function after major reconstructive procedures. However, the evaluation of shoulder function is difficult due to the biomechanical complexity of the joint. Utilizing a rating scale currently being evaluated by the Musculoskeletal Tumor Society and well established biomechanical means, a system was devised for the assessment of each patient with reference to the performance index of normal subjects and the contralateral uninvolved upper extremity. It is hoped that this system will also serve in predicting potential function based on the surgical procedures performed. The patient assessment includes shoulder strength, measured by a Cibex II Dynamometer, and shoulder mobility, assessed by utilizing a Biplanar Video System that allows digitization and computerization of the shoulder motion with respect to the trunk. It affords the opportunity to evaluate shoulder mobility requirements for daily activities such as opposing the other shoulder, mouth, and back of the head as well as the capacity to reach the lower back and buttocks area. The *sum* of these data is referred to as the functional arc; each patient's capacity to meet this standard was documented.

Recognizing the inadequacy of a universal evaluation scheme for skeletal reconstruction after tumor resection, the Musculoskeletal Tumor Society has developed a rating system that encompasses the specific parameters unique to the major joint undergoing reconstruction. The system, as it applies to the shoulder, considers combined active motion, pain, stability, strength, capacity to perform activities of daily living, and complications. A rating of good implies that five of the six parameters must meet that standard or better.

Considering all the procedures performed, 63 percent of results would be considered good or excellent and 26 percent fair by the criteria set forth by the Musculoskeletal Tumor Society. Thirteen of 24 patients managed active mobility within the functional range with sufficient strength to perform simple tasks. Six patients were subjected to scapulectomy, two partial and four total. Partial scapulectomy allows retention of shoulder articulations, para-articular soft tissues and nerve supply to the shoulder rotators and stabilizers and is therefore compatible with good functional results. However, scapulectomy demands greater sacrifice of soft tissue and severely compromises active mobility of the joint.

Four of our patients underwent Tikhor-Linberg procedures for tumors requiring extracapsular resections due to their proximity to the glenohumeral joint. The conventional procedure recommended by Linberg and Pack approximated the remaining humerus and arm musculature to the anterolateral chest wall. Modifications recommended by Saltzer, which we endorse, entail using a ceramic prosthesis or intramedullary nail as a spacer which is secured into the remaining clavicle or chest wall. This affords the opportunity of advancing soft tissue into the prosthesis while maintaining the length of the extremity, improving cosmetic appearance and allowing greater stability for elbow function. However, as anticipated, only fair results may be expected after this procedure, with no one achieving a functional range.

Two patients were given fibular struts used as intercalary grafts for segmental defects of the proximal humerus. The good results obtained with these patients are attributable to the preservation of the articulating humeral head. However, delayed union, nonunion, absorption and fatigue fractures continue to represent significant contraindications to the use of an articulating single fibular graft for the proximal humerus.

Nine patients underwent proximal humeral resection and reconstruction with proximal humeral megaprosthesis. The functional results of these patients are contingent on the degree of soft tissue sacrifice at the time of en bloc resection. Low grade intraosseous lesions allowed retention of the para-articular muscles with the exclusion of the anterior third of the deltoid and the long head of the biceps. However, sufficient soft tissue existed to encapsulate the prosthesis, rendering a stable functional articulation. Extraosseous low grade or high grade lesions necessitated further soft tissue resection, eliminating both encapsulation of the prosthesis and advancement of soft tissue into the proximal aspect of the prosthesis. Thus, the shoulder rotators were rendered inactive.

The discrepancy in functional status between patients subjected to these two different procedures was dramatized by their performance. The success of using conventional proximal humeral replacements is therefore contingent on the preservation of soft tissue. However, removal of the tumor en bloc with wide margins should not be compromised in an effort to maintain function.

Complications other than local recurrence, metastases and death were unique to patients subjected to proximal humeral replacement for high grade extracompartmental tumors. These included subluxation and dislocation in four cases, two of which were subjected to revision. Two patients experienced loosening of the prosthesis, one of which necessitated revision. It has become obvious that conventional endoprostheses tend to fail in those patients with extracompartmental lesions. We have therefore designed a series of prostheses that are fashioned to compensate for deficits created by radical oncological surgery. This is a modular system based on conical self-lock coupling components made of titanium, chosen for its light weight, high fatigue strength and fiber metal coating capacity. Situations that allow for preservation of periarticular soft tissues such as aggressive benign or low grade intracompartmental malignancies would articulate freely with a titanium humeral head that resembles the natural anatomic configuration and allows for soft tissue apposition to the component. We have designated this the Mayo Design. Wide resection for a high grade extraosseous lesion is not compatible with restoration of functional shoulder mobility or stability. Our second model, designated the Mayo Campanacci Design, allows for rotation at the shaft head junction while stabilizing the polyethylene head component to the acromion or glenoid with fascia lata or nonabsorbable suture. The prosthesis therefore serves only as a spacer to allow active rotation and passive positioning of the extremity to facilitate forearm and hand use.

In summary, local procedures for primary bone sarcomas of the shoulder girdle have been found to be safe, with rates of recurrence comparable to those of ablative procedures. Of the various anatomical areas suitable for limb salvage, the shoulder appears to enjoy the greatest success, with a recurrence rate of 4 percent as opposed to 10 percent for the knee, 21 percent for the pelvis and 12 percent for the hip. We have also shown that limb salvage attempts have afforded maintenance of extremity function. The morbidity of patients with high grade extracompartmental lesions attests to the fact that we cannot apply conventional reconstructive concepts to this patient population.

SURGICAL PATHOLOGY IN CHRONIC SHOULDER PAIN

P. PAAVOLAINEN, M.D., P. SLÄTIS, M.D., and K. AALTO, M.D.

During recent years there has been increasing interest in chronic shoulder pain because of the prevalence of the disorder. Thus, Hammond[6] stated that shoulder pain is, after low back pain, the most frequent cause of orthopedic consultations; similar conclusions were drawn from a large scale survey on the incidence of musculoskeletal complaints in primary health care by Borchgrevink[3].

Surgical attempts at relieving intractable shoulder pain have been hampered by lack of information regarding the pathology of the shoulder joint, inconclusive methods of examination and lack of a system of classification. In his article Kessel[8] quotes Burns and Ellis:[4] "Painful shoulders form an important part of orthopedic practice, but their obscurity, uncertain prognosis, and the fact that they present so few definite signs and symptoms, render their classification into types difficult on clinical grounds" and adds that there have been few important advances in our understanding of common soft-tissue disorders of the shoulder.

There is unanimous agreement that the rotator cuff plays an important role in the puzzling etiology of shoulder joint pain. The coalescence of several muscles on the facets of the greater and lesser tubercles, and the stabilizing spacer function of the coracohumeral ligament interposed between the musculotendinous parts form a dynamic unit susceptible to repetitive trauma in the anterior area of the supraspinatus tendon. Furthermore degenerative changes are apt to occur in the anterior area; an avascular zone close to the insertion of the supraspinatus muscle has been repeatedly demonstrated[9,10,14,15] and clearly contributes to the increasing incidence of degenerative tears in higher age groups. To this may be added the wear on the anterior aspects of the rotator cuff due to daily microtrauma caused by strain on the shoulder during work with the arms elevated.[2,5,7] The deleterious effect of the impact of the head of the humerus against the coracoacromial arch has been pointed out by Neer[11,12] in which the majority of tears of the rotator cuff are initiated by impingement wear rather than by circulatory impairment or trauma.

The present report was prompted by some surgical notes on different types of cuff tears and on the observation that the shoulder impingement syndrome, with or without concomitant cuff tears, is frequently associated with pathological conditions of the biceps tendon and its gliding mechanism.

MATERIALS AND METHODS

From 1979 to 1982 a total of 224 patients were referred to the Shoulder Service of the Division of Orthopaedic Surgery and Traumatology of the Surgical Hospital, Helsinki.

The predominant complaint in all was longstanding pain in the shoulder, resistant to repeated conservative treatment periods. On 119 patients a total of 126 arthrotomies of the shoulder joint were made. The series comprised 78 males and 41 females. Sixty percent of the patients attributed their condition to trauma. All patients underwent preoperative arthrographies in addition to plain radiography. Those cases with recurrent luxation or fracture of the shoulder girdle were excluded from the series.

A delta-splitting incision was used in all cases and in a few instances extended into a transacromial approach.[8] The coracoacromial ligament was resected together with the anterior part of the acromion;[11] this gives a good exposure of the underlying rotator cuff.

In cases with a tear of the rotator cuff, exploration of the joint proceeded as follows. The inferior aspect of the acromial arch was inspected, with due attention to the following points: the bursa and any enlargement of the acromioclavicular joint, with encroachment upon the underlying supraspinatus tendon; the rotator cuff and any adhesions to the pericapsular tissue; the size of the rotator cuff tear and the thickness of the adjacent part of the cuff; the condition of the coracohumeral ligament, especially at its insertion on the greater and lesser tubercles where this ligament guides the movements of the biceps tendon; the condition of the biceps tendon as seen when lifted gently while extending the humerus; and the condition of the joint cartilage, the synovial lining and the rim of the labrum.

In cases with an intact rotator cuff a similar exploration was made by dividing the rotator cuff in the borderline between the anterior part of the supraspinatus tendon and the posterior part of the coracohumeral ligament, extending the incision from the musculotendinous junction to the anterior facet of the greater tuberosity about 3 mm lateral to the intertubercular groove. If examination of the biceps revealed gross thickening, synovitis and fraying of the tendon, the intertubercular groove was exposed by extending the incision along the lateral wall of the sulcus, thus exposing the tendon along its course and allowing inspection of the groove. If on initial inspection the biceps tendon appeared normal, the sulcus was not opened.

The stability of the joint was assessed by extreme outward and backward rotation of the humeral head; only a clear tendency to subluxate or the presence of the Bankart lesion was accepted as evidence of a subluxating joint.

RESULTS

The preoperative findings at these 126 arthrotomies are compiled in Table 1. The thickness of the coracoacromial ligament varied considerably. In several cases it could be considered very tight, but on inspection there were no signs of wear on the surface of the ligament facing the rotator cuff. Arthritic changes in the acromioclavicular joint were seldom sizable enough to warrant resection of the distal end of the clavicle or smoothing of the undersurface of the joint. Adhesions were regularly seen around the rotator cuff.

Changes in the Rotator Cuff

Complete cuff tears were divided into small, moderate, large and massive.[13] There were five patients with small tears, 13 with moderate, 28 with large and five with massive tears. In the long-standing cases, the edges of the rupture were thin and the retracted rotator cuff thickened. A common feature in the retracted part of the cuff was synovial folding due to scarring of the cuff. On exploration of the incomplete cuff tears the undersurface of the supraspinatus and infraspinatus tendons was often rugose with degenerative changes in the insertion area of the tendon proper. These were confined predominantly to the supraspinatus and infraspinatus area. In two cases virtually no firm tendinous tissue was left at the point of attachment to the humeral head, although the cuff was intact enough to prevent leakage of the contrast medium in arthrography. All these findings were considered indicative of a ruptured rotator cuff; there were 51 arthrotomies in this group (Tab. 2).

In the remaining 75 arthrotomies, the cuff was considered intact. There was no leakage of contrast medium in the arthrograms, no tear on exploration of the cuff, and no hidden rupture on inspection of the interior of the tendinous capsule. In many of these arthrotomies, however, the cuff showed clear degenerative changes, with edema and thickening of the tendon, as seen in the early stages of the impingement syndrome, or with incrustation of calcified deposits or fibrous thickening of the tendon, as in the late stages of the impingement syndrome.

TABLE 1 Preoperative Diagnosis in 126 Arthrotomies Made for Chronic Shoulder Pain

Rupture of the rotator cuff	51
Degeneration or impingement on the rotator cuff	24
Tendinitis of the biceps tendon	38
Subluxation of the glenohumeral joint	11
Arthrosis of the acromioclavicular joint	2
Total	126

TABLE 2 Incidence of Concomitant Pathological Changes in the Biceps Tendon in the Operated Cases With and Without Rupture of the Rotator Cuff

A. Rotator cuff ruptured (51 cases)	
biceps tendinitis	31
medial dislocation of the biceps tendon	12
rupture of the biceps tendon	3
	46
B. Rotator cuff intact (75 cases)	
biceps tendinitis	38
medial dislocation of the biceps tendon	9
rupture of the biceps tendon	5
	52

Changing the Bicipital Tendon and the Intertubercular Groove

Inspection of the tendon of the long head of the biceps muscle and the intertubercular groove revealed pathological changes in 98 arthrotomies; thus in only 28 shoulders arthrotomized because of chronic pain were the synovium and tendon considered to be quite normal. The incidence of bicipital changes was slightly higher in shoulders with a ruptured cuff (Tab. 2). Here, bicipital tenosynovitis was observed in 31 cases, medial dislocation of the tendon in 12 cases and rupture of the tendon in three cases. The corresponding values for the shoulders with an intact rotator cuff were 38, 9 and 5 cases, respectively.

Assessment of the etiology in the various manifestations of bicipital pathology showed that contributory factors are lesions in the following parts: the rotator cuff, the coracohumeral ligament and the intertubercular groove. The function of the biceps tendon depends on one or other of these factors, or all three together. It should further be noted that at operation the tendon may be seen in different stages of the disease.

Impingement Tendinitis

This category of tenosynovitis is the most common, but not usually the most severe. It is encountered in cases with a tear of the rotator cuff located in the anterior part of the cuff in such a way that on elevation of the arm the tendon is pinched between the head of the humerus below and the acromion above. The tendon becomes thickened because of edema, and fibrous changes may cause a continual broadening of the tendon proper; however, the synovium is not usually inflamed. Fraying of the tendon is seldom seen and is mostly confined to the area close to the intertubercular groove (Fig. 3B, 4).

Subluxation of the Biceps Tendon

Normally, the tendon of the long head of the biceps muscle lies in the intertubercular groove surrounded by the synovial pouch. On elevation of the arm, the intra-articular portion of the tendon is only a few centimeters long; on extension about 4 cm. The tendon is fixed at the supraglenoid rim; thus, the head of the humerus moves against the

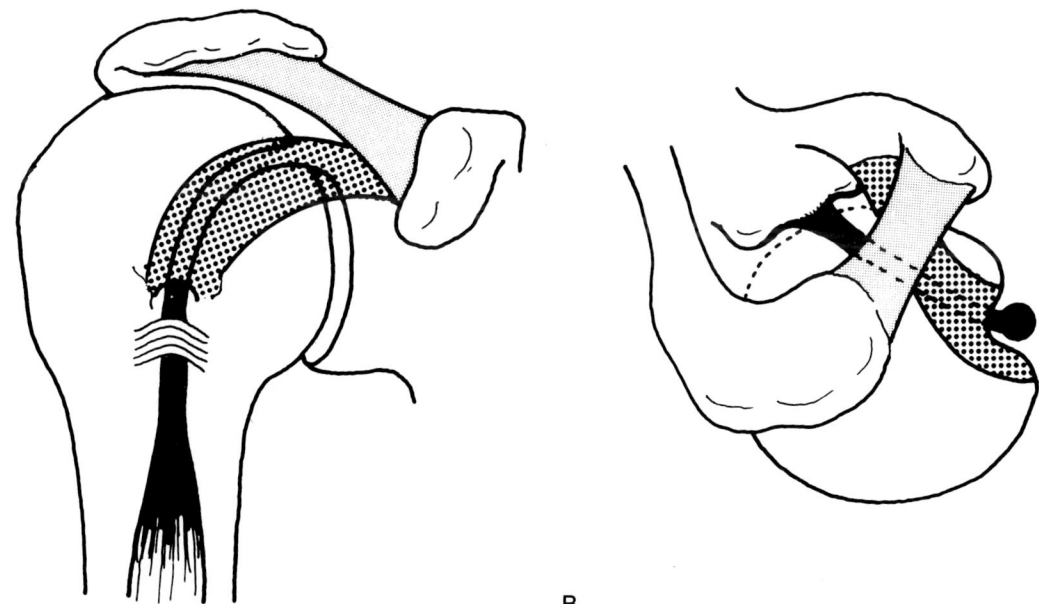

Figure 1 Diagram of the anterior (A) and craniocaudal (B) aspects of the right glenohumeral joint. The biceps tendon is drawn in black and the shaded area is the coracohumeral ligament. The coracohumeral ligament is that part of the rotator cuff which is interposed between the subscapularis and supraspinatus muscles (A). The biceps tendon glides in the intertubercular groove between the medial and lateral attachments of the ligament (B) and it is chiefly the coracohumeral ligament that keeps it aligned in the sulcus.

tendon on elevation and extension (Fig. 1, A to B). The gliding mechanism of the tendon is guided by the coracohumeral ligament (Fig. 2). A lesion to the medial portion of the ligament disturbs the normal gliding mechanisms and the tendon is gradually displaced medially.[16] The lesion may be hidden, but it is usually concomitant to moderate or massive tears extending into the anterior part of the cuff. A fully displaced bicipital tendon lies in a sling of the ruptured cuff, and may in the early phases slip in and out of the groove; but as the sulcus gradually fills with scar tissue, the groove becomes shallower, and finally the tendon remains in its medially dislocated position. In the early phases, the synovium of the tendon is inflamed by the to and fro movement; later the inflammatory reaction may subside, but the impaired function of the joint persists (Fig. 3B).

Attrition Tendinitis

The intertubercular groove seems to adjust its width and depth according to the size of the tendon, and not to the size of the humeral head.[1] In 14 arthrotomies a localized process was seen causing narrowing of the sulcus and impingement of the tendon. In these cases the synovial reaction was usually impressive, with edema, swelling and intense redness of the synovium. In the sulcus area the tendon was frequently frayed and thinned, whereas the intra-articular portion was as a rule unaffected by the nearby reaction. The sulcus was narrow and deep, and in plain radiographs osteophytes could be seen in the aperture of the groove. This type of bicipital tendinitis seemed to be the most painful and seemed to be the commonest cause of complete rupture of the tendon (Fig. 3C).

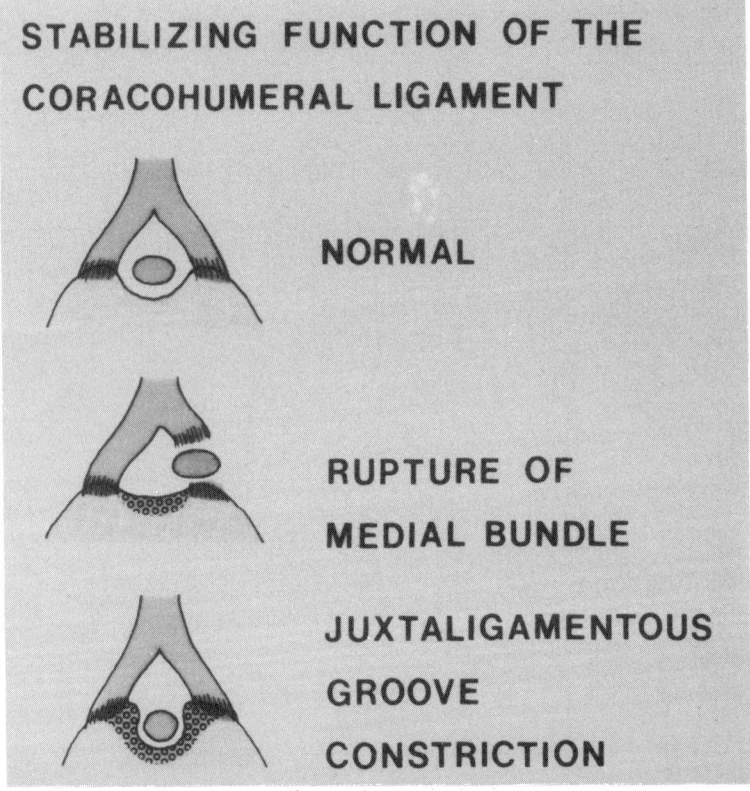

Figure 2 Stabilizing mechanism of the coracohumeral ligament. The ligament has two distal attachments in the humeral head: one lateral in the greater tubercle and the other medial in the lesser tubercle. Any tear in the cuff that extends into these attachments will affect the normal gliding mechanism and lead to medial displacement of the tendon of the long head of the biceps muscle. Local new bone and connective tissue formation can lead to stenosis of the bicipital groove and the tendon lies squeezed in its narrow sulcus.

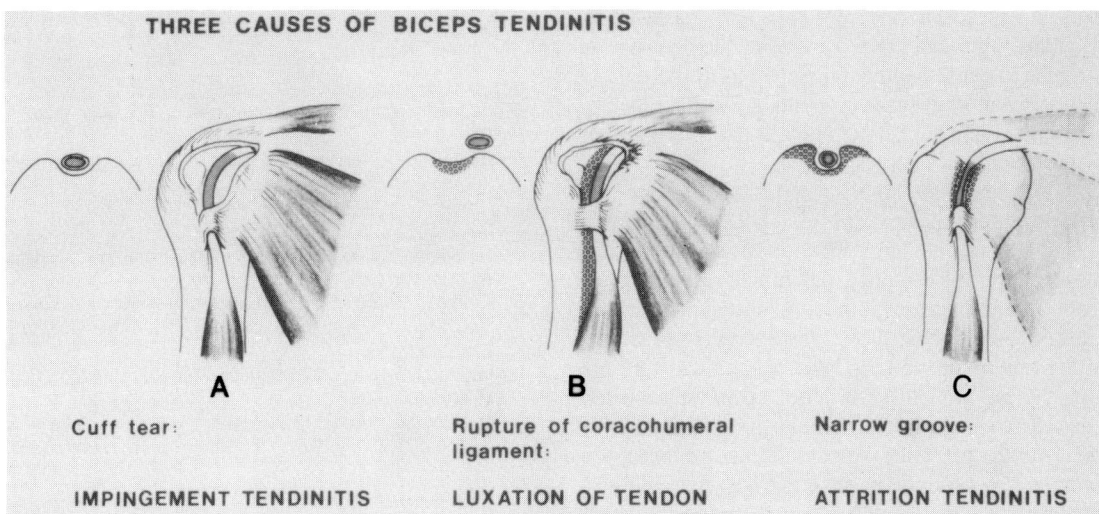

Figure 3 Pathological conditions in the mechanism stabilizing the biceps tendon can lead to tendinitis in at least three different ways: A. Rupture of the rotator cuff exposes the tendon to compression between the acromion above and the humeral head below. The tendon lies normally in its groove. B. A tear in the medial portion of the coracohumeral ligament causes luxation and medial displacement of the tendon from the bicipital groove. C. Local new bone and connective tissue formation causes stenosis of the bicipital groove leading to attrition of the tendon of the long head of the biceps muscle.

DISCUSSION

Neer[12] has pointed out that inclination of the acromion may contribute to the development of an impingement syndrome by increasing the pressure against the anterior part of the cuff on elevation of the arm. Herberts[7] reported a significantly higher rate of shoulder pain in welders, who often work with elevated arms, than in clerks. Both observations point to the importance of impingement on the anterior capsule as a cause of gradual derangement of the cuff and persistent pain.

The surgical observations in this study confirmed earlier reports of the high prevalence of cuff ruptures in the supraspinatus area, corresponding to the area of impingement. In addition to this, preoperative findings revealed a high incidence of bicipital pathology which in our opinion may be an important factor contributing to persistent shoulder pain.

The relationship between impingement of the humeral head against the acromion and the anterior edge of the coracoacromial ligament is not fully understood. Neer considers impingement to be an important causative factor in chronic shoulder pain and even in most cuff tears.[12] Two other factors can be added: firstly, extension of a rupture onto the medial portion of the coracohumeral ligament, which instantly alters the mechanics of gliding properties of the tendon;[16] secondly, constriction of the intertubercular groove, which causes attrition tendinitis. The mechanism of the latter needs further data. We gained the impression that avulsion trauma, as caused by forcible external rotation-abduction of the arm, causes hemorrhage in the insertion of the coracohumeral ligament and subsequent reactive formation of bone and con-

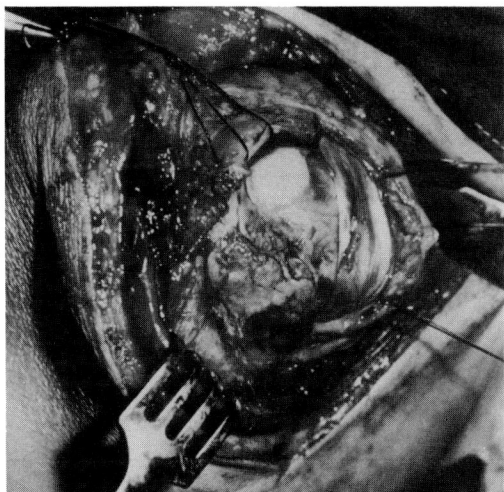

Figure 4 Classical vast rupture of the rotator cuff with concomitant pathological lesions of the biceps tendon. The tendon can be seen to be badly inflamed and swollen. In this case, tendinitis and fraying are caused by compression of the tendon between the acromion and the humeral head.

nective tissue. The incongruence between the tendon and the available space in the groove is thought to cause segmental ischemia in the tendon and surrounding synovia, with a strong reactive synovitis, which leads eventually to total rupture of the tendon.

Injuries to the anterior part of the rotator cuff are more apt to cause chronic shoulder pain than cuff tears confined to the more lateral parts. The reason for this is partly the higher incidence of tears in the juxtaosseus zone of the supraspinatus tendon, but especially the susceptibility to injury of the tendon of the long head of the biceps in this area. Even clinically, tenderness is more often elicited from the intertubercular groove than over the lateral cuff tear. Accumulating radiographic data and peroperative observations may be expected gradually to clarify the pathology in each individual case.

REFERENCES

1. Ahovuo J. Radiographic anatomy of the intertubercular groove of the humerus. Eur J Radiol (in press).
2. Bateman J. The shoulder and neck. Toronto: WB Saunders, 1978.
3. Borchgrevink CF, Brekke TH, Ogar B. Skjelett/muskelsykdommer i almenpraksis. Tidssk Nor Laegerforen 1980; 100(7):439–445.
4. Burns BH, Ellis VH. Recent advances in orthopaedic surgery. London: J and A Churchill, 1937; 151.
5. Codman EA. The Shoulder. Boston: Privately printed, 1934.
6. Hammond G, Torgerson W, Dotter W, Leach R. The painful shoulder. Instructional Course Lectures. Amer Acad Orthop Surg St. Louis: CV Mosby, 1971; 20:83–90.
7. Herberts P, Kadefors R, Andersson G, Petersen, I. Shoulder pain in industry: an epidemiological study on welders. Acta Orthop Scan 1981; 52:299–306.
8. Kessel L, Watson M. The painful arch syndrome. Clinical classification as a guide to management. J Bone Joint Surg 1977; 59B:166–172.
9. Macnab I. Rotator cuff tendinitis. Ann Roy Coll Surg Engl 1973; 53:271–287.
10. Moseley HF, Goldie I. The arterial pattern of the rotator cuff of the shoulder. J Bone Joint Surg 1963; 45B:780–789.
11. Neer CS II. Anterior acromionplasty for the chronic impingement syndrome in the shoulder. J Bone Joint Surg 1972; 54A:41–50.
12. Neer CS II. Impingement lesions. Clin Orthop 1983; 173:70–77.
13. Post M, Silver R, Singh M. Rotator cuff tear. Diagnosis and treatment. Clin Orthop 1983; 173:78–91.
14. Rathbun JB, Macnab I. The microvascular pattern of the rotator cuff. J Bone Joint Surg 1970; 52B:540–553.
15. Rothman RH, Parke WW. The vascular anatomy of the rotator cuff. Clin Orthop 1965; 41:176–182.
16. Slätis P, Aalto K. Medial dislocation of the tendon of the long head of the biceps brachii. Acta Orthop Scand 1979; 50:73–77.

PYOGENIC ARTHRITIS OF THE GLENOHUMERAL JOINT FOLLOWING THE INTRA-ARTICULAR INJECTION OF CORTICOSTEROID

TAKEHIKO TORISU, M.D., SHOGO MASUMI, M.D., and MASATERU SHINDO, M.D.

Pyogenic arthritis of the glenohumeral joint is usually blood-borne and demonstrates acute pain, swelling and heat of the lesion. Laboratory examination reveals an elevated erythrocyte sedimentation rate and increased leukocytes. If an infectious organism is identified from the purulent joint fluid, a diagnosis of pyogenic arthritis may be easily confirmed. However, it is not always possible to recover an infecting organism from the joint fluid following an intra-articular corticosteroid injection. Diagnosis is difficult when, despite suspicion of infection by plain roentgenography or arthrography, the joint fluid is not cloudy in appearance and culture of the joint fluid produces no bacterial growth.

The purpose of this paper is to describe those clinical manifestations of pyogenic arthritis of the glenohumeral joint following intra-articular injection of corticosteroid which have been encountered at our hospital, and to present some problems in diagnosis.

CASES AND FINDINGS

During a period of only one year since the opening of the Medical College Hospital of Oita in 1981, five cases of pyogenic arthritis of the glenohumeral joint were referred to our hospital. They consisted of four men and one woman, ranging in age from 54 to 70. One was affected in the right shoulder and four in the left shoulder. At the time of the initial physical examination elsewhere, four had been diagnosed as periarthritis because of shoulder pain without any roentgen manifestation. One had been suspected of rotator cuff tear. Their treatment consisted of physical therapy and intra-articular corticosteroid injections. Fifteen to 60 months had passed since the first notice of shoulder pain until they were referred to our hospital. The onset time of infection could not be determined from acute shoulder pain, probably because the underlying painful condition already existed or the patients had always experienced some pain in the local area after the injections. There was no predisposed systemic illness except diabetes mellitus in one patient. There was also no history of oral administration of corticosteroid.

Physical examination on admission revealed swelling around the shoulder in three cases and heat in two but reddening in none. Local tenderness, pain and limited motion of the shoulder were found in all. Two of them were capable of 90 degrees of forward elevation and 80 degrees of abduction of the shoulder. The remaining three were entirely unable to elevate the affected upper limb.

On laboratory examination, as shown in Table 1, the joint fluid aspirated from the glenohumeral joint was turbid only in Case 1 and nearly clear in the remaining four cases. Bacterial culture of the joint fluid on admission showed Staphylococcus aureus in Case 1 but proved negative in the four other cases. Among these negative cases Staphylococcus epidermidis was isolated in Case 2 by culture of the homogenate of granulation tissue from the intramedullary cavity of the humeral neck.

Plain roentgenograms demonstrated abnormalities, including demineralization in four of five cases, joint space loss in two, bone atrophy and blurring at the greater tubercle in four, superior migration of the humeral head in one and inferior subluxation of the humeral head in two (Table 2).

Shoulder arthrograms revealed a small dependent pouch, synovial irregularities and extravasation into the subacromial bursa in all. Lymphatic drainage was visualized in two. Radioisotope ex-

TABLE 1 Laboratory Examination

Case	Age	Sex	Systemic Disorders	ESR	Leukocyte	RA	CRP	Synovial Fluid	Fluid Culture	Synovia Culture	Histology
1	59	M	Diabetes	50	8500	−	+ +	turbid	+	+	not done
2	71	M	—	16	7200	−	+	nearly clear	−	+	+ +
3	70	M	—	18	7200	−	+ + +	nearly clear	−	−	+
4	54	F	—	18	7500	−	−	nearly clear	−	−	+
5	56	M	—	18	6800	−	±	nearly clear	−	−	+

amination was performed on three, in all of whom the increased bone concentration of ^{99m}Tc-phosphate was noted.

Synovectomy, debridement and repair of the rotator cuff were carried out in all cases, followed by closed suction irrigation for one or two weeks. Histological examination was performed in four cases in whom culture of the joint fluid was negative. There were marked villous proliferation and hyperplasia of the synovial tissue with bleeding and hypervascularity. However, cell infiltration was slight without polymorphonuclear leukocytes. On the other hand, the granulation tissue with marked infiltration of polymorphonuclear leukocytes invaded the cartilage and penetrated into the medullary cavity. Histological diagnosis was suppurative arthritis with osteomyelitis.

Case Reports

Case 2: A 70-year-old man was referred to our hospital for persistent pain, loss of motion of the left shoulder and abnormality of roentgenograms on October 24, 1981. This patient had suffered from left shoulder pain insidiously since around 1978. Since then intra-articular injection of corticosteroid and physical therapy had been given

TABLE 2 Radiographic Findings

Plain Films	
Demineralization	4/5
Joint space loss	2/5
Humeral head erosion	4/5
Superior subluxation of humeral head	1/5
Inferior subluxation of humeral head	2/5
Arthrograms	
Small dependent pouch	5/5
Synovial irregularities	5/5
Rotator cuff tears	5/5
Visualized lymphatic drainage	2/5

with some relief. The pain increased from the beginning of October, 1981.

At the time of our initial examination, the erythrocyte sedimentation rate was 16 mm per hour, leukocyte count was 7200 per cubic millimeter, RA test was negative, C-reactive protein was 1 plus and Mantoux test was negative. Repeated culture of the joint fluid grew no infectious organism.

On roentgenography, cystic osteolytic lesions with slight marginal sclerosis were disclosed in the humeral neck and glenoid. The articular surface of the humeral head itself was preserved (Fig. 1a). The distance between the humeral head and the acromion was conspicuously widened and the humeral head was in a state of inferior subluxation. Arthrography revealed the extravasation of the contrast material into the subacromial and subdeltoid bursae with multiple filling defects (Fig. 1b). At the time of surgery, the Gram smear of the joint fluid and synovial homogenate showed negative. Staphylococcus epidermidis was recovered from the culture of the homogenate of pathological granulation tissue that penetrated into the intramedullary cavity.

Case 3: A 70-year-old man with a history of right shoulder pain for 4 to 5 years was referred to our hospital on March 5, 1982. At our out-patient clinic, the erythrocyte sedimentation rate was 18 mm per hour, leukocyte count was 7200 per cubic millimeter, RA test was negative and C-reactive protein was negative. The joint fluid seemed to be normal in appearance. No infectious organism was grown from the joint fluid.

On roentgenographic examination, superior migration of the humeral head was noted and a new joint was formed between the acromion and humeral head (Fig. 2c). Arthrograms demonstrated marked proliferation of synovia and adhesion of the glenohumeral joint. Lymphatic channels and

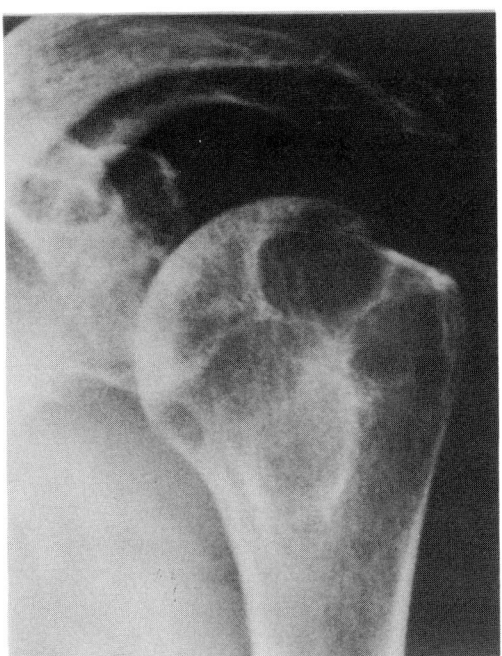 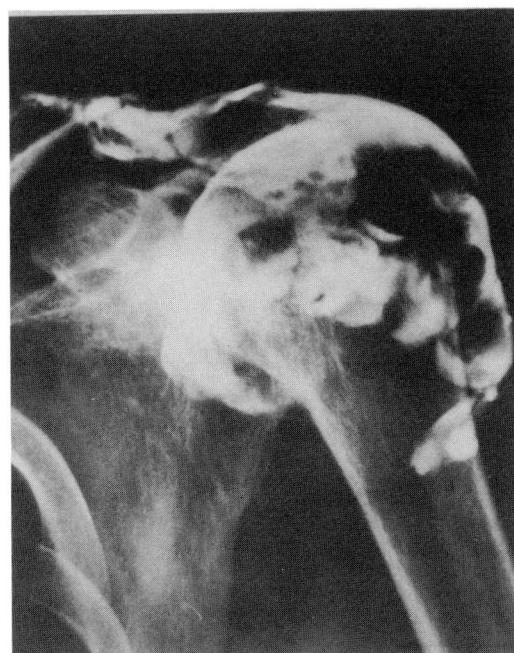

Figure 1a Roentgenogram showing cystic osteolytic lesions with slight marginal sclerosis in the humeral neck and glenoid. The articular surface of the humeral head itself was preserved. The humeral head was in a state of inferior subluxation.

Figure 1b Arthrogram revealing the extravasation of the contrast material into the subacromial and subdeltoid bursae with multiple filling defects.

rotator cuff tear were also visualized (Fig. 2d). Cuff tear arthropathy was most *suspected*. Although no infectious organism was recovered from the joint fluid and synovial homogenate at the time of surgery, the histological diagnosis was suppurative arthritis with osteomyelitis.

By careful review of the laboratory and x-ray records of the clinic where the patient had been previously taken care of, an elevated erythrocyte sedimentation rate and a positive C-reactive protein were disclosed. In addition, roentgenograms had shown transient bone atrophy and blurring of the greater tubercle corresponding to elevation of the erythrocyte sedimentation rate and positive C-reactive protein (Figs. 2a, 2b). There was no history of antibiotic administration.

DISCUSSION

Roentgenographic examination is helpful in alerting clinicians to the possibility of pyogenic arthritis, because clinical evidence of synovial inflammation of the shoulder joint is hidden. The important initial signs are bone atrophy and blurring of the greater tubercle. Another possibility never to be overlooked is superior or inferior subluxation of the humeral head. Armbuster and his associates[1] noted inferior subluxation of the humeral head in one of their five cases of pyogenic arthritis of the glenohumeral joint. Master and his colleagues[7] showed it in one of their six cases. Two of our five cases had the inferiorly subluxated humeral head. The etiology of this manifestation is unclear but it may be due to hypotony of the deltoid and rotator cuff muscle as a result of necrotic mass filling the subacromial and deltoid bursae.[4]

Arthrography of the shoulder is also helpful in evaluation of synovial proliferation. Synovial irregularity in the capsular attachment is not a pathognomonic but a meaningful finding for hypertrophy of the synovium. Adhesion of the joint cavity is clarified by a small dependent pouch and obliteration of the subscapular bursa. The presence of the rotator cuff was confirmed in all of our cases as indicated by extravasation of the contrast medium into the subacromial bursa. Kelly et al[5] described a patient with septic arthritis of the glenohumeral joint by initial normal radiography, which, however, showed superior migration of the humeral head on subsequent examinations. Arm-

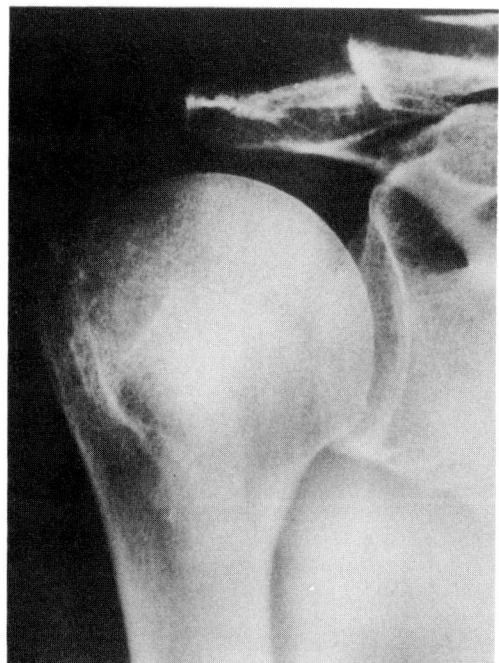

Figure 2a Roentgenogram taken on July 20, 1981 showing normal.

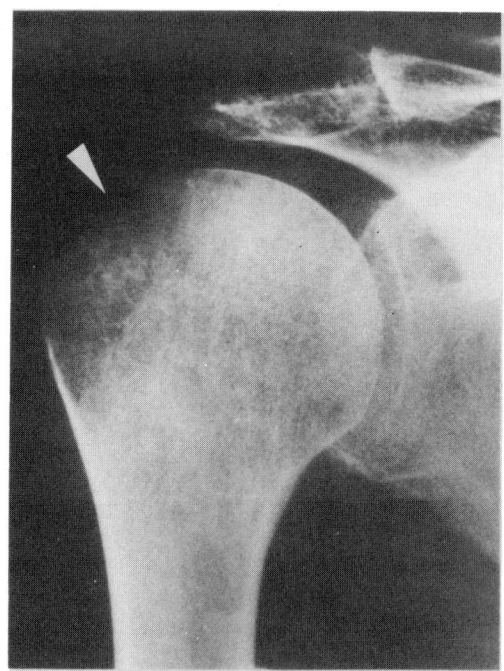

Figure 2b Roentgenogram taken on Oct 9, 1981 revealing the localized bone atrophy and lysis of the greater tubercle of the humeral head.

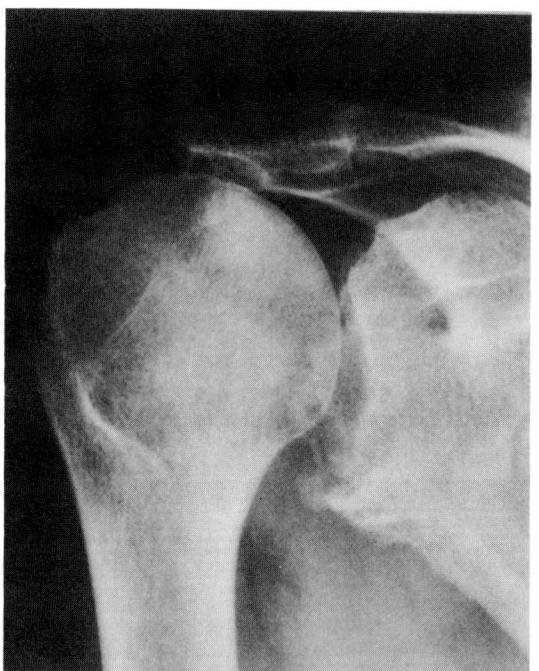

Figure 2c Roentgenogram, taken at our hospital on March 2, 1982, disclosing an increased bone density with marginal sclerosis of the greater tubercle.

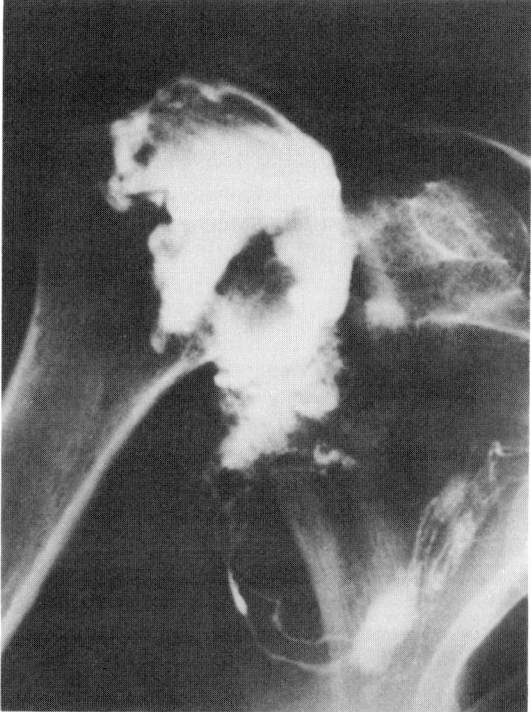

Figure 2d Arthrograms demonstrating marked proliferation of synovia and adhesion of the glenohumeral joint. Lymphatic channels and rotator cuff tear were also visualized.

buster et al[1] reported five cases of septic arthritis with rotator cuff tear.

Another outstanding feature of shoulder arthrography is the visualization of lymphatic channels. De Smet et al[2] reported that arthrographic visualization of lymphatic drainage, as observed at a high incidence (31%) in their 13 cases, was suggestive of rheumatoid arthritis. However, in our previous report on 10 cases of rotator cuff arthropathy with repeated, marked effusion in the subacromial bursa, three patients gave visualization of lymphatic channels on shoulder arthrography.[8] We, therefore, consider that visualization of lymphatic channels just demonstrates a sign of hyperpermeability of the synovial membrane.[6]

We now discuss some problems in relation to the joint fluid. Diagnosis of pyogenic arthritis may be regarded as conclusive by microbiological determination of an infectious agent in the joint fluid. The appearance of the joint fluid, mucin clot, leukocyte count and sugar content in the joint fluid may suggestively support a diagnosis of pyogenic arthritis, even if the culture results are negative.

In addition to these routine tests, Gupta and his associates[3] advocated nitroblue tetrazolium test of the synovial fluid to be a simple and useful method for early detection of pyogenic arthritis. We carried out an experimental study in rabbits to confirm Gupta's data. At 12 and 24 hours after injection of 9×10^8 Staphylococcus aureus into the knee joint of rabbits, polymorphonuclear leukocytes in the joint fluid were counted and treated with a nitroblue tetrazolium solution. Ninety to 100 percent of the polymorphonuclear leukocytes were confirmed having distinct deposits of blue formazan granules in the cells (Table 3). However, by simultaneous intra-articular injection of 9×10^8 Staphylococcus aureus and 0.2 g/kg of dexamethazone, only 30 to 40 percent of the polymorphonuclear leukocytes were deposited with blue formazan granules. This indicates the difficulty in the diagnosis of pyogenic arthritis pretreated with intra-articular corticosteroid administration.

CONCLUSIONS

Five patients with pyogenic arthritis involving the glenohumeral joint were described. An infectious organism was identified in two cases. Three other cases were diagnosed by histological data. This report calls attention to the evidence that while positive culture indicates infection, negative culture does not dismiss the diagnosis from consideration. This paper also presented some problems in relation to difficulty and importance of differential diagnosis.

We stressed that careful review of the laboratory and roentgenographic records of previous clinics was meaningful for diagnosis, and that histological examination should be routinely carried out at the time of surgery in suspected cases of pyogenic arthritis. Experimental evaluation of nitroblue tetrazolium test of joint fluid from rabbits with pyogenic arthritis confirmed only a minor role of this test method in the diagnosis of pyogenic arthritis after corticosteroid administration.

REFERENCES

1. Armbuster TG et al. Extra-articular manifestations of septic arthritis of glenohumeral joint. Am J Roentgenol 1977; 129:667–672.
2. DeSmet AA et al. Shoulder arthrography in rheumatoid arthritis. Diagnostic Radiol 1975; 116:601–605.
3. Gupta RC et al. Nitroblue tetrazolium test in the diagnosis of Pyogenic arthritis. Ann Int Med 1974; 80:723–726.
4. Iwabuchi A et al. Some problems of Hanging cast. The Shoulder Joint 1977; 1:77–79. (in Japanese).
5. Kelly PJ et al. Bacterial arthritis of the shoulder. Mayo Clin Proc 1965; 40:695–699.
6. Lewin JR et al. Lymphatic visualization during contrast arthrography of the knee. Diag Radiol 1972; 103:577–579.
7. Master R et al. Septic arthritis of the glenohumeral joint. Arthr and Rheum 1977; 20:1500–1506.
8. Torisu T et al. Rotator cuff tear with chronic effusion in subacromial bursa—diagnostic and therapeutic problems. J of West Japanese Soc of Orthop and Traumatology. (in press, in Japanese).

TABLE 3   Nitroblue Tetrazolium Test on Pyogenic Arthritis of Knee Joints of Rabbits

Injection	Post Injection Hours	Leukocyte Count	NBT Test
S. aureus	12	23.1×10^4	90–100%
	24	36.2×10^4	
S. aureus and corticosteroid	12	47.4×10^4	30–40%
	24	31.5×10^4	

CRUTCHWALKER'S SHOULDER

ROBERT G. PRINGLE, M.B., Ch.B., F.R.C.S.

In this paper two patients are presented in whom the sudden need to use crutches appears to have led to the development of aseptic necrosis of the humeral head. A further case is described where osteoarthritis of the shoulder appears to have developed as a secondary phenomenon following aseptic necrosis of the humeral head in a patient using a walking aid over a long term.

Case 1

This patient is a slim, healthy woman who was 73 when in 1979 she fell from a stage sustaining an isolated intertrochanteric fracture of the neck of the femur. She was admitted to hospital and her fracture was fixed the following day. Recovery was uneventful and after twelve days she was discharged walking with elbow crutches which she used for a further six weeks before progressing to sticks.

One month after injury she became aware of the gradual onset of pain in the contralateral shoulder. This persisted and three months post injury, when seen in the clinic, the picture on examination was that of a mild capsulitis. Radiographs at that time were passed as normal although in retrospect early changes of aseptic necrosis were visible. In fact, as the radiographs were passed as normal, the shoulder was manipulated and injected under anaesthetic. A full range of adhesion–free movement was present and there was an effusion in the joint. Physiotherapy was prescribed. Relief from these measures was short lived and four months later the clinical picture was unchanged. The radiographs at that time showed clear evidence of aseptic necrosis of the humeral head.

Serum proteins and electrophoresis, lipids and lipid electrophoresis, calcium, phosphate, alkaline phosphatase, urea and uric acid, and whole body scan were normal apart from increased uptake in the scan in the humeral head and a little around the hip fracture. In retrospect there was no evidence of fat embolism having occurred.

Without further treatment there was slow symptomatic improvement and over a two year period the area of aseptic necrosis healed without deformity. When seen four years from injury she continued to have terminal restriction of movement and some night pain in the shoulder. There was no tenderness, wasting, weakness or pain on resisted movement and all other joints were normal. Her general health remained good. Radiographs after four years revealed no deterioration in the shoulder joint.

Case 2

This patient is a slim healthy headmistress who was 59 when in 1979 she slipped on a polished floor and sustained an intertrochanteric femoral neck fracture. She was admitted to hospital and her fracture was fixed the same day. Union was uneventful. Her convalescence was uneventful and she was discharged home with elbow crutches after twelve days. She continued under Out-patient review and discontinued the use of crutches after three months. At that time she commenced hydrotherapy for her hip.

Seven months after injury she commented in passing that the hydrotherapy had cured her shoulder pain also. On further questioning she admitted to the gradual onset of ipsilateral shoulder pain one month after her fracture, reaching a peak after four months before waning and ultimately resolving completely.

Radiographs of the shoulder seven months after injury revealed an area of aseptic necrosis of the humeral head. Clinically the shoulder was normal with the exception of terminal restriction of movement. No treatment was offered. The lesion healed radiologically over a twelve month period. After four years she remains well in herself, and her shoulder is symptom–free and clinically normal. Radiologically the shoulder is normal.

The shoulder lesions in these two patients appeared similar to those resulting from aseptic necrosis from other causes and it was clear that neither patient had injured her shoulder in falling.

While there are lesser contributions from the posterior circumflex humeral artery and in some cases the rotator cuff, the main blood supply to the humeral head is derived as a constant branch from the anterior circumflex humeral artery. It commonly enters the bone at the top of the bicipital groove, thence running posteromedially in the bone just below the epiphyseal line. From it vessels branch at right angles towards the articular surface. The area of humeral head involved in aseptic necrosis clearly is at the end of the arterial line.

Radiographs of a normal shoulder in a young adult paraplegic revealed no change in the glenohumeral relationship between non-weight bearing and full weight bearing when lifting up. Radiographs of the affected shoulder of Case 2 revealed significant upwards displacement of the humeral head relative to the glenoid in the change from non–weight bearing to weight bearing as she leaned on a crutch. It is suggested that this upwards shift may stretch the capsular structures and impede the blood supply to the humeral head sufficiently to cause aseptic necrosis in an aging shoulder on which the task of weight bearing has been imposed abruptly.

Case 3

This patient, now aged 81, underwent a left McKee Farrar hip replacement in 1971. The hip remains mobile and pain free, but from the time of the operation she has had a Trendelenburg gait and has used a stick in the right hand. Two years ago she developed a progressively painful right shoulder with the radiological appearance of localized glenohumeral arthritis and deformity suggestive of previous aseptic necrosis. She does not suffer from generalized arthritis and her other shoulder is normal.

The changes appear so localized to the glenohumeral joint that it is postulated that this is the end result of aseptic necrosis in the weight bearing shoulder of an elderly patient who persisted with her walking aid.

Summary

The cases presented suggest that aseptic necrosis of the humeral head may result from the use of walking aids in the elderly. While the condition is uncommon, the symptoms are so low grade that the condition may be overlooked or passed off as capsulitis in some cases. If walking aids are discarded the condition may be self-limiting, but it may be the precursor of osteoarthrosis if the long term use of walking aids is necessary. The weight bearing shoulder is worthy of closer study.

ROENTGENOGRAPHICAL EXAMINATION OF THE TILTED ANGLE OF THE SCAPULA IN THREE DIMENSIONS IN THE RELAXED STANDING POSITION

TAKEHIKO TORISU, M.D. and SHINKICHI HIMENO, M.D.

The shoulder has an almost global range of motion. This wide range of mobility is provided by delicate coordination of the muscles and the adjacent joints.[3] Impairment of any part of this coordinated mechanism is directly reflected in the total performance of the arm and trunk mechanism.[9,10] Clear understanding and evaluation of normal anatomy and function in a relaxed standing position are extremely important towards better recognition of the pathological conditions of the shoulder.[6]

Anatomically the scapula is located obliquely behind the thoracic wall at specific angles. What is the tilted angle of the scapula in a relaxed standing position? The purpose of this paper is to present, by means of roentgenographical examination in the relaxed standing position, the degrees of tilted angles of the scapula in three dimensions.

MATERIALS AND METHODS

Fifty–six normal subjects were examined bilaterally by using the roentgenogram for the purpose of evaluating the degree of the tilted angle of the scapula in the standing position. They were asymptomatic volunteers with an age range of 12 to 80 years. The sex ratio was approximately 1:1. These subjects were divided into five age groups: < 19 years, 20–39 years, 40–59 years, 60–79 years, and > 80. The average degrees of the tilted angles of the scapula in three dimensions were analysed and compared in each group.

Method of Roentgenography

As illustrated in Figure 1, each subject was requested to stand relaxed in front of the film cassette with the back slightly touching the cassette in an anteroposterior projection. The focus-film distance was 150 centimeters. The central ray was directed at the point of seven centimeters caudad to the upper margin of the sternum in median line. Each shoulder was viewed at thirty degrees oblique position, as shown in Figure 1. A 30° foam wedge was placed behind the back of the shoulder for ensuring the exact position. Central ray was directed towards the mid-point of the scapula.

Designation of the X and Y Coordinates

Five points were selected as landmarks in order to measure the X and Y coordinate in each roentgenogram. These landmarks were as follows (Fig. 2): The first landmark was fixed on the midpoint of the acromioclavicular joint, the second on the intersection of the medial border and the spine of the scapula, the third on the lower edge of the glenoid, the fourth on the middle point of the sternoclavicular joint, and the fifth on the tip of the lower angle of scapula. An origin O was fixed at the midpoint of the first thoracic vertebra. The direction of gravity was designated the Y-axis on the roentgenogram. The axis at right angle to the Y-axis on the frontal plane was designated the X-axis. the axis perpendicular to the frontal plane was designated the Z-axis.

The landmarks on the anteroposterior and oblique roentgenograms were then transfered to tracing paper; X and Y coordinates were measured in millimeters.

Measurement of the X and Y Coordinates

The distance between the origin O and each landmark on the anteroposterior roentgenogram was measured and recorded as X′, Y′. The dis-

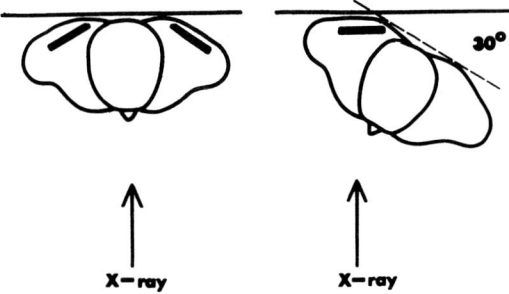

Figure 1 Bilateral roentgenograms were taken in the standard anteroposterior at 30° of oblique projection. A 30° foam wedge was placed at the back of the shoulder to ensure exact positioning.

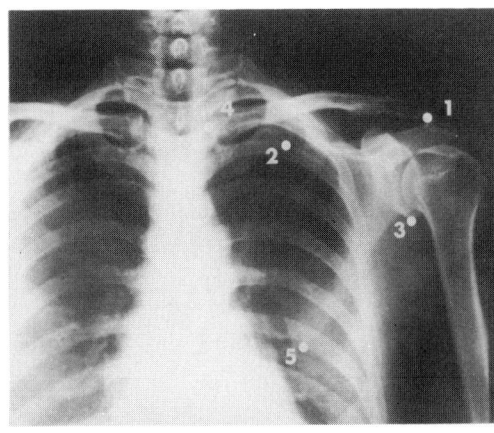

Figure 2 Five landmarks were selected in order to measure the X and Y coordinates in each roentgenogram. The X, Y and Z axes were designated.

tance between the origin O and each landmark on the oblique roentgenogram was measured and recorded as X″, Y″. By utilizing these measured values, the real X, Y and Z coordinates of the tilted scapula were calculated by using the equation: X = X′, Y = (Y′ + Y′)/2, Z = X″ − 3X′.

Since the focus-film distance was 150 centimeters, the x-ray beam is not exactly parallel and a slight adjustment is required in strict calculation. Extremely sophisticated knowledge of geometric principles is required in order to revise the data. However, this degree of correction is not clinically significant and the x-ray beams were considered to be parallel in our clinical study.

Determination of Tilted Angles

Connecting the following three landmarks, the middle of acromioclavicular joint, the intersection of the medial border and the spine of the scapula, and the tip of the inferior angle of the scapula, forms a plane. If this plane were considered to be the actual plane of the scapula were calculated and determined using the direction of the three vectors which were defined as follows.

$$U = (\cos\theta x, \cos\theta y, \cos\theta z)$$
$$a = (X1.5., Y1.5., Z1.5.)$$
$$b = (X2.5., Y2.5., Z2.5.)$$

where U
is a directional unit vector perpendicular to the plane of scapula composed of landmark 1, 2 and 5.
a, b are vectors which combine landmark 1 and 5, landmark 2 and 5, respectively.
θx is an angle between the directional unit vector U and X axes, as are also θy, θz.

$X_{i,j}$ is (X coordinate of landmark i) − (X coordinate of landmark j), as is the case of $Y_{i,j}$, $X_{i,j}$.

Three equations can be deduced directly.
A directional unit vector has a unit length.
$$U \cdot U = 1 \quad \ldots \ldots \ldots \ldots \quad 1$$
Any lines in the plane of scapula are perpendicular to the directional unit vector.
$$a \cdot U = 0 \quad \ldots \ldots \ldots \ldots \quad 2$$
$$b \cdot U = 0 \quad \ldots \ldots \ldots \ldots \quad 3$$

The angles between the directional unit vector (U) and X, Y and Z axes were determined by solving these equations.

RESULTS

Medial Tilt of the Scapula

The face of the scapula is directed toward the sagittal plane at a specific angle. This specific angle composed of the frontal plane and the face of the scapula was termed the medial tilt of the scapula. The average angle of medial tilt of the scapula in both sexes was 32.1° ± 7.0° on the right and 31.9° ± 8.0° on the left. There was considerable variance within individuals. The average angle of medial tilt of the scapula in both sides was 29.9° ± 7.7° in male and 34.0° ± 6.5° in females (Tables 1 and 2). The average angle in each age group in both sexes was as follows: Group 1 35.1° ± 6.1°, Group 2 32.5° ± 6.9°, Group 3 31.9° ± 6.7°, Group 4 31.3° ± 8.0° and

TABLE 1 The Average Tilted Angle of the Male Scapula (in degrees)

Group	Number	Medial Mean	Tilt S.D.	Downward Mean	Tilt S.D.	Upward Mean	Rotation S.D.
1	4	33.2	(±7.9)	2.9	(±6.4)	6.2	(±3.5)
2	22	31.3	(±6.3)	9.0	(±9.7)	9.1	(±5.9)
3	22	30.1	(±7.0)	14.3	(±12.0)	10.8	(±7.0)
4	8	27.0	(±8.6)	16.3	(±10.1)	10.9	(±6.1)
5	2	18.2	(±18.6)	48.0	(±3.9)	17.6	(±0.2)
Total	58	29.9	(±7.7)	12.9	(±12.7)	10.1	(±6.3)

Group 5 18.2° ± 18.6° (Tab. 3). The average angle in Group 1 was larger than those in Group 2, 3 or 4 (P 0.005). The average angle in Groups 2, 3 and 4 was larger than that in Group 5 (P 0.005). These results mean that the average angle of medial tilt of the scapula tends to decrease with advancing age.

Downward Tilt of the Scapula

The face of the scapula is directed downward to the horizontal plane at a specific angle. This specific angle composed of the frontal plane and the face of the scapula was termed the downward tilt of the scapula. The average angle of downward tilt of the scapula in both sexes was 11.5° ± 12.5° in the right and 12.3° ± 11.1° in the left. There was considerable variance within individuals and no statistical significance was found. The average angle of the downward tilt in both sides was 12.9° ± 12.7° in males and 10.8° ± 10.7° in females (Tables 1 and 2). Excluding Group 5, which included only male subjects, there was no statistical significance between the sexes. The average angle in each age group was as follows: Group 1 1.7° ± 9.1°, Group 2 8.6° ± 10.2°, Group 3 13.8° ± 9.5°, Group 4 15.2° ± 11.2° and Group 5 48.0° ± 3.9° (Tab. 3). These results mean that the average angle of the downward tilt of the scapula tends to increase with age with statistically positive correlation ($r = 0.34$).

Correlation Between the Medial and the Downward Tilt

The correlation between the medial and the downward tilt of the scapula was computed. Negative correlation was identified ($r = 0.42$). With the increase of the angle of downward tilt of the scapula, the angle of the medial tilt of the scapula has a tendency to decrease.

Rotation of the Scapula

The rotation of the scapula occurs on an axis perpendicular to the face of the scapula. The specific angle between the Y-axis and the line connecting the second landmark and the fifth landmark was measured (Tab. 3). The average of this specific angle in each age group of both sexes was as follows: Group 1 5.9° ± 3.1°, Group 2 9.7° ± 6.2°, Group 3 10.5° ± 6.4°, Group 4 11.5° ± 5.7° and Group 5 17.6° ± 0.2°. The results revealed that the scapula shows upward rotation with advancing age.

TABLE 2 The Average Tilted Angle of the Female Scapula (in degrees)

Group	Number	Medial Mean	Tilt S.D.	Downward Mean	Tilt S.D.	Upward Mean	Rotation S.D.
1	6	36.4	(±5.0)	0.9	(±11.1)	5.7	(±3.1)
2	16	34.2	(±7.5)	8.1	(±11.2)	10.5	(±6.7)
3	14	34.7	(±5.3)	13.0	(±3.0)	10.0	(±5.5)
4	18	33.2	(±7.1)	14.7	(±11.9)	12.1	(±5.7)
5	—	—	—	—	—	—	—
Total	54	34.0	(±6.5)	10.8	(±10.7)	10.4	(±5.9)

TABLE 3 The Average Tilted Angle of the Scapula in Both Sexes (in degrees)

Group	Number	Medial Mean	Tilt S.D.	Downward Mean	Tilt S.D.	Upward Mean	Rotation S.D.
1	10	35.1	(±6.1)	1.7	(±9.1)	5.9	(±3.1)
2	38	32.5	(±6.9)	8.6	(±10.2)	9.7	(±6.2)
3	36	31.9	(±6.7)	13.8	(±9.5)	10.5	(±6.4)
4	26	31.3	(±8.0)	15.2	(±11.2)	11.7	(±5.7)
5	2	18.2	(±18.6)	48.0		17.6	(±0.2)
Total	112	32.0	(±7.4)	11.9	(±11.8)	10.2	(±6.1)

DISCUSSION

The morphological changes of the scapula were brought about by alterations in posture, from the pronograde to the orthograde, and the highly specialized functional requirements of a prehensile limb during the evolution of the human being.[4,5] Obvious morphological modification occurred simultaneously in the thorax. The human thoracic cage shows anteroposterior flattening more than the pronograde does.[1] The scapula was considered to be transposed more dorsally and the glenoid came to face more laterally during these morphological modifications.

The scapula is a large, flattened, triangular bone located on the posterolateral aspect of the thorax overlapping parts of the second to the seventh ribs. The scapula forms with the frontal plane at a specific angle in three dimensions. What is the tilted angle of the scapula at a relaxed standing position? According to Kapandi[7] and Steindler,[11] the scapula is formed by the frontal plane at an angle of 30°. Von Lanz[8] reported that to be an angle of 40°. These authors reported neither the method of evaluation used nor the variation in sexes and age.

As the scapula is located on the posterolateral aspect of the thorax, the face of the scapula is directed toward the sagittal plane at a specific angle. This angle which was composed of the frontal plane and the face of the scapula was termed the medial tilt of the scapula. The average angle of medial tilt of the scapula was determined to be 32.1° ± 7.0° on the right and 31.9° ± 8.0° on the left. The medial tilt of the scapula tends to decrease with age, that is, the scapula moves dorsally with age. Furthermore, the face of the scapula is directed downward to the horizontal plane at a specific angle in addition to the medial tilt. This angle composed of the frontal plane and the face of the scapula was identified as the downward tilt of the scapula. The average angle of downward tilt was demonstrated to be approximately 10°. The downward tilt of the scapula was shown to increase with age.

Calliet[2] reported that aging impaired the range of shoulder motion because of the altered position of the scapula due to increased dorsal spinal kyphosis. His illustration only presented the increased downward tilt of the scapula. He mentioned that this increased downward tilt of the scapula was regarded to be a cause of impingement of the humerus against the coracoacromial arch during abduction of the arm. Our study supported his finding. Further, our study demonstrated that restricted rotation of the scapula was one of the major causes of restricted abduction of the scapula in the aged.

REFERENCES

1. Bateman JE. The shoulder and neck. Philadelphia: WB Saunders, 1972.
2. Cailliet P. Shoulder pain. Philadelphia: FA, Davis, 1966.
3. Codman EA. The shoulder. Boston: Thomas Toss, 1934.
4. Hojo T. Secular changes in the form of the Japanese scapula compared with other races. Kumamoto Igakukai Zoshi 1970; 44:937.
5. Inman VT et al. Observations on function of shoulder joint. J Bone Joint Surg 1944; 26:1.
6. Johnston TB. The movements of the shoulder-joint—A plea for the use of the plane of the scapula as the plane of the reference for movements occurring at the humero-scapular joint. Br J Surg 1937; 23:252.
7. Kapandji IA The physiology of the joints. Vol. 1. New York: Churchill Livingstone, 1970:9.
8. Von Lanz T, Wachsmuth W. Prektische Anatomie. Berlin: Springer-Verlag, 1935.
9. Saha AK. Theory of Shoulder Mechanism: Descriptive and applied. Springfield Illinois: Charles C Thomas, 1961:14.
10. Sasaki N, Torisu T, Nakayama A, and Tagawa Y. Shoulder movements during abduction and adduction of quadriplegic patients. J Jpn Orthop Ass 1980; 54:431.
11. Steindler A. Kinesiology of human body under normal and pathological conditions. Springfield Illinois: Charles C. Thomas 1955:457.

CLASSIFICATION AND ASPECTS OF TREATMENT OF FRACTURES OF THE PROXIMAL HUMERUS

R. P. JAKOB, M.D., T. KRISTIANSEN, M.D., K. MAYO, M.D., R. GANZ, M.D., and M. E. MÜLLER, M.D.

Fracture classifications are formulated to facilitate the understanding and management of fractures in a specific anatomic region. The utility of these classifications should be continuously reviewed. To be meaningful, each classification system should denote the morphology of the fracture, describe the biological and mechanical short-term behavior, provide therapeutic guidelines, and discuss expected long-term clinical outcomes.

Several important factors should be considered when classifying fractures of the proximal humerus. The paramount consideration is the vascular supply of the articular segment, which is determined by the number of fragments and the degree of displacement by fracture force and muscular pull. The pivotal role of vascularity derives from the infrequent but devastating complication of osteonecrosis. A related concern is the level of the fracture, with the capsular insertion at the anatomic neck being the important landmark. The stability of the fracture is determined by the related considerations of impaction, angulation, and displacement. Since fracture dislocations are common, this factor must be included if the system is to be representative. Thus biological concerns should be ideally integrated with morphology in a classification which then provides prognostic and therapeutic guidelines.

Historically, Kocher[10] and Böhler[3,4] introduced classifications based on anatomic location of the fracture (Fig. 1). These have been criticized to be of little assistance in depicting displaced fractures where more than one level is often involved. Furthermore, a classification based merely upon the level of the fracture permits a nondisplaced lesion to be grouped with one of marked displacement. Fracture classifications by Watson Jones,[17] Dehne,[6] and Knight and Mayne[9] offered varied emphases on anatomic and mechanistic considerations, yet none of these added significantly to understanding of the natural history of these injuries or their clinical management.

In 1934, Codman[5] was the first to formalize the recognition that fractures of the proximal humerus take place in 1 or more of 4 essentially discreet anatomic segments (Fig. 2). These are the articular component delineated by the anatomic neck, the greater tuberosity, the lesser tuberosity, and the shaft. This 4-part partitioning has provided the foundation for all subsequent fracture classifications. A significant advance was provided in 1965 by de Anquin[1] in his discussion of complex fractures of the proximal humerus which emphasizes vascular considerations and underscores the importance of 3-part and 4-part fractures for the first time.

In 1970, Neer[12] published his now classic study of proximal humerus fractures which included a classification also based on the 4-segment scheme (Fig. 3). He discussed in detail the fracture pattern with particular regard to soft-tissue determinants such as rotator cuff and capsular insertions. He reemphasized vascular considerations. These, combined with functional concerns, provided the basis for defining segment displacement as occurring with greater than 45 degrees of angulation or more than 10 mm of separation between segments. His classification system consisted of 6 groups encompassing the primary 2-part fractures and separate categories for minimal displacement fractures and fracture dislocations. Subgroups were included for the 3- and 4-part fractures and articular surface impression fractures. He outlined fully the optimal radiographic evaluation of these injuries and, based on the literature and his own series of patients, provided detailed prognostic and therapeutic guidelines. This was the first truly comprehensive work in this area, integrating fracture biomechanics and biology with diagnosis and therapeutics.

Special Considerations / **331**

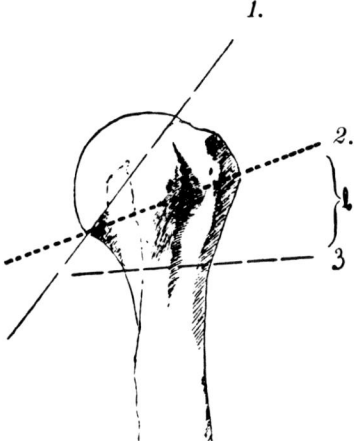

a) **Fracturae supratuberculares.**
1. Fractura colli anatomici.
   b) **Fracturae infratuberculares.**
2. Fractura pertubercularis.
   (Fractura epiphysaria*)
3. Fractura subtubercularis.
   Fractura colli chirurgici.

Figure 1 Classification of proximal humerus fractures according to anatomic level by Kocher, 1896. (By permission, G. Sallmann Verlag, Basel)

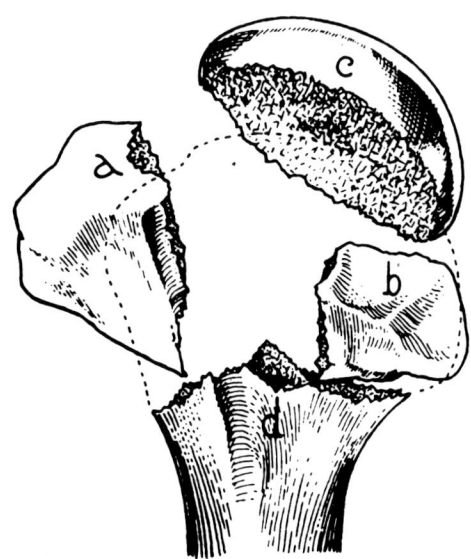

Figure 2 Classification dividing the proximal humerus into 4 parts by Codman, 1934. (By permission, G. Miller & Co. Medical Publishers, New York)

Nevertheless, there are a few deficiencies in the Neer classification system that emerge with routine use. First, we have observed a number of valgus impaction 4-part fractures which appear to have a natural history different from more displaced forms. The therapeutic implication here is that there is a subgroup of 4-part fractures where endoprosthetic replacement may not be necessary because of continued articular segment viability or acceptable function despite avascular necrosis. This group is not discussed by Neer.

Next, the general organization of the classification tends to underemphasize the severity of the displaced anatomic neck fracture. Placement between the relatively benign undisplaced fractures and 2-part surgical neck fractures belies the disastrous complication of osteonecrosis which is virtually universal in this fortunately infrequent fracture.

Thirdly, the Neer classification does not provide adequate subgrouping for detailed analysis and documentation. This is important not only for initial evaluation and treatment recommendations but also for any systematic long-term follow-up studies.

Lastly, the foundation for the Neer displacement criteria has not been truly established either clinically or experimentally. These criteria address two concerns. The first is allowable deformity as dictated by long-term functional considerations; the second and more important aspect is vascular supply to the fracture segments with its implications for fracture healing and osteonecrosis. As standards for allowable deformity, the Neer criteria would appear reasonable, though not well documented. However, we have no information that ensures that less than 10 mm separation or 45 degrees angulation assures vascular continuity between fragments.

THE AO CLASSIFICATION

It is the purpose of this paper to outline an expanded classification of proximal humerus fractures, based on Neer's scheme but taking into account most of the above considerations. Unfortunately, we can provide no answers for the dilemma of displacement criteria. These must come from more detailed clinical evaluations and fracture biology investigations.

The clinical basis for this classification was provided by a radiographic analysis of 930 surgically treated fractures of the proximal humerus on file at the AO documentation center. 200 cases were excluded because of poor radiograph quality, incomplete records, or open epiphyses, leaving a final data base of 730 fractures. The standard AO

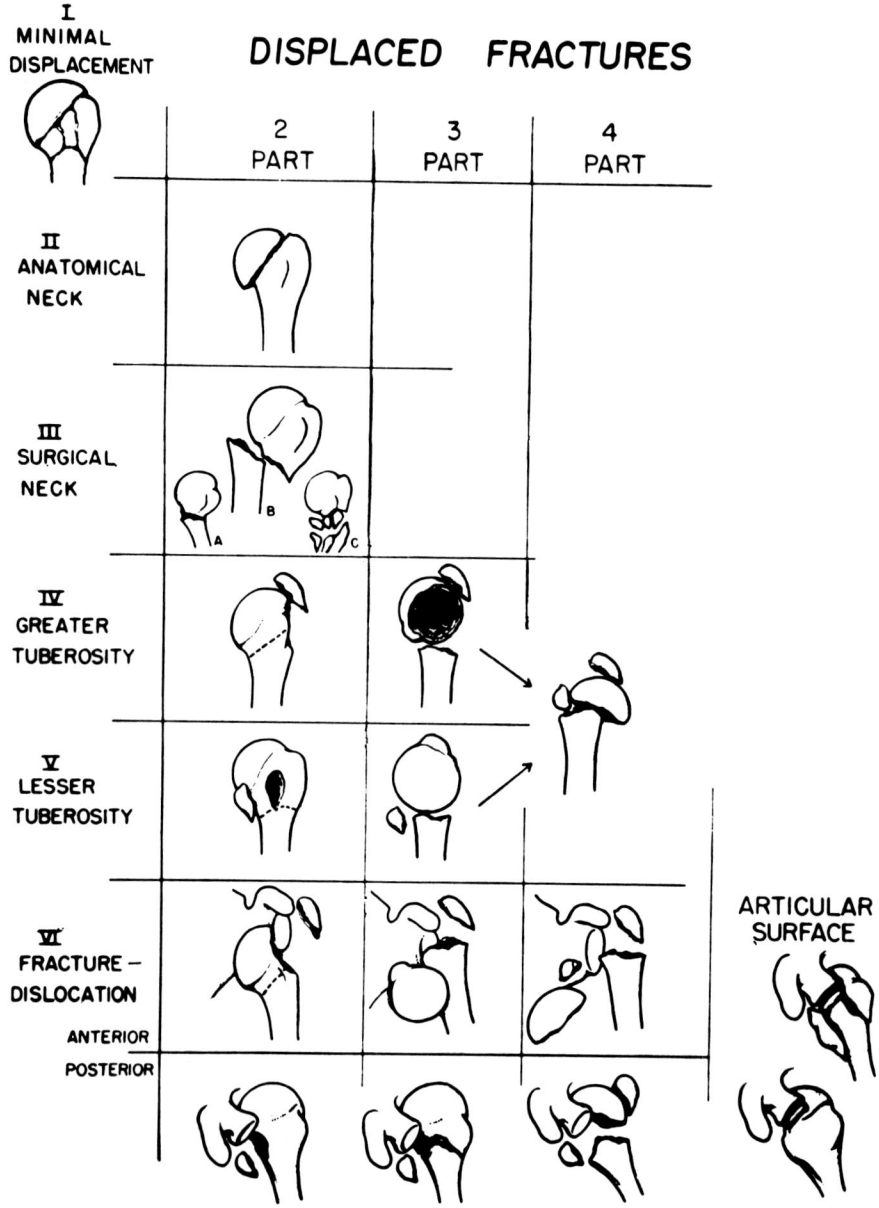

Figure 3 2-, 3-, 4-part classification by Neer, 1970. (By permission, J Bone Joint Surg, Boston)

alpha numerical system has been adopted to this application following the interrelated themes of fracture anatomy and vascular status of the articular segment. The classification recognizes both displaced (Neer criteria) and undisplaced fractures and provides adequate specificity for documentation as part of the AO documentation system for all fractures. In addition, it provides a framework for more detailed therapeutic and prognostic guidelines.

As mentioned, the central focus of this system is the vascular status of the articular segment. The status of the small vessels derived from the posterior humeral circumflex artery and the ascending branch of the anterior humeral circumflex artery (arcuate artery) can presumably be determined on the basis of the fracture pattern (Fig. 4). Therefore, if either tuberosity and its cuff attachment remain in continuity with the articular segment, the vascular supply is probably sufficient.

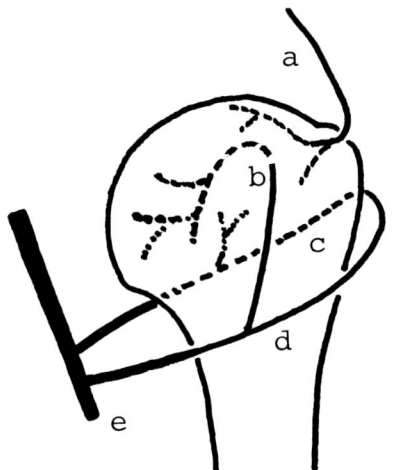

Figure 4 Vascular supply to the humeral head. (a) Vessels from the rotator cuff; (b) arcuate artery; (c) posterior humeral circumflex artery; (d) anterior humeral circumflex artery; (e) axillary artery.

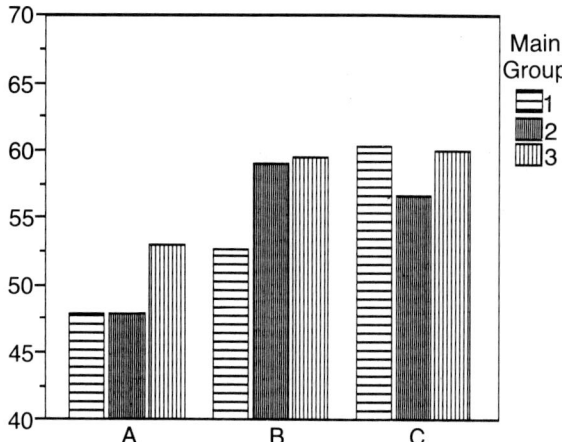

Figure 5 Age distribution of 730 fractures of the proximal humerus according to the main groups of A, B and C fractures. The bars represent the mean age for each fracture subgroup.

An outline of the major fracture groups is given below along with the salient features of each group. The alpha numerical system provides an index of injury severity. Type A fractures are less severe than type B and these are less severe than type C. In addition, each alphabetical group is subgrouped numerically with higher numbers generally reflecting greater severity.

Group A:
  Fracture without vascular isolation of the articular segment
  Avascular necrosis unlikely
  Extracapsular
  2 of the 4 primary segments involved
Group B:
  Fracture with partial vascular isolation of the articular segment
  Low risk of avascular necrosis
  Partially intracapsular
  3 of the 4 primary segments involved
Group C:
  Fracture with total vascular isolation of the articular segment
  High risk of avascular necrosis
  Intracapsular
  All 4 primary segments involved

In this system, as a general rule, subgroup 1 includes the undisplaced or minimally displaced fractures, subgroup 2 the displaced fractures, and subgroup 3 the displaced fractures with an additional complicating factor.

Since the clinical base for this classification includes only surgically treated fractures, the numbers in each category do not allow conclusions regarding the general distribution of these fractures by type. The epidemiology of humeral fractures has been published elsewhere (Horak,[8] Rose[14]).

There were 338 fractures in group A (47%), 115 fractures in group B (16%), and 277 in group C (37%). In the following section, the number of each fracture subgroup is shown as well as the percentage of the total series. Since fractures of the A1-type are usually treated nonsurgically, they appear in very small numbers in our statistics.

The age distribution in the main groups shows that most fractures of the A type occur near age 50, whereas the mean age for B and C type fractures is between 55 and 60 years of age (Fig. 5). With the discussion of each subgroup below please refer to the corresponding diagrams (Fig. 6).

Group A

A1 (Undisplaced 2- and 3-part fractures)
By virtue of intact soft-tissue attachments, these fractures are always stable and there is no risk of vascular embarassment of the articular fragment. Therefore they have a good prognosis and should be treated by closed methods with early mobilization.

A = EXTRACAPSULAR OR TWO SEGMENTS INVOLVED

— A1 Undisplaced
— A2 Displaced
— A3 Displaced with additional complicating factor

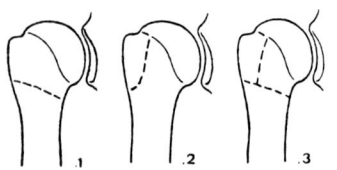
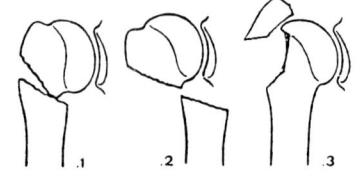
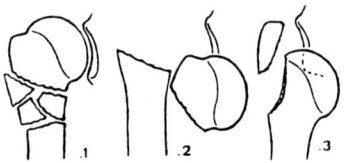

.1 Surgical neck
.2 Tuberosity
.3 Surgical neck and Tuberosity

.1 Surgical neck angulated
.2 Surgical neck completely displaced
.3 Tuberosity displaced

.1 Surgical neck and metaphyseal comminution
.2 Surgical neck with dislocation
.3 Tuberosity displaced with dislocation

B = PARTIALLY INTRACAPSULAR OR THREE SEGMENTS INVOLVED

— B1 One of three segments undisplaced
— B2 Three segments displaced
— B3 Three segments displaced with additional complicating factor

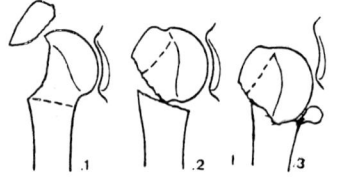
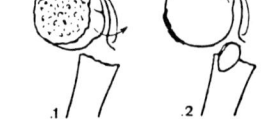
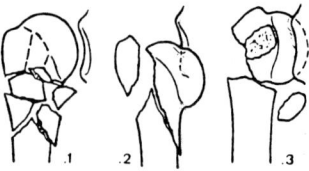

.1 Tuberosity displaced, surgical neck undisplaced
.2 Surgical neck displaced, tuberosity undisplaced
.3 Surgical neck varus impaction, lesser tuberosity displaced

.1 Surgical neck and greater tuberosity displaced
.2 Surgical neck and lesser tuberosity displaced

.1 Metaphyseal comminution involving greater or lesser tuberosity
.2 Surgical neck and greater tuberosity displaced w. dislocation
.3 Surgical neck and lesser tuberosity displaced w. dislocation

C = INTRACAPSULAR OR FOUR SEGMENTS INVOLVED

— C1 A. neck
— C2 Four segments impacted or displaced
— C3 Four segments displaced with additional complicating factor

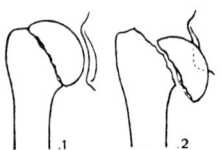
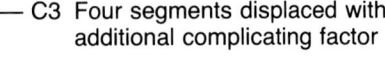
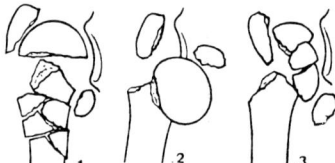

.1 Anatomical neck undisplaced or displaced
.2 Anatomical neck dislocated

.1 Moderate valgus impaction, greater tuberosity displaced
.2 Severe valgus impaction, tuberosity displaced
.3 Anatomical neck and tuberosities displaced

.1 Anatomical neck and tuberosities displaced, metaphyseal comminution
.2 Anatomical neck and tuberosities displaced, dislocation
.3 Anatomical neck and tuberosities displaced, comm. articulation

Figure 6 Proposed AO-classification for fractures of the proximal humerus.

A2 (Displaced 2-part fractures)
A2.1 Angulated surgical neck fractures:
n = 84/730 (11%)

The shaft here engages the head fragment but the fracture is not truly impacted which differentiates this group from B1.3. In our series of 84 cases, angulation at the fracture was primarily apex anterior in 40 and a combination of apex anterior and apex lateral in 35. These fractures often require manipulative closed reduction which is facilitated by the periosteum usually being intact posteriorly and medially. The maneuver of manipulation consists of traction in 90 degrees abduction combined with pressure on the proximal humeral shaft from anterior to posterior. This corrects the primary apex anterior deformity; in more unstable cases percutaneous pin fixation is warranted.

A2.2 Surgical neck fracture with complete displacement: n = 94/730 (12%)

This is the historical "abduction fracture" (Watson-Jones).[17] These are often high energy injuries; associated neurovascular damage is not uncommon. In this group we have included patterns with both medial and lateral shaft displacement, with the latter associated with the more marked soft–tissue disruption.

Many methods have been advocated for internal fixation of unstable fracture at the surgical neck. When plate fixation is selected, one has to be aware that the holding power of the screws in the proximal fragment may be poor in the elderly patient. Since 1978, we have used percutaneous pinning for most of these cases, following the technique outlined by Böhler[3] in 1964 for the epiphyseal fracture separation in the child.

Technique

Under biplane image intensifier control (anterior-posterior and axial views with the arm in 70–90 degrees of abduction), the humeral shaft should be manipulated into a position of slight lateral displacement with progressive traction. Anterior pressure on the proximal shaft allows correction of residual apex anterior angulation after initial reduction. Four 2.5 mm terminally threaded pins are then inserted through the distal fragment cortex from the level of the deltoid insertion into the humeral head. Two pins are directed from the lateral aspect and one from the frontal aspect of the shaft (Fig. 7). One must avoid entrance below the insertion of the deltoid muscle because of danger of radial nerve injury. Each pin position is

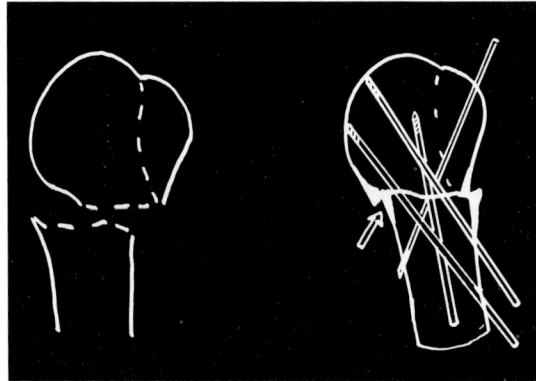

Figure 7 Technique of percutaneous pinning.

carefully evaluated using biplane fluoroscopy. A final pin may be inserted from the greater tuberosity, engaging the medial cortex of the distal fragment. The pins are cut off beneath the skin and the arm is secured in a soft Velpeau dressing. As the swelling subsides, further shortening of the pins may be needed one or two weeks after injury to avoid local irritation of the soft tissues. The proximal pin may be removed three weeks after the injury when careful pendulum exercises are begun. The distal pin should not be removed until six weeks after injury when early evidence of the fracture union usually appears on radiographs. Only at this time is more active physiotherapy allowed.

Since 1978, we have treated 40 displaced fractures of the proximal humerus by percutaneous pinning. Thirty-five have proceeded to uneventful healing with only minimal deformity. Although this technique may appear deceptively simple on radiographic case review, it is indeed very demanding and should only be used by an experienced surgical team as a useful alternative to open reduction and internal fixation.

A2.3 Displaced fracture of the greater or lesser tuberosity: n = 44/730 (6%)

We have followed the pattern of previous authors in subdividing this group. The following subgroups are differentiated:

Mild to moderate displacement of the greater tuberosity (22/44). Displacement is 5–10 mm, but the tuberosity remains in an acceptable position for nonoperative treatment. Because of the risk of secondary displacement, active physiotherapy should not be commenced before healing is well advanced. This must be assessed on an individual basis, but three to four weeks is normally the minimum safe interval.

Marked superior displacement of the greater tuberosity (11/44). This is due to unopposed pull of the supraspinatus tendon; the fragment may be retracted into the subacromial bursa. Operative reattachment is required. A limited deltoid splitting approach is utilized. Interfragmentary screws provide the best combination of insertion ease and fixation stability, although cerclage wire and nonabsorbable osseous sutures are alternatives, especially when there is more than one fragment.

Comminution of greater tuberosity (3/44). Watson-Jones[17] attributes this to a direct blow injury. We found this comminution more commonly with A3.3-fractures (13/38). Immobilization on an abduction frame for six weeks is our preferred treatment modality in cases without significant displacement.

Inferior and posterior displacement of the greater tuberosity (6/44). This occurs because of unopposed pull of the teres minor and infraspinatus musculature as described by Olivier.[13] This displacement is made possible by a longitudinal tear in the rotator cuff between the supraspinatus and infraspinatus. It may appear deceptively benign on the anterior-posterior roentgenogram, but the axillary view shows the true degree of displacement. Marked displacement represents an indication for open reduction and internal fixation. Minimal exposure by a lateral deltoid splitting approach with or without acromial osteotomy followed by minimal internal fixation is recommended as discussed above.

Also included in this group are the displaced fractures of the lesser tuberosity (2/730). Because of the rarity of this lesion it is not possible to provide unequivocal treatment guidelines based on a wide clinical experience. Neer maintained that this fracture could be treated nonoperatively without sequelae. It is our feeling that with displacement of greater than 1–1.5 cm, open reduction and internal fixation is warranted for optimum functional result.

It should be remembered that displaced fractures of either tuberosity are accompanied by an obligatory tear in the rotator cuff. In most cases, this tear propagates through the rotator interval and reduction of the tuberosity fragment reapproximates the cuff and obviates the need for formal repair. However, with cases of marked displacement or in more complex fracture patterns as discussed below, full exploration of the rotator cuff lesion and appropriate repair are essential.

A3 Displaced 2-part fractures with additional complicating factors

A3.1 Surgical neck fracture plus comminution of the metaphyses: n = 47/730 (6%)

Frequently, a large metaphyseal fragment is displaced medially by pull of the pectoralis major. This injury can be treated by overhead olecranon pin or screw traction with careful monitoring of rotational alignment. Open reduction and plate fixation (Fig. 8) may be warranted in the polytrauma patient to facilitate nursing care and general medical management. It is a demanding procedure; in many cases the degree of comminution precludes anatomic reduction. In these cases, the plate spans the area of comminution, where great care is taken to preserve all possible remaining soft-tissue attachments. Primary bone grafting may be needed, especially when there is a significant medial cortical defect. Postoperative mobilization is dictated by the security of fixation.

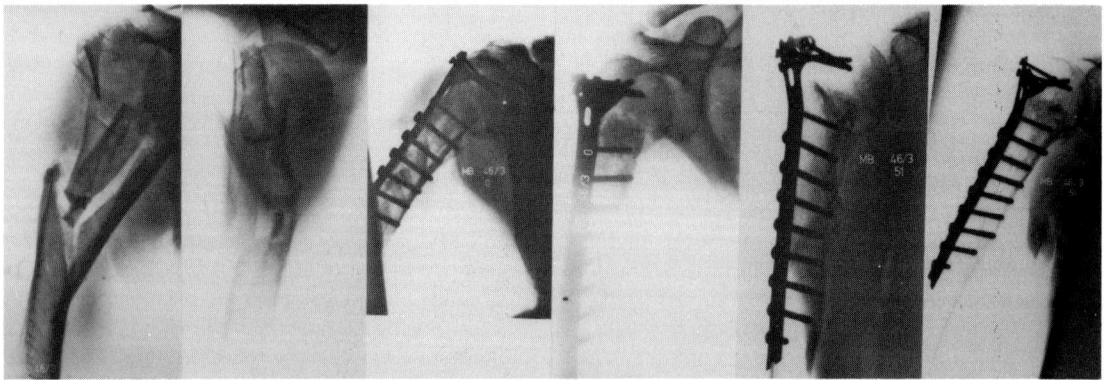

Figure 8 Fracture of the surgical neck with marked metaphyseal comminution (A 3.1), treated by internal fixation with a long cloverleaf plate. Follow-up 1 year postop.

A3.2 Displaced surgical neck fracture with anterior dislocation: n = 4/730 (0.6%)

This is a rare and interesting lesion. Watson-Jones described a method by which closed reduction is occasionally possible. However, since the head is usually trapped by the conjoint coraco-biceps tendon, we would strongly advocate open reduction of this fracture dislocation to avoid further soft-tissue damage. Plate or pin fixation are both acceptable.

A3.3 Displaced fracture of the greater or lesser tuberosity with associated gleno-humeral dislocation: n = 38/730 (5%)

Fifteen to 30 percent of anterior dislocations are associated with fractures of the greater tuberosity (Tondeur,[16] Watson-Jones).[17] Comminution is frequent (13/33); the lesser tuberosity remains intact. The mechanism of injury either produces a Hill-Sachs type impression fracture, or under concomitant pull of the external rotators, a propagation into an avulsion fracture of the greater tuberosity (Fig. 9). Due to the high energy nature of this injury, damage to the neurovascular structures may be observed. Its prognosis is generally good, although pericapsular ossification may complicate the course in a small percentage of cases. Treatment consists of manipulative reduction followed by surgical reattachment of the greater tuberosity if marked displacement persists (see A2.3).

In posterior dislocations, which are most often seen after electroconvulsive therapy, grand mal seizures, or electrical injuries, the lesser tuberosity is occasionally fractured (5/38). Associated peripheral nerve injuries are not uncommon. There is frequently an associated vertical fracture of the articular surface (Duparc).[7] De Morgues[11] has reported a series of 13 posterior fracture dislocations with recommendation for either closed or open emergent treatment and reattachment of the lesser tuberosity if necessitated by significant displacement. We concur with these recommendations. In addition, emphasis should be given to the problem associated with the articular impression fracture. Neer states that lesions involving more than 20 percent of the articular surface predispose to redislocation. These cases are best managed by subscapularis transplantation into the defect. With a defect greater than 50 percent, prosthetic replacement or fusion are indicated because of refractory instability despite subscapularis transfer.

Group B

B1 3-part fracture, 1-part undisplaced
B1.1 Undisplaced fracture of surgical neck plus displaced fracture of either tuberosity:
n = 6/730 (0.8%)

The greater tuberosity was involved in all 6 of our cases. Closed treatment is satisfactory unless marked displacement is present. The guidelines for treatment of the greater tuberosity component are as outlined for A2.3.

B1.2 Displaced surgical neck fracture plus nondisplaced fracture of either tuberosity:
n = 20/730 (3%)

This type may occur with the surgical neck component similar to subgroup A2.1 (angulated) or A2.2 (displaced). The treatment guidelines are essentially the same. As with all displaced 3-part fractures, the primary blood supply to the articular segment is through the uninvolved tuberosity. Operative intervention should be carried out in a manner that carefully protects this supply as well as all remaining capsular sources.

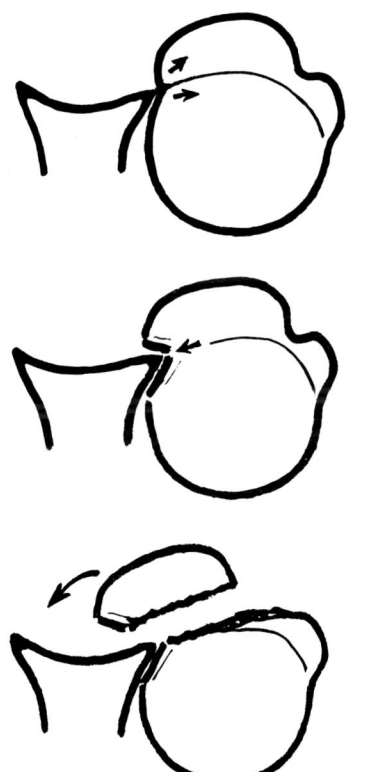

Figure 9 Mechanism of Hill-Sachs impression fracture and its extension into a displaced fracture of the greater tuberosity.

B1.3 Surgical neck fracture with varus impaction: n = 10/730 (1.5%)

In fact, this fracture pattern combines an extension (apex anterior) deformity with varying degrees of impaction. It corresponds to the "impacted adduction fracture" of Watson-Jones. The lesser tuberosity is crushed. Typically, there is some inferior subluxation of the humeral head. This may be due in part to a transient weakness of the deltoid and rotator cuff musculature subsequent to injury. However, true supraspinatus insufficiency may be manifested secondary to the varus positioning of the head and an effective shortening of the distance between origin and insertion of the muscle. Although, a part of the inferior subluxation may resolve with improved muscle tone during the first few weeks after injury, a certain component may persist and result in loss of function as well as a predisposition to post-traumatic arthrosis. Furthermore, a combination of relative supraspinatus insufficiency with the altered greater tuberosity profile may lead to subacromial impingement and hinder motion, particularly in forward elevation and abduction.

This fracture is stable and if articular congruity is satisfactory, closed treatment may be adequate. If marked inferior subluxation and incongruity are present, reduction of the fracture by an abduction maneuver is recommended. Since this disimpaction creates instability in the fracture, internal fixation is then necessary. Treatment options include percutaneous pinning followed by abduction splint immobilization or open reduction and internal fixation with pins and a tension band wire or with a plate acting as a tension band (Fig. 10).

B2 3-part displaced fractures with rotation
B2.1 Displaced fractures of the surgical neck and greater tuberosity: n = 10/730 (1.5%)

This fracture, discussed in detail by Neer, allows the articular segment to be internally rotated with the unopposed pull of the subscapularis. The articular segment faces posteriorly. Open reduction and internal fixation are indicated, once again taking care to preserve blood supply to the head through the remaining muscular attachment. Fixation should be minimal as previously outlined (Sturzenegger).[15] Rotator cuff repair is usually necessary. Failure to recognize and properly treat this fracture leads to malunion or nonunion in nearly all cases.

B2.2 Displaced fractures of the surgical neck and lesser tuberosity: n = 25/730 (3%)

This fracture represents the complement of B2.1. The lesser tuberosity is displaced by the pull of the subscapularis and the head is abducted and often externally rotated by the pull of the spinati and teres minor. The treatment guidelines are the same as for B2.1. Open reduction, rotator cuff repair, and minimal adequate internal fixation are necessary (Sturzenegger).[15]

B3 3-part displaced fractures with additional complicating factor
B3.1 Metadiaphyseal comminution involving either tuberosity: n = 10/730 (1.5%)

This fracture is similar to A3.1, but with an extension into one tuberosity. Despite this extension, the tuberosity remained functionally intact in our cases. The rotational problems associated with B2 fractures therefore do not enter into discussion here. The treatment concerns are nearly identical to those outlined for A3.1, although there is some additional element of risk to surgical exposure with a potentially compromised blood supply to the articular segment.

B3.2 Displaced fractures of the surgical neck and greater tuberosity with dislocation:
n = 28/730 (4%)

This fracture was described by Duparc[7] and earlier by Autin[2] ("fracture verticale"). The head is dislocated anteriorly. The greater tuberosity may be minimally or markedly displaced. This pattern is differentiated from A3.3 not only by the displaced surgical neck component but also by significant incidence of posterior articular surface impression fractures. The primary remaining blood supply to the head goes through the muscular attachment of the lesser tuberosity. Open reduction and internal fixation through a deltopectoral approach are recommended with concommitant rotator cuff repair.

B3.3 Displaced fractures of the surgical neck and lesser tuberosity with dislocation:
n = 6/730 (0.8%)

This pattern consists of posterior glenohumeral dislocation with a displaced fractured lesser tuberosity and often an impression fracture of the anterior humeral articular surface. Once again, open reduction and internal fixation are mandatory. Concerns regarding management of the articular surface lesion have been previously outlined.

Group C

C1 Anatomical neck
C1.1 Displaced or undisplaced anatomic neck fractures: n = 2/730 (0.3%)

These fractures are quite rare and if undis-

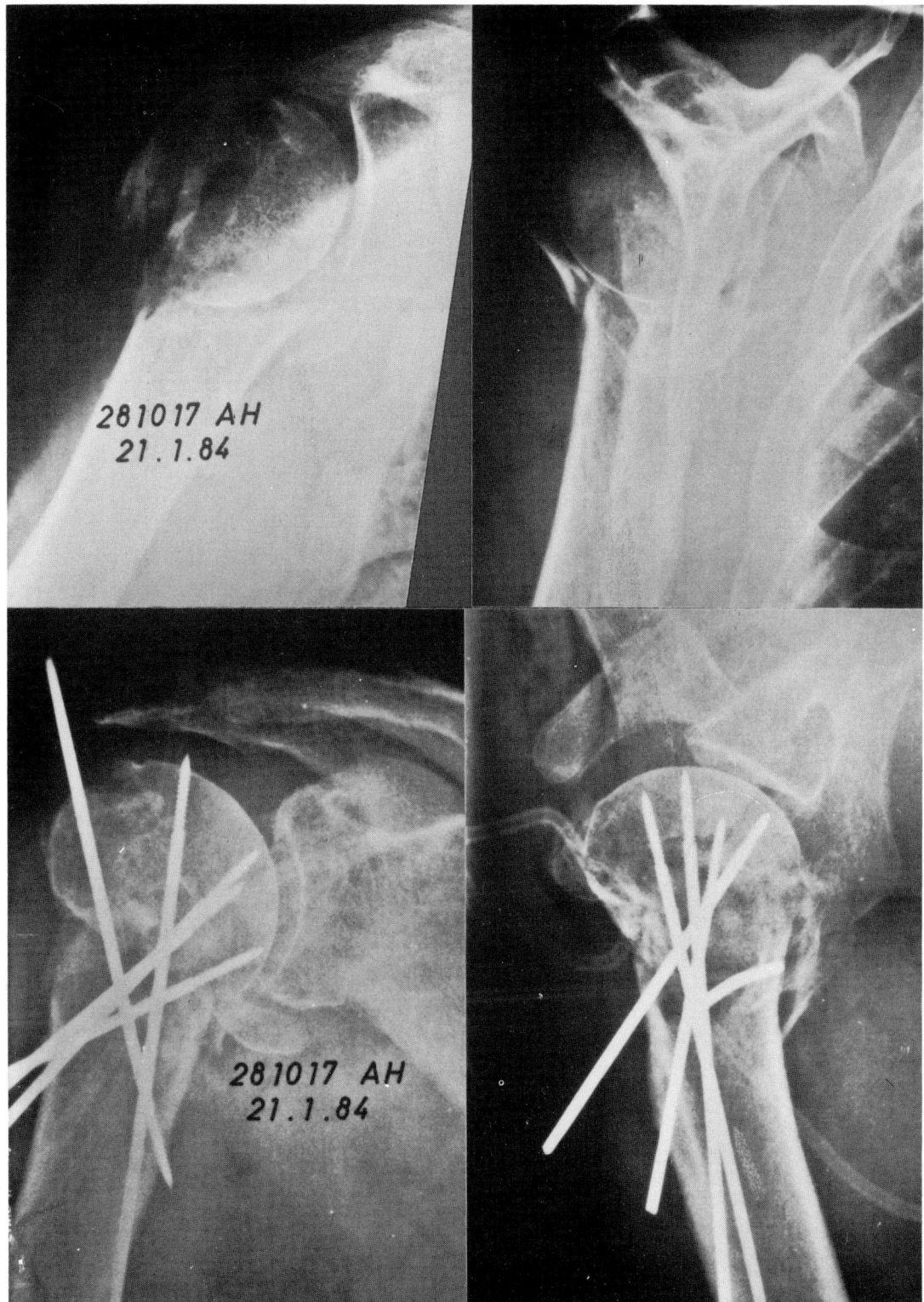

Figure 10 A variant of the true varus displacement is presented as an example where the head is impacted in the shaft. In this 67-year-old patient, open exposure through a deltopectoral incision only allowed the disimpaction and reduction of the fracture. The lesser tuberosity was avulsed; the greater tuberosity shows a fissure line. Percutaneous pinning and postoperative immobilization on a 45° abduction wedge.

placed frequently escape notice on routine roentgenograms. Malunion and avascular necrosis are the major complications of displaced fractures. Despite the fact that there is little to offer the patient with this fracture therapeutically, the diagnosis is crucial in terms of prognostic discussions.

C1.2 Displaced anatomic neck fractures with dislocation: n = 4/730 (0.6%)

Fortunately, this lesion is also quite rare. It is always attended by avascular necrosis. Thus, it is an indication for prosthetic replacement in the elderly. In the younger patient, open reduction and minimal internal fixation may be attempted with the hope that collapse secondary to avascular necrosis may be minimal and a prolonged period of adequate function obtained. A less attractive but definite alternative is early arthrodesis, especially in the young manual worker.

C2 4-part fractures
C2.1 Surgical neck fractures with mild to moderate valgus impaction and displaced greater tuberosity fracture: n = 36/730 (5%)

This fracture type is not included in Neer's classification. It has been mentioned by Duparc ("fracture céphalo-tubérositaire engrenée") and by de Anquin ("impacted fracture with inferior subluxation") and appears to be a relatively frequent pattern. The head is positioned in valgus and there is typically some superior widening of the glenohumeral joint. This group is distinguished from C2.2 by acceptable glenohumeral congruity. Since disimpaction carries with it the risk of further devascularization, we advocate leaving the articular segment in a less than perfect but acceptable impacted position and reattaching the greater tuberosity in a more distal position, to prevent subsequent impingement and restore the lever arm for abduction. Since portions of the vascular supply to the articular segment through intact posterior capsular attachments and the lesser tuberosity may be preserved, the prognosis is reasonably good.

C2.2 Surgical neck fractures with severe valgus impaction and displaced greater tuberosity: n = 63/730 (9%)

Here the impaction is more severe and the joint congruity unacceptable. This is a common fracture pattern. The articular surface, in addition to being displaced into valgus, is inferiorly subluxed secondary to a combination of rotator cuff insufficiency with the tuberosity fracture and also bone loss secondary to impaction between the anatomical and surgical neck levels. The overall appearance of the proximal humerus, therefore, takes the configuration of an ice cream cone. Although this fracture may be regarded as stable, conservative treatment leads to a poor result due to distortion of the articular anatomy and persistent inferior subluxation (Fig. 11). Despite this being a 4-part fracture, primary prosthetic replacement

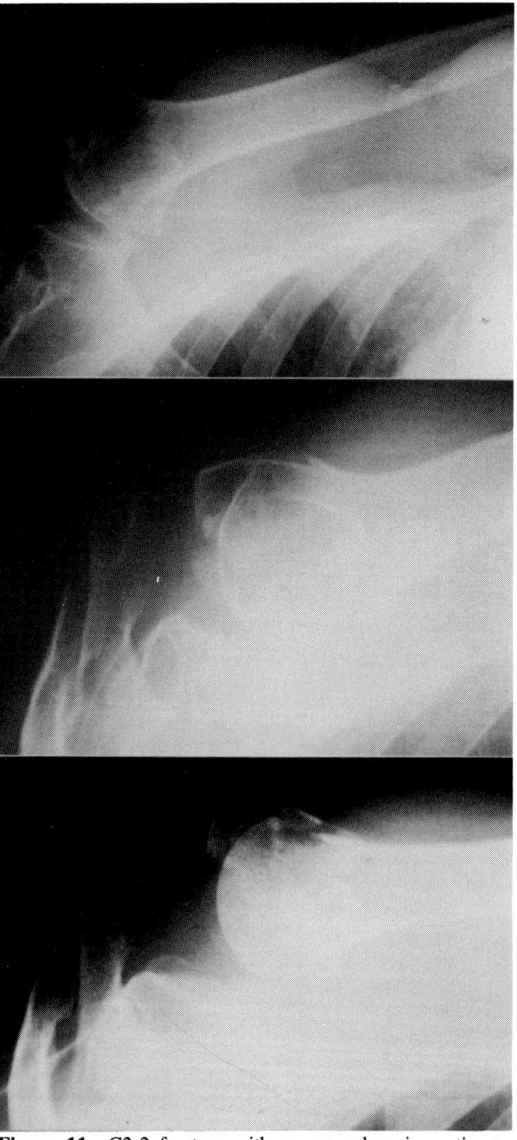

Figure 11 C2.2 fracture with severe valgus impaction and displaced tuberosities. The radiographic sequence is over 2 years showing persistent inferior subluxation and advanced arthrosis. This patient required subsequent prosthetic replacement because of intractable pain and loss of function.

probably represents overtreatment in many cases. As with the partial valgus impaction (C2.1), some vascular supply may remain intact through posterior capsular vessels and impacted lesser tuberosity. We therefore strongly advocate careful exposure through a deltopectoral or a deltoid splitting approach to elevate and reposition the head fragment using an impactor (Fig. 12). With gentle retraction of the greater tuberosity, one will suddenly feel and hear the articular fragment move back into position against the glenoid. The greater tuberosity is then reduced and secured to the metaphysis with one or two screws or percutaneous pins. With this fixation, insertion of a bone graft is usually unnecessary. With this management, we have observed an articular segment survival rate of approximately 50 percent in this very specific but frequent type of 4-part fracture (Fig. 13). Furthermore, even in the event of avascular necrosis, function often remains astonishingly good, perhaps due to restoration of the anatomy.

C2.3 Displaced fractures of the anatomic neck and both tuberosities: n = 78/730 (11%)

In this lesion, the articular segment is usually completely avascular. In patients over 60, prosthetic replacement is recommended. In young patients, an attempt at reconstruction may be warranted with approximation of the tuberosities and fixation of the articular segment to the oblique surface of the metaphysis. Minimal internal fixation is preferable. Truly stable fixation is generally not achievable; vigorous effort toward this goal may further devitalize bony fragments. Despite avascular necrosis with varying degrees of collapse, functional results in many cases have been gratifying, and endoprosthetic replacement has been at the very least forestalled.

C3 4-part fractures with additional complicating factor
C3.1 Displaced fractures of the anatomic neck and both tuberosities with metaphyseal comminution: n = 9/730 (1.5%)

This is a devastating lesion. The articular segment is avascular and the comminution may preclude prosthetic replacement. Dependency traction for 3 to 4 weeks followed by progressive motion may provide a surprisingly adequate functional result, particularly for the patient with limited functional demands. In the remaining patients, a delayed prosthetic replacement or arthrodesis are the only alternatives and both present numerous technical problems.

C3.2 Displaced fractures of the surgical neck and both tuberosities with dislocation: n = 67/730 (9%)

In this group, the articular segment is devascularized as well. Primary prosthetic replacement is probably best in the healthy elderly individual despite what may be a compromised functional result secondary to rotator cuff insufficiency. In the younger patient, we prefer an attempt at open reduction and internal fixation despite the expected avascular necrosis (see C2.3).

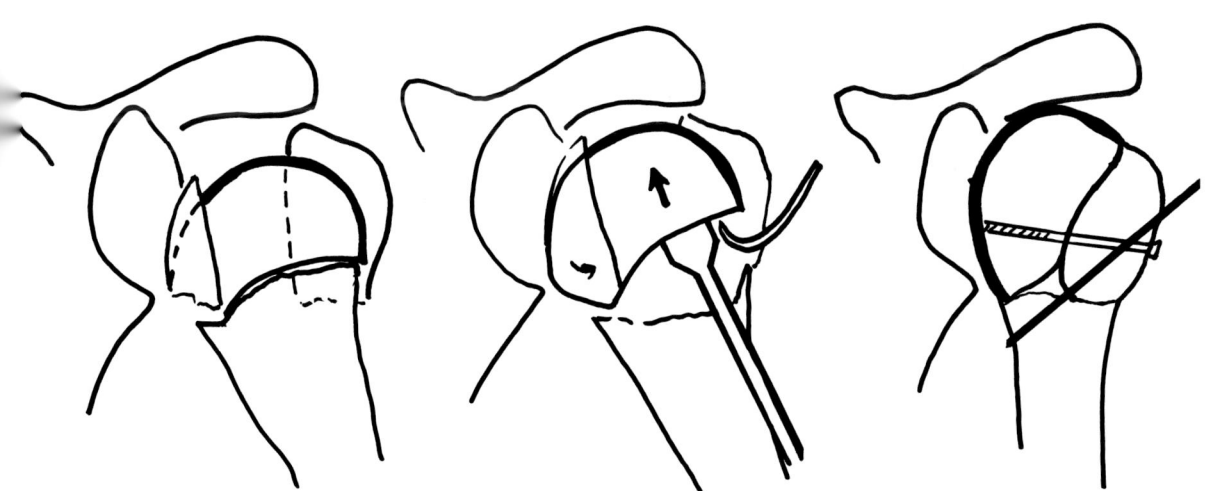

Figure 12   Scheme of advocated treatment for a C2.2 fracture.

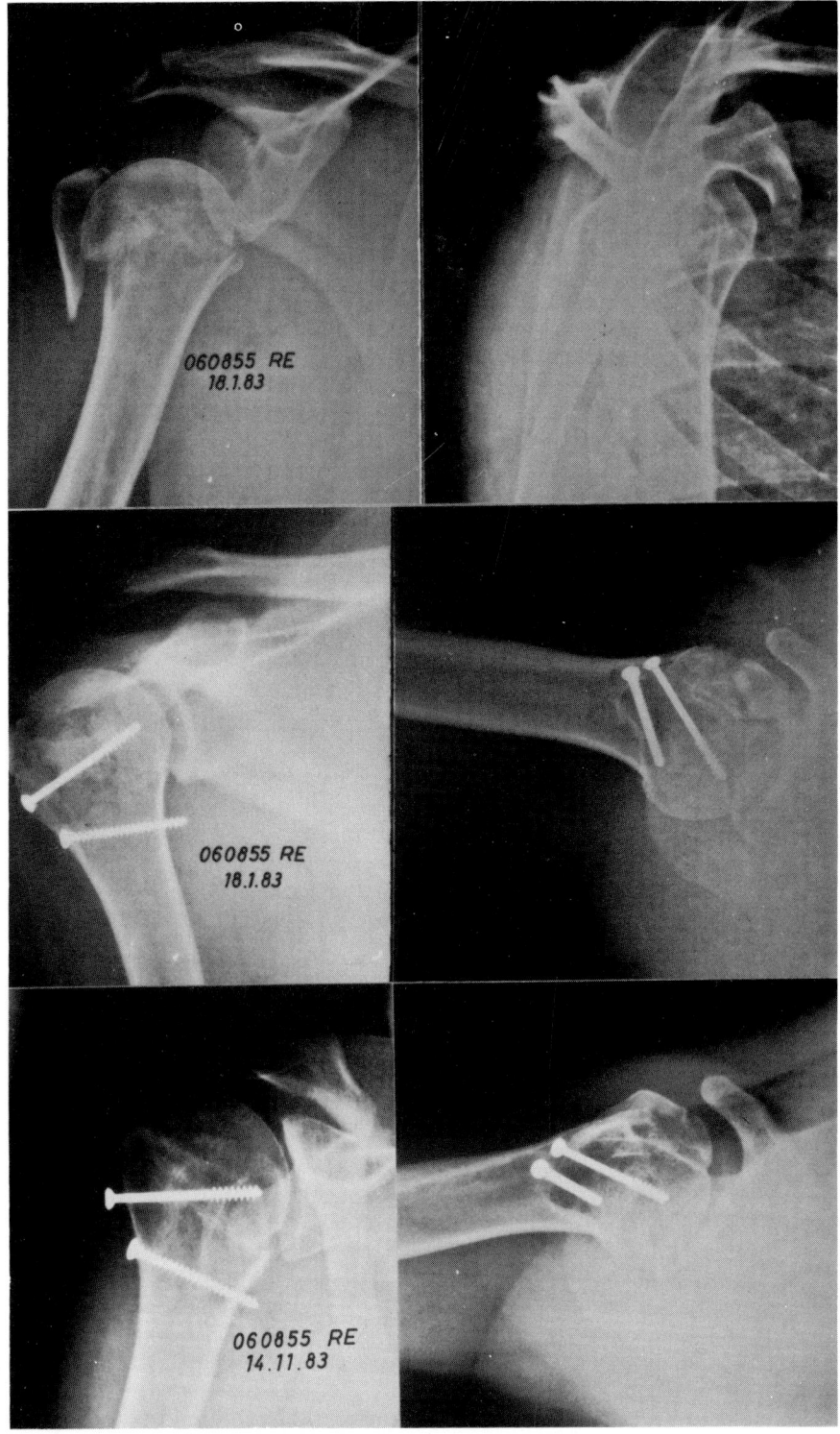

Figure 13 C2.2 fracture in 40-year-old male treated using the previously outlined technique (Fig. 12). Radiographs 10 months postop are the last follow-up.

C3.3 Displaced fractures of the anatomical neck and both tuberosities plus comminution of the articular segment: n = 18/730 (2.5%)

These fractures are probably caused by the central impaction mechanism described by Dehne[6] in which the head is driven directly against the glenoid fossa with one or the other or both surfaces injured. The comminution is frequently greater than can be appreciated on standard radiographs. This type of fracture occurs primarily in the older patient with considerable osteoporosis. When the general medical condition will allow, consideration can be given to prosthetic replacement, but a number of these patients with low level functional demands have done well with minimal treatment as outlined under C3.1.

DISCUSSION

This classification represents a modification and expansion of the classifications of Neer and others. In addition, it has been formulated in such a way as to allow easy integration into the overall AO-documentation system. The tiered structure of the classification follows a general progression in terms of increasing severity of the injury and prognosis. Emphasis is given to 4-part fractures, where an elderly subgroup may require treatment by prosthetic replacement. However, other types of 4-part injuries mandate a more differentiated therapeutic approach, especially in the patient under 60 years of age where there is a significant chance of preserving a functional joint through carefully planned open reduction and internal fixation.

In order to effectively use this classification, it is mandatory that adequate radiographs be obtained. These ideally include an anterior-posterior radiograph of the glenohumeral joint, a lateral view of the scapula, and an axillary view. These views allow the true relationship of the fragments to be appreciated. It is not our intention that this classification system be memorized. Once the system is understood, however, it should be relatively easy to communicate, stating only the main group to which a fracture belongs (A, B, C). Subsequent subgrouping can be carried out with the aid of printed diagrammatic classification sheets for standardized documentation purposes. This is the successful general scheme by which AO documentation has functioned now for more than 20 years.

The following steps are recommended when using this classification:

1) Obtain an adequate radiologic survey.
2) Describe: (a) the size and number of fragments; (b) major fragment impaction as well as displacement and angulation; and (c) degree of vascular isolation of the articular segment and its relation to the glenoid articular surface.
3) Classify the fracture using the detailed diagrams.
4) Select an appropriate form of treatment, taking into account the fracture type and the age and functional demands of the patient.
5) Document for later analysis and comparison.

REFERENCES

1. de Anquin CL, de Anquin A. Prosthetic replacement in the treatment of serious fractures of the proximal humerus. In: Shoulder Injury. Bayley I, Kessel L, eds. Berlin: Springer Verlag, 1965:206–217.
2. Autin A. Traitement des fractures de l'ESH. Thèse médicine, no 840. Paris, 1960.
3. Böhler J. Les fractures récentes de l'épaule. Acta Orthop Belg 1964; 30:235–242.
4. Böhler L. The Treatment of Fractures. 5th ed. New York: Grune and Stratton, 1956.
5. Codman EA. The Shoulder: Rupture of the Supraspinatous Tendon and Other Lesions in or about the Subacromial Bursa. Brooklyn: G. Miller Publishers, 1934.
6. Dehne Ernst. Fractures of the upper end of the humerus. A classification based on the etiology of the trauma. Surg Clin N Am 1945; 25:28–47.
7. Duparc J, Lagier A. Les luxations-fractures de l'extrémité supérieure de l'humérus. Rev Chir Orthop 1976; 62:91–110.
8. Horak J, Nilsson BE. Epidemiology of fractures of the upper end of the humerus. Clin Orthop 1975; 112:250.
9. Knight RA, Mayne JA. Comminuted fractures and fracture dislocations involving the articular surface of the humeral head. J Bone Joint Surg 1957; 39A:1343–1355.
10. Kocher T. Beiträge zur Kenntnis einiger praktisch wichtiger Fracturenformen. Basel: Carl Sallman Verlag, 1896.
11. de Morgues G, Fisher L, Schul JF. Les fractures-luxations postérieures de l'extrémité supérieure de l'humérus. Rev Chir Orthop 1974; 60:365–376.
12. Neer CS. Displaced proximal humerus fractures. J Bone Joint Surg 1970; 52A:1077–1103.
13. Olivier H, Dufour G, Duparc J. Les fractures du trochiter. Rev Chir Orthop 1976; 62:8.
14. Rose SH, Melton J, Morrey BF, Ilstrup DM, Riggs BL. Epidemiologic features of humerus fractures. Clin Orthop 1982; 168:24.
15. Sturzenegger M, Fornaro E, Jakob RP. Results of surgical treatment of multifragmented fractures of the humeral head. Arch Orthop Trauma Surg 1982; 100:249–259.
16. Tondeur G. Les fractures récentes de l'épaule. Acta Orthop Belg 1964; 30:1–144.
17. Watson-Jones R. Fractures and Joint Injuries. 4th ed. Baltimore: Williams and Wilkins, 1955; 2:473–476.

INDEX

Numbers in *italics* refer to accompanying illustrations; numbers followed by t refer to accompanying tables.

Abduction, shoulder, 18–21, *18–20*
  after arthroplasty, 221, 225, 226t, 231
  after surgery for deltoid muscle contracture, 259
  after thoracic scapulopexy, 256t
  in rotator cuff repairs, 196
Acromioclavicular joint,
  abnormalities in athletes, 140–141. *See also names of specific abnormalities.*
  degenerative changes of, 138
  distally-pointing osteophytes and supraspinatus tendon, 129–133, *130–132*
  treatment of acute complete dislocation, 67–78, *68–69,* 71t, *74–78*
ACS. *See* Adhesive capsulitis of the shoulder.
Acromion process,
  in impingement syndrome, 141
  relation to rotator cuff tendons, 134–139, *135–137*
Acromioplasty, anterior. *See* Anterior acromioplasty technique.
Acropole prosthesis, 200–201
Adhesive capsulitis of the shoulder, 154–156
  arthroscopic observations, 41, *41*
  in missed posterior dislocations, 118
Anterior acromioplasty technique, for rotator cuff tears, 162–164, *162–164,* 204–205, *204–205*
Anteroinferior vulnerable point of glenoid rim, 94–99, *95–98*
A.O. technique. *See* ASIF technique.
Arm elevation, and scapula movement, 12–16, *13–15*
Arthritis,
  arthrodesis of shoulder, A.O. (ASIF) technique, 207–210, *208–209*
  arthroplasty for, 229–233, *230–232*
    bipolar implant, 211–223, *213, 215–219, 221–223*
  Neer total shoulder replacement for, 224, 228, *226–228*
  pyogenic, 319–323, *320–322*
  rheumatoid, 243
  surgery for, 269–280, *270–280*
Arthrodesis, A.O. (ASIF) technique, 207–210, *208–209*
  for rheumatoid arthritis, 278
Arthroplasty,
  bipolar implant, 211–223, *213, 215–219, 221–223*
  for rheumatoid arthritis, 278–279, *279–280*
  total, and associated disease of the rotator cuff, 229–233, *230–232*
  unconstrained, 234–239, *235–238,* 240–245, *241–243*
Arthroscopy,
  in shoulder surgery, 41–50, *41–44, 47,* 48t
  of shoulder joint, 34–40, *35–40*
Arthrotomography,
  computed, in unstable shoulder, 306–309, *307–308*
  double contrast, in diagnosis of rotator cuff tears, 126–128, *127–128*
  in location of posterior dislocations, 118
  in shoulder subluxation studies, 26–27, 31, 33, *27–32*
Aseptic necrosis of humeral head, 324–325
ASIF (A.O.) technique, of shoulder arthrodesis, 207–209, *208–209*

Athletes,
  chronic shoulder pain, 79–83, *80–82*
  shoulder impingement syndrome, 140–142
Avascular necrosis, 58
  in shoulder replacement, 242, 297
Axial tomography, and shoulder subluxation studies, 26–27, 31, 33, *27–33*

Bankart lesion, 41–42
  arthroscopic identification of, 35, *36,* 39, *39*
  arthrotomographic identification of, 27, *27*
  computer tomographic identification of, 84, *85*
Bankart's procedure, 98, *98*
  in failed repair for shoulder instability, 114, *115*
  on recurrent anterior dislocations, 91–93, *91–92*
  on shoulder dislocation, 305
Biceps brachii,
  free graft, 174, *174*
  role of the tendon of the long head,
    in anterior subluxation, 104–105
    in impingement syndrome, 140–142
    in chronic shoulder pain, 315–316, *315–317*
  rupture, 165
Biceps tendinitis. *See* Tendinitis, biceps.
Bipolar implant shoulder arthroplasty, 211–223, *213, 215–219, 221–223*
Bone tumors of shoulder, limb salvage procedures, 310–312
Bosworth method of screw fixation, 73, *75*
Bristow-Latarjet procedure on recurrent anterior dislocations, 87–90, *88–89*
Bursae, subacromial, 121–125, *122–124*
Bursogram, 121–123, *123*

C-arm fluoroscopy, in study of glenohumeral subluxations, 22–25, *24*
Chronic shoulder pain,
  from rotator cuff tears, 126–128, *127–128*
  in athletes, 78–83, *80–82*
  surgical pathology, 313–318, *314–317*
Clicking shoulder. *See* Bankart lesion.
Closed reduction procedure,
  comparison with open reduction, 56, 57t
  in acromioclavicular dislocations, 73, *76*
  in posterior shoulder dislocations, 119
Computerized tomography,
  axial, and shoulder subluxation studies, 26–27, *27–33,* 31,33
  on recurrent shoulder dislocation, 84–86, *85*
  of unstable shoulder, 306–309, *307–308*
Coracoacromial ligament, as cause of impingement syndrome, 141
Coracohumeral ligament, stabilizing function, *316*
Coracoid process, as cause of impingement syndrome, 142
Corticosteroid injections, causing pyogenic arthritis of glenohumeral joint, 319–323, *320–322*
Crutchwalker's shoulder, 324–325

345

CT scan. *See* Computerized tomography.
CYBEX II, isokinetic dynamometer in shoulder studies, 1–5, *2–4*

Dead arm syndrome,
  in shoulder dislocations, 306, 309
  in glenohumeral subluxations, 22
  in recurrent subluxations, 26
Deltoid muscle contracture, surgery for, 259–268, *260–268*
Dewar and Barrington dynamic technique, in treatment of complete acromioclavicular dislocations, 73, *75*
Dislocations,
  early and late, as complications of unrestrained shoulder replacement, 237
  of acromioclavicular joint, treatment, 67–78, *68–69*, 68–69t, 71t, *74–78*
  posterior, missed, 117–120, *119*
  recurrent,
    bone lesions, 303–305
    computer tomography, 84–86, *85*
  recurrent anterior,
    arthroscopic observations, 35, *35*
    operative treatment,
      Bristow-Latarjet procedure, 87–90, *88–89*
      Bankart's procedure, 91–93, *91–92*
      Oudard-Iwahara procedure, 106–110, *107–109*
Dye technique,
  use in studies of surface contact between cuff tendons and acromion process, 134–139, *135–137*
  use in treatment of partial thickness tears of rotator cuff, 145, *147*
Dynamometry, isokinetic, of the shoulder, 1–5, *2–4*

Electromyography, in shoulder studies, 6, 8, *7–11*
Exercise. *See* Physiotherapy.

Facioscapulohumeral dystrophy, thoracoscapular fusion, 247–251, *248–250*, 255–258, *256–258*
Failed repair for shoulder instability, 111–116, *112–116*
Fluoroscopy, C-arm, in study of glenohumeral subluxations, 22–25, *24*
Fractures,
  classification, 54
  glenoid, arthroscopic observations, 48
  glenoid fossa, 63–66, *64–65*
  proximal humeral,
    prognostic factors, 51–59, *52–57*
    treatment by Neer hemiarthroplasty, 60–62, *61*, 61–62t
Freeze-dried rotator cuff graft technique, 175–176, *175–176*
Frozen shoulder. *See* Adhesive capsulitis of the shoulder.

Gallium scintigraphy, in diagnosis of synovitis, 277, *278*
Glenohumeral joint,
  pyogenic arthritis from corticosteroids, 319–323, *320–322*
  subluxations,
    C-arm fluoroscopic evaluation, 22–25, *24*
    failed repair analysis, 111–116, *112–115*
Glenoid,
  arthroscopic observations, 39, *39–40*
  arthrotomographic observations, 27, *84*
  CT scanning observations, 84, *85*, 86

effect of bone lesions, 304
fractures,
  arthroscopic observations, 48
  types, 63–66, *64–65*, 84, *85*
osteotomy, for loose shoulder, 100–103, *101–102*
rim, anteroinferior vulnerable point, 94–99, *95–98*
role of rotator cuff in shoulder, 17–21, *18–20*
Glenoid fossa, fractures, 63–66, *64–65*
Global rotator cuff tears, trapezius transfer procedure, 196–199, *197–199*
Grafts,
  cancellous iliac crest, 247
  fascia lata, 168, 194
  free biceps, 174, *174*
  freeze-dried rotator cuff, 151, 175–176, *175–176*
  in repair of rotator cuff tears, 194
  Oudard-Iwahara's procedure, 106–110, *107–109*
  tibial cortical, in thoracoscapular fusion technique, 247–251, *248–250*
Grammont, PM, Acropole prosthesis, 200–201, 279–280, *279*

Hemiarthroplasty, Neer, 60–62, *61*, 61–62t
Hill-Sachs lesion,
  arthroscopic observations, 39, *39*, *41*, *42*
  computer tomography of, 84, *85*
  in shoulder instability, 23, 27
Humerus, proximal,
  prognostic factors in comminuted and dislocated, 51–59, *52–57*
  treatment of fractures by Neer hemiarthroplasty, 60–62, *61*, 61–62t
  unconstrained shoulder arthroplasty, 242–243

Impingement syndrome. *See* Shoulder impingement syndrome.
Implants,
  Acropole prosthesis, 200–201, 279–280, *279*
  bipolar, 211–223, *213*, *215–219*, *221–223*
  Kölbel prosthesis, 279, 281, 283, *282–292*, 292–293
  Mayo prosthesis, 311–312
  Mayo Campanacci prosthesis, 312
  Neer total shoulder replacement, 224–228, *226–228*, 294–302, *295–301*
  St. George Mark II prosthesis, 236
  survival of, 229–233, *230–232*
  unconstrained shoulder arthroplasty, 234–239, *235–238*, 240–245, *241–243*
  Zippel prosthesis, 279
Infection,
  in arthroscopic surgery, 48
  in dislocated fractures, 52
  in recurrent anterior dislocations, 92
  in rotator cuff tear surgery, 164
Instability of shoulder. *See* Shoulder instability.
Isokinetic dynamometry of the shoulder, 1–5, *2–4*

Keloids, prevention of, 266, *267*
Kenny-Howard support, for acromioclavicular dislocations, 73, *76*
Kinesiology of the shoulder, 6, 8, *7–11*
Kirschner pins, use in dislocations, 73, *74*
Kirschner wires, use in proximal humerus fractures, 51

Kocher procedure for unconstrained shoulder replacement, 234–239, *235–238*
Kölbel prosthesis, 279, 281, 283, *282–292*, 292–293

Labrum syndrome, 94, 105
Labrum lesions, 96, *97*
Larksen-Dahle-Eek, rheumatoid shoulder stages, 269, *270–272*
Lesions,
 Bankart. See Bankart lesion.
 Hill-Sachs. See Hill-Sachs lesion.
 in traumatic recurrent dislocations, 303–305
 of the anteroinferior glenoid rim, 95, *95–97*
 of the labrum, 96, *97*
 soft tissue, 41–42, *41*
Limb salvage procedures for primary bone tumors, 310–312
Locking technique, in reconstruction of the anteroinferior buttress, 98, *98–99*
Loose shoulder syndrome,
 arthroscopic observations, 35, *36*
 glenoid osteotomy for, 100–103, *101–102*

Magnuson-Stack procedure,
 in failed repair for instability, 114, *115*
 in glenohumeral subluxations, 25
Mayo design prostheses, 311–312
McLaughlin, HL,
 classification of rotator cuff tears, 193
 lesion, 31
 technique for rotator cuff tears, 164, 175, *175*
Meniscectomy, in treatment of acromioclavicular dislocation, 70
Muscular dystrophy, facioscapulohumeral type, thoracic scapulopexy, 255–258, *256–258*

Neer, CS,
 anterior acromioplasty technique for rotator cuff tears, 162–164, *162–164*
 hemiarthroplastic treatment of proximal humerus fractures, 60–62, *61*, 61–62t
 prognostic factors in proximal humerus fractures, 53, 53t
 rotator cuff damage classification, 79, *80*, 161
 total shoulder replacement technique, 224–228, *226–228*, 294–302, *295–301*
Nitroblue tetrazolium test, for pyogenic arthritis, 323, 323t
Notch defect, of the humerus, 304

Open reduction procedure,
 compared to closed reduction, 56, 57t
 in acromioclavicular dislocations, 73
 in humeral fractures, 51–58, *52–57*
Osteoarthritis, following aseptic necrosis of the humeral head, 324–325
Osteotomy,
 double, for rheumatoid arthritis, 277–278
 glenoid, for loose shoulder, 100–103, 101–102
Oudard-Iwahara procedure for recurrent anterior dislocation, 106–110, *107–109*

Pain, chronic shoulder,
 in athletes, 79–83, *80–82*

 surgical pathology, 313–318, *314–317*
Painful arc syndrome, arthroscopic observation, 35, *36*
Paralysis, A.O. (ASIF) technique of shoulder arthrodesis for, 207–210, *208–209*
Paresis,
 serratus anterior, 6, *8*
 trapezius, 6, *8*
Pectoralis minor transposition, in serratus anterior paralysis, 252–254, *254*
Periarthritis, arthroscopic observations, 48–49
Physiotherapy,
 after arthroplasty, 219–220, 241
 after rotator cuff tear surgery, 180–184, *181–184*
 Codman's rotation, 150–151
 for chronic shoulder pain in the athlete, 79–80
Prostheses. See under names of individual prostheses; Arthroplasty; Implants.
Proximal humeral fractures, arthroplastic techniques, 243
Putti-Platt procedure,
 for recurrent anterior dislocation, 87
 in glenohumeral subluxations, 25
 in failed repair for instability, 114, *115*

Radiologic techniques,
 in identification of pyogenic arthritis, 320–322, *321–322*
 in missed posterior dislocations, 118
 in Neer total shoulder replacement, 227–228, 298–299, *300–301*
 in scapular examination, 326–329, *327–329*
 in shoulder subluxation studies, 26–27, 31, 33, *27–33*
 in studies of dislocations, 303–304
 in studies of implants, 222–223
 in studies of scapula movement, 12–16, *13–15*
 in studies of shoulder arthroplasty, 231–232, *232*
 in studies of the acromioclavicular joint, 67–68, *68*
 in subacromial joint studies, 134, *136–137*
 in supraspinatus tendon rupture studies, 129–133, *130–132*
 in treatment of rheumatoid shoulder, 269, *270–272*
Recurrent dislocation. See Dislocation, recurrent.
Reduction procedures. See Open reduction procedure; Closed reduction procedure.
Rehabilitation. See Physiotherapy.
Rheumatoid arthritis. See Arthritis, rheumatoid.
Rotator cuff,
 chronic pain in, 79, 81, 314
 decompression, in treatment of impingement syndrome, 140–142
 disease, and total shoulder arthroplasty, 229–233, *230–232*
 relation of cuff tendons to acromion process, 134–139, *135–137*
 role as stabilizing mechanism of the shoulder, 17–21, *18–20*
 surgery. See Rotator cuff tears, surgery
Rotator cuff tears,
 arthroscopic observations, 35, *36*, 38–39, *38*, 46
 arthrotomographic diagnosis of, 126–128, *127–128*
 as cause of chronic shoulder pain, 79–81, *80*, 313–318, *314–317*
 causes of, 151–152
 classification of, 143–144, 144t, 147t, 159t
 in athletes, *80*, 82
 in the young, 157–160, 158–159t
 partial thickness, 143–148, 144t, *145–147*

surgery, 161–166, *162–164*, 192–195, 202–206, *203–205*
    Acropole prosthesis, 200–201
    arthroscopic, 43, *44, 46*
    chronic tears, 172–179, *173–177*
    complete tears, 149–153, 167–171
    global tears, trapezius transfer, 196–199, *197–199*
    McLaughlin repair, 164, 175, *175*
    rehabilitation following, 180–184, *181–184*
    use of synthetic fabrics, 185–191, *186–190*
Rowe modification, 73–74, *76*
Rupture,
    of the biceps, 165
    of the supraspinatus tendon, 129–133, *130–132*

Scapula,
    fractures involving glenoid fossa, 63–66, *64–65*
    movement during elevation of the arm, 12–16, *13–15*
    roentgenographical examination of tilt, 326–329, *327–329*
    winging,
        due to deltoid muscle contracture, 259–268, *260–268*
        due to facioscapulohumeral muscular dystrophy, 247–251, *248–250*, 255–258, *256–258*
        due to serratus anterior paralysis treatment, 252–254, *254*
Scapulohumeral rhythm, 17–18, 21
Scapulopexy, thoracic. *See* Thoracoscapular fusion.
Serratus anterior paralysis, pectoralis minor transposition, 252–254, *254*
Shoulder,
    anatomy, 12, 17, 211
    arm elevation and angle of scapula, 12–16, *13–18*
    arthroscopic diagnosis of disorders, 34–37, *35–36*
    glenohumeral subluxations, 22–25, *24*
    instability. *See* Shoulder instability.
    kinesiology, 6, 8, *7–11*
    missed posterior dislocations, 117–120, *119*
    power during movement, 1–5, *2–4*
    rotator cuff as stabilizing mechanism, 17–21, *18–20*
Shoulder impingement syndrome,
    and arthroscopic surgery, 46
    and subacromial bursae, *123*, 125
    in athletes, 79, 80, 81, 140–142
    Neer stages, 161
Shoulder instability,
    arthroscopic observations, 47
    failed repair analysis, 111–116, *112–115*
    joint replacement implants, 281–293, *282–292*
    role of rotator cuff, 17–21
Shoulder replacement technique, Neer total, 224–228, *226–228*, 294–302, *295–301*
Snow cap phenomenon, 100, *101*
Steroids, in treatment of impingement syndrome, 80
Stereophotogrammetric shoulder studies, 6, 8, *7–11*

St. George Mark II prosthesis, 236
Subacromial bursae, 121–125, *122–124*
Subacromial joint, contact areas, 134–139, *135–137*
Subluxation,
    anterior, role of biceps tendon, 104–105, 315–316, *315–316*
    glenohumeral, C-arm fluoroscopic evaluation, 22–25, *24*
    recurrent, 26–33, *27–32*
Supraspinatus tendon,
    arthroscopic observations, 34–35, *35–36*
    effect of subacromial bursae, 122, *122*
    ruptures due to distally-pointing acromioclavicular osteophytes, 129–133, *130–132*
    testing for weakness of, 79, *80*
Synthetic fabrics, use in surgery on rotator cuff tears, 185–191, *186–190*
Synovectomy, on rheumatoid shoulder, 276–277, *277–278*

Teflon, use in rotator cuff surgery, 185–191, *186–190*
Tendinitis, biceps,
    attrition, 316, *317*
    causes, *317*
    impingement, 315, *317*
    of the rotator cuff, 79
    subacromial bursae, 124–125, *124*
Tendon shortening procedures. *See* Magnuson-Stack procedure; Putti-Platt procedure.
Tendon transfer technique, in rotator cuff surgery, 176–177, *177–178*
Thoracic scapulopexy. *See* Thoracoscapular fusion.
Thoracoscapular fusion, 247–251, *248–250*
Tikhott-Lindberg procedure, 311
Tomography, axial, and shoulder subluxation studies, 26–27, 31, 33, *27–33*
Tomography, computer. *See* Computerized tomography.
Total shoulder arthroplasty, and associated disease of the rotator cuff, 229–233, *230–232*
Total shoulder replacement, Neer technique, 294–228, *226–228*, 284–302, *295–301*
Transacromial anterior deltoid technique, in rotator cuff surgery, 186, *187*, 192
Trapezius transfer procedure, in repair of global rotator cuff tears, 196–199, *197–199*
Tuberosities, as cause of impingement syndrome, 142
Tumors, of primary shoulder bones, limb salvage procedures, 310–312

Winging scapula. *See* Scapula, winging.

Zippel prosthesis, 279